Neonatology Questions and Controversies
The Newborn Lung

Neonatology Questions and Controversies
The Newborn Lung
Fourth Edition

Series Editor
Richard A. Polin, MD
William T. Speck Professor of Pediatrics
Executive Vice Chair Department of Pediatrics
Vagelos College of Physicians and Surgeons
Columbia University
New York, New York
United States

Other Volumes in the Neonatology Questions and Controversies Series
GASTROENTEROLOGY AND NUTRITION

HEMATOLOGY AND TRANSFUSION MEDICINE

RENAL, FLUID AND ELECTROLYTE DISORDERS

INFECTIOUS DISEASE, IMMUNOLOGY, AND PHARMACOLOGY

NEONATAL HEMODYNAMICS

NEUROLOGY

4th Edition

Neonatology Questions and Controversies

The Newborn Lung

Edited by

Eduardo H. Bancalari, MD
Emeritus Professor of Pediatrics
University of Miami Miller School of Medicine
Miami, Florida
United States

Martin Keszler, MD, FAAP
Professor of Pediatrics
Alpert Medical School, Brown University;
Director of Respiratory Services
Pediatrics
Women and Infants Hospital of Rhode
Island
Providence, Rhode Island
United States

Peter G. Davis, MBBS, MD, FRACP
Professor of Neonatology
The Royal Women's Hospital
Melbourne, Victoria
Australia

Consulting Editor

Richard A. Polin, MD
William T. Speck Professor of Pediatrics
Executive Vice Chair Department of Pediatrics
Vagelos College of Physicians and Surgeons
Columbia University
New York, New York
United States

ELSEVIER

Elsevier
1600 John F. Kennedy Blvd.
Ste 1800
Philadelphia, PA 19103-2899

Content Development Manager: Ranjana Sharma
Content Strategist: Sarah E. Barth
Senior Content Development Specialist: Vaishali Singh
Publishing Services Manager: Shereen Jameel
Project Manager: Vishnu T. Jiji
Senior Designer: Margaret M. Reid

Printed in India

Last digit is the print number: 9 8 7 6 5 4 3 2 1

Working together
to grow libraries in
developing countries

www.elsevier.com • www.bookaid.org

CONTRIBUTORS

Steven H. Abman, MD
Professor of Pediatrics
University of Colorado Health Sciences Center;
Director
Pediatric Health Lung Center
The Children's Hospital
Aurora, Colorado
United States

Eduardo H. Bancalari, MD
Emeritus Professor of Pediatrics
University of Miami Miller School of Medicine
Miami, Florida
United States

Jeanie L.Y. Cheong, MBBS, MD, FRACP
Professor of Neonatal Services
Royal Women's Hospital;
Professor of Obstetrics and Gynaecology
University of Melbourne;
Professor of Clinical Sciences
Murdoch Children's Research Institute
Melbourne, Victoria
Australia

Nelson Claure, MSc, PhD
Professor of Pediatrics and Biomedical Engineering
Director of Neonatal Respiratory Physiology
   Laboratory
Department of Pediatrics, Division of Neonatology
University of Miami Miller School of Medicine
Miami, Florida
United States

Peter G. Davis, MBBS, MD, FRACP
Professor of Neonatology
The Royal Women's Hospital
Melbourne, Victoria
Australia

Elizabeth R. Fisher, BMed, MMed(Clin Epi)
Fellow
Neonatology
Royal North Shore Hospital, St Leonards;
Clinical Associate Lecturer
Department of Obstetrics, Gynaecology and
   Neonatology, Northern Clinical School
University of Sydney
Sydney, New South Wales
Australia

Martin Kluckow, MBBS, FRACP, PhD
Professor
Division of Women's, Children's & Family Health
University of Sydney;
Senior Staff Specialist
Department of Neonatology
Royal North Shore Hospital
Sydney, New South Wales
Australia

Daniele De Luca, MD, PhD
Full Professor of Neonatology,
Paris Saclay University and APHP
"A.Beclere" Hospital
Paris
France

Juliann M. Di Fiore, BS
Research Engineer III
Department of Pediatrics
Case Western Reserve University
Cleveland, Ohio
United States

Lex W. Doyle, MD
Professor Emeritus of Neonatal Medicine
Department of Obstetrics and Gynaecology
University of Melbourne
Melbourne, Victoria
Australia

Kate A. Hodgson, MBBS(Hons), BMedSci, FRACP
Neonatal Consultant
Newborn Services
Royal Women's Hospital
Melbourne, Victoria
Australia

Stuart Brian Hooper, BSc(Hons), PhD
Professor
The Ritchie Centre
Hudson Institute for Medical Research;
Professor of Obstetrics and Gynaecology
Monash University
Melbourne, Victoria
Australia

Thomas Alexander Hooven, MD
Assistant Professor
Department of Pediatrics
University of Pittsburgh School of Medicine
Pittsburgh, Pennsylvania
United States

Alan H. Jobe, MD, PhD
Professor of Pediatrics
Pulmonary Biology, Neonatology
Cincinnati Children's Hospital Medical Center
Cincinnati, Ohio
United States

Suhas G. Kallapur, MD
Professor of Pediatrics
Division of Neonatology and Developmental Biology
David Geffen School of Medicine, University of
    California Los Angeles
Los Angeles, California
United States

Martin Keszler, MD, FAAP
Professor of Pediatrics
Alpert Medical School, Brown University;
Director of Respiratory Services
Pediatrics
Women and Infants Hospital of Rhode Island
Providence, Rhode Island
United States

Satyan Lakshminrusimha, MD, MBBS, FAAP
Dennis & Nancy Marks Professor and Chair
Department of Pediatrics
UC Davis;
Pediatrician-in-Chief
UC Davis Children's Hospital;
Co-Chair
Clinical Funds Flow Committee
UC Davis Health
Sacramento, California
United States

Brett J. Manley, MBBS, FRACP, PhD
Neonatologist
Newborn Research
The Royal Women's Hospital;
Associate Professor
Department of Obstetrics and Gynaecology
The University of Melbourne;
Honorary Fellow
Murdoch Children's Research Institute
Melbourne, Victoria
Australia

Richard J. Martin, MBBS
Professor of Pediatrics, Reproductive Biology, and
    Physiology & Biophysics
Case Western Reserve University School of Medicine;
Drusinsky-Fanaroff Chair in Neonatology
Pediatrics/Neonatology
Rainbow Babies & Children's Hospital
Cleveland, Ohio
United States

Cindy T. McEvoy, MD, MCR
Professor of Pediatrics
Department of Pediatrics
Oregon Health & Science University
Portland, Oregon
United States

Amit Mukerji, MD, FRCP(C)
Associate Professor of Paediatrics
McMaster University
Hamilton, Ontario
Canada

Namasivayam Ambalavanan, MBBS, MD
Professor
Division of Neonatology, Department of Pediatrics
University of Alabama at Birmingham
Birmingham, Alabama
United States

Cristina T. Navarrete, MD
Associate Professor of Clinical Pediatrics
Division of Neonatology, Department of Pediatrics
University of Miami
Miami, Florida
United States

Leif D. Nelin, MD
Chief
Division of Neonatology
Nationwide Children's Hospital;
Professor
Department of Pediatrics
The Ohio State University
Columbus, Ohio
United States

Shahab Noori, MD, MS CBTI
Professor of Pediatrics
Fetal and Neonatal Institute, Division of Neonatology
Children's Hospital Los Angeles;
Department of Pediatrics
Keck School of Medicine
University of Southern California
Los Angeles, California
United States

Howard B. Panitch, MD
Director
Technology Dependence Center
Division of Pulmonary and sleep medicine
The Children's Hospital of Philadelphia;
Professor Emeritus of Pediatrics
Perelman School of Medicine at The University
   of Pennsylvania
Philadelphia, Pennsylvania
United States

Peter A. Dargaville, MD
Professorial Research Fellow
Menzies Institute for Medical Research
University of Tasmania;
Staff Specialist
Neonatal and Paediatric Intensive Care Unit
Paediatrics
Royal Hobart Hospital
Hobart, Tasmania
Australia

Erik A. Jensen, MD
Assistant Professor of Pediatrics
Department of Pediatrics
Children's Hospital of Philadelphia
Philadelphia, Pennsylvania
United States

Oluwateniayo O. Okpaise, MD
Acute Medicine
Medway Maritime hospital
Gilligham
United Kingdom

Won Soon Park, MD, PhD
Clinical Professor
Department of Pediatrics
Gangnam Cha Hospital
Seoul
Korea

Richard A. Polin, MD
William T. Speck Professor of Pediatrics
Executive Vice Chair Department of Pediatrics
Vagelos College of Physicians and Surgeons
Columbia University
New York, New York
United States

Rodrigo Ruano, MD, PhD
Professor
Chief of the Maternal-Medicine Division
Director of U Health Jackson Fetal Care Center
Co-Director of the Labor & Delivery Unit
Department of Obstetrics and Gynecology
University of Miami
Miami, Florida
United States

Augusto F. Schmidt, MD, PhD
Associate Professor
Department of Pediatrics, Division of Neonatology
University of Miami Miller School of Medicine
Miami, Florida
United States

Barbara Schmidt, MD, MSc
Professor (Part-time)
Health Research Methods, Evidence, and Impact
McMaster University
Hamilton, Ontario
Canada;
Professor Emeritus of Pediatrics
University of Pennsylvania
Philadelphia, Pennsylvania
United States

Arun Sett, MBBS (Hons), CCPU (Neonatal and Neonatal Lung), FRACP
Neonatal Research Fellow
Newborn Research Centre
The Royal Women's Hospital;
Honorary Research Fellow
Neonatal Research
Murdoch Children's Research Institute;
Neonatologist
Newborn Services
Joan Kirner Women's and Children's, Western Health;
PhD Candidate
Department of Obstetrics and Gynaecology
University of Melbourne
Melbourne, Victoria
Australia

Robin H. Steinhorn, MD
Professor and Vice Dean
Pediatrics
Rady Children's Hospital and University of California
   San Diego
San Diego, California
United States

Daniel T. Swarr, MD
Assistant Professor of Pediatrics
Division of Neonatology & Pulmonary Biology
Cincinnati Children's Hospital Medical Center
Cincinnati, Ohio
United States

Bernard Thebaud, MD, PhD
Pediatrics
Children's Hospital of Eastern Ontario
Regenerative Medicine
Ottawa Hospital Research Institute
Ottawa, Ontario
Canada

David Gerald Tingay, MBBS, DCH, FRACP, PhD
Group Leader
Neonatal Research
Murdoch Children's Research Institute, Parkville;
Principal Fellow
Department of Pediatrics
The University of Melbourne, Melbourne;
Neonatologist
Department of Neonatology
The Royal Children's Hospital
Parkville, Victoria
Australia

Rose M. Viscardi, MD
Professor Emeritus of Pediatrics
University of Maryland School of Medicine
Baltimore, Maryland
United States

Gary Marshall Weiner, MD
Clinical Professor of Neonatal-Perinatal Medicine
University of Michigan;
Medical Director
Neonatal Intensive Care
C.S. Mott Children's Hospital
Ann Arbor, Michigan
United States

Jeffrey A. Whitsett, MD
Professor of Pediatrics
Perinatal Institute
Cincinnati Children's Hospital Medical Center
Cincinnati, Ohio
United States

Myra H. Wyckoff, MD
Professor of Pediatrics
UT Southwestern Medical Center;
Director of Newborn Resuscitation Services
Parkland Health and Hospital Systems
Dallas, Texas
United States

Karen Cecile Young, MD
Professor of Pediatrics
Pediatrics/Neonatology
University of Miami Miller School of Medicine
Davie, Florida
United States

SERIES FOREWORD

"To study the phenomena of disease without books is to sail an uncharted sea, while to study books without patients is not to go to sea at all."

"Medicine is learned by the bedside and not in the classroom. Let not your conceptions of disease come from the words heard in the lecture room or read from the book. See and then reason and compare and control. But see first."

William Osler

Before the invention of the movable type by Johannes Gutenberg in the 15th century, physicians learned medicine by serving an apprenticeship with individuals considered experienced. There were no printed textbooks, and medical journals were not published until the beginning of the 19th century. By apprenticing yourself to a physician over a period of years, one learned how to be a competent practitioner. Internships in the United States evolved from those apprenticeships in the 18th century. The term *residency* was chosen because the physicians in training had a "residence" at the hospital. Modern-day internships began at Johns Hopkins Hospital in 1904. The Johns Hopkins Hospital was founded by Osler, Halstead, Welch, and Kelly. Halstead is credited with creating the first surgical residency and coined the phrase "see one, do one, teach one" (SODOTO). That educational philosophy has been adopted by nearly every specialty in medicine, including neonatology.

Modern-day trainees in neonatology still learn how to care for critically ill infants and how to perform procedures by watching, assisting, and listening to more experienced individuals at the bedside. The SODOTO approach is considered a fundamental educational tool. However, over a 3-year period, much of education occurs remote from the bedside during teaching rounds and conferences. The teaching is often more theoretical, and by design, rounds in the nursery and conferences are passive learning exercises. In those settings, trainees listen but do not take an active role in the educational process. Learning is always more effective when the recipient takes an active role in their own education. Ideally, they should be questioning what they hear, reading pertinent literature, and, when the opportunity arises, teaching others. Unfortunately, much of the information transmitted in those settings is not usually followed by an active phase of questioning and reading by the trainee.

Most graduates of fellowship programs turn out to be excellent practitioners, but once they leave the fellowship program, new information is acquired only intermittently either at conferences or from journals and textbooks. As a source of new information, journals provide access to the most up-to-date information. However, that information is unfiltered, and the conclusions of a study may not be appropriate (or perhaps risky) for a critically ill infant. Textbooks like *Neonatology Questions and Controversies* series offer an opportunity to hear from experts in neonatal-perinatal medicine who have synthesized (and filtered) the existing literature and can provide up-to-date recommendations.

The fourth edition of the Questions and Controversies series will also have seven volumes. Each of them has been extensively revised, and we have added several new editors: Terri Inder has joined Jeffrey Perlman for the Neurology volume, James Wynn joined William Benitz and P. Brian Smith as a coeditor for the Infectious Disease, Immunology and Pharmacology volume, and Patrick McNamara is now a coeditor with Martin Kluckow for the Neonatal Hemodynamics volume. The reader will find many completely new chapters; however, like the last edition, each of them is focused on day-to day clinical decisions encountered by neonatologists. Nothing will replace the teaching that occurs at the bedside when confronted with a critically ill neonate, and the SODOTO educational approach still has an important role in education. Procedures are best learned by simulations and guidance by experienced practitioners at the bedside. However, expertise as a practitioner can only be enhanced by reading and incorporating new information into daily practice, once proven safe and effective. Perhaps SODOTO should be changed to LQRT (listen, question, read, and teach). Questions and Controversies is a unique source to learn from experts in the field who have been through the LQRT process many times. Osler's quotes at the top of this preface suggest that both bedside teaching and journals/textbooks have a synergistic role in physician education, and neither alone is sufficient.

As with all prior editions, I am indebted to an exceptional group of volume editors who chose the content and authors and edited the manuscripts. I also want to thank Sarah Barth (Publisher) as well as Vasowati Shome and Vaishali Singh (Senior Content Development Specialists) at Elsevier, who have guided the development of this series.

Richard A. Polin

PREFACE

We are very pleased to introduce the fourth edition of *The Newborn Lung*.

Chapters from leading experts provide the reader with the most current developments in the pathophysiology, diagnosis, and management of the most common neonatal respiratory problems.

While there are important advances in respiratory management that have been implemented to reduce lung damage and long-term sequelae in extremely premature infants, the incidence of complications of neonatal intensive care remains unacceptably high. Ongoing and future research will seek to improve our understanding of injury mechanisms and focus on intact survival, not only survival itself.

The fourth edition of *The Newborn Lung* emphasizes those areas where there have been major new developments in recent years, and several chapters deal with strategies that may reduce lung damage and some of the consequences of neonatal respiratory failure and its management.

We are certain that the reader will enjoy learning as much as we have from each of these chapters, and we hope that the new knowledge will contribute to improved outcomes for babies treated in their units.

We are most grateful to all authors who have taken the time to share their expertise in this new edition of *The Newborn Lung*.

Eduardo H. Bancalari, MD
Peter G. Davis, MBBS, MD, FRACP
Martin Keszler, MD, FAAP

CONTENTS

1. Perinatal Events and Their Influence on Lung Development and Injury 1
   Suhas G. Kallapur and Alan H. Jobe

2. Respiratory and Cardiovascular Support in the Delivery Room 29
   Gary Marshall Weiner, Stuart Brian Hooper, Peter G. Davis, and Myra H. Wyckoff

3. Vascular Development and Pulmonary Hypertension 51
   Robin H.Steinhorn, Steven H. Abman, and Satyan Lakshminrusimha

4. Airway Microbiome and Lung Injury 75
   Rose M. Viscardi and Namasivayam Ambalavanan

5. Ventilator-Associated Pneumonia 93
   Thomas Alexander Hooven and Richard A. Polin

6. Noninvasive Respiratory Support for Preterm Infants: An Alternative to Mechanical Ventilation 107
   Brett J. Manley, Kate A. Hodgson, Amit Mukerji, and Peter G. Davis

7. Newer Strategies for Surfactant Delivery 133
   Peter A. Dargaville

8. Respiratory Control and Oxygen Instability in Premature Infants 151
   Juliann M. Di Fiore, Richard J. Martin, Nelson Claure, and Eduardo H. Bancalari

9. Pulmonary-Cardiovascular Interaction 165
   Shahab Noori, Elizabeth R. Fisher, and Martin Kluckow

10. Ventilator Strategies to Reduce Lung Injury and Duration of Mechanical Ventilation 189
    Martin Keszler and Nelson Claure

11. Prenatal and Postnatal Steroids and Pulmonary Outcomes 205
    Augusto F. Schmidt and Alan H. Jobe

12. Cell-Based Therapy for Neonatal Lung Diseases 221
    Karen Cecile Young, Bernard Thebaud, and Won Soon Park

13. Definitions and Diagnostic Criteria of Bronchopulmonary Dysplasia: Clinical and Research Implications 235
    Eduardo H. Bancalari, Nelson Claure, Erik A. Jensen, and Alan H. Jobe

14. A Physiology-Based Approach to the Respiratory Care of Children With Severe Bronchopulmonary Dysplasia 249
    Leif D. Nelin, Steven H. Abman, and Howard B. Panitch

15. Long-Term Pulmonary Outcome of Preterm Infants 279
    Jeanie L.Y. Cheong and Lex W. Doyle

16. Perinatal Nutrition and the Lung 291
    Cindy T. McEvoy and Cristina T. Navarrete

17. Caffeine—Respiratory Stimulant or Magic Bullet? 313
    Barbara Schmidt

18. The Neonatal Lung: Lung Imaging Using Ultrasound and Electric Impedance Tomography 323
    Arun Sett, David Gerald Tingay, and Daniele De Luca

19. Genetic Disorders of Alveolar Formation and Homeostasis 337
    Daniel T. Swarr and Jeffrey A. Whitsett

20. Fetal Intervention in Congenital Malformations of the Respiratory System 349
    Rodrigo Ruano and Oluwateniayo O. Okpaise

Index 359

Perinatal Events and Their Influence on Lung Development and Injury

Suhas G. Kallapur and Alan H. Jobe

Chapter Outline

Overview of Lung Development and Perinatal Events

Lung Development: The Substrate for Adverse Events

Lung Maturation

Antenatal Infection/Inflammation

Overview of Fetal Inflammation

Diagnosis of Chorioamnionitis

Clinical Pulmonary Outcomes of Fetal Exposure to Inflammation/Infection

Experimental Results: The Link Between Fetal Exposure to Inflammation and Lung Maturation, Lung Remodeling

Mediators that Induce Fetal Lung Inflammatory Responses

Early Gestational Fetal Lung Responses to Inflammation

Mechanisms of Inflammation-Mediated Lung Maturation

Experimental Chronic Chorioamnionitis

Immune Response and Modulation from Fetal Exposures to Inflammation

Immune Changes in Preterm Infants Exposed to Chorioamnionitis

Inflammatory Mediators and Bronchopulmonary Dysplasia

Interactions Between Antenatal Corticosteroid Treatments and Chorioamnionitis

Intrauterine Growth Restriction/Small for Gestational Age (SGA)

Environmental Factors and Lung Disease

Summary: The Complexities

Key Points

- Multiple antenatal exposures exert effects on the fetal lung—some adverse and other beneficial for postnatal survival.
- Antenatal exposures can alter lung development and interact with postnatal exposures.
- Early gestational lung maturation is common and promoted by both antenatal steroids and fetal exposure to inflammation.
- Antenatal steroid is a common exposure that may interact with postnatal care practices in presently unknown ways.
- Sepsis with chorioamnionitis is an infrequent event in term and near-term infants.

- Fetal exposure to inflammation/chorioamnionitis results in complex immunomodulation which may alter postnatal exposures.
- Growth restriction, tobacco and alcohol alter fetal lung development with effects on post-delivery outcomes.

Overview of Lung Development and Perinatal Events

Lung growth and development are the substrates on which all lung outcomes ultimately depend. This chapter emphasizes four categories of events that can modulate fetal and subsequent postnatal lung

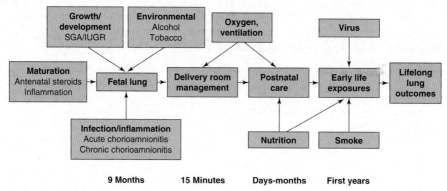

Fig. 1.1 Sketch of factors that modulate the fetal lung development and function. Some effectors that alter lung development after delivery also are indicated. *IUGR*, Intrauterine growth restriction; *SGA*, small for gestational age.

development and thus alter lung outcomes for a life-time (Fig. 1.1). Antenatal corticosteroids as a potent antenatal intervention demonstrated to mature fetal lung are discussed elsewhere in this book. McElrath and colleagues[1] propose that there are two pathologic pathways that result in deliveries at very early gestational age (GA): intrauterine inflammation that is often chronic and aberrations of placentation/vascular development. Other examples of clinically relevant modulators of lung development are small for gestational age/intrauterine growth restriction (SGA/IUGR) and environmental exposures such as maternal tobacco and alcohol use. Lung maturation is a late phase of lung development that can be accelerated by antenatal corticosteroids and by fetal exposure to inflammation. Although infection can induce lung maturation, fetal exposures to acute or chronic chorioamnionitis also can injure the lung. There are two "elephants in the room" for this discussion of events that influence lung development. The first is the concept of what is "normal." Any discussion of premature lungs is complicated by the lack of a normal comparison group with which to evaluate the impact of the perinatal event of interest. Although the words *all* or *never* should be sparingly used in biology and medicine, all very-low-birth-weight (VLBW) deliveries must be regarded as adverse pregnancy outcomes. The 24-week GA newborn who does not have respiratory distress syndrome (RDS) is a true wonder of nature.

The second "elephant" is the complexity of the entangled pathways that regulate lung development, injury, and repair for any perinatal event that affects

the lung. These three cellular and molecular response programs share signaling pathways that are superimposed simultaneously or sequentially on the immature lung. This complexity confounds simple interpretations about what mediator is causing which outcome. Finally, outcomes such as bronchopulmonary dysplasia (BPD) and asthma/airway disease in childhood and later life may be initiated by fetal events that then are modulated by postnatal responses of the lungs. An example is early life exposures to viral infections.[2] This biologic complexity generates inconsistencies in clinical data and controversies. In this chapter, we provide our current understanding of how prenatal exposure to various conditions can change postnatal lung function based on both clinical information and animal models.

Lung Development: The Substrate for Adverse Events

Lung development is programmed by the fetus to be sufficiently mature to adapt rapidly to air breathing at birth. The timing of the structural development of the lung in Fig. 1.2 is given as weeks from last menstrual period and from conception to emphasize the 2-week difference. Infants born by elective cesarean section as early term infants (38 weeks postmenstrual age) have more problems with pulmonary adaptation than infants born at 40 weeks postmenstrual age.[3] Late preterm infants have more lung adaptation problems and more RDS for each week of birth prior to 37 weeks.[4] Finally, lung adaptation abnormalities, RDS, and

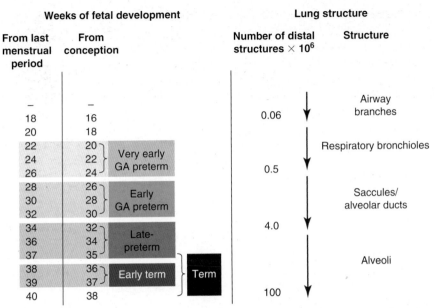

Fig. 1.2 Timing of fetal lung development, emphasizing the 2-week difference in weeks between postmenstrual age and conceptional age. The lung progressively branches from airways to alveoli with a large increase in distal structures. The adult lung contains about 500 × 10^6 alveoli. *GA,* Gestational age. (Data from Avery ME, Mead J. Surface properties in relation to atelectasis and hyaline membrane disease. *AMA J Dis Child.* 1959;97(5, Part 1): 517-523.)

subsequently BPD become increasingly frequent as GA decreases into the early GA and very early GA categories of preterm infants.[5] Lung development includes development of the structural elements as well as functional maturation of fluid clearance pathways and the surfactant system. The major structural events are the completion of airway branching by about 18 weeks of gestation, followed by three generations of airway divisions to form respiratory bronchioles, and three more divisions to form alveolar ducts to about 32 to 36 weeks.[6] Subsequently, secondary septation or alveolarization occurs to term and for several years after birth. Septation events are dynamic with about 0.06 × 10^6 distal structures at 18 to 20 weeks that increase to about 100 × 10^6 alveoli at term—a 1700-fold increase. Alveolar numbers increase only about fivefold from the term birth lung to the adult lung.[7] There is essentially no information about the variability of the timing of normal septation in the human lung. It is also not known whether very early lung maturation changes the timing of the later gestational septation events that generate respiratory bronchioles and alveolar ducts. Some forms of pulmonary

hypoplasia may result from altered septation and airway development. The injury and repair associated with BPD do inhibit and delay alveolarization of the developing lung.[8]

Recent human anatomic and experimental data demonstrate that the healthy lung probably grows new alveoli and loses old alveoli continuously at a very slow rate.[9,10] Empirically, very preterm infants with a BPD-associated "arrest" in alveolar septation must be able to grow alveoli or they could not grow and survive. These lungs may "catch up" to have lung volumes or alveolar numbers equivalent to normal lungs.[11] The questions for the future include how alveoli grow after very preterm birth and how lung injury can be prevented.

Lung Maturation

From the clinical perspective, questions about lung maturation have focused on RDS and the surfactant system since the seminal report from Avery and Mead[12] in 1959 that the lungs of infants who died of RDS had less surfactant. Lung maturation also includes epithelial development of ion/water regulation, thinning of the alveolar capillary barrier, and microvascular development. The first challenge is to define the timing of normal lung maturation, which is not an easy task if one assumes that most preterm infants are abnormal. In the 1970s, amniotic fluid was sampled from women with relatively normal gestations to test for lung maturation using surfactant components.[13] The lecithin/sphingomyelin (L/S) ratio was less than 2 until after 34 to 35 weeks of gestation, and phosphatidylglycerol was seldom detected prior to 34 weeks of gestation in normal pregnancies.[14] The true time course and the variability for the timing for normal lung maturation are not known with any precision for the human. However, lung maturity testing and inadvertent experiences with nonindicated cesarean sections prior to 37 weeks demonstrate that lung maturation, defined as absence of RDS, normally occurs after about 34 to 36 weeks in normal pregnancies.

The diagnosis of RDS for very early GA preterm infants has been confounded in clinical series and epidemiologic studies by intubation and ventilation with or without surfactant treatment shortly after birth. These intubated and ventilated infants likely carry the diagnosis RDS even if they are not receiving supplemental oxygen.[15] Furthermore, if these infants have infection, transient tachypnea of the newborn, a degree of pulmonary hypoplasia, or apnea requiring ventilatory support, they likely will be said to have RDS. The successful use of continuous positive airway pressure (CPAP) to minimize lung injury in very early GA infants demonstrates that many very preterm infants do not have enough RDS to need surfactant or mechanical ventilation.[16-18] Infants born at 24 to 25 weeks of GA without RDS are surprisingly common.[19] Because lung maturation (and RDS) is a continuum from severe immaturity to sufficient maturation to avoid RDS, we think that most very preterm infants have some degree of induced lung maturation.[20] The infant born at 24 to 26 weeks of gestation with severe respiratory failure and a poor response to surfactant and who dies soon after birth is an infant with "normal" 25-week lungs or an infant with RDS-plus (RDS plus infection or pulmonary hypoplasia, for example). Very few infants die of RDS in the United States unless they are of extremely low GA.

At the margin of lung maturity in preterm sheep, a surfactant pool size of about 4 mg/kg is sufficient to support normal gas exchange with CPAP,[21] demonstrating that a small amount of surfactant is sufficient to protect the preterm lung from RDS. We have no good tests to quantify the lung maturation status prior to or soon after delivery. The L/S ratio or phosphatidylglycerol measurements in amniotic fluid are no longer commonly available, and other tests such as lamellar body number in amniotic fluid are imprecise. Samples of fetal lung fluid (intubated infants) or gastric aspirates soon after birth could provide information about surfactant and inflammation, but they are not used routinely. An evaluation of the messenger RNA (mRNA) in amniotic fluid may provide a maturation profile for multiple fetal organs in the future.[22] A clinical controversy is: Which very preterm infant should receive surfactant/ventilation or CPAP after birth? The controversy is based on the perceived risk for RDS and the ability of these infants to transition if treated by CPAP. The clinical trials demonstrate that the two approaches yield similar outcomes that marginally favor an initial trial of CPAP.[23] However, individualized treatments could be given if the functional potential of the very preterm lung could be assessed prior to delivery. Clearly, very preterm delivery is an event that profoundly changes the developing lung. However, there is no good information about how preterm delivery and breathing, independent of oxygen exposure and injury, change the trajectory of subsequent lung development. Lung stretch from breathing and the striking changes in hormone milieu alter lung development in experimental models.[24,25] The implication is that independent of injury, lung structure at 40 weeks will be different for infants born at 25 weeks or 35 weeks from those for infants born at 40 weeks.[26]

Antenatal Infection/Inflammation

OVERVIEW OF FETAL INFLAMMATION

The human fetus is normally considered to be in an environment protected from infection. However, the human fetus can be exposed to a variety of pathogens, which may initiate an inflammatory process in the placenta, chorioamnion, or fetus. For example, human fetuses are exposed to viral pathogens as a consequence of maternal viremia. The patterns of injury to agents such as varicella and cytomegalovirus depend on the period of gestation during which the infection occurs. Similarly, the fetus can acquire a spirochete infection with syphilis or a parasitic infection with toxoplasmosis secondary to maternal infection, and each causes characteristic syndromes depending on the gestational timing of exposure. These infections are not generally viewed as predominantly inflammatory, although the fetal injury and immune responses have inflammatory characteristics. Asphyxia with injury to fetal tissue also causes inflammation as part of the injury and the repair process. Similarly, normal labor is associated with an increase in proinflammatory mediators.[27] Both innate and acquired inflammatory responses of the fetus are generally considered to be less robust than those in the child or adult because the response systems in the fetus are immature and pregnancy is an immune-suppressive environment.[28] For example, fetal inflammatory responses to pathogens such as group B streptococcus and *Listeria monocytogenes* are blunted, resulting in severe infection and often death of the fetus or newborn. The most common fetal infectious exposure is to chorioamnionitis, which is associated with preterm labor and delivery.[29] In this section, we identify the questions and controversies about the associations of chorioamnionitis with a range of effects on the fetal and newborn lung.

DIAGNOSIS OF CHORIOAMNIONITIS

Chorioamnionitis can be either a clinical syndrome or a silent, indolent process. The clinical diagnosis of chorioamnionitis is made when a pregnant woman has a constellation of findings that include fever, a tender uterus, an elevated blood granulocyte count, and bacteria and/or inflammatory cells in amniotic fluid and often preterm labor or prolonged rupture of membranes (PROM).[30] Clinical chorioamnionitis is an imprecise diagnosis that has little prognostic or treatment value. In an attempt to decrease misclassification, a National Institute of Child Health and Human Development (NICHD) workshop recommended replacing the terminology of chorioamnionitis with "triple I" (intrauterine infection or inflammation) with categories of isolated fever, suspected triple I, and confirmed triple I.[31] The diagnosis of clinical chorioamnionitis is frequently made for near-term or term labors, and occasionally infection can be caused by highly virulent organisms. Before 30 weeks of gestation, *clinical chorioamnionitis* is most often diagnosed after attempts to delay preterm delivery or with preterm PROM. Another method to diagnose chorioamnionitis is by histopathology of the chorioamnion with inflammation, indicating *histologic chorioamnionitis*. The amount of infiltration of the chorioamnion by inflammatory cells and the intensity of secondary changes are used to grade the severity of the fetal exposure to inflammation.[32] Inflammation of the cord, called *funisitis*, is generally considered to indicate a more advanced inflammatory process that involves the fetus.[33] Another diagnostic approach is to culture amniotic fluid or fetal membranes for organisms or to assay amniotic fluid for inflammatory mediators such as tumor necrosis factor α (TNFα) and interleukin-1 (IL-1) and IL-6.[34] With the recognition that only a minority of organisms in the human biome can be cultured, polymerase chain reaction (PCR) and DNA sequencing techniques are being used to demonstrate that chorioamnionitis is often polymicrobial with organisms that cannot be cultured.[35] Technologies to identify multiple proteins in biologic fluids also are being adapted to develop proteomic biomarkers for chorioamnionitis in amniotic fluid.[36] These technologies have the potential to rapidly diagnose inflammation and to identify specific organisms. Such approaches will change the understanding of fetal exposures to inflammation and pathology related to specific organisms.

The chorioamnion is fetal tissue, and the amniotic fluid surrounding the fetus is in direct contact with the fetal gut, skin, and lung.[33] Therefore, the fetus will be exposed to inflammation if there is histologic chorioamnionitis or if the amniotic fluid contains mediators of inflammation. The Venn diagram in Fig. 1.3 illustrates the diagnostic conundrum. Clinical chorioamnionitis does not correlate well with the subsequent diagnosis of histologic chorioamnionitis, and an amniotic fluid diagnosis of infection may or may not predict chorioamnionitis associated with preterm delivery. PCR-based analyses of amniotic fluid call into question the assumption that fetal colonization with organisms is abnormal and will cause preterm delivery. Gerber and associates[37] demonstrated that 11% of 254 presumably normal

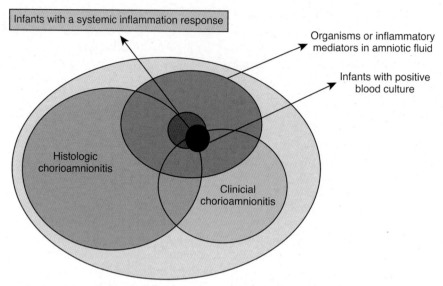

Fig. 1.3 Venn diagram illustrating the overlapping relationships among different ways to diagnose chorioamnionitis and the outcomes of sepsis and systemic inflammatory syndromes. The *outer circle* represents preterm deliveries prior to 30 weeks of gestation.

amniotic fluid samples collected at 15 to 19 weeks of gestation for genetic analysis were PCR-positive for *Ureaplasma urealyticum*. Although 17 of the 29 *Ureaplasma*-positive pregnancies had preterm labor, only 2 fetuses were delivered before 34 weeks of gestation. Perni and colleagues[38] analyzed 179 amniotic fluid samples, finding 13% positive for *Ureaplasma* and 6% positive for *Mycoplasma hominis*; however, 28 of the 33 pregnancies with positive amniotic fluid samples did not deliver preterm. Deep sequencing of the microbial genome reveal "colonization" of the amniotic fluid in some women without apparent adverse effects suggesting the presence of amniotic biome.[39,40] Attempts to extensively culture the placenta/chorioamnion have recovered multiple organisms of low virulence that include vaginal flora.[41] The severity of the chorioamnionitis does not correlate well with the organisms but tends to be more severe with *Ureaplasma* and *Mycoplasma* species.[42-44] Furthermore, in many preterm deliveries, polymicrobial organisms are recovered by culture or PCR from the amniotic fluid. The unknowns are the association of organisms with pregnancies that do not deliver preterm and the variety of organisms that can be identified by PCR. For example, Steel and coworkers[45] used a fluorescent probe for a common 16s ribosomal RNA bacterial sequence and identified organisms deep

within the membranes of all preterm deliveries and many term deliveries. These results suggest that the human pregnancy can tolerate colonization/infection with low-pathogenicity organisms. The provocative question is if the fetus needs exposure to a biome for normal development.

There is no clear answer to the question, "what is chorioamnionitis?" The multiple ways to make the diagnosis are not necessarily congruent. Furthermore, if one accepts that chorioamnionitis results from colonization/infection, then the diagnosis is imprecise in the extreme in relation to how infectious diseases are generally diagnosed. The diagnosis of an infection includes the identity of the organism, an estimate of the duration of infection, its intensity, and specific sites of involvement. The diagnosis of chorioamnionitis contains none of these elements. Research is now linking genetically determined inflammatory response characteristics of the mother and fetus with prematurity.[46] The chronic indolent chorioamnionitis associated with prematurity may result from the interaction of the environment and the genetically determined immunomodulatory characteristics of the mother and fetus. Challenges for the future are how to better diagnose and to understand what makes patients susceptible to chorioamnionitis, and how to

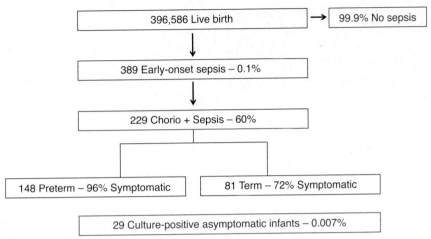

Fig. 1.4 Culture-proven sepsis—infrequent and usually symptomatic. The flow diagram is for almost 400,000 deliveries with assessments for early-onset sepsis by blood culture. The overall occurrence of sepsis was only 0.1% and the majority of the septic infants were premature and symptomatic. (Data from Wortham JM, Hansen NI, Schrag SJ, et al. Chorioamnionitis and culture-confirmed, early-onset neonatal infections. *Pediatrics*. 2016;137(1):e20152323.)

quantify the severity potential for fetal injury from the chorioamnionitis.[31]

CLINICAL PULMONARY OUTCOMES OF FETAL EXPOSURE TO INFLAMMATION/INFECTION

An important perspective is how infrequent severe sepsis and pneumonia occur in populations where the diagnosis of clinical chorioamnionitis affects 5% to 10% of the population. A clinical experience from Dallas is representative: of 23,321 deliveries, 7% (1660) were diagnosed as clinical chorioamnionitis and 1571 infants were asymptomatic.[47] Only 61 (0.26%) were ultimately thought to be sick and needed NICU care, primarily for respiratory and sepsis symptoms. The occurrence of culture-proven sepsis is very infrequent, and of 396,586 infants, 389 or 0.1% had early-onset sepsis with 60% of them having clinical chorioamnionitis. Most of the infants with sepsis were born preterm and symptomatic (Fig. 1.4).[48] Another concern is a sepsis/pneumonia risk for infants born as preterm infants after PROM. Should women with PROM have immediate delivery on presentation or expectant management with maternal treatment with antibiotics? A recent trial demonstrated that expectant management was associated with fewer cesarean sections, less RDS, and no difference in neonatal sepsis.[49] While a risk of

infection is associated with chorioamnionitis, the risk is very low for asymptomatic infants and overtreatment with antibiotics is prevalent.

The fetal effects of chorioamnioitis are much more frequent in preterm populations. This preterm population is also frequently exposed to other common exposures (Table 1.1). A decreased incidence of RDS was associated with preterm PROM, a surrogate marker for chorioamnionitis, as early as 1974.[50] Watterberg and associates[51] reported in 1996 that ventilated preterm infants exposed to histologic chorioamnionitis had a lower incidence of RDS but a higher incidence of BPD than infants not exposed to chorioamnionitis. Furthermore, the initial tracheal aspirates from infants exposed to chorioamnioitis contained proinflammatory mediators such as IL-1, IL-6, and IL-8, indicating that the lung inflammation was of antenatal origin. Other reports support that association.[52,53] Clinical chorioamnionitis was associated with decreased death in all infants born at or before 26 weeks of gestation in the United Kingdom and Ireland in 1995.[54] Hannaford and colleagues[55] identified *U. urealyticum* as an organism of fetal origin that was associated with a decreased risk of RDS. Lahra and coworkers[56] noted, in a population of 724 preterm infants, that RDS was decreased for

TABLE 1.1   Characteristics of Antenatal Variables for 22 to 28 Weeks Gestational Age Infants Cared for in NICHD Neonatal Research Network Centers[a]

Characteristic	Percentage of Population Affected from 1993 to 2012 (%)	Percentage Change from 1993 to 2012
Antenatal corticosteroids	80	Increased by 62%
Antenatal antibiotics	66	Increased by 33%
Cesarean delivery	56	Increased by 19%
Small for gestational age	7	No change
Multiple births	24	Increased by 8%

[a]34,636 infants receiving care from 2003 to 2012 at the National Institute of Child Health and Human Development centers.

Data from Stoll BJ, Hansen NI, Bell EF, et al. Trends in Care Practices, Morbidity, and Mortality of Extremely Preterm Neonates, 1993-2012. *JAMA.* 2015;314(10):1039-1051.

infants exposed to histologic chorioamnionitis (odds ratio [OR] 0.49, 95% confidence interval [CI] 0.31–0.78) or chorioamnionitis plus funisitis (OR 0.23, 95% CI 0.15–0.35) relative to no chorioamnionitis. This group also reported a 13-year experience that histologic chorioamnionitis (with or without funisitis) was associated with a decreased risk of BPD (OR 0.58, 95% CI 0.51–0.67).[57] A recent systematic meta-analysis showed that histologic chorioamnionitis was associated with increased BPD, but there was low confidence in the findings because of evidence of publication bias.[58]

In contrast, there are other reports associating chorioamnionitis with poor pulmonary and other outcomes. Hitti and associates,[59] for example, reported that high levels of TNFα in amniotic fluid predicted prolonged postnatal ventilation, suggesting early and persistent lung injury from chorioamnionitis. Ramsey and colleagues[60] also demonstrated that chorioamnionitis increased neonatal morbidities. Laughon and coworkers,[61] after extensively evaluating and culturing the placentas of 1340 infants born before 28 weeks of gestation, found no association between histologic chorioamnionitis, funisitis, or specific organisms and the initial oxygen requirements of the infants or subsequent development of BPD. The Canadian Neonatal Network also reported that clinical chorioamnionitis was not predictive of RDS or BPD.[62]

These discrepant reports need to be understood within the complexities of the diagnosis of chorioamnionitis as well as the factors contributing to the diagnosis of RDS or BPD. Van Marter and associates[63] evaluated the outcomes of ventilated VLBW infants and found that chorioamnionitis was associated with a decreased incidence of BPD (OR 0.2). However, BPD was increased if the infant had been exposed to chorioamnionitis and either was mechanical ventilated for more than 7 days (OR 3.2) or had postnatal sepsis (OR 2.9). Lahra and coworkers[57] noted the same associations in an unselected population of 761 infants with gestation less than 30 weeks. BPD was lower in infants exposed to histologic chorioamnionitis than in infants without chorioamnionitis, as noted previously. However, the combination of histologic chorioamnionitis and postnatal sepsis increased the risk for BPD (OR 1.98, 95% CI 1.15–3.39). These reports demonstrate that antenatal and postnatal exposures interact to change outcomes such as BPD. Been and colleagues[64,65] reported that newborns exposed to chorioamnionitis with fetal involvement had more severe RDS and impaired surfactant treatment responses. In contrast, infants exposed to chorioamnionitis without fetal involvement had minimal lung disease. The severity of the chorioamnionitis and postnatal interventions confound simple correlations between chorioamnionitis and outcomes such as RDS and BPD.

Other studies have explored the associations of antenatal inflammation with postnatal lung outcomes with measurements of proinflammatory cytokines in umbilical cord plasma and tracheal aspirates collected shortly after birth. In general, cord plasma from early gestational deliveries had higher proinflammatory cytokine levels than cord plasma from term deliveries, but the median values were not greatly different,[66] suggesting little useful resolution between the preterm and term populations. Although Ambalavanan and coworkers[67] could detect differences in blood cytokines collected within 4 hours of birth for infants in whom BPD developed from those without BPD, the resolution between the populations was not clinically useful for the prediction of risk of BPD. Similarly, Paananen and associates[68] found higher selected cord

TABLE 1.2 Pulmonary and Systemic Outcomes for Consecutively Treated Infants Born Before 30 Weeks of Gestation and Exposed to Infection[a]

	PERCENTAGE OF POPULATION (%)		
Histologically Diagnosed Chorioamnionitis	Yes	No	*P* value
Respiratory distress syndrome	61	73	0.008
Bronchopulmonary dysplasia	17	17	NS
Fetal inflammatory response syndrome	44	18	<0.001
Positive result of cord blood culture	Yes	No	*P* value
Respiratory distress syndrome	66	65	NS
Bronchopulmonary dysplasia	27	10	0.001
Fetal inflammatory response syndrome	41	26	0.007

[a]A comparison of fetal exposures diagnosed by histologic chorioamnionitis or positive results of cord blood cultures for *Urea-plasma* or *Mycoplasma*.
Data from Andrews WW, Goldenberg RL, Faye-Petersen O,
 et al. The Alabama Preterm Birth study: polymorphonuclear and mononuclear cell placental infiltrations, other markers of inflammation, and outcomes in 23- to 32-week preterm newborn infants. *Am J Obstet Gynecol.* 2006;195(3):803-808; and Goldenberg RL, Andrews WW, Goepfert AR, et al. The Alabama Preterm Birth Study: umbilical cord blood *Ureaplasma urealyticum* and *Mycoplasma hominis* cultures in very preterm newborn infants. *Am J Obstet Gynecol.* 2008; 198(1):43.e41-e45.

plasma cytokine levels in infants exposed to severe chorioamnionitis. The cord cytokine levels decreased with age for infants at lower risk for BPD, but cord cytokine levels were not reliable predictors of BPD. De Dooy and colleagues[52] predicted chorioamnionitis from IL-8 levels in tracheal aspirates collected soon after birth, but the clinical utility of that information also is unclear. Been and colleagues[64] did find that vascular endothelial growth factor levels in initial tracheal aspirates were predictive of BPD. However, there is no compelling evidence that measurements of pro-inflammatory mediators in cord plasma or tracheal aspirates will predict either RDS or BPD.

The inconsistent clinical correlates most likely result from the imprecise nature of the diagnosis of chorioamnionitis and its association with different populations of infants. An example of the inconsistency is the diagnosis of fetal exposures by histologic chorioamnionitis or by blood culture for *Ureaplasma* collected from the cord at delivery and the outcomes of RDS and BPD for the same cohort of consecutive patients (Table 1.2).[69,70] The associations with histologic chorioamnionitis and culture positivity for *Ureaplasma* for BPD are the *opposite* of those for RDS in the same cohort of patients. The diagram in Fig. 1.5 may help frame the question about the variable outcome. A progressive chorioamnionitis caused by virulent organisms may cause severe postnatal

lung and systemic inflammation with the outcomes of more severe RDS, BPD, or sepsis/death. Such outcomes are relatively infrequent in VLBW infants who are not stillborn. Fewer than 2% of VLBW infants have positive blood culture results at birth.[71] Chronic, indolent chorioamnionitis caused by organisms such as *Ureaplasma* can induce lung maturation (less RDS), but that early maturation may be associated with more BPD.[51] These associations may depend on how the diagnosis of chorioamnionitis is made (clinical, histopathologic, other) and the population of infants studied (ventilated only, all VLBW infants, other selected populations). In an attempt to better establish a cause-and-effect relationship, Viscardi and associates[72] correlated the intensity of the inflammatory response to chorioamnionitis in the fetal membranes with the clinical outcome of BPD (Fig. 1.6). More severe chorioamnionitis at delivery predicted a higher incidence and greater severity of BPD.

EXPERIMENTAL RESULTS: THE LINK BETWEEN FETAL EXPOSURE TO INFLAMMATION AND LUNG MATURATION, LUNG REMODELING

Animal models have consistently demonstrated that fetal exposure to inflammation causes lung injury and induces lung maturation. In a strict sense, lung maturation should probably be called "dysmaturation" since the beneficial effects of improved lung mechanics are

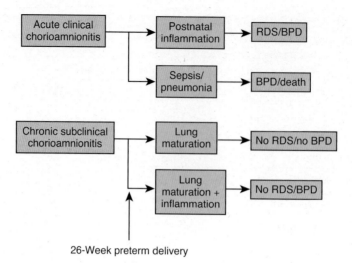

Fig. 1.5 Overview of outcomes of acute clinical or chronic subclinical chorioamnionitis. Acute chorioamnionitis with virulent organisms is likely to cause severe lung disease or death. In contrast, chronic chorioamnionitis may improve lung outcomes by inducing lung maturation. However, bronchopulmonary dysplasia *(BPD)* may occur if the inflammation in the fetal lung is increased by postnatal exposures to oxygen, ventilation, or postnatal sepsis. *RDS*, Respiratory distress syndrome.

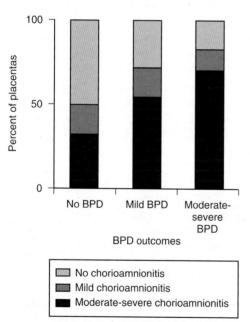

Fig. 1.6 Relationship of severity of chorioamnionitis by histologic grading with the severity of bronchopulmonary dysplasia *(BPD)*. Infants with moderate-to-severe BPD were more likely to have been exposed to more severe histologic chorioamnionitis. (Data from Viscardi RM, Muhumuza CK, Rodriguez A, et al. Inflammatory markers in intrauterine and fetal blood and cerebrospinal fluid compartments are associated with adverse pulmonary and neurologic outcomes in preterm infants. *Pediatr Res.* 2004;55:1009-1017.)

also accompanied by altered lung development. Bry and colleagues[73] first demonstrated in 1997 that inflammation induced lung maturation by intraamniotic injection of IL-1α. Our group found that intraamniotic injection of the proinflammatory mediator endotoxin from *Escherichia coli* in sheep caused chorioamnionitis (inflammatory cells and increased IL-1β and IL-6 mRNA expression in the chorioamnion), inflammatory cells in amniotic fluid, and increased IL-8 protein levels in amniotic fluid.[74,75] The chorioamnionitis was accompanied by inflammation of the fetal lung, as demonstrated by recruitment of granulocytes to the fetal lung tissue and air spaces within 24 hours and expression of multiple proinflammatory mediators (Fig. 1.7).[76,77] Apoptosis of lung cells increased at 24 hours, and proliferation increased at 3 days. This lung inflammation/injury sequence included multiple indicators of lung microvascular injury—epithelial nitric oxide synthase and vascular endothelial growth factor decreased, and medial smooth muscle hypertrophied.[77] Thus, intraamniotic endotoxin caused lung inflammation and an injury sequence that resulted in lung remodeling.

There are very few studies of respiratory muscle function in preterm babies. Recently, Song et al. reported that intraamniotic endotoxin exposure in preterm fetal lambs resulted in transient inflammation in

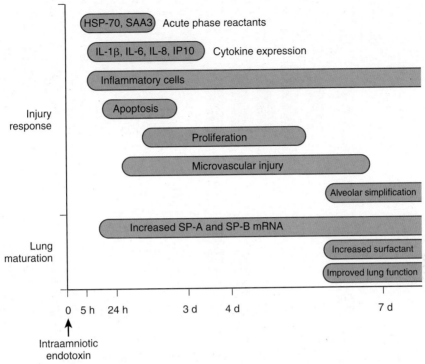

Fig. 1.7 Time course of lung injury and lung maturation responses in fetal sheep to an intraamniotic injection of endotoxin. The lung initially has an inflammation and injury response, which are followed by lung maturation. *d*, Day(s); *h*, hour(s); *HSP-70*, heat shock protein 70; *IL*, interleukin; *IP10*, interferon gamma–inducing protein 10; *mRNA*, messenger RNA; *SP*, surfactant protein.

fetal diaphragm followed by atrophic gene expression resulting in impaired diaphragm contractility.[78]

Inflammation was associated with the induction of the mRNAs for the surfactant proteins within 12 to 24 hours, persistent elevation of those mRNAs for weeks, and an increase in alveolar surfactant proteins and lipids with improved lung function within 5 to 7 days.[74,79] The improvement in lung function was accompanied by a decrease in mesenchymal tissue and an increase in potential gas volume in the fetal lung. The residual effects of the injury at 7 days were greater thickness of the pulmonary microvessels and a reduction in secondary septation of the alveoli.[77,80] However, the net effect was a lung that was easier to ventilate because of improved compliance and that had better gas exchange (Fig. 1.8). Of note, the lung injury followed by maturation sequence did not result from "fetal stress," because fetal blood cortisol levels did not increase. An elegant new single-cell

RNA-seq study in fetal rhesus macaques provides an unprecedented resolution of mechanisms of lung injury. Fetal rhesus macaques in the saccular stage exposed to intraamniotic lipopolysaccharide (LPS) demonstrated extensive injury to alveolar type I cells, specialized alveolar capillary endothelium including endothelial progenitors in the lung resulting in loss of secondary alveolar septae.[81] Intraamniotic endotoxin also increased surfactant protein mRNA in the primate.[82] Lung inflammation results in accelerated lung maturation.

To understand whether the signal for lung inflammation or lung maturation during chorioamnionitis is systemic versus local, Moss and colleagues[83] isolated the lung from the amniotic fluid surgically with collection of the fetal lung fluid in a bag placed in the amniotic cavity. Intraamniotic endotoxin, without exposure to fetal lung, induced chorioamnionitis but not lung inflammation or lung maturation. In contrast, a

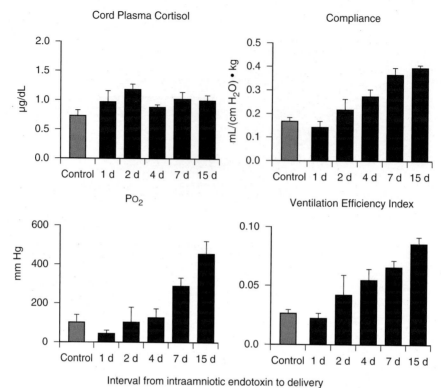

Fig. 1.8 Cord plasma cortisol values and lung function following intraamniotic injections of endotoxin for intervals from 1 to 15 days before preterm delivery and mechanical ventilation of lambs. Plasma cortisol values did not increase from the low fetal values. Lung function increased progressively following the intraamniotic injection of endotoxin. (Redrawn from Jobe AH, Newnham JP, Willet KE, et al. Endotoxin-induced lung maturation in preterm lambs is not mediated by cortisol. *Am J Respir Crit Care Med.* 2000;162(5):1656-1661.)

24-hour tracheal infusion of endotoxin induced both lung inflammation and lung maturation. This same result also was achieved with a fetal tracheal infusion of IL-1 as the proinflammatory agonist.[84] Therefore, the sequence from fetal lung inflammation to maturation did not result from a lung response to a systemic fetal inflammatory response. Also, new mediators resulting from the chorioamnionitis were not required for the response. Rather, direct contact of the fetal lung—presumably the airway epithelium—with endotoxin or IL-1 given by intraamniotic injection or tracheal infusion induced the lung maturation. The initial inflammation is thought to result from responses to the mediators by the airway epithelium, because the airways express the acute-phase reactants heat shock protein 70 (Hsp70) and serum amyloid A3 (SAA3), and there are very few monocytes/macrophages present in the fetal lung to initiate an inflammatory

response. However, in chronic chorioamnionitis, the inflammatory products of the chorioamnionitis or organisms in the amniotic fluid probably are mediating the responses of the fetal lungs.

MEDIATORS THAT INDUCE FETAL LUNG INFLAMMATORY RESPONSES

Innate immune responses are signaled by a family of pattern recognition molecules called the Toll-like receptors (TLRs). TLR4 recognizes endotoxin from gram-negative organisms, TLR2 signals gram-positive organisms, and TLR3 recognizes double-stranded RNA from viral pathogens, for example. The chorioamnion has TLRs, but there is very little information about the pattern of responses or the expression of the TLRs in the human fetus.[85] The inflammatory cells in the chorioamnion are likely of maternal origin when organisms localized between the endometrium and chorioamnion initiate the inflammation.[86] The fetal rabbit lung expresses low levels of TLR2 and TLR4, and mRNA levels remain unchanged for the last third of gestation in the fetal mice and sheep.[87,88] Empirically, *E. coli* endotoxin induces a rapid inflammatory response in the fetal sheep lung, as does IL-1, a cytokine that signals inflammation through a receptor that shares receptor elements and the signaling pathways with endotoxin. A high dose of a TLR2 agonist given by intraamniotic injection in sheep induced less inflammation than did endotoxin and had inconsistent effects on lung maturation. Blood monocytes from preterm sheep also do not respond as well as monocytes from adult sheep to challenge with TLR agonists.[89] The fetus may not respond uniformly to different TLR agonists.

Ureaplasma given by intraamniotic injection in sheep can colonize the amniotic fluid and fetal lung as early as 50 days of gestation (term is 150 days) and cause low-grade chronic lung inflammation and lung maturation (Table 1.3).[90] In fetal sheep, the innate inflammatory response to *Ureaplasma* is modest, with an increase in neutrophils by 3 days and persistent increase in lymphocyte populations in the lung.[91] The organism is not cleared from the fetal lungs. Colonization with *Ureaplasma* also does not cause fetal death or injury, a result similar to the outcomes of human pregnancies in which amniotic fluid samples were PCR-positive for *Ureaplasma* at 15 to 19 weeks of gestation.[37,38] However, the fetal lungs have increased surfactant and persistent elevations in mRNAs for surfactant proteins. This model of chronic colonization or infection of the fetal lung with *Ureaplasma* may closely resemble the clinical effects of *Ureaplasma* associated with preterm deliveries in humans.

These experiments demonstrate that fetal sheep can respond to a variety of proinflammatory agonists and can be colonized with *Ureaplasma*, the organisms most frequently associated with preterm delivery in the human. However, fetal responses do not simply replicate responses in the adult. For example, fetal sheep do not respond to intraamniotic or intravascular injections of sheep recombinant TNFα,[92] and as noted previously, responses to TLR2 agonist were insufficient to consistently induce lung maturation. The spectrum of the response potential of the fetus and the fetal lung to the multiple mediators of innate immune responses remains to be studied. Clinical responses also may reflect the polymicrobial nature of the chorioamnionitis. Questions that remain relate to receptor expression, the cell localization of that expression, the response potential of the signaling pathways, and the maturity of the integration of innate and acquired immune responses.

EARLY GESTATIONAL FETAL LUNG RESPONSES TO INFLAMMATION

The interval from fetal exposure to chorioamnionitis and lung inflammation or lung maturation is not known in the human, primarily because of the lack of precision about the diagnosis of chorioamnionitis. In fetal sheep, significant lung maturation is not detected until 4 to 7 days after an intraamniotic injection of endotoxin.[79] Lung maturation is striking if the interval between intraamniotic endotoxin injection and preterm delivery is 15 days. Intraamniotic *Ureaplasma*

TABLE 1.3 Measurements After Intra-Amniotic Injection of *Ureaplasma Parvum* in Sheep Fetuses[a]

	Controls	*Ureaplasma* Group
Culture for *Ureaplasma*	Negative	Positive
Plasma cortisol (mg/dL)	0.43 ± 0.05	0.54 ± 0.06
Measurements in Bronchiolar Lavage Fluid[b]		
Inflammatory cells (×10⁶/kg)	0.1 ± 0.06	6.7 ± 1.2
Protein (mg/kg)	85 ± 21	34 ± 3
Saturated phosphatidylcholine (mmol/kg)	6.7 ± 3.0	0.2 ± 0.1
Lung gas volume (mL/kg)	11.2 ± 1.5	28.5 ± 2.8

[a]Intraamniotic injection of 2×10^7 colony-forming units of *Ureaplasma parvum* at 67 days gestational age (GA) for sheep fetuses; measurements made at 124 days GA.
[b]Values per kg are expressed per kg body weight; all values for the *Ureaplasma* animals are different from those in controls except plasma cortisol.
Data from Moss TJ, Nitsos I, Kramer BW, et al. Intra-amniotic endotoxin induces lung maturation by direct effects on the developing respiratory tract in preterm sheep. *Am J Obstet Gynecol.* 2002;187(4):1059-1065.

did not induce lung maturation within 7 days but did induce lung maturation when given 14 to 45 days before preterm delivery.[90] Intraamniotic endotoxin given at 60 days of gestation (40% of gestation) to fetal sheep resulted in a doubling of lung-saturated phosphatidylcholine, increased SP-A, SP-B, and SP-C mRNA, and improved in lung function 65 days later.[93] The fetal sheep lung can respond to intraamniotic endotoxin/chorioamnionitis across a wide range of GAs. The question how early in gestation an inflammatory stimulus can modulate fetal lung development remains unanswered in the clinical context. However, the frequent occurrence of early lung maturation and chorioamnionitis suggests that inflammation is the major mediator of lung maturation in the very preterm infant.

MECHANISMS OF INFLAMMATION-MEDIATED LUNG MATURATION

The mechanisms responsible for inflammation-induced lung maturation are not well understood. The minimal amount of *E. coli* endotoxin given by intraamniotic injection that will induce lung maturation in the fetal sheep is 1 to 4 mg, and doses as high as 100 mg induce lung maturation without increasing the amount of lung inflammation or causing fetal injury or preterm delivery.[75,79] In general, the amount of lung inflammation induced by chorioamnionitis correlated with the amount of lung maturation. Our group used a monoclonal antibody to the integrin CD18 to block endotoxin-induced lung inflammation, which also prevented lung maturation (Fig. 1.9).[94] In contrast, inflammation and lung maturation induced by IL-I was not blocked by this anti-CD18 antibody. This experiment directly links inflammation to lung maturation and further demonstrates that different proinflammatory agonists can recruit inflammatory cells to the fetal lungs by different mechanisms.

This inflammation-maturation relationship was further examined with an IL-1 receptor blocker.[95] IL-1α or IL-1β are potent inducers of chorioamnionitis, lung inflammation, and lung maturation. When the IL-1 receptor antagonist IL-1ra was given into the amniotic fluid, about 80% of the lung inflammatory response to intraamniotic endotoxin was blocked, and lung maturation decreased. Since IL-1β is a potent cytokine, its secretion is exquisitely controlled in the cytoplasm by inflammasomes—a collection of interacting proteins that ultimately activate caspase-1, which cleaves pro–IL-1β to active IL-1β. In mice, whose inflammasome NLRP3 was knocked out, there was a significant reduction of lung IL-1β of neonatal mice in response to hyperoxia challenge with a corresponding protection against BPD-like changes in response to hyperoxia.[96] These experiments demonstrate that lung inflammation in response to multiple stimuli is mediated, at least in part, by IL-1 signaling and that lung inflammation can drive lung maturation response. There currently is no information about what products of lung inflammation signal lung maturation. Presumably, mediators produced locally in the distal lung parenchyma, possibly by granulocytes and/or monocytes, induce a signaling cascade resulting in the mesenchymal and type II cell changes that result in lung maturation. Insight into this signaling sequence may provide clues for the development of clinically practical strategies to induce lung maturation.

EXPERIMENTAL CHRONIC CHORIOAMNIONITIS

Although the majority of VLBW infants may be exposed to chronic chorioamnionitis, the duration and the intensity of the inflammatory exposure to the fetus remain undefined. A single proinflammatory exposure from intraamniotic injections of endotoxin in fetal lambs caused acute lung inflammation, mild microvascular injury, and an arrest in alveolar septation by 7 days.[77,80] Low-grade inflammation (increased inflammatory cells) persisted for weeks. Live *Ureaplasma* caused mild inflammation despite prolonged persistence in the fetal lung.[90] The clinically relevant question is how the fetal lung copes with prolonged exposures to inflammatory agonists such as endotoxin. Surprisingly, few VLBW infants seem to have severe pneumonia after preterm birth despite exposure to infection or inflammation. Although a single intrauterine exposure to endotoxin caused histologic changes consistent with a mild BPD phenotype in experimental animals, infants are not born with BPD. A possible exception is the rapid development of the BPD variant described by radiologic changes as the Wilson-Mikity syndrome, which has been associated with chorioamnionitis.[97] However, in general, severe lung injury and pneumonia

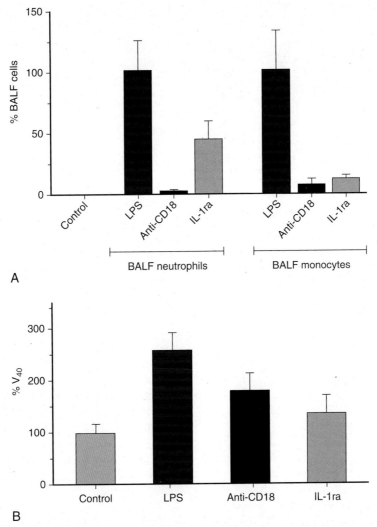

Fig. 1.9 Anti-CD18 antibody and IL-1 receptor antagonist *(IL-1ra)* block lung inflammation and maturation in fetal sheep. A, Fetal sheep were given an anti-CD18 antibody by intramuscular injection or IL-1ra into the amniotic fluid 3 hours before intraamniotic lipopolysaccharide *(LPS)*. Both treatments decreased the numbers of neutrophils and monocytes in bronchoalveolar lavage fluid *(BALF)*, indicating almost complete blockade of the endotoxin-induced lung inflammation at 2 days. B, The treatments also decreased lung gas volumes, measured at 40 cm H_2O pressure (V_{40}) relative to LPS, indicating decreased lung maturation. (Data from Kallapur SG, Moss JTM, Newnham JP, et al. Recruited inflammatory cells mediate endotoxin-induced lung maturation in preterm fetal lambs. *Am J Respir Crit Care Med.* 2005;172(10):1315-1321; and Kallapur SG, Nitsos I, Moss TJ, et al. IL-1 mediates pulmonary and systemic inflammatory responses to chorioamnionitis induced by lipopolysaccharide. *Am J Respir Crit Care Med.* 2009;179(10):955-961.)

are infrequent after the histologic chorioamnionitis associated with preterm birth.

Our group has modeled chronic endotoxin-induced chorioamnionitis with repeated weekly intraamniotic injections of endotoxin and with osmotic pumps that deliver endotoxin continuously over 28 days to the amniotic fluid. A prolonged fetal exposure resulting from a 28-day intraamniotic infusion of endotoxin from 53% to 72% of gestation caused striking lung maturation and increases in surfactant with decreased alveolar septation at 125 days (83% of gestation).[93] When the lungs of the fetal sheep were examined at 138 days of gestation, low-grade inflammation persisted 30 days after the end of endotoxin administration and surfactant was increased

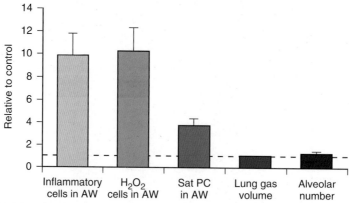

Fig. 1.10 Residual effects at 138 days of gestation of the intraamniotic infusion of 1 mg/day of endotoxin for 28 days of gestation, from day 80 to day 108, in fetal sheep. All measurements are expressed relative to the control group, which was normalized to 1.0 *(dashed line)*. Residual indicators of inflammation were the number of inflammatory cells in bronchoalveolar lavage *(BAL)* and their ability to produce hydrogen peroxide *(H₂O₂)*. Although the amount of saturated phosphatidylcholine *(Sat PC)* in alveolar wash (AW) was increased, lung structure was not altered. (Data from Kallapur SG, Nitsos I, Moss TJM, et al: Chronic endotoxin exposure does not cause sustained structural abnormalities in the fetal sheep lungs. *Am J Physiol Lung Cell Mol Physiol.* 2005;288:L966-L974.)

as a residual effect of the induced lung maturation (Fig. 1.10).[98] Remarkably, all anatomic indicators of the arrest of alveolar septation seen at 125 days of gestation had disappeared. There also were no biochemical or histologic indicators of microvascular injury.

Weekly intraamniotic injections with 10 mg endotoxin given at 100 days, 107 days, 114 days, and 121 days of gestation resulted in the persistence of inflammatory cells in the bronchoalveolar lavage, just prior to term.[98] The mRNA for the proinflammatory cytokine IL-1β in lung tissue was higher than in controls, as was the amount of surfactant, but there were no changes in the lung architecture or microvasculature. These results demonstrate that the fetal lung can adapt to chronic inflammation and that despite a brief interference with alveolar septation and microvascular development, the fetal lung corrects the deficits and can continue to develop. *Ureaplasma* also causes subtle alterations in lung structure after a 14-day exposure, but the changes do not persist with more chronic exposures.[91,99]

IMMUNE RESPONSE AND MODULATION FROM FETAL EXPOSURES TO INFLAMMATION

A central question is how the naïve immune system of the fetus responds to an intrauterine inflammatory challenge. In a rhesus macaque model of chorioamnionitis, inlammatory cytokines IL-17(+) and IL-22(+),

CD4(+) expressing T cells increased in the spleen of endotoxin-exposed fetuses, and the normally antiinflammatory regulatory T cell (Treg) frequency decreased.[100] Compounding the decrease in Tregs, larger proportions of the normally antiinflammatory Tregs expressed the proinflammatory cytokine 1L-17 (IL-17(+)FOXP3(+)) designated inflammatory Tregs. The emergence of inflammatory Tregs was largely dependent on IL-1 signaling. These results demonstrate that a prenatal inflammatory environment can lead to inadequate Treg generation in the thymus with a switch of splenic Tregs toward an inflammatory phenotype.

The sentinel immune cell of the lung is the alveolar macrophage. In adult humans and animals, macrophages are located in the airspaces directly in contact with the alveolar hypophase. Fetuses do not normally have alveolar macrophages. In mice, macrophages can be detected in the lung interstitium from early gestation, while in other species, including nonhuman primates and sheep, very few mature macrophages are found in the fetal lung. In all species, mature alveolar macrophages begin populating the lung in large numbers postnatally with the onset of air breathing. Immature lung monocytes from preterm sheep have a minimal IL-6 secretory response to an in vitro challenge to endotoxin and do not respond to TNFα.[101] However, intraamniotic endotoxin matures the lung monocytes by stimulating GM-CSF and PU.1 expression in the fetal

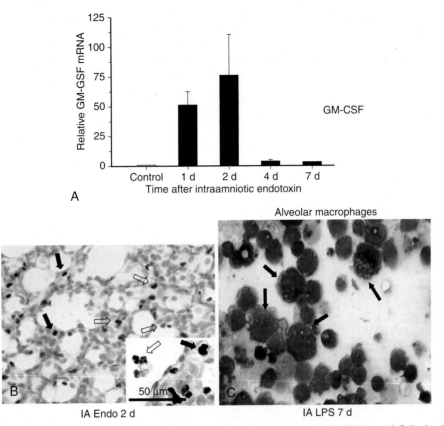

Fig. 1.11 Intraamniotic administration of lipopolysaccharide *(LPS)* matures alveolar macrophages in the fetal lungs. A, Following the intraamniotic injection *(IA)* of 10 mg LPS, granulocyte-monocyte colony-stimulating factor *(GM-CSF)* is induced in the fetal lung and (B) PU.1-positive cells appear in the lung, indicating maturation from monocytes to macrophages. Expression is localized to nuclei of monocyte cells *(filled arrows)* and neutrophils *(open arrows).* C, By 7 days *(d)*, mature-appearing alveolar macrophages *(arrows)* are in high numbers in alveolar washes. *mRNA*, Messenger RNA. (Data from Kramer BW, Joshi SN, Moss TJ, et al. Endotoxin-induced maturation of monocytes in preterm fetal sheep lung. *Am J Physiol Lung Cell Mol Physiol.* 2007;293:L345-L353.)

lung (Fig. 1.11). These monocytes migrate into the fetal alveolar spaces and respond vigorously to both endotoxin and TNFα in vitro.[101] Thus exposure to a proinflammatory agonist in the amniotic fluid is a potent stimulus for maturation and responsiveness of monocytes in the lung. Single-cell RNA-seq experiments in the fetal rhesus macaque lung exposed to LPS demonstrated that the myeloid cell subsets participating in lung inflammation include neutrophils, interstitial macrophages, inflammatory monocytes, and alveolar macrophages. Furthermore, matrix fibroblasts in addition to myeloid cells mediate the injury response via CXC and CC family of chemokines/cytokines. Blockade of IL-1

and TNF reduced CCL and CXCL cytokine expression, and promoted continued alveologenesis, although the directs effects on myeloid cells were only modest.[81,102]

Intraamniotic endotoxin also can cause an innate immune tolerance in the fetus. In adult animals and humans, endotoxin tolerance is the suppression of endotoxin signaling caused by a complex reprogramming of inflammatory responses. As part of endotoxin tolerance, proinflammatory cytokine expression is downregulated, while there is no change or an increase in the expression of antiinflammatory genes, antimicrobial genes, and genes mediating phagocytosis. In the preterm fetal sheep, exposure to intraamniotic endotoxin 2 days before delivery induces a robust expression to cytokines in the fetal lung. However, if the fetus is exposed to two intraamniotic endotoxin injections of the same dose 7 days and 2 days prior to delivery, the fetal lung is refractory to the second endotoxin injection.[103] Interestingly, both lung and blood monocytes are refractory to an in vitro challenge with endotoxin.

The phenomenon of innate immune tolerance is not just restricted to exposure to endotoxin. Exposure to intraamniotic *Ureaplasma parvum* almost completely abolished responsiveness of the fetal lung to endotoxin implying a profound immune paralysis in the fetal lung induced by *Ureaplasma* exposure.[104] The lung and blood monocytes from fetal sheep exposed to two injections of intraamniotic endotoxin were also refractory to stimulation by other TLR agonists, indicating a cross-tolerance.[105] Other interactive phenomena between antenatal endotoxin and postnatal inflammatory insults have also been reported. Intraamniotic endotoxin alone induced aberrant lung development and pulmonary hypertension in rats similar to that in sheep. When fetal mice exposed to endotoxin were exposed as newborns to moderate hyperoxia, the lung abnormalities were no longer evident. However, exposure to severe hyperoxia as newborns further enhanced the pulmonary abnormalities induced by antenatal endotoxin.[106] Thus the interactive phenomena between different inflammatory insults can be complex and either increase or reduce lung injury responses. The innate immune tolerance is time-dependent; thus it is not clear how these immune phenomena will translate into clinical scenarios where the timing of exposure to different inflammatory insults is not known. Although the precise mechanisms of innate immune tolerance are not known, the expression of the negative regulator of Toll/IL-1 signaling, IRAK-M was increased in both the lung and blood monocytes,[103] suggesting a possible mechanism for innate immune tolerance in the fetus.

IMMUNE CHANGES IN PRETERM INFANTS EXPOSED TO CHORIOAMNIONITIS

There are limited studies on immune changes in response to chorioamnionitis in humans. In 2010, the National Institutes of Health initiated a collaborative network of five major academic centers in the United

States (Prematurity and Respiratory Outcomes Program [PROP]) to understand the epidemiology and pathogenesis of BPD and to facilitate biomarker discovery.[107] As part of PROP, studies were conducted to identify immunological alterations that might predispose to BPD. In a study of 35 extremely low-birthweight (ELBW) infants, adverse ratios of the antiinflammatory Treg to the proinflammatory Th17 cells in the peripheral blood were detected in ELBW infants exposed to funisitis but not to BPD.[108] The infants with severe BPD had increased expression of IL-4 mRNA in peripheral blood mononuclear cells in response to stimulation. However, another study suggested involvement of Tregs in the pathogenesis of BPD.[109] A proinflammatory CD4(+) T-cell status was noted in preterm infants exposed to chorioamnionitis and those developing BPD, but those developing BPD also had decreased numbers of the antiinflammatory Tregs.[109] In another study from the PROP cohort, CD8+ T cells from the more immature infants had a loss of regulatory co-receptor CD31 and greater effector differentiation than the more mature infants. This may place preterm neonates at unique risk for CD8+ T-cell–mediated inflammation and impaired T-cell memory formation.[110]

INFLAMMATORY MEDIATORS AND BRONCHOPULMONARY DYSPLASIA

To understand the pathogenesis of BPD, NICHD enrolled a cohort of 1067 VLBW infants at multiple Neonatal Research Network sites in the United States.[67] Dried blood spots were collected from these infants serially over the first 21 days of life. Plasma cytokines in infants surviving without BPD were compared to those developing BPD or who died. In early samples from the BPD group (0–3 days), IL-8 and IL-10 were increased and RANTES and IL-17 were decreased. In the late samples (14–21 days), IL-6 and interferon gamma were increased in infants who later had BPD. These data were recently reanalyzed for the surviving infants with BPD by D'Angio et al.[111] using the different respiratory patterns identified by Laughon et al.[61] The premise of this analysis was that since BPD is a heterogenous disease, better insights might be gained by comparing cytokines in infants who developed BPD and had persistently high oxygen needs for the first 14 days (classic BPD) versus those needing very low oxygen for the first 14 days of life (new BPD); IL-6, IL-8, IL-10, IL-18, C-reactive protein, MIP-1a, and MMP9 were increased in new versus classic BPD. Increased IL-8 and ICAM1 and decreased RANTES, VEGF, and MMP1 were demonstrated in plasma from infants developing BPD/death versus those surviving without BPD in another report.[112] Thus these different studies, while suggesting that inflammatory pathways underlie BPD, do not identify a particular inflammatory pathway. A limitation of these studies is that the inflammatory mediators associated with BPD may be missed because the expression and effect may be restricted to the lungs and not be present in the blood. Tissue cannot be sampled clinically. Since multiple different etiologies contribute to BPD (e.g., oxygen, mechanical ventilation, antenatal inflammation, postnatal infections), the complexity of inflammatory pathways induced may preclude identification of common pathways leading to BPD.

INTERACTIONS BETWEEN ANTENATAL CORTICOSTEROID TREATMENTS AND CHORIOAMNIONITIS

Antenatal corticosteroids and lung maturation are discussed in detail elsewhere in this book. In this section, we will focus on interactions between two seemingly opposite fetal exposures of corticosteroids and prenatal inflammation. Corticosteroids are given antenatally to more than 80% of the women at risk for preterm delivery before 30 weeks of gestation, and the majority of these women have undiagnosed (histologic) chorioamnionitis.[30,61] The majority of women with preterm rupture of membranes have histologic chorioamnionitis. Thus, preterm rupture of membranes is a surrogate marker for chorioamnionitis. The current recommendation is to give antenatal corticosteroids with preterm rupture of membranes, because the treatment reduces the incidences of RDS, intraventricular hemorrhage, and death.[113] In clinical series, antenatal corticosteroids are of benefit for preterm deliveries that in retrospect had associated histologic chorioamnionitis.[114] A 2011 meta-analysis of observational studies identified benefit of corticosteroid treatment in infants from women with chorioamnionitis (Table 1.4).[115] Antenatal corticosteroids also decrease the fetal inflammatory response syndrome in preterm infants exposed to histologic chorioamnionitis.[114]

TABLE 1.4 Meta-Analysis of Observational Studies of Antenatal Corticosteroid Treatments for Women With Chorioamnionitis

	Odds Ratio	95% Confidence Interval
Histologic Diagnosis of Chorioamnionitis (Five Studies)		
Mortality of newborn	0.45	0.30–0.68
Respiratory distress syndrome	0.53	0.40–0.71
Bronchopulmonary dysplasia	0.79	0.35–1.83
Severe intraventricular hemorrhage	0.39	0.19–0.82
Clinical Diagnosis of Chorioamnionitis (Four Studies)		
Mortality of newborn	0.77	0.36–1.65
Respiratory distress syndrome	0.73	0.48–1.12
Bronchopulmonary dysplasia	0.80	0.37–1.74
Severe intraventricular hemorrhage	0.29	0.10–0.89

Data from Been JV, Degraeuwe PL, Kramer BW, et al. Antenatal steroids and neonatal outcome after chorioamnionitis: a meta-analysis. *BJOG.* 2011;118(2):113-122.

Although there is no specific clinical information available about how corticosteroids influence chorioamnionitis, the corticosteroids might suppress inflammation—a potential benefit—or increase the risk of progressive inflammation—a potential risk. Both outcomes seem possible on the basis of the small amount of information available from experimental studies. Maternal treatment with betamethasone suppressed the inflammation caused by intraamniotic endotoxin in the chorioamnion and lungs of fetal sheep (Fig. 1.12).[116,117] Inflammatory cells and proinflammatory cytokine expression were suppressed for about 2 days after the betamethasone treatment, but subsequently inflammation was *increased* in the lungs of lambs exposed to both maternal betamethasone and intraamniotic endotoxin in comparison with lambs exposed to endotoxin alone 5 and 15 days after the exposures. Lung maturation was greater in lambs exposed at the same time to both betamethasone and endotoxin than to either treatment alone (Fig. 1.13).[118] A surprising result was that growth restriction

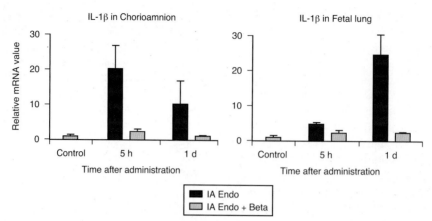

Fig. 1.12 Maternal betamethasone suppressed the inflammation induced by intraamniotic *(IA)* administration of endotoxin in the chorioamnion and fetal lung. The expression of interleukin-1β *(IL-1β)* messenger RNA *(mRNA)* was decreased to control values by maternal betamethasone given to sheep 3 hours *(h)* before IA endotoxin. *d*, Days. (Data from Newnham J, Kallapur SG, Kramer BW, et al. Betamethasone effects on chorioamnionitis induced by intra-amniotic endotoxin in sheep. *Am J Obstet Gynecol.* 2003;189:1458-1466; and Kallapur SG, Kramer BW, Moss TJ, et al. Maternal glucocorticoids increase endotoxin-induced lung inflammation in preterm lambs. *Am J Physiol Lung Cell Mol Physiol.* 2003;284:L633-L642.)

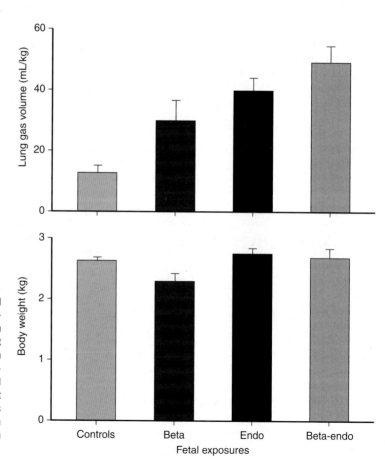

Fig. 1.13 Lung gas volumes and body weights of fetal sheep 7 days after exposure to maternal betamethasone *(Beta)*, intraamniotic endotoxin *(Endo)*, or both *(Beta-endo)*. Maximal lung gas volume measured at an airway pressure of 40 cm H$_2$O, increased with either treatment but was largest with both treatments. Only maternal betamethasone decreased fetal weight, and this effect was prevented by concurrent endotoxin exposure. (Redrawn from Newnham JP, Moss TJ, Padbury JF, et al. The interactive effects of endotoxin with prenatal glucocorticoids on short-term lung function in sheep. *Am J Obstet Gynecol.* 2001;185(1):190-197.)

induced by betamethasone did not occur with concurrent endotoxin exposure. These results in fetal sheep support the clinical observations that betamethasone can further decrease RDS in the presence of histologic chorioamnionitis.[114] In fetal sheep, the lung maturational response to endotoxin was larger and more uniform than the response to betamethasone. A distinct difference in the responses is the improvement in lung function within 15 hours after betamethasone and the delay for an improvement in lung function of at least 4 days following intraamniotic endotoxin.[119,120] Betamethasone also can augment the lung maturation induced by chronic fetal *Ureaplasma* colonization.[121]

The increased inflammation in the fetal sheep lungs that occurs 5 to 15 days after combined betamethasone and endotoxin exposures is a potential concern. A potential mechanism to explain the increased inflammation is that both betamethasone and the endotoxin "mature" an immature innate immune system. Blood monocytes from fetal sheep have decreased responses in vitro to endotoxin stimulation in comparison with monocytes from adult sheep.[89] However, 7 days after the fetal exposures, the monocytes respond to endotoxin in vitro similarly to monocytes from adult sheep. Maternal betamethasone also initially suppresses the fetal monocyte, but function is increased 7 days after the maternal treatment.[122] These results illustrate just how clinically complex interactions between these two clinically relevant exposures may be.

These experiments in fetal sheep describe simultaneous exposures to betamethasone and chorioamnionitis. The more likely clinical scenarios are the superposition of maternal betamethasone treatments on chronic, subclinical chorioamnionitis or maternal betamethasone treatments followed by the acute onset of chorioamnionitis. In fetal sheep, exposure to endotoxin 14 days followed by betamethasone 7 days before preterm delivery qualitatively induced the largest lung maturation response.[123] There is no information about how timing of exposures may alter clinical outcomes. Repetitive courses of betamethasone treatments may be a concern, particularly when chorioamnionitis is present. The clinical dilemma is that histologic chorioamnionitis is a retrospective diagnosis of a process that is frequently clinically silent.

Intrauterine Growth Restriction/Small for Gestational Age (SGA)

Fetuses identified to have IUGR on the basis of estimates of fetal size and Doppler flow patterns of the fetal circulation and infants born SGA according to standardized growth charts are overlapping populations with varied causes for the inadequate growth. For the preterm segment of this population, the majority of infants result from pregnancies with associated hypertension or preeclampsia,[124] excluding genetic and chromosomal abnormalities. Lung disease after term or near-term delivery has not been well studied but is not appreciated as a clinical problem. In contrast, preterm growth-restricted infants and infants of preeclamptic pregnancies have an increased risk for RDS, despite the severe chronic stress experienced by the fetuses.[125,126] Jelin and associates[127] also reported that preeclampsia with onset early in pregnancy increased the risk for SGA infants (OR 3.9, 59% CI 2.5–6.2) and for RDS (OR 1.5, 95% CI 1.1–2.2). In a prospective multicenter study of 587 preterm infants <34 weeks, maternal preexisting hypertension was identified as an independent risk factor for bronchopulmonary dysplasia, with a twofold increased risk.[128] The concept has been that fetal stress will increase fetal cortisol levels and induce lung maturation, but the stresses causing fetal growth restriction and preeclampsia do not decrease RDS relative to the comparison populations of preterm infants. We suspect that the comparison group simply illustrates one "elephant in the room," in that the comparison population may be enriched for infants exposed to chorioamnionitis, which is less frequent in IUGR/SGA infants. This interpretation suggests decreased RDS in both populations relative to a theoretical population of "normal" preterm infants. A reasonable conclusion is that preeclampsia/IUGR/SGA preterm infants are not protected from respiratory problems soon after birth, as captured by the diagnosis of RDS.

These small infants are at increased risk for mortality and BPD. In one study, IUGR or SGA status at birth raised mortality for infants at all gestations, and increased the need for respiratory support at 28 days of age primarily for infants born at 26 to 29 weeks GA.[129] Reiss and colleagues[130] reported an increased risk in BPD for infants with birth weights below the

10th percentile (OR 3.8, 95% CI 2.1–6.8). This relationship of increased BPD with low birth weight for GA is a continuum that includes less BPD at high birth weights for GA (Fig. 1.14).[124] Bose and coworkers[131] also demonstrated an increased risk of BPD with logistic regression models for 1241 infants who were born prior to 28 weeks of gestation and survived to 36 weeks GA. The predictors of BPD were GA and birth weights for GA below −1 Z score (OR 3.2, 95% CI 2.1–5.0) or −2 Z scores (OR 4.4, 95% CI 2.2–8.2). There are several possible explanations for the increased risk of BPD in infants born SGA. The somewhat trivial explanation is that the respiratory and nutritional care of smaller infants are more difficult technically than that for larger infants. For example, the 600g 27-week infant may be kept on a ventilator because of perceived fragility longer than the 1000g 27-week infant, with the consequence being increased BPD. However, biologic explanations likely contribute to this association. McElrath and associates[1] hypothesize that most severe prematurity results from either inflammation/infection or vascular developmental abnormalities that may progress from implantation. These vascular abnormalities (preeclampsia) are highly associated with fetal growth failure and an increased risk for BPD.[132] Therefore, the clinical data are consistent with the likelihood that small infants may have abnormal lung vascular development.

IUGR may interact with hypoxemia to cause adverse outcomes in preterm infants. In a secondary analysis of the SUPPORT trial designed to evaluate optimal oxygen targeting, and less invasive respiratory support to decrease BPD, Walsh et al. report that the unexpected finding of increased mortality in infants randomized to the low oxygen targeting group was almost exclusively in the IUGR population.[133] Collectively, these studies highlight the importance of intrauterine growth as a potent modulator for the risk of BPD or death in preterm infants.

Antenatal corticosteroids decrease fetal growth in animal models and can decrease fetal growth with repetitive treatments in humans.[134] Thus, the combined effects of antenatal corticosteroid treatments on growth-restricted fetuses could be adverse. There are no targeted randomized trials of antenatal corticosteroids for these at-risk pregnancies, although antenatal corticosteroids are routinely used for pregnancies with preeclampsia and at risk for preterm delivery.[129] Data from the early randomized trials show no adverse effects of corticosteroid use with maternal hypertension or for SGA infants.[135] The available data from clinical series do not suggest that antenatal corticosteroids are of benefit for growth-restricted fetuses.[136] Thus, there remain questions about the benefit of antenatal corticosteroids for the growth-restricted fetus.

Experimental models demonstrate clear effects of decreased fetal growth on lung development. Fetal sheep become growth restricted if placental implantation sites are decreased prior to pregnancy. Lipsett and colleagues[137] reported that fetal growth restriction caused a reduction in the gas exchange surface density of the fetal lung with smaller alveoli. Growth-restricted preterm fetal sheep had reduced surfactant protein levels, indicating delayed lung maturation despite high fetal cortisol levels.[138] Similarly, fetal growth restriction caused by an hypoxic environment in mice decreased mRNA expression of the surfactant proteins.[139] Exposure of growth-restricted fetal sheep to corticosteroids altered cardiovascular responses and increased indicators of brain injury relative to normally grown comparison groups.[140,141] Although the causes of fetal growth restriction in humans differ

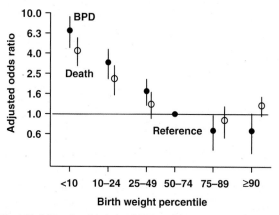

Fig. 1.14 Odds ratios *(circles)* and 95% confidence intervals *(lines)* for bronchopulmonary dysplasia *(BPD)* and mortality for infants grouped by birth weight percentiles adjusted for gestational ages. The risks for BPD and mortality increase as birth weight percentiles decrease from the reference group for the 50 to 74 percentiles. The risks of BPD and death are lower for the larger infants. (Data from Zeitlin J, El Ayoubi M, Jarreau PH, et al. Impact of fetal growth restriction on mortality and morbidity in a very preterm birth cohort. *J Pediatr.* 2010;157:733-739 e731.)

from those in the animal models, the lungs may have abnormal structure and maturation. Multiple questions remain about the mechanisms by which growth restriction increases BPD.

Environmental Factors and Lung Disease

Multiple environmental factors could modulate lung development in the fetus and have consequences after birth. Fetal and early neonatal exposures that may increase risks for asthma in children and chronic lung diseases in adults are included in the research on early origins of adult diseases and the hygiene hypothesis. Studies have focused primarily on term infant populations, and these subjects are beyond the scope of this review. However, we briefly explore two fetal exposures that may be underappreciated modulators of fetal lung development and that have not been adequately explored in relation to lung diseases in preterms. In a perspective written in 2001, Pierce and Nguyen[142] itemized the multiple effects of maternal cigarette smoking on fetal and newborn lung growth and function in animal models. These include decreased lung size and volume, changes in lung collagen and elastin, greater alveolar size, and increased type II cell numbers. Maternal smoking induced airway remodeling in fetal mice,[143] the presumed substrate for the airway disease reported in infants exposed to environmental smoke.[144] Maternal smoking was associated with increases in tests of lung maturation and cortisol in amniotic fluid in humans,[145] and nicotine altered developmental programs in the fetal lungs of rats.[146] In fetal monkeys, prenatal exposure to nicotine also caused lung hypoplasia and increased collagen deposition around large airways and vessels.[147] Infants who were exposed to maternal smoking and who died of sudden infant death syndrome had fewer alveolar attachment points on airways.[148] In a prospective multicenter study of 587 preterm infants <34 weeks, maternal smoking was identified as an independent risk factor for poor respiratory outcomes with a twofold increased for bronchopulmonary dysplasia, increased need for respiratory support at 36 weeks corrected GA, and respiratory disease up to 2 years of age.[128] A striking example of prevention of adverse lung function in infants born to mothers smoking cigarettes is maternal treatment with vitamin C. In a randomized,

double-blind trial enrolling 159 newborns of pregnant smokers, supplemental vitamin C improved newborn pulmonary function tests and decreased wheezing through 1 year.[149] These observations are consistent with the hypothesis that maternal smoking may alter lung structural and maturational development in both term and preterm infants, an effect that should be reflected in disease incidences of RDS, BPD, and more frequent airway reactivity in childhood. Populations of very preterm infants have not been evaluated for such effects.

A less studied exposure with possible effects on the preterm lung is maternal alcohol use. The fetal alcohol syndrome that includes fetal growth restriction and impaired neurodevelopment is well described. Exposure of fetal sheep to alcohol for the last third of gestation decreased surfactant protein mRNA expression but increased extracellular matrix deposition.[150] Changes in cytokine levels in the fetal lungs could result in altered immune status. Alcohol abuse alters the redox state of the adult lung, in which adult RDS is more likely to develop with an injury.[151] The effects of maternal alcohol abuse on lung function and injury in preterm infants remain unexplored.

Summary: The Complexities

Premature delivery is an abnormal event, and the preterm infant must have sufficiently developed lungs to survive, often with the help of multiple interventions such as antenatal corticosteroids, surfactant, and mechanical ventilation. The experimental literature relating to lung development and maturity is vast and informative, but the story becomes quite messy when clinical experiences are considered. There are just too many variables that influence the status of the preterm lung at delivery. GA and birth weight are the overriding predictors of outcomes. Maternal/fetal diseases such as preeclampsia and chorioamnionitis have potent effects on the fetal lung, but both have a spectrum of effects, from decreased risks to increased risks of RDS or BPD. Antenatal corticosteroids clearly benefit preterm infants overall, but how they further modulate the pregnancy abnormalities resulting in preterm delivery probably differs for each abnormality and with the timing of the fetal exposures. Environmental exposures such as smoke and alcohol are seldom considered relative to lung disease in the preterm. Other factors, such as genetic background, race, and fetal sex, are not discussed in this chapter. Finally, the diagnoses of RDS and BPD are imprecise and also represent spectrums of severity. The pathophysiology that accompanies RDS or BPD results in large part from how the preterm is managed clinically. As clinicians, we can understand populations of infants, but we are poor at predicting the outcomes for individual very preterm infants. Our failures result from a lack of a basic understanding of how lung developmental programs interact with injury programs and repair programs that are superimposed during the fetal period on the abnormalities that result in preterm delivery. The fetus then is assaulted by postnatal events—oxygen, mechanical ventilation, and infection. It is a wonder of nature that VLBW infants can survive and that most of the survivors have relatively normal lung function in childhood.

REFERENCES

1. McElrath TF, Hecht JL, Dammann O, et al. Pregnancy disorders that lead to delivery before the 28th week of gestation: an epidemiologic approach to classification. *Am J Epidemiol.* 2008; 168(9):980-989.
2. Berry CE, Billheimer D, Jenkins IC, et al. A distinct low lung function trajectory from childhood to the fourth decade of life. *Am J Respir Crit Care Med.* 2016;194(5):607-612.
3. Tita AT, Landon MB, Spong CY, et al. Timing of elective repeat cesarean delivery at term and neonatal outcomes. *N Engl J Med.* 2009;360(2):111-120.
4. Consortium on Safe Labor, Hibbard JU, Wilkins I, et al. Respiratory morbidity in late preterm births. *JAMA.* 2010;304(4): 419-425.
5. Stoll BJ, Hansen NI, Bell EF, et al. Trends in care practices, morbidity, and mortality of extremely preterm neonates, 1993-2012. *JAMA.* 2015;314(10):1039-1051.
6. Burri P. *Structural Aspects of Prenatal and Postnatal Development and Growth of the Lung.* New York: Marcel Dekker, Inc; 1997.
7. Ochs M, Nyengaard JR, Jung A, et al. The number of alveoli in the human lung. *Am J Respir Crit Care Med.* 2004;169(1): 120-124.
8. Coalson JJ, Winter V, deLemos RA. Decreased alveolarization in baboon survivors with bronchopulmonary dysplasia. *Am J Respir Crit Care Med.* 1995;152(2):640-646.
9. Burri PH. Structural aspects of postnatal lung development: alveolar formation and growth. *Biol Neonate.* 2006;89(4):313-322.
10. Schittny JC, Mund SI, Stampanoni M. Evidence and structural mechanism for late lung alveolarization. *Am J Physiol Lung Cell Mol Physiol.* 2008;294(2):L246-L254.
11. Narayanan M, Beardsmore CS, Owers-Bradley J, et al. Catch-up alveolarization in ex-preterm children: evidence from (3)He magnetic resonance. *Am J Respir Crit Care Med.* 2013;187(10): 1104-1109.
12. Avery ME, Mead J. Surface properties in relation to atelectasis and hyaline membrane disease. *AMA J Dis Child.* 1959;97 (5, Part 1):517-523.
13. Gluck L, Kulovich MV, Borer Jr RC, et al. Diagnosis of the respiratory distress syndrome by amniocentesis. *Am J Obstet Gynecol.* 1971;109(3):440-445.
14. Hallman M, Kulovich M, Kirkpatrick E, et al. Phosphatidylinositol and phosphatidylglycerol in amniotic fluid: indices of lung maturity. *Am J Obstet Gynecol.* 1976;125(5):613-617.
15. Bancalari EH, Jobe AH. The respiratory course of extremely preterm infants: a dilemma for diagnosis and terminology. *J Pediatr.* 2012;161(4):585-588.
16. Morley CJ, Davis PG, Doyle LW, Brion LP, Hascoet JM, Carlin JB. Nasal CPAP or intubation at birth for very preterm infants. *N Engl J Med.* 2008;358(7):700-708.
17. Finer NN, Carlo WA, Walsh MC, et al. Early CPAP versus surfactant in extremely preterm infants. *N Engl J Med.* 2010; 362(21):1970-1979.
18. Verder H, Albertsen P, Ebbesen F, et al. Nasal continuous positive airway pressure and early surfactant therapy for respiratory distress syndrome in newborns of less than 30 weeks' gestation. *Pediatrics.* 1999;103(2):E24.
19. Ammari A, Suri M, Milisavljevic V, et al. Variables associated with the early failure of nasal CPAP in very low birth weight infants. *J Pediatr.* 2005;147(3):341-347.
20. Jobe AH. "Miracle" extremely low birth weight neonates: examples of developmental plasticity. *Obstet Gynecol.* 2010; 116(5):1184-1190.
21. Mulrooney N, Champion Z, Moss TJ, Nitsos I, Ikegami M, Jobe AH. Surfactant and physiologic responses of preterm lambs to continuous positive airway pressure. *Am J Respir Crit Care Med.* 2005;171(5):488-493.
22. Kamath-Rayne BD, Du Y, Hughes M, et al. Systems biology evaluation of cell-free amniotic fluid transcriptome of term and preterm infants to detect fetal maturity. *BMC Med Genomics.* 2015;8(1):67.
23. Schmolzer GM, Kumar M, Pichler G, Aziz K, O'Reilly M, Cheung PY. Non-invasive versus invasive respiratory support in preterm infants at birth: systematic review and meta-analysis. *BMJ.* 2013;347:f5980.
24. Bland RD, Ertsey R, Mokres LM, et al. Mechanical ventilation uncouples synthesis and assembly of elastin and increases apoptosis in lungs of newborn mice. Prelude to defective alveolar septation during lung development? *Am J Physiol Lung Cell Mol Physiol.* 2008;294(1):L3-L14.
25. Mokres LM, Parai K, Hilgendorff A, et al. Prolonged mechanical ventilation with air induces apoptosis and causes failure of alveolar septation and angiogenesis in lungs of newborn mice. *Am J Physiol Lung Cell Mol Physiol.* 2010;298(1):L23-L35.
26. Hjalmarson O, Sandberg K. Abnormal lung function in healthy preterm infants. *Am J Respir Crit Care Med.* 2002;165(1): 83-87.
27. Stjernholm-Vladic Y, Stygar D, Mansson C, et al. Factors involved in the inflammatory events of cervical ripening in humans. *Reprod Biol Endocrinol.* 2004;2:74.
28. Marshall-Clarke S, Reen D, Tasker L, Hassan J. Neonatal immunity: how well has it grown up? *Immunol Today.* 2000; 21(1):35-41.
29. Goldenberg RL, Culhane JF, Iams JD, Romero R. Epidemiology and causes of preterm birth. *Lancet.* 2008;371(9606):75-84.
30. Goldenberg RL, Hauth JC, Andrews WW. Intrauterine infection and preterm delivery. *N Engl J Med.* 2000;342(20):1500-1507.

31. Higgins RD, Saade G, Polin RA, et al. Evaluation and management of women and newborns with a maternal diagnosis of chorioamnionitis: summary of a workshop. *Obstet Gynecol.* 2016;127(3):426-436.

32. Redline RW, Wilson-Costello D, Borawski E, Fanaroff AA, Hack M. Placental lesions associated with neurologic impairment and cerebral palsy in very-low-birth-weight infants. *Arch Pathol Lab Med.* 1998;122(12):1091-1098.

33. Romero R, Espinoza J, Chaiworapongsa T, Kalache K. Infection and prematurity and the role of preventive strategies. *Semin Neonatol.* 2002;7(4):259-274.

34. Yoon B, Romero R, Jun J, et al. Amniotic fluid cytokines (interleukin-6, tumor necrosis factor-alpha, interleukin-1 beta, and interleukin-8) and the risk for the development of bronchopulmonary dysplasia. *Am J Obstet Gynecol.* 1997; 177(4):825-830.

35. DiGiulio DB, Romero R, Amogan HP, et al. Microbial prevalence, diversity and abundance in amniotic fluid during preterm labor: a molecular and culture-based investigation. *PloS One.* 2008;3(8):e3056.

36. Buhimschi IA, Christner R, Buhimschi CS. Proteomic biomarker analysis of amniotic fluid for identification of intraamniotic inflammation. *BJOG.* 2005;112(2):173-181.

37. Gerber S, Vial Y, Hohlfeld P, Witkin SS. Detection of Ureaplasma urealyticum in second-trimester amniotic fluid by polymerase chain reaction correlates with subsequent preterm labor and delivery. *J Infect Dis.* 2003;187(3):518-521.

38. Perni SC, Vardhana S, Korneeva I, et al. Mycoplasma hominis and Ureaplasma urealyticum in midtrimester amniotic fluid: association with amniotic fluid cytokine levels and pregnancy outcome. *Am J Obstet Gynecol.* 2004;191(4):1382-1386.

39. Combs CA, Gravett M, Garite TJ, et al. Amniotic fluid infection, inflammation, and colonization in preterm labor with intact membranes. *Am J Obstet Gynecol.* 2014;210(2):125.e1-125.e15.

40. DiGiulio DB. Diversity of microbes in amniotic fluid. *Semin Fetal Neonatal Med.* 2012;17(1):2-11.

41. Onderdonk AB, Delaney ML, DuBois AM, Allred EN, Leviton A. Detection of bacteria in placental tissues obtained from extremely low gestational age neonates. *Am J Obstet Gynecol.* 2008;198(1):110.e1-110.e7.

42. Hecht JL, Onderdonk A, Delaney M, et al. Characterization of chorioamnionitis in 2nd-trimester C-section placentas and correlation with microorganism recovery from subamniotic tissues. *Pediatr Dev Pathol.* 2008;11(1):15-22.

43. Oh KJ, Lee KA, Sohn YK, et al. Intraamniotic infection with genital mycoplasmas exhibits a more intense inflammatory response than intraamniotic infection with other microorganisms in patients with preterm premature rupture of membranes. *Am J Obstet Gynecol.* 2010;203(3):211.e1-211.e8.

44. Sweeney EL, Kallapur SG, Gisslen T, et al. Placental infection with ureaplasma species is associated with histologic chorioamnionitis and adverse outcomes in moderately preterm and late-preterm infants. *J Infect Dis.* 2016;213(8):1340-1347.

45. Steel JH, Malatos S, Kennea N, et al. Bacteria and inflammatory cells in fetal membranes do not always cause preterm labor. *Pediatr Res.* 2005;57(3):404-411.

46. Reiman M, Kujari H, Ekholm E, et al. Interleukin-6 polymorphism is associated with chorioamnionitis and neonatal infections in preterm infants. *J Pediatr.* 2008;153(1):19-24.

47. Shalak LF, Laptook AR, Jafri HS, Ramilo O, Perlman JM. Clinical chorioamnionitis, elevated cytokines, and brain injury in term infants. *Pediatrics.* 2002;110(4):673-680.

48. Wortham JM, Hansen NI, Schrag SJ, et al. Chorioamnionitis and culture-confirmed, early-onset neonatal infections. *Pediatrics.* 2016;137(1):e20152323.

49. Morris A, Meaney S, Spillane N, O'Donoghue K. The postnatal morbidity associated with second-trimester miscarriage. *J Matern Fetal Neonatal Med.* 2016;29(17):2786-2790.

50. Richardson CJ, Pomerance JJ, Cunningham MD, Gluck L. Acceleration of fetal lung maturation following prolonged rupture of the membranes. *Am J Obstet Gynecol.* 1974; 118(8):1115-1118.

51. Watterberg KL, Demers LM, Scott SM, Murphy S. Chorioamnionitis and early lung inflammation in infants in whom bronchopulmonary dysplasia develops. *Pediatrics.* 1996;97(2):210-215.

52. De Dooy J, Colpaert C, Schuerwegh A, et al. Relationship between histologic chorioamnionitis and early inflammatory variables in blood, tracheal aspirates, and endotracheal colonization in preterm infants. *Pediatr Res.* 2003;54(1):113-119.

53. Groneck P, Goetze-Speer B, Speer CP. Inflammatory bronchopulmonary response of preterm infants with microbial colonisation of the airways at birth. *Arch Dis Child Fetal Neonatal Ed.* 1996;74(1):F51-F55.

54. Costeloe K, Hennessy E, Gibson AT, Marlow N, Wilkinson AR. The EPICure study: outcomes to discharge from hospital for infants born at the threshold of viability. *Pediatrics.* 2000;106(4):659-671.

55. Hannaford K, Todd DA, Jeffrey H, John E, Byth K, Gilbert GL. Role of ureaplasma urealyticum in lung disease of prematurity. *Arch Dis Child Fetal Neonatal Ed.* 1999;81:F162-F167.

56. Lahra MM, Beeby PJ, Jeffery HE. Maternal versus fetal inflammation and respiratory distress syndrome: a 10-year hospital cohort study. *Arch Dis Child Fetal Neonatal Ed.* 2009;94(1): F13-F16.

57. Lahra MM, Beeby PJ, Jeffery HE. Intrauterine inflammation, neonatal sepsis, and chronic lung disease: a 13-year hospital cohort study. *Pediatrics.* 2009;123(5):1314-1319.

58. Hartling L, Liang Y, Lacaze-Masmonteil T. Chorioamnionitis as a risk factor for bronchopulmonary dysplasia: a systematic review and meta-analysis. *Arch Dis Child Fetal Neonatal Ed.* 2012;97(1):F8-F17.

59. Hitti J, Krohn MA, Patton DL, et al. Amniotic fluid tumor necrosis factor-alpha and the risk of respiratory distress syndrome among preterm infants. *Am J Obstet Gynecol.* 1997;177:50-56.

60. Ramsey PS, Lieman JM, Brumfield CG, Carlo W. Chorioamnionitis increases neonatal morbidity in pregnancies complicated by preterm premature rupture of membranes. *Am J Obstet Gynecol.* 2005;192(4):1162-1166.

61. Laughon M, Allred EN, Bose C, et al. Patterns of respiratory disease during the first 2 postnatal weeks in extremely premature infants. *Pediatrics.* 2009;123(4):1124-1131.

62. Soraisham AS, Singhal N, McMillan DD, Sauve RS, Lee SK. A multicenter study on the clinical outcome of chorioamnionitis in preterm infants. *Am J Obstet Gynecol.* 2009;200(4):372. e1-372.e6.

63. Van Marter LJ, Dammann O, Allred EN, et al. Chorioamnionitis, mechanical ventilation, and postnatal sepsis as modulators of chronic lung disease in preterm infants. *J Pediatr.* 2002; 140(2):171-176.

64. Been JV, Rours IG, Kornelisse RF, Jonkers F, de Krijger RR, Zimmermann LJ. Chorioamnionitis alters the response to surfactant in preterm infants. *J Pediatr.* 2010;156(1):10-15.e1.

65. Been JV, Rours IG, Kornelisse RF, et al. Histologic chorioamnionitis, fetal involvement, and antenatal steroids: effects on neonatal

outcome in preterm infants. *Am J Obstet Gynecol.* 2009; 201(6):587.e1-587.e8.

66. Matoba N, Yu Y, Mestan K, et al. Differential patterns of 27 cord blood immune biomarkers across gestational age. *Pediatrics.* 2009;123(5):1320-1328.

67. Ambalavanan N, Carlo WA, D'Angio CT, et al. Cytokines associated with bronchopulmonary dysplasia or death in extremely low birth weight infants. *Pediatrics.* 2009;123(4):1132-1141.

68. Paananen R, Husa AK, Vuolteenaho R, Herva R, Kaukola T, Hallman M. Blood cytokines during the perinatal period in very preterm infants: relationship of inflammatory response and bronchopulmonary dysplasia. *J Pediatr.* 2009;154(1):39-43.e3.

69. Andrews WW, Goldenberg RL, Faye-Petersen O, Cliver S, Goepfert AR, Hauth JC. The Alabama Preterm Birth study: polymorphonuclear and mononuclear cell placental infiltrations, other markers of inflammation, and outcomes in 23- to 32-week preterm newborn infants. *Am J Obstet Gynecol.* 2006;195(3):803-808.

70. Goldenberg RL, Andrews WW, Goepfert AR, et al. The Alabama Preterm Birth Study: umbilical cord blood Ureaplasma urealyticum and Mycoplasma hominis cultures in very preterm newborn infants. *Am J Obstet Gynecol.* 2008;198(1):43. e1-43.e5.

71. Stoll BJ, Hansen N, Fanaroff AA, et al. Changes in pathogens causing early-onset sepsis in very-low-birth-weight infants. *N Engl J Med.* 2002;347(4):240-247.

72. Viscardi RM, Muhumuza CK, Rodriguez A, et al. Inflammatory markers in intrauterine and fetal blood and cerebrospinal fluid compartments are associated with adverse pulmonary and neurologic outcomes in preterm infants. *Pediatr Res.* 2004; 55(6):1009-1017.

73. Bry K, Lappalainen U, Hallman M. Intraamniotic interleukin-1 accelerates surfactant protein synthesis in fetal rabbits and improves lung stability after premature birth. *J Clin Invest.* 1997;99(12):2992-2999.

74. Kallapur SG, Willet KE, Jobe AH, Ikegami M, Bachurski CJ. Intra-amniotic endotoxin: chorioamnionitis precedes lung maturation in preterm lambs. *Am J Physiol Lung Cell Mol Physiol.* 2001;280(3):L527-L536.

75. Kramer BW, Moss TJ, Willet KE, et al. Dose and time response for inflammation and lung maturation after intra-amniotic endotoxin in preterm lambs. *Am J Respir Crit Care Med.* 2001; 164:982-988.

76. Kramer BW, Kramer S, Ikegami M, Jobe AH. Injury, inflammation, and remodeling in fetal sheep lung after intra-amniotic endotoxin. *Am J Physiol Lung Cell Mol Physiol.* 2002;283(2):L452-L459.

77. Kallapur SG, Bachurski CJ, Le Cras TD, Joshi SN, Ikegami M, Jobe AH. Vascular changes after intra-amniotic endotoxin in preterm lamb lungs. *Am J Physiol Lung Cell Mol Physiol.* 2004;287(6):L1178-L1185.

78. Song Y, Karisnan K, Noble PB, et al. In utero LPS exposure impairs preterm diaphragm contractility. *Am J Respir Cell Mol Biol.* 2013;49(5):866-874.

79. Jobe AH, Newnham JP, Willet KE, et al. Endotoxin-induced lung maturation in preterm lambs is not mediated by cortisol. *Am J Respir Crit Care Med.* 2000;162(5):1656-1661.

80. Willet KE, Jobe AH, Ikegami M, Newnham J, Brennan S, Sly PD. Antenatal endotoxin and glucocorticoid effects on lung morphometry in preterm lambs. *Pediatr Res.* 2000;48(6):782-788.

81. Toth A, Steinmeyer S, Kannan P, et al. Inflammatory blockade prevents injury to the developing pulmonary gas exchange surface in preterm primates. *Sci Transl Med.* 2022; 14(638):eabl8574.

82. Kallapur SG, Presicce P, Rueda CM, Jobe AH, Chougnet CA. Fetal immune response to chorioamnionitis. *Semin Reprod Med.* 2014;32(1):56-67.

83. Moss TJ, Nitsos I, Kramer BW, Ikegami M, Newnham JP, Jobe AH. Intra-amniotic endotoxin induces lung maturation by direct effects on the developing respiratory tract in preterm sheep. *Am J Obstet Gynecol.* 2002;187(4):1059-1065.

84. Sosenko IR, Jobe AH. Intraamniotic endotoxin increases lung antioxidant enzyme activity in preterm lambs. *Pediatr Res.* 2003;53(4):679-683.

85. Kim YM, Romero R, Chaiworapongsa T, et al. Toll-like receptor-2 and -4 in the chorioamniotic membranes in spontaneous labor at term and in preterm parturition that are associated with chorioamnionitis. *Am J Obstet Gynecol.* 2004;191(4): 1346-1355.

86. Steel JH, O'Donoghue K, Kennea NL, Sullivan MH, Edwards AD. Maternal origin of inflammatory leukocytes in preterm fetal membranes, shown by fluorescence in situ hybridisation. *Placenta.* 2005;26(8-9):672-677.

87. Harju K, Glumoff V, Hallman M. Ontogeny of Toll-like receptors Tlr2 and Tlr4 in mice. *Pediatr Res.* 2001;49(1):81-83.

88. Hillman NH, Moss TJ, Nitsos I, et al. Toll-like receptors and agonist responses in the developing fetal sheep lung. *Pediatr Res.* 2008;63(4):388-393.

89. Kramer BW, Ikegami M, Moss TJ, Nitsos I, Newnham JP, Jobe AH. Endotoxin-induced chorioamnionitis modulates innate immunity of monocytes in preterm sheep. *Am J Respir Crit Care Med.* 2005;171(1):73-77.

90. Moss TJ, Nitsos I, Ikegami M, Jobe AH, Newnham JP. Intrauterine Ureaplasma infection accelerates fetal lung maturation and causes growth restriction in sheep. *Am J Obstet Gynecol.* 2005;192:1179-1186.

91. Collins JJ, Kallapur SG, Knox CL, et al. Inflammation in fetal sheep from intra-amniotic injection of Ureaplasma parvum. *Am J Physiol Lung Cell Mol Physiol.* 2010;299(6):L852-L860.

92. Ikegami M, Moss TJ, Kallapur SG, et al. Minimal lung and systemic responses to TNF-alpha in preterm sheep. *Am J Physiol Lung Cell Mol Physiol.* 2003;285:L121-L129.

93. Moss TJ, Newnham JP, Willett KE, Kramer BW, Jobe AH, Ikegami M. Early gestational intra-amniotic endotoxin: lung function, surfactant, and morphometry. *Am J Respir Crit Care Med.* 2002;165(6):805-811.

94. Kallapur SG, Moss TJ, Ikegami M, Jasman RL, Newnham JP, Jobe AH. Recruited inflammatory cells mediate endotoxin-induced lung maturation in preterm fetal lambs. *Am J Respir Crit Care Med.* 2005;172(10):1315-1321.

95. Kallapur SG, Nitsos I, Moss TJ, et al. IL-1 mediates pulmonary and systemic inflammatory responses to chorioamnionitis induced by lipopolysaccharide. *Am J Respir Crit Care Med.* 2009;179(10):955-961.

96. Liao J, Kapadia VS, Brown LS, et al. The NLRP3 inflammasome is critically involved in the development of bronchopulmonary dysplasia. *Nat Commun.* 2015;6:8977.

97. Hodgman JE. Relationship between Wilson-Mikity syndrome and the new bronchopulmonary dysplasia. *Pediatrics.* 2003;112(6 Pt 1):1414-1415.

98. Kallapur SG, Nitsos I, Moss TJ, et al. Chronic endotoxin exposure does not cause sustained structural abnormalities in the fetal sheep lungs. *Am J Physiol Lung Cell Mol Physiol.* 2005; 288(5):L966-L974.

99. Polglase GR, Hillman NH, Pillow JJ, et al. Ventilation-mediated injury after preterm delivery of Ureaplasma parvum colonized fetal lambs. *Pediatr Res.* 2010;67(6):630-635.

100. Rueda CM, Presicce P, Jackson CM, et al. Lipopolysaccharide-induced chorioamnionitis promotes IL-1-dependent inflammatory FOXP3+ CD4+ T cells in the fetal rhesus macaque. *J Immunol.* 2016;196(9):3706-3715.

101. Kramer BW, Joshi SN, Moss TJ, et al. Endotoxin-induced maturation of monocytes in preterm fetal sheep lung. *Am J Physiol Lung Cell Mol Physiol.* 2007;293(2):L345-L353.

102. Jackson CM, Demmert M, Mukherjee S, et al. A potent myeloid response is rapidly activated in the lungs of premature Rhesus macaques exposed to intra-uterine inflammation. *Mucosal Immunol.* 2022;15(4):730-744.

103. Kallapur SG, Jobe AH, Ball MK, et al. Pulmonary and systemic endotoxin tolerance in preterm fetal sheep exposed to chorioamnionitis. *J Immunol.* 2007;179(12):8491-8499.

104. Kallapur SG, Kramer BW, Knox CL, et al. Chronic fetal exposure to Ureaplasma parvum suppresses innate immune responses in sheep. *J Immunol.* 2011;187(5):2688-2695.

105. Kramer BW, Kallapur SG, Moss TJ, Nitsos I, Newnham JP, Jobe AH. Intra-amniotic LPS modulation of TLR signaling in lung and blood monocytes of fetal sheep. *Innate Immun.* 2009;15(2):101-107.

106. Tang JR, Seedorf GJ, Muehlethaler V, et al. Moderate postnatal hyperoxia accelerates lung growth and attenuates pulmonary hypertension in infant rats after exposure to intra-amniotic endotoxin. *Am J Physiol Lung Cell Mol Physiol.* 2010;299(6):L735-L748.

107. Pryhuber GS, Maitre NL, Ballard RA, et al. Prematurity and respiratory outcomes program (PROP): study protocol of a prospective multicenter study of respiratory outcomes of preterm infants in the United States. *BMC Pediatr.* 2015;15:37.

108. Jackson CM, Wells CB, Tabangin ME, Meinzen-Derr J, Jobe AH, Chougnet CA. Pro-inflammatory immune responses in leukocytes of premature infants exposed to maternal chorioamnionitis or funisitis. *Pediatr Res.* 2017;81(2):384-390.

109. Misra RS, Shah S, Fowell DJ, et al. Preterm cord blood CD4(+) T cells exhibit increased IL-6 production in chorioamnionitis and decreased CD4(+) T cells in bronchopulmonary dysplasia. *Hum Immunol.* 2015;76(5):329-338.

110. Scheible KM, Emo J, Yang H, et al. Developmentally determined reduction in CD31 during gestation is associated with CD8+ T cell effector differentiation in preterm infants. *Clin Immunol.* 2015;161(2):65-74.

111. D'Angio CT, Ambalavanan N, Carlo WA, et al. Blood cytokine profiles associated with distinct patterns of bronchopulmonary dysplasia among extremely low birth weight infants. *J Pediatr.* 2016;174:45-51.e5.

112. Bose C, Laughon M, Allred EN, et al. Blood protein concentrations in the first two postnatal weeks that predict bronchopulmonary dysplasia among infants born before the 28th week of gestation. *Pediatr Res.* 2011;69(4):347-353.

113. Harding JE, Pang J, Knight DB, Liggins GC. Do antenatal corticosteroids help in the setting of preterm rupture of membranes? *Am J Obstet Gynecol.* 2001;184(2):131-139.

114. Goldenberg RL, Andrews WW, Faye-Petersen OM, Cliver SP, Goepfert AR, Hauth JC. The Alabama preterm birth study: corticosteroids and neonatal outcomes in 23- to 32-week newborns with various markers of intrauterine infection. *Am J Obstet Gynecol.* 2006;195(4):1020-1024.

115. Been JV, Degraeuwe PL, Kramer BW, Zimmermann LJ. Antenatal steroids and neonatal outcome after chorioamnionitis: a meta-analysis. *BJOG.* 2011;118(2):113-122.

116. Kallapur SG, Kramer BW, Moss TJ, et al. Maternal glucocorticoids increase endotoxin-induced lung inflammation in preterm lambs. *Am J Physiol Lung Cell Mol Physiol.* 2003;284(4):L633-L642.

117. Newnham JP, Kallapur SG, Kramer BW, et al. Betamethasone effects on chorioamnionitis induced by intra-amniotic endotoxin in sheep. *Am J Obstet Gynecol.* 2003;189(5):1458-1466.

118. Newnham JP, Moss TJ, Padbury JF, et al. The interactive effects of endotoxin with prenatal glucocorticoids on short-term lung function in sheep. *Am J Obstet Gynecol.* 2001;185(1):190-197.

119. Ikegami M, Polk D, Jobe A. Minimum interval from fetal betamethasone treatment to postnatal lung responses in preterm lambs. *Am J Obstet Gynecol.* 1996;174(5):1408-1413.

120. Jobe AH, Newnham JP, Willet KE, et al. Effects of antenatal endotoxin and glucocorticoids on the lungs of preterm lambs. *Am J Obstet Gynecol.* 2000;182(2):401-408.

121. Moss TJ, Nitsos I, Knox CL, et al. Ureaplasma colonization of amniotic fluid and efficacy of antenatal corticosteroids for preterm lung maturation in sheep. *Am J Obstet Gynecol.* 2009;200(1):96.e1-96.e6.

122. Kramer BW, Ikegami M, Moss TJ, Nitsos I, Newnham JP, Jobe AH. Antenatal betamethasone changes cord blood monocyte responses to endotoxin in preterm lambs. *Pediatr Res.* 2004;55(5):764-768.

123. Kuypers E, Collins JJ, Kramer BW, et al. Intra-amniotic LPS and antenatal betamethasone: inflammation and maturation in preterm lamb lungs. *Am J Physiol Lung Cell Mol Physiol.* 2012;302(4):L380-L389.

124. Zeitlin J, El Ayoubi M, Jarreau PH, et al. Impact of fetal growth restriction on mortality and morbidity in a very preterm birth cohort. *J Pediatr.* 2010;157(5):733-739.e1.

125. Chang EY, Menard MK, Vermillion ST, Hulsey T, Ebeling M. The association between hyaline membrane disease and preeclampsia. *Am J Obstet Gynecol.* 2004;191(4):1414-1417.

126. Tyson JE, Kennedy K, Broyles S, Rosenfeld CR. The small for gestational age infant: accelerated or delayed pulmonary maturation? Increased or decreased survival? *Pediatrics.* 1995;95(4):534-538.

127. Jelin AC, Cheng YW, Shaffer BL, Kaimal AJ, Little SE, Caughey AB. Early-onset preeclampsia and neonatal outcomes. *J Matern Fetal Neonatal Med.* 2010;23(5):389-392.

128. Morrow LA, Wagner BD, Ingram DA, et al. Antenatal determinants of bronchopulmonary dysplasia and late respiratory disease in preterm infants. *Am J Respir Crit Care Med.* 2017;196(3):364-374.

129. Garite TJ, Clark R, Thorp JA. Intrauterine growth restriction increases morbidity and mortality among premature neonates. *Am J Obstet Gynecol.* 2004;191(2):481-487.

130. Reiss I, Landmann E, Heckmann M, Misselwitz B, Gortner L. Increased risk of bronchopulmonary dysplasia and increased mortality in very preterm infants being small for gestational age. *Arch Gynecol Obstet.* 2003;269(1):40-44.

131. Bose C, Van Marter LJ, Laughon M, et al. Fetal growth restriction and chronic lung disease among infants born before the 28th week of gestation. *Pediatrics.* 2009;124(3):e450-e458.

132. Hansen AR, Barnes CM, Folkman J, McElrath TF. Maternal preeclampsia predicts the development of bronchopulmonary dysplasia. *J Pediatr.* 2010;156(4):532-536.

133. Walsh MC, Di Fiore JM, Martin RJ, Gantz M, Carlo WA, Finer N. Association of oxygen target and growth status with increased mortality in small for gestational age infants: further analysis of the surfactant, positive pressure and pulse oximetry randomized trial. *JAMA Pediatr.* 2016;170(3):292-294.

134. Murphy KE, Hannah ME, Willan AR, et al. Multiple courses of antenatal corticosteroids for preterm birth (MACS): a randomised controlled trial. *Lancet.* 2008;372(9656):2143-2151.

135. Roberts D, Dalziel S. Antenatal corticosteroids for accelerating fetal lung maturation for women at risk of preterm birth. *Cochrane Database Syst Rev.* 2006;3:CD004454.

136. Torrance HL, Derks JB, Scherjon SA, Wijnberger LD, Visser GH. Is antenatal steroid treatment effective in preterm IUGR fetuses? *Acta Obstet Gynecol Scand.* 2009;88(10):1068-1073.

137. Lipsett J, Tamblyn M, Madigan K, et al. Restricted fetal growth and lung development: a morphometric analysis of pulmonary structure. *Pediatr Pulmonol.* 2006;41(12):1138-1145.

138. Orgeig S, Crittenden TA, Marchant C, McMillen IC, Morrison JL. Intrauterine growth restriction delays surfactant protein maturation in the sheep fetus. *Am J Physiol Lung Cell Mol Physiol.* 2010;298(4):L575-L583.

139. Gortner L, Hilgendorff A, Bahner T, Ebsen M, Reiss I, Rudloff S. Hypoxia-induced intrauterine growth retardation: effects on pulmonary development and surfactant protein transcription. *Biol Neonate.* 2005;88(2):129-135.

140. Miller SL, Chai M, Loose J, et al. The effects of maternal betamethasone administration on the intrauterine growth-restricted fetus. *Endocrinology.* 2007;148(3):1288-1295.

141. Miller SL, Supramaniam VG, Jenkin G, Walker DW, Wallace EM. Cardiovascular responses to maternal betamethasone administration in the intrauterine growth-restricted ovine fetus. *Am J Obstet Gynecol.* 2009;201(6):613.e1-613.e8.

142. Pierce RA, Nguyen NM. Prenatal nicotine exposure and abnormal lung function. *Am J Respir Cell Mol Biol.* 2002;26(1):10-13.

143. Blacquiere MJ, Timens W, Melgert BN, Geerlings M, Postma DS, Hylkema MN. Maternal smoking during pregnancy induces airway remodelling in mice offspring. *Eur Respir J.* 2009; 33(5):1133-1140.

144. Hylkema MN, Blacquiere MJ. Intrauterine effects of maternal smoking on sensitization, asthma, and chronic obstructive pulmonary disease. *Proc Am Thorac Soc.* 2009;6(8): 660-662.

145. Lieberman E, Torday J, Barbieri R, Cohen A, Van Vunakis H, Weiss ST. Association of intrauterine cigarette smoke exposure with indices of fetal lung maturation. *Obstet Gynecol.* 1992; 79(4):564-570.

146. Rehan VK, Wang Y, Sugano S, et al. In utero nicotine exposure alters fetal rat lung alveolar type II cell proliferation, differentiation, and metabolism. *Am J Physiol Lung Cell Mol Physiol.* 2007;292(1):L323-L333.

147. Sekhon HS, Jia Y, Raab R, et al. Prenatal nicotine increases pulmonary alpha7 nicotinic receptor expression and alters fetal lung development in monkeys. *J Clin Invest.* 1999; 103(5):637-647.

148. Elliot JG, Carroll NG, James AL, Robinson PJ. Airway alveolar attachment points and exposure to cigarette smoke in utero. *Am J Respir Crit Care Med.* 2003;167(1):45-49.

149. McEvoy CT, Schilling D, Clay N, et al. Vitamin C supplementation for pregnant smoking women and pulmonary function in their newborn infants: a randomized clinical trial. *JAMA.* 2014;311(20):2074-2082.

150. Sozo F, O'Day L, Maritz G, et al. Repeated ethanol exposure during late gestation alters the maturation and innate immune status of the ovine fetal lung. *Am J Physiol Lung Cell Mol Physiol.* 2009;296(3):L510-L518.

151. Joshi PC, Guidot DM. The alcoholic lung: epidemiology, pathophysiology, and potential therapies. *Am J Physiol Lung Cell Mol Physiol.* 2007;292(4):L813-L823.

Chapter 2

Respiratory and Cardiovascular Support in the Delivery Room

Gary Marshall Weiner, Stuart Brian Hooper, Peter G. Davis, and Myra H. Wyckoff

Chapter Outline

Understanding the Transition to Newborn Life

Anticipating and Preparing for Neonatal Resuscitation

Rapid Assessment After Birth

Initial Steps for Non-vigorous and Preterm Newborns

Effective Ventilation: The Key!

Chest Compressions During Resuscitation in the Delivery Room

Medications During Resuscitation in the Delivery Room

Discontinuing Resuscitative Efforts

Key Points

- After birth, lung aeration and an increase in pulmonary blood flow are closely linked.
- Although it is possible to identify deliveries of infants at increased risk of requiring resuscitation, appropriately trained personnel should be present at every birth.
- Establishing effective ventilation is the key to successful neonatal resuscitation. A very small number of newborns require chest compressions or emergency medications.
- Routine tracheal suction for nonvigorous newborns with meconium-stained amniotic fluid is not recommended.
- Air should be used for resuscitation of term and late preterm infants, and oxygen supplementation should be guided by pulse oximetry.
- Laryngeal masks are an effective alternative to face mask ventilation and endotracheal intubation.
- The two-thumb technique should be used to deliver chest compressions.
- Discontinuing resuscitative efforts may be reasonable if the newborn's heart rate remains undetectable around 20 minutes after birth despite all recommended interventions and exclusion of reversible causes.

Understanding the Transition to Newborn Life

What is the primary trigger that facilitates cardiopulmonary transition in the newly born infant?

The transition from fetal to newborn life represents one of the greatest physiologic challenges that humans encounter. During fetal life, the lungs are liquid-filled and at birth this liquid must be rapidly cleared from the airways to allow the entry of air and the onset of pulmonary gas exchange. Pulmonary blood flow (PBF) must markedly increase, and several specialized vascular shunts must also close to separate the pulmonary and systemic circulations. While it is often considered that these events are independent, we now know that they are intimately linked. Lung aeration is the primary trigger that not only facilitates the onset of pulmonary gas exchange but also stimulates an increase in PBF, which in turn initiates the cardiovascular changes.[1] The fact that lung aeration triggers the physiologic transition at birth underpins the well-established tenet that establishing effective pulmonary ventilation is the key step in neonatal resuscitation.

How is airway liquid removed from the newborn infant's lung?

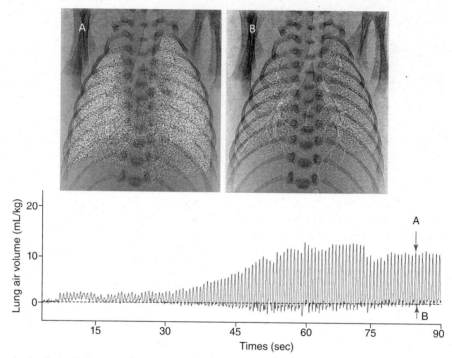

Fig. 2.1 Phase-contrast radiographic images and a plethysmograph recording of a preterm newborn rabbit immediately after birth ventilated from birth in the absence of a positive end-expiratory pressure (PEEP). In the absence of PEEP, preterm rabbits failed to develop a functional residual capacity (FRC), resulting in liquid reentry or airway collapse at end-expiration. Phase-contrast radiographic images (A and B) were recorded at each time point on the plethysmograph trace. Image A was acquired at end inspiration, whereas image B was acquired at FRC.

Radiographic imaging studies have demonstrated that lung aeration can occur rapidly (in three to five breaths) and mostly occurs during inspiration in spontaneously breathing newborns or during positive-pressure inflations in ventilated newborns (Fig. 2.1).[2,3] The hydrostatic pressure gradients generated by inspiration, or positive-pressure inflations, drive liquid from the airways into the surrounding lung tissue.[2,3] However, as the interstitial tissue compartment of the lung has a fixed volume, the clearance of airway liquid into this compartment during lung aeration increases lung interstitial tissue pressures. Thus, immediately following lung aeration, the neonatal lung is essentially edematous, which affects lung tissue mechanics and increases the likelihood of liquid reentering the airways during expiration. Use of positive end-expiratory pressure (PEEP) during assisted ventilation opposes liquid reentry and ensures that distal airways and gas exchange units remain aerated at end-expiration (Fig. 2.2).[4] As a result, PEEP allows gas exchange to continue throughout the respiratory cycle.

How does the timing of umbilical cord clamping affect the cardiovascular transition at birth?

Before birth, most of the right ventricular output bypasses the lung and flows through the ductus arteriosus into the systemic circulation mainly because pulmonary vascular resistance (PVR) is high.[1] In the fetus, PBF is low and contributes little to venous return and the supply of preload for the left ventricle. Instead, this mainly comes from umbilical venous return via the ductus venosus and foramen ovale. Thus, blood flow through the placenta is vital not only for oxygen and nutrients supply during fetal life but also for delivering left ventricle preload. Clamping the umbilical cord at birth immediately decreases preload, thereby causing a large reduction in cardiac output.[5] Furthermore, cardiac output remains low until the

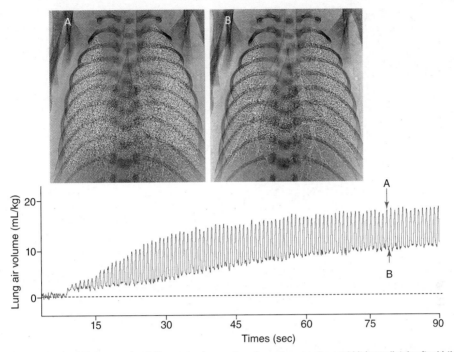

Fig. 2.2 Phase-contrast radiographic images and a plethysmograph recording of a preterm newborn rabbit immediately after birth ventilated from birth with a positive end-expiratory pressure (PEEP) of 5 cm H_2O. With this level of PEEP, preterm rabbits gradually develop a significant functional residual capacity (FRC) with most distal airways (not all, see basal lung regions) remaining aerated at FRC. Phase-contrast x-ray images (A and B) were recorded at each time point on the plethysmograph trace. Image A was acquired at end inspiration, whereas image B was acquired at FRC

lungs aerate and PBF increases to restore preload for the left ventricle. Recognition of this shift in dependence from umbilical venous return to pulmonary venous return for sustaining ventricular preload at birth has led to the concept of physiology-based cord clamping.[6] That is, if cord clamping is delayed until after the lungs have aerated and PBF has increased, then PBF can immediately replace umbilical venous return as the major source of left ventricular preload as soon as the cord is clamped, with no diminution in supply. This procedure greatly mitigates the large changes in cardiac output associated with umbilical cord clamping before the onset of ventilation.[5] It also greatly reduces the instantaneous increase in arterial blood pressure associated with cord clamping caused by the removal of the low-resistance placental vascular bed.[5] As a redistribution of cardiac output and increased blood flow to the brain is critical for protecting the fetal brain from hypoxia, any constraint on

cardiac output caused by a lack of venous return at birth is potentially catastrophic. However, because uterotonic medications given to the mother at birth to contract the uterus also reduce umbilical blood flows (Fig. 2.3), uterotonic administration prior to cord clamping can mitigate some of the benefits of physiological-based cord clamping.[7]

Is pulmonary blood flow increased only in the aerated portions of the newborn's lung?

At birth, lung aeration triggers the increase in PBF required for facilitating pulmonary gas exchange. As noted earlier, lung aeration is important for replacing left ventricular preload and maintaining cardiac output potentially lost following cord clamping. Imaging studies have shown that partial lung aeration after birth is sufficient to stimulate a global increase in PBF (Fig. 2.4).[8,9] While oxygen can enhance this response, it is not oxygen dependent.[8,9] Although partial aeration has the potential

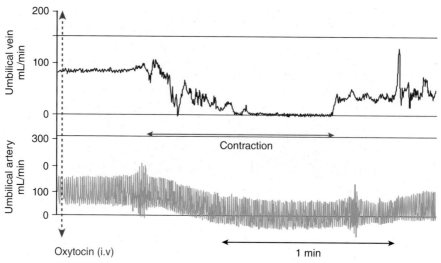

Fig. 2.3 Effect of oxytocin-induced uterine contraction on umbilical venous and arterial blood flows. Blood flow in the umbilical vein ceases during the contraction, whereas flow in the umbilical artery becomes bidirectional, with blood flowing away from the placenta during diastole. (Data redrawn from Stenning FJ, Polglase GR, Te Pas AB, et al. Effect of maternal oxytocin on umbilical venous and arterial blood flows during physiological-based cord clamping in preterm lambs. *PLoS One.* 2021;16(6):e0253306.)

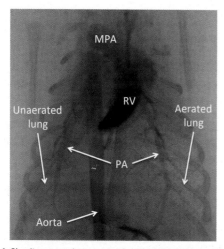

Fig. 2.4 Simultaneous phase-contrast and angiographic radiographic image of a near-term rabbit kitten following partial ventilation of the right lung. Aerated lung regions can be seen as "speckle" in the image and are due to refraction at the air/water interface. Although only part of the right lung is aerated, pulmonary blood flow is increased in both lungs equally. *MPA*, Main pulmonary artery; *PA*, pulmonary artery; *RV*, right ventricle.

to cause large ventilation-perfusion mismatches in the lung at birth, as the high PBF is vital for maintaining cardiac output, this response has major benefits during transition. Indeed, by not limiting the increase in PBF to the degree of lung aeration, venous return and cardiac output are not limited by the degree of lung aeration.

Anticipating and Preparing for Neonatal Resuscitation

How often are resuscitative interventions needed after birth?

The incidence of stabilization and resuscitative interventions after birth varies based on setting and gestational age. Within 30 seconds of birth, most newly born term and late preterm infants initiate respirations spontaneously or in response to drying and tactile stimulation.[10] In a population-based study of all births in three Norwegian hospitals (n = 1507 liveborn infants), 4% received positive-pressure ventilation (PPV), 0.4% were intubated, and a very small number received either chest compressions (0.2%) or intravenous epinephrine (0.1%).[11] The probability of requiring resuscitative interventions increases with decreasing gestational age. In the study, 21% of newborns < 34 weeks' gestation received PPV and 54% of those < 28 weeks' gestation were intubated.[11] Others have demonstrated that even late preterm newborns (34–36 weeks) have a twofold risk of receiving PPV compared with term newborns.[12]

Can the need for resuscitation be anticipated before birth?

Although the likelihood of requiring resuscitation is higher in the presence of identified risk factors (Table 2.1),[13] individual risk factors and scoring systems that combine risk factors have limited discriminatory power. They identify many births as high risk where subsequently no interventions are needed. Moreover, some newborns require intervention in the absence of any risk factors. In two Canadian cohort studies, approximately 14% of newborns considered low risk and 7% of normal term deliveries without identified risk factors received PPV in the delivery room.[14,15] Even among very low-birth-weight newborns, antenatal risk factors have low discriminatory power to identify those that will require extensive resuscitation.[16] In a multicenter case-control study of term and late preterm newborns, Berazategui incorporated 10 antenatal and intrapartum risk factors in a multivariate regression model to predict the need for tracheal intubation, chest compressions, or emergency medications in the delivery room.[17] The final

model correctly predicted the need for these advanced intervention with 72% sensitivity and 93% specificity. Because the model used a case control design, the results could not be used to directly predict the need for advanced resuscitation in an unselected population. Subsequently, the authors performed a series of bootstrap simulations with the original dataset and have published an online calculator to predict the need for advanced neonatal resuscitation among term and late preterm newborns (https://medicine.ouhsc.edu/Academic-Departments/Pediatrics/Sections/Neonatal-Perinatal-Medicine/Research/Risk-Calculator).[18] Because the need for resuscitative interventions cannot always be predicted, trained personnel must be available at every birth to assess the newborn and initiate resuscitation without delay. If the need for advanced resuscitation can be anticipated, a trained team proficient in all steps of resuscitation should be present at the time of birth.

What ambient temperature should be maintained in the delivery room?

The ideal delivery room or operating room ambient temperature that prevents neonatal and maternal hypothermia without increasing the risk of hyperthermia or interfering with medical staff performance has not been established. The World Health Organization (WHO) recommends maintaining the newborn's temperature between 36.5°C (97.7°F) and 37.5°C (99.5°F).[19] Among term and late preterm newborns delivered by cesarean birth, an operating room temperature of 23°C (74°F) compared to 20°C (68°F) modestly increased admission temperature (mean difference 0.3°C) and decreased the probability of moderate hypothermia (relative risk 0.26).[20] Among extremely low-birth-weight newborns, where hypothermia significantly increases mortality, an environmental delivery room/operating room temperature of 23°C (74°F), in addition to other adjuncts, prevents admission hypothermia.[21] For anticipated births of newborns < 32 weeks' gestation, the International Liaison Committee on Resuscitation (ILCOR) suggests an ambient temperature between 23°C (74°F) and 25°C (77°F) in combination with adjuncts such as warm blankets, polyethylene plastic bags or wraps, and head caps.[22] In a recent Consensus on Science and Treatment Recommendation (COSTR) update,

TABLE 2.1 Risk Factors for Neonatal Resuscitation	
Moderate Risk	**High Risk**
Late preterm (34–36 weeks' gestation)	Preterm (<34 weeks' gestation)
Fetal anemia	Birth weight < 2 kg
Polyhydramnios	Major fetal anomalies or hydrops
Intrauterine growth restriction	Fetal bradycardia
Gestational diabetes mellitus	Acute or severe labor complication
Chorioamnionitis	
Placental abruption	
Cord prolapse	
Maternal general anesthesia	
Meconium-stained amniotic fluid	
Category II or III fetal heart rate	
Instrumented delivery (forceps or vacuum)	
Emergency cesarean birth	
Shoulder dystocia	
Abnormal fetal position	

Adapted from Sawyer T, Lee HC, Aziz K. Anticipation and preparation for every delivery room resuscitation. *Semin Fetal Neonatal Med.* 2018;23(5):312-320.

ILCOR suggested maintaining a room temperature of 23°C (74°F) for infants $\geq$ 34 weeks' gestation.[23] For those at low risk of needing resuscitation, skin-to-skin care is suggested immediately after birth. Although WHO recommends a higher (25°C–28°C) environmental temperature, surgeons performing cesarean deliveries report discomfort at this temperature and concern that it would negatively impact their performance.[20]

Rapid Assessment After Birth

When should the umbilical cord be clamped?

As noted, delaying umbilical cord clamping may improve cardiovascular transition after birth by providing additional preload for the left ventricle until it can be replaced with pulmonary venous return. For most term and preterm newborns, international guidelines recommend delaying cord clamping for at least 30 to 60 seconds after birth.[22] Among preterm newborns (< 34 weeks' gestation) who do not require immediate resuscitation, evidence suggests that delaying cord clamping for at least 30 to 60 seconds improves cardiovascular transition, improves mean arterial blood pressure during the first 12 hours of life, decreases the need for inotropes during the first 24 hours of life, increases peak hematocrit after birth, decreases the need for blood transfusions, and may improve survival.[24] Among vigorous term and late preterm newborns, evidence suggests that delayed cord clamping for at least 30 seconds increases hematocrit during the first 7 days of life but has no apparent effect on the probability of anemia at 4 to 6 months.[25] While milking the intact umbilical cord from the placenta toward the newborn three to four times may be an alternative to improve hematologic measures during the first week of life if delayed umbilical cord clamping is not feasible, it is not recommended for preterm newborns less than 28 weeks' gestation because of a potential increased risk of severe intraventricular hemorrhage.[26]

How should the newborn be assessed immediately after birth?

Immediately after birth, a rapid initial assessment is performed to determine if the newborn can remain skin-to-skin with the mother to complete transition or should be moved to a radiant warmer for the initial steps of newborn care.[27] This can be performed during the interval between birth and umbilical cord clamping. Within 10 to 30 seconds of birth, approximately 85% of term newborns are vigorous with good muscle tone and strong respiratory effort, and an additional 10% become vigorous as they are dried and stimulated.[10] Regardless of the appearance of the amniotic fluid, vigorous term newborns with good tone and respiratory effort should be placed skin-to-skin on the mother's chest or abdomen and covered with a warm, dry blanket to complete the initial steps of newborn care, thermal management, and ongoing assessment.[27]

After vaginal birth and delayed cord clamping, the healthy, term newborn's heart rate remains above 100 beats per minute (bpm). Using a dry electrode capable of recording the newborn's heart rate within seconds of birth, Bjorland demonstrated that the median (interquartile range) heart rate increased from 122 (98–146) bpm to 168 (146–185) bpm during the first 30 seconds and peaked at 175 (157–189) bpm at 1 minute.[28] Over the first minutes of life, the newborn's skin and mucous membrane color should gradually become pink. However, clinical judgment of the newborn's color is notoriously difficult and is not an accurate predictor of arterial oxygenation.[29] If a vigorous term newborn remains cyanotic or develops respiratory distress, pulse oximetry is indicated to assess oxygenation. When measured by preductal pulse oximetry, the healthy newborn's oxygen saturation increases gradually from a median of near 60% at 1 minute of life to around 90% by 5 to 10 minutes of life.[30] For the first 5 minutes after cesarean birth, infants have oxygen saturation values approximately 10% lower than vaginally born infants.[31] With delayed cord clamping ($\geq$ 60 seconds), oxygen saturation increases more rapidly. Among healthy, vaginally born infants with delayed cord clamping, the median oxygen saturation plateaus above 90% by 3 to 4 minutes after birth.[32]

Should clear amniotic fluid be suctioned from the healthy newborn's mouth and nose?

There is no evidence that normal lung liquid and secretions obstruct the newly born infant's airway. If the infant is crying vigorously, there is no need for routine oral, nasal, or pharyngeal suction. In an updated consensus statement, the ILCOR neonatal task force reviewed 10 studies (8 randomized controlled trials [RCTs] and 2 observational studies) enrolling healthy, low-risk term newborns and found no evidence to support routine suctioning of clear amniotic fluid from the newborn infant's mouth or nose.[33] Clearing secretions with a suction device should be reserved for those infants who have evidence of airway obstruction or cannot clear secretions on their own. Deep, vigorous, or prolonged suctioning is rarely helpful. It can traumatize tissues and induce vagal responses that are counterproductive during transition.

Initial Steps for Nonvigorous and Preterm Newborns

The steps of neonatal stabilization and resuscitation for nonvigorous and preterm newborns are described on a single algorithm based on an international science consensus (Fig. 2.5).[22,27] Infants who are not vigorous after birth and those who are born preterm should be taken to a radiant warmer for assessment, the initial steps of newborn care, and possible resuscitative interventions. In some settings, this may be performed on a purpose-built resuscitation trolley placed adjacent to the mother, allowing the steps to be performed without dividing the umbilical cord.[34]

What steps should be performed to maintain normal body temperature?

Immediately after birth, the initial steps of care focus on preventing hypothermia by warming and drying the newborn. Wet newborns rapidly lose heat and become hypothermic. For newly born, nonasphyxiated infants, the goal is to maintain normothermia (36.5°C–37.5°C) while avoiding both hypothermia and hyperthermia.[35] Cold stress in nonasphyxiated newborns is associated with multiple adverse outcomes, including hypoglycemia, metabolic acidosis, late-onset sepsis, lower arterial oxygen tension, and increased mortality.[36] Receive infants who do not qualify for routine care in warm blankets, place them under a preheated radiant warmer, remove the wet blankets, and continue drying with additional warm, dry blankets. Preventing hypothermia is particularly important for preterm newborns. Large cohort studies have repeatedly demonstrated an inverse relationship between admission temperature and in-hospital mortality among preterm newborns across a range of settings and gestational ages.[37,38] The updated ILCOR

scientific consensus has confirmed the importance of using a combination of interventions, such as radiant warmers, plastic wraps, hats, and thermal mattresses, to prevent hypothermia in newborns less than 32 weeks' gestation.[22] When using a combination of interventions, the temperature of the newborn baby must be monitored to prevent unintended hyperthermia because perinatal hyperthermia (>38°C) is also associated with respiratory depression and other complications.[39]

Should routine laryngoscopy and tracheal suction be performed for nonvigorous newborns with meconium-stained amniotic fluid?

The approach to meconium-stained amniotic fluid (MSAF) has evolved over several decades but remains controversial. Based on physiologic plausibility and nonrandomized observational studies in the 1970s, oropharyngeal suction at the perineum before delivery of the shoulders and tracheal suction immediately after birth were recommended to reduce the incidence and severity of meconium aspiration syndrome (MAS). As the level of evidence progressed in the early 2000s from observational studies to large RCTs, both oropharyngeal suction and routine tracheal suction of vigorous newborns were shown to be ineffective and were no longer recommended. Routine intubation and tracheal suction of nonvigorous newborns with MSAF immediately after birth was an intervention that was difficult to study rigorously and was still commonly practiced. Beginning in 2015, the ILCOR neonatal life support task force recommended against routine laryngoscopy and tracheal suction because of the lack of high-quality evidence supporting this invasive procedure.[40] A meta-analysis of four small RCTs showed no benefit for the prevention of MAS or improvement in survival to discharge.[41] The certainty of evidence in the meta-analysis was low, or very low, largely because the study personnel in the RCTs could not be blinded to the intervention, and the total number of newborns enrolled in the trials (n = 571) was below the optimal information size. The recently updated North American and European guidelines continue to recommend against routine laryngoscopy and tracheal suction.[35,42] Retrospective cohort studies examining the incidence of neonatal intensive care unit (NICU) admission for respiratory distress and MAS before and after the practice change have arrived at conflicting conclusions.[43-48]

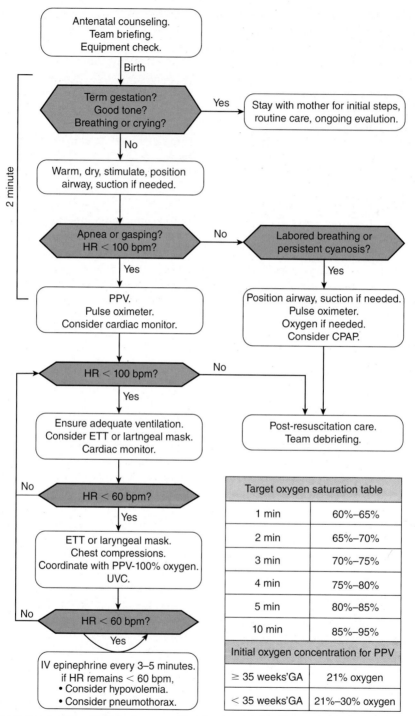

Fig. 2.5 Neonatal resuscitation algorithm. *CPAP*, Continuous positive airway pressure; *ECG*, electrocardiograph; *ETT*, endotracheal tube; *HR*, heart rate; *IV*, intravenous; *O₂*, oxygen; *PPV*, positive-pressure ventilation; *Spo₂*, oxygen saturation measured by pulse oximetry; *UVC*, umbilical venous catheter. Reprinted with permission. (From Weiner GM, Zaichkin J. *Textbook of Neonatal Resuscitation.* 8th ed. Itasca, IL: American Academy of Pediatrics; 2021.)

Although most found no difference in outcomes, two retrospective chart reviews found an increase in respiratory admissions to the NICU after stopping routine laryngoscopy and tracheal suction.[43,48] One of these, a single-center retrospective chart review, also found an increase in the incidence of MAS, but the authors elegantly demonstrated how their conclusions could change by simply altering the denominator (all births, all births with MSAF, nonvigorous births with MSAF, all NICU admits with MSAF) for several outcomes.[48] A well-designed and adequately powered RCT is still needed to answer this question.

Is tactile stimulation an effective intervention for an apneic newly born infant?

Although tactile stimulation is commonly recommended as an intervention to stimulate respirations in an apneic newborn, the evidence informing this practice is remarkably scarce. Current recommendations are based largely on historical practice, rational conjecture, and extrapolation from fetal vibroacoustic stimulation studies, newborn animal studies, and the postnatal treatment of apnea of prematurity. Given the contemporary focus on supporting preterm newborns with noninvasive ventilation, the potential role of tactile stimulation has received increased attention. Recent systematic reviews have identified a small number of observational studies and RCTs evaluating whether tactile stimulation improves respiratory effort in the immediate newborn period.[49,50] Most of the studies had low or critically low certainty of evidence because of the lack of a nonstimulated control group, the potential for confirmation bias (preferentially stimulating hypotonic and apneic newborns), and the potential for confounding by indication (preferentially stimulating well newborns and starting PPV immediately in hypotonic and apneic newborns). The systematic reviews found that stimulation was used inconsistently, the first episode of stimulation was often delayed, and the method and duration of stimulation varied widely. Among apneic newborns, the reported success of tactile stimulation for preventing the need for PPV ranged from 9% to 50%. When used for preterm newborns who were already receiving continuous positive airway pressure (CPAP), one observational study suggested that tactile stimulation may decrease the risk of needing tracheal intubation (7% stimulated vs. 18% not stimulated).[51] In a small RCT,

repetitive stimulation during the first 4 minutes of life compared with "standard" stimulation for preterm newborns (27–32 weeks) resulted in a modest increase in oxygen saturation at the end of the stabilization period but no difference in the need for PPV or the duration of PPV.[52] A small RCT suggested that rubbing the newborn's back and trunk may be more effective than flicking the foot, but there is no conclusive evidence.[53] Although additional RCTs are needed, the practical challenges of defining the control group, including what care is allowed in the nonstimulated group (is drying allowed), avoiding performance bias because of the inability to blind providers to the intervention, and the lack of equipoise for enrolling a truly nonstimulated control group have made this basic intervention difficult to study. Current North American and European guidelines do recommend gentle stimulation as part of the initial steps for apneic newborns but caution about the potential for prolonged stimulation to delay the initiation of PPV and the potential for aggressive stimulation to cause cutaneous injury.[35,42,54]

Effective Ventilation: The Key!

PPV should be started for any newborn who does not establish spontaneous respiratory effort after the initial steps or who remains bradycardic (heart rate <100 bpm) by 1 minute after birth.[22] Effective ventilation of the lungs is the single most important and effective action to stabilize a newborn infant who is compromised following delivery. Respiratory support alone (PPV and/or CPAP) is sufficient for more than 90% of newborns that require resuscitative interventions.[11] The goal is to provide aeration and ventilation to achieve gas exchange without causing lung injury.

What device should be used for positive-pressure ventilation during neonatal resuscitation?

Pressure can be generated using a self-inflating bag, flow-inflating bag, T-piece resuscitator, or a neonatal ventilator. Each device has advantages and disadvantages, and the choice of device may be made based on cost; availability of compressed gas; the desire to deliver sustained inflation, PEEP, and CPAP; or personal preference. Self-inflating bags are always ready for immediate use and re-expand without a compressed gas source. Inadvertent high peak pressures have been demonstrated with self-inflating bags when operators use only a pop-off safety valve. However, if providers use an appropriately designed manometer, they can accurately achieve the targeted peak inflation pressure.[55] Self-inflating bags are not routinely used to administer free-flow oxygen or CPAP. Even when outfitted with a PEEP valve, traditional self-inflating bags do not reliably deliver PEEP through the face mask.[56] A novel PEEP valve designed to work with a self-inflating bag in resource-limited settings without an external gas source may be effective.[57] The flow-inflating bag requires more time and practice to set up and a compressed gas source. Because the bag does not inflate unless there is a tight seal, large mask leaks are easy to identify. PEEP and CPAP can be generated by balancing the gas flow into the bag and the amount of gas leaking out of a control valve; however, this adjustment requires experience. T-piece resuscitators more accurately and consistently deliver set inflation pressures and PEEP than the other devices, but they require a compressed gas source and changing the inflation pressures during resuscitation is more difficult.[58] Based on evidence from a mechanical lung model, there is a risk of inadvertent PEEP when using a T-piece resuscitator for infants with an inflation rate > 50 breaths per minute, high airway resistance, and compliant lungs (e.g., an intubated term infant with normal lung compliance).[59]

A recent systematic review identified five RCTs (n = 1247 term and preterm infants) and one prospective cohort study (n = 1962 preterm infants) addressing this topic.[60] Pooled analyses of four RCTs comparing T-piece resuscitators with self-inflating bags showed that while there was no important difference in mortality, infants managed with the T-piece resuscitator had lower rates of bronchopulmonary dysplasia (BPD). Although use of the T-piece resuscitator was associated with some benefits, the authors did not make a strong recommendation in favor of the device due to the low certainty of evidence for most outcomes. Whichever PPV device is chosen, the most important thing is to become proficient using and troubleshooting the selected device.

What are common barriers to achieving effective ventilation with a face mask?

Most newborns who require resuscitation improve promptly with assisted ventilation alone.[11] The best sign that the lungs are being effectively aerated and

ventilated is a rapid rise in heart rate, followed by improvement in oxygen saturation and the infant's tone. To achieve effective ventilation via face mask, the provider must first open the airway by placing the infant in the neutral "sniffing" position. To achieve a good seal, the mask should rest on the chin and snugly cover the mouth and nose, but not the eyes to avoid trauma and a vagal response. Holding the face mask with two hands while another provider operates the PPV device may be more effective than attempting to hold the mask with one hand (Fig. 2.6).[61] If the heart rate has not increased within approximately 15 seconds of initiating PPV, the most likely reason is that the lungs are not being adequately ventilated because of an airway obstruction or large mask leak. A delivery room study of mask ventilation of premature infants documented that up to 25% of breaths had evidence of airway obstruction and 75% had significant mask leak.[62] Among apneic newborns, laryngeal adduction may be an important cause of airway obstructive and ineffective noninvasive ventilation.[63]

A series of ventilation corrective steps described with the mnemonic MR. SOPA (mask adjustment, reposition head and neck, suction mouth and nose, open the mouth, pressure increase, alternative airway) is commonly recommended to improve noninvasive ventilation.[27] A small observational study using a respiratory function monitor showed the corrective steps improved delivered tidal volume in some cases, and bradycardia resolved after nearly half of corrective

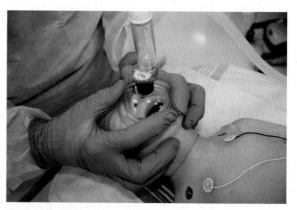

Fig. 2.6 Two-hand face mask hold. A colorimetric capnometer (CO_2 detector) turns yellow when gas exchange is detected.

steps, but the corrective steps could introduce new leaks and obstructions.[64] If the heart rate remains less than 60 bpm despite face mask ventilation that achieves chest movement, or if chest movement cannot be achieved with the corrective steps, insertion of an alternative airway (laryngeal mask or endotracheal tube) is strongly recommended.

Should capnography or a respiratory function monitor be used during neonatal resuscitation?

Even experienced providers have difficulty identifying obstruction, leak, changes in compliance, and the tidal volume of their manual ventilations. Simple disposable capnometers (CO_2 detectors) or continuous capnography may help confirm airway patency and effective lung aeration during face mask ventilation (Fig. 2.6).[65] Accurate measurement of delivered tidal volume may enable providers to avoid the pitfalls of ineffective and excessive ventilation. Sophisticated respiratory function monitors can detect airway obstruction, mask leak, and delivered tidal volume.[66] O'Currain reported that in the simulation setting, the use of a respiratory function monitor as an adjunct to standard resuscitation training improved newborn face mask ventilation skills.[67] A systematic review identified three RCTs (n = 443 infants) comparing outcomes of preterm infants resuscitated using a respiratory function monitor in conjunction with clinical assessment with clinical assessment alone.[68] The authors found no important differences in mortality or the proportion of inflations in the desired tidal volume range. However, they noted that use of the respiratory function monitor was associated with a reduction in rates of brain injury (any intraventricular hemorrhage or periventricular leukomalacia). Respiratory function monitoring remains a promising tool in the delivery room. However, the costs of the devices and the ongoing education required to use them effectively remain potential barriers to their widespread uptake.[69]

Should sustained inflations be used to establish functional residual capacity and improve aeration of the newborn lung?

In animal models, prolonged initial sustained inflations of 10 to 20 seconds have been shown to achieve functional residual capacity (FRC) faster and to improve lung function without adverse circulatory effects.[70,71] However, the largest RCT of this intervention, the SAIL trial, was stopped early

because of a higher rate of early mortality in infants managed using a sustained inflation.[72] In 2020, a pooled analysis of nine RCTs (n = 1406 infants) showed no difference in neonatal mortality and no evidence of a beneficial effect of sustained inflations on any secondary outcome.[73] Alternative methods to facilitate lung aeration are under investigation. A more gradual approach using an escalating PEEP strategy shows promise in the neonatal lamb model but needs to be tested in large RCTs enrolling preterm infants.[74]

What is the role of CPAP in the delivery room for preterm newborns?

If a newly born infant is breathing spontaneously but has labored breathing or persistently low oxygen saturation, CPAP may help establish and maintain an FRC. For premature infants, applying CPAP shortly after birth with subsequent selective surfactant administration has been recommended as an alternative to routine intubation with prophylactic surfactant administration.[75] Pooled analysis of four RCTs in preterm infants (<32 weeks) showed a significant benefit for the combined outcome of death or BPD for infants treated with nasal CPAP (risk difference –0.04, 95% confidence interval –0.08 to –0.00).[76] The current ILCOR treatment recommendation suggests that for spontaneously breathing preterm newborn infants with respiratory distress, the initial use of CPAP is preferred over intubation and intermittent PPV.[22] Although CPAP may help establish and maintain an FRC, thus improving respiratory distress, it should not be used in place of PPV when the infant is apneic or bradycardic.

Can a laryngeal mask be used in place of either a face mask or endotracheal tube?

A laryngeal mask is a type of supraglottic airway device that includes a small elliptical mask attached to an airway tube. The device is inserted into the baby's mouth and the mask is placed in the posterior pharynx where it makes a low-pressure seal just above the laryngeal inlet (Fig. 2.7). Insertion of a laryngeal mask does not require instruments or the operator to visualize the vocal cords. Most laryngeal masks are designed for infants greater than 2000 g, but a high rate of rapid and successful insertion has been reported across a wide range of gestational ages (29–35 weeks' gestation).[77] A Cochrane systematic review found that PPV

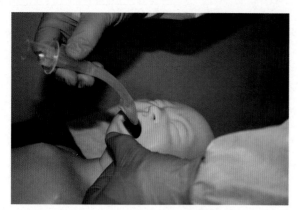

Fig. 2.7 Insertion of a cuffless laryngeal mask.

administered in the delivery room with a laryngeal mask was more effective than PPV with a face mask.[78] Use of a laryngeal mask was associated with a decreased need for endotracheal intubation and a shorter duration of PPV. These authors also reported that, in most cases, the use of a laryngeal mask when infants were not responding to face mask ventilation prevented the need for endotracheal intubation. Subsequently, in a large RCT (n=1163 infants), Pejovic found that a cuffless laryngeal mask could be safely and successfully inserted with minimal training by midwives in a limited resource setting.[79] The updated ILCOR consensus on science suggests that, where resources and training are available, a laryngeal mask may be used in place of a face mask as the initial device to provide PPV in the delivery room.[80]

Intubation is a difficult skill to acquire and requires extensive training to become proficient. Changes in practice have led to fewer infants being intubated in the delivery room and trainees having fewer opportunities to acquire this skill.[81] As a result, resident physicians take longer to complete the procedure, require multiple attempts, are successful in less than half of attempts, and repeated attempts are associated with adverse events.[82] Although the Cochrane review found no difference in first attempt success between endotracheal intubation and laryngeal mask placement, the first attempt intubation success rate was significantly higher in the included studies than typically reported.[78] Overall, the time required for laryngeal mask insertion was short, the first attempt success rate was high, and minimal training was required for

successful use in the delivery room. A laryngeal mask is an effective alternative to intubation and may be a life-saving device during an unanticipated airway emergency. When intubation is either unsuccessful or unfeasible, a laryngeal mask should be inserted.[27]

What concentration of oxygen should be used during neonatal resuscitation?

Use of 100% oxygen was routine for newborn resuscitation until resuscitation guidelines were changed in 2010. Although the optimal starting concentration of oxygen is unknown, the available evidence suggests that resuscitation of late preterm and term infants should be started with air (21% oxygen).[22] The ideal oxygen saturation range at each minute of life has not been defined, but a reasonable goal is to target a preductal oxygen saturation within the interquartile range for healthy term infants (Fig. 2.5). There is evidence from both animal and human studies of significant oxidative tissue damage in the lung and brain following asphyxia that is exacerbated by subsequent hyperoxygenation. In one study, hyperoxemia (arterial partial pressure of oxygen >100 mm Hg) during the first hour of recovery from perinatal asphyxia was associated with a higher incidence of hypoxic-ischemia encephalopathy and abnormal findings on magnetic resonance imaging of the brain.[83] Several cohort studies reporting an association of delivery room oxygen exposure with increased risk for childhood cancer raise additional concern about the risks of hyperoxygenation in the delivery room.[84-86] Meta-analyses of trials comparing oxygen with air for newborns during delivery room resuscitation suggest that term and near-term infants resuscitated with air begin spontaneous breathing faster, reach acceptable oxygen saturation values just as quickly, have less evidence of oxidative damage, and, most importantly, lower mortality.[87-90]

Preterm infants are deficient in antioxidant protection and face potential adverse effects of oxygen toxicity, such as chronic lung disease, retinopathy of prematurity, and necrotizing enterocolitis. A recent meta-analysis of 10 studies in preterm infants (< 35 weeks) demonstrated no benefit to initiating resuscitation with a high (fraction of inspired oxygen [FiO_2] 0.51–1.0) compared with a low (FiO_2 0.21–0.50) oxygen concentration.[91] The authors noted that nearly all infants born ≤ 32 weeks' gestation required oxygen supplementation to meet oxygen saturation targets. Based on a goal of limiting additional oxygen exposure without evidence of benefit, the current international guidelines for preterm infants born at less than 35 weeks' gestation recommend starting resuscitation with 21% to 30% oxygen and titrating the oxygen concentration using pulse oximetry.[22,35,42] Among preterm newborns (< 32 weeks), achieving a minimum oxygen saturation of 80% by 5 minutes has been associated with a lower risk of severe intraventricular hemorrhages and death.[92,93]

There is currently little evidence to guide how much oxygen should be administered during neonatal chest compressions (cardiopulmonary resuscitation [CPR]). There are no human studies available and those in animals have not shown any consistent advantage to the use of 100% oxygen during CPR.[94] Once the newborn has reached the point of requiring CPR, however, return of circulation has not occurred despite ventilation with a low oxygen concentration, and pulse oximetry may not be providing a reliable signal. With the lack of evidence in mind, the current European and North American guidelines make the cautious recommendation to use 100% oxygen until the heart rate has recovered (>60 bpm) and pulse oximetry is functioning.[35,42] Subsequently, the oxygen should be weaned as quickly as possible while maintaining saturation goals.

Chest Compressions During Resuscitation in the Delivery Room

When should chest compressions be initiated?

Regardless of gestational age, most newborns requiring resuscitation have primary respiratory failure and only require effective PPV. If gas exchange is impaired for a prolonged period, myocardial energy stores may become sufficiently depleted to depress cardiac function to the point that assisted ventilation alone will not be sufficient.[95] Chest compressions (CPR) increase coronary artery perfusion and help to restore cardiac function by increasing the diastolic pressure gradient between the aorta and coronary sinus.[131] The current guidelines continue to recommend CPR for a newborn infant with a heart rate less than 60 bpm despite at least 30 seconds of ventilation that aerates and ventilates the lung.[27,35] Because

effective ventilation is the critical step in newborn resuscitation and compressions are likely to interfere with effective ventilation, resuscitation providers are strongly encouraged to optimize assisted ventilation via placement of an advanced airway such as endotracheal tube or laryngeal mask before initiation of CPR. The optimal interval of ventilation before initiation of CPR is unknown. Rationally, there needs to be a balance between ensuring there is adequate ventilation in the hope of avoiding the need for CPR altogether and the risk of additional hypoxic/ischemic injury if circulation is not assisted in a timely manner. A study in a neonatal animal model of asphyxia-induced asystole found that under conditions of asystole, there was no advantage or disadvantage in delaying initiation of CPR for 1 minute rather than an initial 30 seconds of room air ventilation; however, when initiation of CPR was delayed for 90 seconds of ventilation, fewer animals were successfully resuscitated.[96] Animals exposed to 90 seconds of initial ventilation before support of the circulation with CPR required more doses of epinephrine to stabilize the heart rate and had lower blood pressures after resuscitation. Whether longer delays in initiation of CPR for bradycardia as opposed to asystole would have the same potential harm is unknown. There are no clinical data to offer guidance.

What technique should be used to administer chest compressions to a newborn?

Chest compressions (CPR) should be centered over the lower third of the sternum to compress most directly over the heart. Animal studies in an asphyxiated newborn pig model confirm that the depth of compressions is associated with changes in hemodynamic parameters during CPR.[97] A compression depth of approximately one-third the anterior-posterior (AP) diameter of the chest should be adequate to produce a palpable pulse. Mathematical modeling based on neonatal chest CT scan dimensions suggests that a compression depth of one-third the AP diameter of the chest should be more effective than one-quarter and safer than one-half the AP chest diameter.[98,99] Although a small case series of six infants suggested that a compression depth of one-half the AP diameter of the chest resulted in higher systolic, mean, and systemic perfusion pressures, this greater depth did not result in better diastolic blood pressure (the critical determinant of coronary perfusion) than a depth of one-third the AP diameter.[98]

The two-thumb method, in which the thumbs compress the sternum while the provider's hands encircle the chest (Fig. 2.8), should be used for neonatal CPR. Compared with the previously recommended two-finger method, the two-thumb method improves the quality and consistency of CPR while decreasing compressor fatigue.[100,101] Even with a lone rescuer, a recent systematic review with meta-analysis found that when CPR is performed on a simulated infant, the two-thumb technique with hands encircling the chest improves compression quality and does not appear to compromise ventilation.[102]

In the past, the two-finger technique was used while umbilical access was obtained so that the compressor's arms would be out of the way. Now it is recommended that once the airway is secured, which should have been completed before initiating CPR, the compressor should move to the head of the bed and continue two-thumb compressions.[27] This position allows unrestricted access to the umbilical stump for another team member to insert a catheter for emergency medication administration (Fig. 2.8).

Why do neonatal resuscitation guidelines recommend a lower compression-to-ventilation ratio compared with other resuscitation guidelines?

The ratio of compressions to ventilations that would truly optimize the dual goals of perfusion and ventilation during neonatal resuscitation from asphyxial arrest is unknown.[103] A compression-to-ventilation

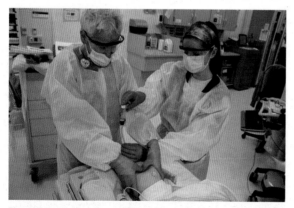

Fig. 2.8 The two-thumb compression technique can be continued from the head of the bed once the airway is secured, leaving ample access to the umbilical stump for emergency placement of an umbilical venous catheter.

ratio of 3:1, such that 90 compressions and 30 breaths are achieved per minute, is currently recommended to optimize ventilation.[35] During adult CPR, continuous chest compressions and infrequent, asynchronous ventilations are recommended; however, the pathophysiology of adult cardiac arrest is different. Most adults have a primary cardiac arrhythmia without respiratory failure, while most neonatal arrests are preceded by respiratory failure. What is known is that asphyxiated, asystolic piglets resuscitated with a combination of chest compressions and ventilations have better outcomes than those resuscitated with ventilations or compressions alone, especially during prolonged resuscitation.[104-106] A physiologic mathematical modeling study suggests that higher compression-to-ventilation ratios would result in underventilation of asphyxiated infants.[107] The model predicts that three to five compressions to one ventilation should be most efficient for newborns. A study comparing 2:1, 3:1, and 4:1 compression-to-ventilation ratios found similar rate of return of spontaneous circulation (ROSC), mortality, oxygen, and epinephrine administration during resuscitation in a porcine model of neonatal asphyxia.[108] Studies have compared 3:1 with 9:3 and 3:1 with 15:2 compression-to-ventilation ratios in piglet models of asystole owing to asphyxia.[109,110] Although the 15:2 ratio provided more compressions per minute without compromising $Paco_2$ and generated statistically higher diastolic blood pressures, the diastolic blood pressure was still inadequate until epinephrine was given, so there was no difference in time to ROSC. At present, there is no evidence from quality human, animal, manikin, or mathematical modeling studies to warrant a change from the current 3:1 compression-to-ventilation ratio.

Why are chest compressions coordinated with ventilations during neonatal resuscitation?

Coordination of chest compressions and ventilations, with three rapid compressions followed by a short pause to interpose one ventilation so that they are not delivered simultaneously, is still recommended, but the evidence for this recommendation is weak.[22] Based on physiologic plausibility, there is historical concern that if compressions and ventilations were delivered at the same time, ventilation might be critically compromised. Small studies using neonatal piglet asphyxia models have compared various synchronized compression-to-ventilation ratios with continuous compressions and asynchronous ventilations.[111-114] Several reported that piglets resuscitated with the asynchronous ventilation method had similar rates of ROSC, survival, and hemodynamic recovery compared to piglets resuscitated by the traditional 3:1 synchronized ratio[111,113]; however, others reported that the continuous compressions with asynchronous ventilation method resulted in improved oxygenation,[112] coronary perfusion pressure, end-tidal CO_2, time to ROSC, and survival.[114] In contrast to the animal models showing possible benefits from continuous compressions with asynchronous ventilations, manikin studies focused on the ergonomic issues found this method provided lower tidal volume breaths and more compressor fatigue.[115-118] Given the current lack of evidence of a consistent significant benefit, ILCOR, the European, and the North American guidelines continue to recommend coordination of compressions and ventilations.[22,35,42] Investigations are ongoing to see if providing a sustained inflation while giving the cardiac compressions might have advantages over the 3:1 synchronized ventilation-to-compression ratio. A clinical pilot trial suggested this technique might reduce time to ROSC.[119] A larger multicenter randomized trial is now underway.[120]

When should the heart rate response to chest compressions be checked?

To avoid critical interruptions in coronary perfusion, the guidelines recommend waiting 60 seconds after starting compressions to check the heart rate response.[27] Because physical examination methods used to assess the newborn's heart rate are inaccurate and the pulse oximeter may not display a reliable signal during cardiovascular collapse, the guidelines recommend using an electronic cardiac monitor to assess the infant's heart rate during compressions.[35]

Is capnography useful during chest compressions?

Frequent repetitive pauses in chest compressions and ventilation make it difficult to achieve and maintain adequate coronary perfusion pressure. Use of end-tidal CO_2 ($ETCO_2$) capnography during CPR may provide a continuous, noninvasive tool to eliminate frequent pauses during CPR to assess the infant's heart rate. $ETCO_2$ values reflect a balance between CO_2 production by cellular metabolism, alveolar ventilation, and pulmonary perfusion. During asystole there

is no cardiac output and CO_2 is not carried to the lungs to be exhaled. During CPR, cellular metabolism and alveolar ventilation are presumed to be at a steady state (provided that PPV is given in a steady manner), so changes in $ETCO_2$ primarily reflect changes in cardiac output. A piglet model of asphyxia-induced asystole has demonstrated that after PPV, $ETCO_2$ falls to near zero with loss of PBF and then increases slightly with initiation of cardiac compressions, reflecting blood being pumped through the lungs by effective CPR.[121] When circulation is restored, there is a sudden increase in $ETCO_2$ as the reestablished perfusion brings CO_2-rich blood back to the lungs. In that animal model, an $ETCO_2$ greater than 15 mm Hg correlated well with return of an audible heart rate higher than 60 bpm. One small study of infants in an intensive care unit found similar $ETCO_2$ cut-offs for ROSC during CPR.[122] Current neonatal resuscitation guidelines do not address the use of capnography during chest compressions.

Medications During Resuscitation in the Delivery Room

When should medications be considered during resuscitation in the delivery room?

When asphyxia is so severe that it results in asystole or agonal bradycardia, the newborn heart has become depleted of energy substrate and can no longer beat effectively.[95] Adequate perfusion of the heart with oxygenated blood must be restored or resuscitation efforts will be unsuccessful. During chest compression, coronary blood flow occurs during diastole, presumably because of increased right atrial pressure during chest compressions. Therefore, coronary perfusion pressure is determined by the aortic diastolic blood pressure minus the right atrial diastolic blood pressure. Cardiac compressions plus adequate systemic vascular resistance must generate diastolic blood pressure adequate to achieve ROSC. Given the profound acidemia and resultant vasodilation induced by asphyxia, a vasopressor agent such as epinephrine is frequently required to achieve an adequate aortic diastolic pressure for sufficient coronary perfusion. A single study in a neonatal piglet model of asphyxial cardiac arrest suggested that vasopressin, a pulmonary vasodilator and systemic vasopressor, may improve survival but no human neonatal data are available.[123]

What is the recommended dose of epinephrine during neonatal resuscitation?

Epinephrine is a catecholamine that stimulates α-adrenergic receptor–mediated vasoconstriction to elevate the diastolic blood pressure and increase the coronary perfusion pressure during chest compressions (Fig. 2.9). Data evaluating the most effective and safest dose for intravenous epinephrine during delivery room CPR are minimal and have been largely based on animal models and extrapolation from clinical trials in older children and adults.[124] Current guidelines recommend that if the heart rate remains less than 60 bpm despite 1 minute of effective PPV with coordinated chest compressions, then 0.01 to 0.03 mg/kg of epinephrine (equal to 0.1–0.3 mL/kg of a 0.1-mg/mL solution) should be given rapidly through a central venous catheter or intraosseous (IO) needle (Table 2.2).[22,27,35] Although the full dosing

range is acceptable, for educational efficiency, the Neonatal Resuscitation Program recommends an initial intravascular dose of 0.02 mg/kg (equal to 0.2 mL/kg of a 0.1 mg/mL solution).[27] The intravascular dose should be followed by a 3-mL saline flush to ensure it reaches the central circulation.[27,125]

What is the preferred route of epinephrine administration during neonatal resuscitation?

Although neonatal health care providers are trained to insert umbilical venous catheters (UVCs), other health care providers may be less comfortable with this procedure. Prehospital providers and emergency department personnel frequently insert IO needles for rapid vascular access. One case series has described 27 newborns ranging from 25 to 41 weeks' gestation who were resuscitated with medications administered through an IO needle.[126] A simulation study using a neonatal manikin model demonstrated that IO needle insertion was faster than UVC placement with no difference in the participants' perceived ease of use.[127]

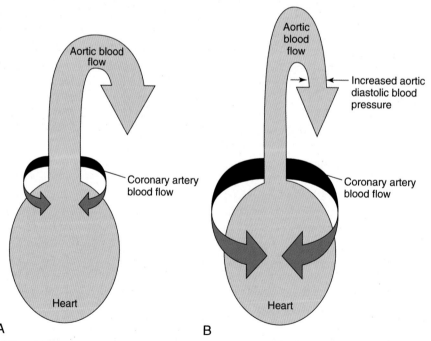

Fig. 2.9 The effect of diastolic blood pressure on coronary blood flow during cardiac compressions. **A,** Cardiac compressions with minimal aortic diastolic blood pressure preferentially send the majority of the cardiac output around the aortic arch to the periphery. **B,** Cardiac compressions with improved aortic diastolic blood pressure send more blood into the coronary arteries to bring oxygenated blood that will help generate adenosine triphosphate to get the heart beating again. (From Wyckoff M. Neonatal cardiopulmonary resuscitation: Critical hemodynamics. *Neoreviews.* 2010;11(3): e123-e129.)

TABLE 2.2 Neonatal Resuscitation Medications

Drug	Dose Mass (Volume)	Administration
Epinephrine IV/IO Concentration 0.1 mg/mL	0.01–0.03 mg/kg (0.1–0.3 mL/kg)	• IV/IO rapid push • Flush with 3 mL 0.9% NaCl • Repeat every 3–5 minutes if heart rate < 60 bpm
Epinephrine ET Concentration 0.1 mg/mL	0.05–0.1 mg/kg (0.5–1 mL/kg)	• Less effective than IV/IO • May administer while vascular access is being established. • No flush. Give PPV to distribute.
Volume expansion IV/IO 0.9% NaCl Type O-negative blood	10 mL/kg	• Give over 5–10 minutes

ET, Endotracheal; *IO*, intraosseous; *IV*, intravenous; *NaCl*, sodium chloride; *PPV*, positive-pressure ventilation.
Adapted from Weiner GM, Zaichkin J. *Textbook of Neonatal Resuscitation*. 8th ed. Itasca, IL: American Academy of Pediatrics; 2021.

Given the importance of administering emergency epinephrine when it is indicated during resuscitation, delivery room resuscitation personnel should have ready access to both of these devices and adequate training to reliably insert them without delay.[128]

Can emergency epinephrine be administered through an endotracheal tube?

While securing vascular access, some providers may consider endotracheal administration of epinephrine; however, newborn transitional physiology does not favor this route for several reasons. Decreased blood flow during cardiac collapse may be insufficient to transport drugs from the alveoli to the central circulation, pulmonary vasoconstriction from acidosis could impede drug absorption, alveolar liquid may dilute the epinephrine, and right-to-left intracardiac shunts could bypass the pulmonary circulation altogether. Newborn animal and human studies indicate that endotracheal epinephrine absorption is unreliable and less effective.[124] If providers choose to administer one dose of endotracheal epinephrine, a higher dose range (0.05–0.1 mg/kg = 0.5 to 1 mL/kg of a 0.1-mg/mL solution) has been recommended (Table 2.2).[22] This higher dose should not be given intravenously.

When should an intravascular volume bolus be considered during resuscitation in the delivery room?

Most asphyxiated, severely depressed newborns are not hypovolemic. Newborns may develop hypovolemic shock from acute blood caused by fetal-maternal hemorrhage, bleeding vasa previa, placental laceration, umbilical cord prolapse, or umbilical cord disruption. Volume should be infused only if the infant does not respond to resuscitation in the setting of acute blood loss and the infant has clinical signs of hypovolemic shock (pallor, weak pulses, poor perfusion) or the infant has signs of hypovolemic shock and there is a clinical suspicion for occult blood loss.[35] The best replacement fluid for shock associated with acute blood loss is type O-negative blood, but an isotonic crystalloid such as normal saline solution is acceptable until blood is available.[27] Emergency volume replacement during resuscitation should be administered in 10-mL/kg aliquots slowly (5–10 minutes) through a UVC or an IO needle (Table 2.2). Additional volume may be required but caution should be used to avoid infusing excessive volume and increasing demands on the already compromised neonatal heart. In an asphyxia-induced hypotension and bradycardia model (without hypovolemia), volume infusion during resuscitation increased pulmonary edema, decreased pulmonary dynamic compliance, and did not improve blood pressure either during or after the resuscitation.[129] Thus, routine volume infusions during delivery room resuscitations not complicated by hypovolemia may be detrimental, exacerbate poor cardiac output, and are not recommended.

Discontinuing Resuscitative Efforts

The decision when to stop resuscitative efforts in the delivery room if the infant is not improving and if there is no detectable heart rate remains controversial.

A recent systematic review examining the outcomes infants with ongoing resuscitative efforts at 10 minutes after birth found that although such infants are at high risk for mortality and moderate-to-severe neurodevelopmental impairment, survival without moderate or severe neurodevelopmental impairment was possible.[130] The authors concluded that no specific duration of resuscitation is likely to consistently and accurately predict survival or survival without moderate-to-severe impairment. Based on this systematic review, the updated ILCOR consensus on science suggested discussion of discontinuing resuscitative efforts with the clinical team and family if despite provision of all recommended steps of resuscitation, and excluding reversible causes, a newborn infant requires prolonged CPR.[22] ILCOR suggested that a reasonable time frame to consider this change in goals of care is around 20 minutes after birth. Ultimately, the decision to initiate and continue resuscitative efforts should be individualized and informed by factors such as gestational age, the presence of congenital anomalies, the timing of perinatal insult (if known), the perceived adequacy of resuscitative interventions, the family's stated preferences and values, and the availability of postresuscitative resources, such as neonatal intensive care, and neuroprotective strategies, such as therapeutic hypothermia. Caution must be taken in global adoption of this treatment recommendation.

REFERENCES

1. Hooper SB, Te Pas AB, Lang J, et al. Cardiovascular transition at birth: a physiological sequence. *Pediatr Res.* 2015;77(5):608-614.
2. Hooper SB, Kitchen MJ, Wallace MJ, et al. Imaging lung aeration and lung liquid clearance at birth. *FASEB J.* 2007;21(12): 3329-3337.
3. Hooper SB, Te Pas AB, Kitchen MJ. Respiratory transition in the newborn: a three-phase process. *Arch Dis Child Fetal Neonatal Ed.* 2016;101(3):F266-F271.
4. Siew ML, Te Pas AB, Wallace MJ, et al. Positive end-expiratory pressure enhances development of a functional residual capacity in preterm rabbits ventilated from birth. *J Appl Physiol (1985).* 2009;106(5):1487-1493.
5. Bhatt S, Alison BJ, Wallace EM, et al. Delaying cord clamping until ventilation onset improves cardiovascular function at birth in preterm lambs. *J Physiol.* 2013;591(8):2113-2126.
6. Hooper SB, Polglase GR, te Pas AB. A physiological approach to the timing of umbilical cord clamping at birth. *Arch Dis Child Fetal Neonatal Ed.* 2015;100(4):F355-F360.
7. Stenning FJ, Polglase GR, Te Pas AB, et al. Effect of maternal oxytocin on umbilical venous and arterial blood flows during physiological-based cord clamping in preterm lambs. *PLoS One.* 2021;16(6):e0253306.
8. Lang JA, Pearson JT, Binder-Heschl C, et al. Increase in pulmonary blood flow at birth: role of oxygen and lung aeration. *J Physiol.* 2016;594(5):1389-1398.
9. Lang JA, Pearson JT, te Pas AB, et al. Ventilation/perfusion mismatch during lung aeration at birth. *J Appl Physiol (1985).* 2014;117(5):535-543.
10. Ersdal HL, Mduma E, Svensen E, et al. Early initiation of basic resuscitation interventions including face mask ventilation may reduce birth asphyxia related mortality in low-income countries: a prospective descriptive observational study. *Resuscitation.* 2012;83(7):869-873.
11. Skare C, Kramer-Johansen J, Steen T, et al. Incidence of newborn stabilization and resuscitation measures and guideline compliance during the first minutes of life in Norway. *Neonatology.* 2015;108(2):100-107.
12. Moreira ME, Pereira AP, Gomes Junior SC, et al. Factors associated with the use of supplemental oxygen or positive pressure ventilation in the delivery room, in infants born with a gestational age >/= 34 weeks. *Reprod Health.* 2016;13(suppl 3):116.
13. Sawyer T, Lee HC, Aziz K. Anticipation and preparation for every delivery room resuscitation. *Semin Fetal Neonatal Med.* 2018;23(5):312-320.
14. Aziz K, Chadwick M, Baker M, Andrews W. Ante- and intrapartum factors that predict increased need for neonatal resuscitation. *Resuscitation.* 2008;79(3):444-452.
15. Aziz K, Chadwick M, Downton G, Baker M, Andrews W. The development and implementation of a multidisciplinary neonatal resuscitation team in a Canadian perinatal centre. *Resuscitation.* 2005;66(1):45-51.
16. Lee J, Lee JH. A clinical scoring system to predict the need for extensive resuscitation at birth in very low birth weight infants. *BMC Pediatr.* 2019;19(1):197.
17. Berazategui JP, Aguilar A, Escobedo M, et al. Risk factors for advanced resuscitation in term and near-term infants: a case-control study. *Arch Dis Child Fetal Neonatal Ed.* 2017;102(1): F44-F50.
18. Szyld E, Anderson M, Shah B, et al. Risk calculator for advanced neonatal resuscitation. *BMJ Paediatrics Open.* 2022;6:e001376.
19. WHO. *Thermal Protection of the Newborn: A Practical Guide.* Geneva; 1997.
20. Duryea EL, Nelson DB, Wyckoff MH, et al. The impact of ambient operating room temperature on neonatal and maternal hypothermia and associated morbidities: a randomized controlled trial. *Am J Obstet Gynecol.* 2016;214(4):505.e1-505.e7.
21. Bhatt DR, Reddy N, Ruiz R, et al. Perinatal quality improvement bundle to decrease hypothermia in extremely low birthweight infants with birth weight less than 1000 g: single-center experience over 6 years. *J Investig Med.* 2020;68(7):1256-1260.
22. Wyckoff MH, Wyllie J, Aziz K, et al. Neonatal Life Support: 2020 International Consensus on Cardiopulmonary Resuscitation and Emergency Cardiovascular Care Science With Treatment Recommendations. *Circulation.* 2020;142(16_suppl_1):S185-S221.
23. de Almeida MF DJ, Ramaswamy VV, Trevisanuto D, et al. *Maintaining Normal Temperature Immediately After Birth in Late Preterm and Term Infants: NLS 5100. ILCOR Consensus on Science with Treatment Recommendations (CoSTR).* Brussels, Belgium: International Liaison Committee on Resuscitation (ILCOR) Neonatal Life Support Task Force; 2022.
24. Seidler AL, Gyte GML, Rabe H, et al. Umbilical cord management for newborns <34 weeks' gestation: a meta-analysis. *Pediatrics.* 2021;147(3):e20200576.
25. Gomersall J, Berber S, Middleton P, et al. Umbilical cord management at term and late preterm birth: a meta-analysis. *Pediatrics.* 2021;147(3):e2020015404.

26. Katheria A, Reister F, Essers J, et al. Association of umbilical cord milking vs delayed umbilical cord clamping with death or severe intraventricular hemorrhage among preterm infants. *JAMA.* 2019;322(19):1877-1886.

27. Weiner GM, Zaichkin J. *Textbook of Neonatal Resuscitation.* 8th ed. Itasca, IL: American Academy of Pediatrics; 2021.

28. Bjorland PA, Ersdal HL, Eilevstjonn J, Oymar K, Davis PG, Rettedal SI. Changes in heart rate from 5 s to 5 min after birth in vaginally delivered term newborns with delayed cord clamping. *Arch Dis Child Fetal Neonatal Ed.* 2021;106(3):311-315.

29. O'Donnell CP, Kamlin CO, Davis PG, Carlin JB, Morley CJ. Clinical assessment of infant colour at delivery. *Arch Dis Child Fetal Neonatal Ed.* 2007;92(6):F465-F467.

30. Dawson JA, Kamlin CO, Vento M, et al. Defining the reference range for oxygen saturation for infants after birth. *Pediatrics.* 2010;125(6):e1340-e1347.

31. Lara-Canton I, Badurdeen S, Dekker J, et al. Oxygen saturation and heart rate in healthy term and late preterm infants with delayed cord clamping. *Pediatr Res.* 2022.

32. Padilla-Sanchez C, Baixauli-Alacreu S, Canada-Martinez AJ, Solaz-Garcia A, Alemany-Anchel MJ, Vento M. Delayed vs immediate cord clamping changes oxygen saturation and heart rate patterns in the first minutes after birth. *J Pediatr.* 2020;227:149-156.e141.

33. Fawke JWJ, Udeata E, Rüdiger M, et al. *Suctioning Clear Amniotic Fluid at Birth: NLS 5120. ILCOR Consensus on Science with Treatment Recommendations (CoSTR).* Brussels, Belgium: International Liaison Committee on Resuscitation (ILCOR) Neonatal Life Support Task Force; 2022.

34. Hutchon D, Pratesi S, Katheria A. How to provide motherside neonatal resuscitation with intact placental circulation? *Children (Basel).* 2021;8(4):291.

35. Aziz K, Lee CHC, Escobedo MB, et al. Part 5: neonatal resuscitation 2020 American Heart Association Guidelines for Cardiopulmonary Resuscitation and Emergency Cardiovascular Care. *Pediatrics.* 2021;147(suppl 1):e2020038505E.

36. McCall EM, Alderdice F, Halliday HL, Jenkins JG, Vohra S. Interventions to prevent hypothermia at birth in preterm and/or low birthweight infants. *Cochrane Database Syst Rev.* 2010;17(3):CD004210.

37. Laptook AR, Bell EF, Shankaran S, et al. Admission temperature and associated mortality and morbidity among moderately and extremely preterm infants. *J Pediatr.* 2018;192:53-59.e52.

38. de Almeida MF, Guinsburg R, Sancho GA, et al. Hypothermia and early neonatal mortality in preterm infants. *J Pediatr.* 2014;164(2):271-275.e271.

39. Cavallin F, Calgaro S, Brugnolaro V, et al. Non-linear association between admission temperature and neonatal mortality in a low-resource setting. *Sci Rep.* 2020;10(1):20800.

40. Perlman JM, Wyllie J, Kattwinkel J, et al. Part 7: Neonatal Resuscitation: 2015 International Consensus on Cardiopulmonary Resuscitation and Emergency Cardiovascular Care Science with Treatment Recommendations (Reprint). *Pediatrics.* 2015;136(suppl 2):S120-S166.

41. Trevisanuto D, Strand ML, Kawakami MD, et al. Tracheal suctioning of meconium at birth for non-vigorous infants: a systematic review and meta-analysis. *Resuscitation.* 2020;149:117-126.

42. Madar J, Roehr CC, Ainsworth S, et al. European Resuscitation Council Guidelines 2021: newborn resuscitation and support of transition of infants at birth. *Resuscitation.* 2021;161:291-326.

43. Chiruvolu A, Miklis KK, Chen E, Petrey B, Desai S. Delivery room management of meconium-stained newborns and respiratory support. *Pediatrics.* 2018;142(6):e20181485.

44. Edwards EM, Lakshminrusimha S, Ehret DEY, Horbar JD. NICU admissions for meconium aspiration syndrome before and after a National Resuscitation Program Suctioning Guideline Change. *Children (Basel).* 2019;6(5):68.

45. Kalra VK, Lee HC, Sie L, Ratnasiri AW, Underwood MA, Lakshminrusimha S. Change in neonatal resuscitation guidelines and trends in incidence of meconium aspiration syndrome in California. *J Perinatol.* 2020;40(1):46-55.

46. Oommen VI, Ramaswamy VV, Szyld E, Roehr CC. Resuscitation of non-vigorous neonates born through meconium-stained amniotic fluid: post policy change impact analysis. *Arch Dis Child Fetal Neonatal Ed.* 2021;106(3):324-326.

47. Myers P, Gupta AG. Impact of the revised NRP meconium aspiration guidelines on term infant outcomes. *Hosp Pediatr.* 2020; 10(3):295-299.

48. Kalra V, Leegwater AJ, Vadlaputi P, Garlapati P, Chawla S, Lakshminrusimha S. Neonatal outcomes of non-vigorous neonates with meconium-stained amniotic fluid before and after change in tracheal suctioning recommendation. *J Perinatol.* 2022;42:769-774.

49. Kaufmann M, Mense L, Springer L, Dekker J. Tactile stimulation in the delivery room: past, present, future. A systematic review. *Pediatr Res.* 2022.

50. Guinsburg R, de Almeida MFB, Finan E, et al. Tactile stimulation in newborn infants with inadequate respiration at birth: a systematic review. *Pediatrics.* 2022;149:e2021055067.

51. Dekker J, Martherus T, Cramer SJE, van Zanten HA, Hooper SB, Te Pas AB. Tactile stimulation to stimulate spontaneous breathing during stabilization of preterm infants at birth: a retrospective analysis. *Front Pediatr.* 2017;5:61.

52. Dekker J, Hooper SB, Martherus T, Cramer SJE, van Geloven N, Te Pas AB. Repetitive versus standard tactile stimulation of preterm infants at birth: a randomized controlled trial. *Resuscitation.* 2018;127:37-43.

53. Cavallin F, Lochoro P, Ictho J, et al. Back rubs or foot flicks for neonatal stimulation at birth in a low-resource setting: a randomized controlled trial. *Resuscitation.* 2021;167:137-143.

54. Kalaniti K, Chacko A, Daspal S. Tactile stimulation during newborn resuscitation: the good, the bad, and the ugly. *Oman Med J.* 2018;33(1):84-85.

55. Rafferty AR, Johnson L, Maxfield D, Dawson JA, Davis PG, Thio M. The accuracy of delivery of target pressures using self-inflating bag manometers in a benchtop study. *Acta Paediatr.* 2016;105(6):e247-e251.

56. Morley CJ, Dawson JA, Stewart MJ, Hussain F, Davis PG. The effect of a PEEP valve on a Laerdal neonatal self-inflating resuscitation bag. *J Paediatr Child Health.* 2010;46(1-2):51-56.

57. Thallinger M, Ersdal HL, Morley C, et al. Neonatal ventilation with a manikin model and two novel PEEP valves without an external gas source. *Arch Dis Child Fetal Neonatal Ed.* 2017; 102(3):F208-F213.

58. Dawson JA, Gerber A, Kamlin CO, Davis PG, Morley CJ. Providing PEEP during neonatal resuscitation: which device is best? *J Paediatr Child Health.* 2011;47(10):698-703.

59. Drevhammar T, Falk M, Donaldsson S, Tracy M, Hinder M. Neonatal resuscitation with T-piece systems: risk of inadvertent PEEP related to mechanical properties. *Front Pediatr.* 2021;9:663249.

60. Trevisanuto D, Roehr CC, Davis PG, et al. Devices for administering ventilation at birth: a systematic review. *Pediatrics.* 2021;148(1):e2021050174.

61. Tracy MB, Klimek J, Coughtrey H, et al. Mask leak in one-person mask ventilation compared to two-person in newborn infant manikin study. *Arch Dis Child Fetal Neonatal Ed.* 2011;96(3):F195-F200.

62. Schmolzer GM, Dawson JA, Kamlin CO, O'Donnell CP, Morley CJ, Davis PG. Airway obstruction and gas leak during mask ventilation of preterm infants in the delivery room. *Arch Dis Child Fetal Neonatal Ed.* 2011;96(4):F254-F257.

63. Crawshaw JR, Kitchen MJ, Binder-Heschl C, et al. Laryngeal closure impedes non-invasive ventilation at birth. *Arch Dis Child Fetal Neonatal Ed.* 2018;103(2):F112-F119.

64. Yang KC, Te Pas AB, Weinberg DD, Foglia EE. Corrective steps to enhance ventilation in the delivery room. *Arch Dis Child Fetal Neonatal Ed.* 2020;105(6):605-608.

65. Leone TA, Lange A, Rich W, Finer NN. Disposable colorimetric carbon dioxide detector use as an indicator of a patent airway during noninvasive mask ventilation. *Pediatrics.* 2006;118(1):e202-e204.

66. Schmolzer GM, Morley CJ, Wong C, et al. Respiratory function monitor guidance of mask ventilation in the delivery room: a feasibility study. *J Pediatr.* 2012;160(3):377-381.e372.

67. O'Currain E, Thio M, Dawson JA, Donath SM, Davis PG. Respiratory monitors to teach newborn facemask ventilation: a randomised trial. *Arch Dis Child Fetal Neonatal Ed.* 2019;104(6):F582-F586.

68. de Medeiros SM, Mangat A, Polglase GR, Sarrato GZ, Davis PG, Schmolzer GM. Respiratory function monitoring to improve the outcomes following neonatal resuscitation: a systematic review and meta-analysis. *Arch Dis Child Fetal Neonatal Ed.* 2022;107:589-596.

69. Fuerch JH RY, Thio M, Halamek LP, et al. *Respiratory Function Monitoring: NLS#806. ILCOR Consensus on Science with Treatment Recommendations (CoSTR).* Brussels, Belgium: International Liaison Committee on Resuscitation (ILCOR) Neonatal Life Support Task Force; 2022.

70. Sobotka KS, Hooper SB, Allison BJ, et al. An initial sustained inflation improves the respiratory and cardiovascular transition at birth in preterm lambs. *Pediatr Res.* 2011;70(1):56-60.

71. te Pas AB, Siew M, Wallace MJ, et al. Effect of sustained inflation length on establishing functional residual capacity at birth in ventilated premature rabbits. *Pediatr Res.* 2009;66(3):295-300.

72. Kirpalani H, Ratcliffe SJ, Keszler M, et al. Effect of sustained inflations vs intermittent positive pressure ventilation on bronchopulmonary dysplasia or death among extremely preterm infants: The SAIL randomized clinical trial. *JAMA.* 2019;321(12):1165-1175.

73. Foglia EE, Te Pas AB, Kirpalani H, et al. Sustained inflation vs standard resuscitation for preterm infants: a systematic review and meta-analysis. *JAMA Pediatr.* 2020;174(4):e195897.

74. Tingay DG, Pereira-Fantini PM, Oakley R, et al. Gradual aeration at birth is more lung protective than a sustained inflation in preterm lambs. *Am J Respir Crit Care Med.* 2019;200(5):608-616.

75. Sweet DG, Carnielli V, Greisen G, et al. European consensus guidelines on the management of respiratory distress syndrome: 2019 update. *Neonatology.* 2019;115(4):432-450.

76. Schmolzer GM, Kumar M, Pichler G, Aziz K, O'Reilly M, Cheung PY. Non-invasive versus invasive respiratory support in preterm infants at birth: systematic review and meta-analysis. *BMJ.* 2013;347:f5980.

77. Wanous AA, Wey A, Rudser KD, Roberts KD. Feasibility of laryngeal mask airway device placement in neonates. *Neonatology.* 2017;111(3):222-227.

78. Qureshi MJ, Kumar M. Laryngeal mask airway versus bag-mask ventilation or endotracheal intubation for neonatal resuscitation. *Cochrane Database Syst Rev.* 2018;3:CD003314.

79. Pejovic NJ, Myrnerts Hook S, Byamugisha J, et al. A randomized trial of laryngeal mask airway in neonatal resuscitation. *N Engl J Med.* 2020;383(22):2138-2147.

80. Yamada NK MC, Quek BH, Rabi Y, et al. *Supraglottic Airways for Neonatal Resuscitation: NLS 5340 ILCOR Consensus on Science with Treatment Recommendations (CoSTR).* Brussels, Belgium: International Liaison Committee on Resuscitation Neonatal Life Support Task Force; 2022.

81. Sawyer T, Johnson K. Neonatal intubation: past, present, and future. *Neoreviews.* 2020;21(5):e335-e341.

82. Foglia EE, Ades A, Sawyer T, et al. Neonatal intubation practice and outcomes: an International Registry Study. *Pediatrics.* 2019;143(1):e20180902.

83. Kapadia VS, Chalak LF, DuPont TL, Rollins NK, Brion LP, Wyckoff MH. Perinatal asphyxia with hyperoxemia within the first hour of life is associated with moderate to severe hypoxic-ischemic encephalopathy. *J Pediatr.* 2013;163(4):949-954.

84. Cnattingius S, Zack MM, Ekbom A, et al. Prenatal and neonatal risk factors for childhood lymphatic leukemia. *J Natl Cancer Inst.* 1995;87(12):908-914.

85. Naumburg E, Bellocco R, Cnattingius S, Jonzon A, Ekbom A. Supplementary oxygen and risk of childhood lymphatic leukaemia. *Acta Paediatr.* 2002;91(12):1328-1333.

86. Spector LG, Klebanoff MA, Feusner JH, Georgieff MK, Ross JA. Childhood cancer following neonatal oxygen supplementation. *J Pediatr.* 2005;147(1):27-31.

87. Davis PG, Tan A, O'Donnell CP, Schulze A. Resuscitation of newborn infants with 100% oxygen or air: a systematic review and meta-analysis. *Lancet.* 2004;364(9442):1329-1333.

88. Tan A, Schulze A, O'Donnell CP, Davis PG. Air versus oxygen for resuscitation of infants at birth. *Cochrane Database Syst Rev.* 2004;(3):CD002273.

89. Rabi Y, Rabi D, Yee W. Room air resuscitation of the depressed newborn: a systematic review and meta-analysis. *Resuscitation.* 2007;72(3):353-363.

90. Welsford M, Nishiyama C, Shortt C, et al. Room air for initiating term newborn resuscitation: a systematic review with meta-analysis. *Pediatrics.* 2019;143(1):e20181825.

91. Welsford M, Nishiyama C, Shortt C, et al. Initial oxygen use for preterm newborn resuscitation: a systematic review with meta-analysis. *Pediatrics.* 2019;143(1):e20181828.

92. Oei JL, Finer NN, Saugstad OD, et al. Outcomes of oxygen saturation targeting during delivery room stabilisation of preterm infants. *Arch Dis Child Fetal Neonatal Ed.* 2018;103(5):F446-F454.

93. Oei JL, Vento M. Is there a "Right" amount of oxygen for preterm infant stabilization at Birth? *Front Pediatr.* 2019;7:354.

94. Garcia-Hidalgo C, Cheung PY, Solevag AL, et al. A review of oxygen use during chest compressions in newborns-a meta-analysis of animal data. *Front Pediatr.* 2018;6:400.

95. Ramachandran S, Wyckoff M. Drugs in the delivery room. *Semin Fetal Neonatal Med.* 2019;24(6):101032.

96. Dannevig I, Solevag AL, Wyckoff M, Saugstad OD, Nakstad B. Delayed onset of cardiac compressions in cardiopulmonary resuscitation of newborn pigs with asphyctic cardiac arrest. *Neonatology.* 2011;99(2):153-162.

97. Bruckner M, O'Reilly M, Lee TF, Neset M, Cheung PY, Schmolzer GM. Effects of varying chest compression depths on carotid blood flow and blood pressure in asphyxiated piglets. *Arch Dis Child Fetal Neonatal Ed.* 2021;106(5):553-556.

98. Meyer A, Nadkarni V, Pollock A, et al. Evaluation of the Neonatal Resuscitation Program's recommended chest compression depth using computerized tomography imaging. *Resuscitation.* 2010;81(5):544-548.

99. Braga MS, Dominguez TE, Pollock AN, et al. Estimation of optimal CPR chest compression depth in children by using computer tomography. *Pediatrics.* 2009;124(1):e69-e74.

100. Christman C, Hemway RJ, Wyckoff MH, Perlman JM. The two-thumb is superior to the two-finger method for administering chest compressions in a manikin model of neonatal resuscitation. *Arch Dis Child Fetal Neonatal Ed*. 2011;96(2):F99-F101.

101. Mildenhall LF, Huynh TK. Factors modulating effective chest compressions in the neonatal period. *Semin Fetal Neonatal Med*. 2013;18(6):352-356.

102. Millin MG, Bogumil D, Fishe JN, Burke RV. Comparing the two-finger versus two-thumb technique for single person infant CPR: a systematic review and meta-analysis. *Resuscitation*. 2020;148:161-172.

103. Solevag AL, Cheung PY, O'Reilly M, Schmolzer GM. A review of approaches to optimise chest compressions in the resuscitation of asphyxiated newborns. *Arch Dis Child Fetal Neonatal Ed*. 2016;101(3):F272-F276.

104. Berg RA, Hilwig RW, Kern KB, Babar I, Ewy GA. Simulated mouth-to-mouth ventilation and chest compressions (bystander cardiopulmonary resuscitation) improves outcome in a swine model of prehospital pediatric asphyxial cardiac arrest. *Crit Care Med*. 1999;27(9):1893-1899.

105. Berg RA, Hilwig RW, Kern KB, Ewy GA. "Bystander" chest compressions and assisted ventilation independently improve outcome from piglet asphyxial pulseless "cardiac arrest". *Circulation*. 2000;101(14):1743-1748.

106. Dean JM, Koehler RC, Schleien CL, et al. Improved blood flow during prolonged cardiopulmonary resuscitation with 30% duty cycle in infant pigs. *Circulation*. 1991;84(2):896-904.

107. Babbs CF, Nadkarni V. Optimizing chest compression to rescue ventilation ratios during one-rescuer CPR by professionals and lay persons: children are not just little adults. *Resuscitation*. 2004;61(2):173-181.

108. Pasquin MP, Cheung PY, Patel S, et al. Comparison of different compression to ventilation ratios (2: 1, 3: 1, and 4: 1) during cardiopulmonary resuscitation in a porcine model of neonatal asphyxia. *Neonatology*. 2018;114(1):37-45.

109. Solevag AL, Dannevig I, Wyckoff M, Saugstad OD, Nakstad B. Extended series of cardiac compressions during CPR in a swine model of perinatal asphyxia. *Resuscitation*. 2010;81(11):1571-1576.

110. Solevag AL, Dannevig I, Wyckoff M, Saugstad OD, Nakstad B. Return of spontaneous circulation with a compression: ventilation ratio of 15:2 versus 3:1 in newborn pigs with cardiac arrest due to asphyxia. *Arch Dis Child Fetal Neonatal Ed*. 2011;96(6):F417-F421.

111. Schmolzer GM, O'Reilly M, Labossiere J, et al. 3:1 compression to ventilation ratio versus continuous chest compression with asynchronous ventilation in a porcine model of neonatal resuscitation. *Resuscitation*. 2014;85(2):270-275.

112. Mendler MR, Maurer M, Hassan MA, et al. Different techniques of respiratory support do not significantly affect gas exchange during cardiopulmonary resuscitation in a newborn piglet model. *Neonatology*. 2015;108(1):73-80.

113. Mendler MR, Weber C, Hassan MA, et al. Effect of different respiratory modes on return of spontaneous circulation in a newborn piglet model of hypoxic cardiac arrest. *Neonatology*. 2016;109(1):22-30.

114. Aggelina A, Pantazopoulos I, Giokas G, et al. Continuous chest compressions with asynchronous ventilation improve survival in a neonatal swine model of asphyxial cardiac arrest. *Am J Emerg Med*. 2021;48:60-66.

115. Solevag AL, Madland JM, Gjaerum E, Nakstad B. Minute ventilation at different compression to ventilation ratios, different ventilation rates, and continuous chest compressions with asynchronous ventilation in a newborn manikin. *Scand J Trauma Resusc Emerg Med*. 2012;20:73.

116. Li ES, Cheung PY, O'Reilly M, Aziz K, Schmolzer GM. Rescuer fatigue during simulated neonatal cardiopulmonary resuscitation. *J Perinatol*. 2015;35(2):142-145.

117. Boldingh AM, Jensen TH, Bjorbekk AT, Solevag AL, Nakstad B. Rescuers' physical fatigue with different chest compression to ventilation methods during simulated infant cardiopulmonary resuscitation. *J Matern Fetal Neonatal Med*. 2016;29(19):3202-3207.

118. Boldingh AM, Solevag AL, Aasen E, Nakstad B. Resuscitators who compared four simulated infant cardiopulmonary resuscitation methods favoured the three-to-one compression-to-ventilation ratio. *Acta Paediatr*. 2016;105(8):910-916.

119. Schmolzer GM, M OR, Fray C, van Os S, Cheung PY. Chest compression during sustained inflation versus 3:1 chest compression:ventilation ratio during neonatal cardiopulmonary resuscitation: a randomised feasibility trial. *Arch Dis Child Fetal Neonatal Ed*. 2018;103(5):F455-F460.

120. Schmolzer GM, Pichler G, Solevag AL, et al. The SURV1VE trial-sustained inflation and chest compression versus 3:1 chest compression-to-ventilation ratio during cardiopulmonary resuscitation of asphyxiated newborns: study protocol for a cluster randomized controlled trial. *Trials*. 2019;20(1):139.

121. Chalak LF, Barber CA, Hynan L, Garcia D, Christie L, Wyckoff MH. End-tidal CO(2) detection of an audible heart rate during neonatal cardiopulmonary resuscitation after asystole in asphyxiated piglets. *Pediatr Res*. 2011;69(5 Pt 1):401-405.

122. Stine CN, Koch J, Brown LS, Chalak L, Kapadia V, Wyckoff MH. Quantitative end-tidal CO2 can predict increase in heart rate during infant cardiopulmonary resuscitation. *Heliyon*. 2019;5(6):e01871.

123. McNamara PJ, Engelberts D, Finelli M, Adeli K, Kavanagh BP. Vasopressin improves survival compared with epinephrine in a neonatal piglet model of asphyxial cardiac arrest. *Pediatr Res*. 2014;75(6):738-748.

124. Isayama T, Mildenhall L, Schmolzer GM, et al. The route, dose, and interval of epinephrine for neonatal resuscitation: a systematic review. *Pediatrics*. 2020;146(4):e20200586.

125. Sankaran D, Chandrasekharan PK, Gugino SF, et al. Randomised trial of epinephrine dose and flush volume in term newborn lambs. *Arch Dis Child Fetal Neonatal Ed*. 2021;106(6):578-583.

126. Ellemunter H, Simma B, Trawoger R, Maurer H. Intraosseous lines in preterm and full term neonates. *Arch Dis Child Fetal Neonatal Ed*. 1999;80(1):F74-F75.

127. Rajani AK, Chitkara R, Oehlert J, Halamek LP. Comparison of umbilical venous and intraosseous access during simulated neonatal resuscitation. *Pediatrics*. 2011;128(4):e954-e958.

128. Granfeldt A, Avis SR, Lind PC, et al. Intravenous vs. intraosseous administration of drugs during cardiac arrest: a systematic review. *Resuscitation*. 2020;149:150-157.

129. Wyckoff M, Garcia D, Margraf L, Perlman J, Laptook A. Randomized trial of volume infusion during resuscitation of asphyxiated neonatal piglets. *Pediatr Res*. 2007;61(4):415-420.

130. Foglia EE, Weiner G, de Almeida MFB, et al. Duration of resuscitation at birth, mortality, and neurodevelopment: a systematic review. *Pediatrics*. 2020;146(3):e20201449.

131. Wyckoff M. Neonatal cardiopulmonary resuscitation: critical hemodynamics. *Neoreviews*. 2010;11(3):e123-e129.

Chapter 3

Vascular Development and Pulmonary Hypertension

Robin H.Steinhorn, Steven H. Abman, and Satyan Lakshminrusimha

Chapter Outline

Development of the Fetal Pulmonary Circulation

Physiology of the Fetal Pulmonary Circulation

Mediators of Fetal Pulmonary Vascular Development

Transitional Circulation and Postnatal Pulmonary Vascular Development

Features of Abnormal Pulmonary Vascular Development

Factors That Disrupt Fetal Pulmonary Vascular Development

   Genetic Factors

   Placental Insufficiency and Maternal Vascular Underperfusion

   Antenatal Ductal Closure

   Maternal Exposures

Clinical Implications and Controversies

   Persistent Pulmonary Hypertension of the Newborn

Perinatal Asphyxia

Congenital Diaphragmatic Hernia

Alveolar Capillary Dysplasia

Acute Pulmonary Hypertension in Preterm Infants

Bronchopulmonary Dysplasia-Associated Pulmonary Hypertension

Pulmonary Vein Stenosis

Pulmonary Hypertension Treatment: Concepts and Controversies

   Oxygen Targets

   Inhaled Nitric Oxide

   Adjunctive and Alternative Therapies

   Blood Pressure Management

   Pulmonary Hypertension Treatment in Preterm Infants

Conclusions

Key Points

- Lung vascular development occurs as highly choreographed sequence, regulated by hypoxia inducible factors, vascular endothelial growth factor, nitric oxide, and other transcription factors and mediators.
- In addition to arterial vessels, pulmonary veins are highly reactive vessels that contribute to the overall regulation of pulmonary vascular resistance in the fetus and newborn.
- Antenatal pulmonary vascular development can be disrupted by events such as placental insufficiency, genetic abnormalities such as Down syndrome, prolonged oligohydramnios, and congenital diaphragmatic hernia.
- Postnatal development of the lung circulation can be disrupted by numerous stresses such as preterm birth, asphyxia, and hypoxia or hyperoxia.
- Therapeutic controversies include optimal oxygenation targets, the role of adjunctive therapies such as cGMP and cAMP phosphodiesterase inhibitors, endothelin receptor antagonists, and prostanoids, the role of cardiac dysfunction (particularly in congenital diaphragmatic hernia), and treatment of acute and chronic pulmonary hypertension in the premature infant.

Development of the Fetal Pulmonary Circulation

The development of the pulmonary vasculature during fetal and neonatal life is highly coordinated with airway growth and plays a key role in normal lung development. In comparison with adult pulmonary vascular disease, disruption of lung vascular development plays a central role in the pathobiology of pulmonary vascular disease and airway development in the neonate and young infant.[1]

Lung development is classically divided into five overlapping stages in humans and rodents based on gross histological features, termed the embryonic (weeks 4–7 of gestation), pseudoglandular (weeks 5–17), canalicular (weeks 16–26), saccular (24–38), and alveolar stages (week 36 to infancy).[2] The development of the pulmonary vasculature is closely correlated with and interacts with airway growth. Lung vascularization initially originates in the mesenchyme, distal to the epithelium. In response to epithelial-derived vascular endothelial growth factor (VEGF), the endothelial cells move toward the epithelium, where they form the epithelium-capillary interface needed for gas exchange.[3] Growth of the lung vasculature continues after birth and into adulthood.

Physiology of the Fetal Pulmonary Circulation

Pulmonary hypertension (PH) is a normal physiologic state during fetal life and permits survival on placental support. Fetal pulmonary vascular resistance (PVR) is high in part due to hypoxic pulmonary vasoconstriction (Fig. 3.1). In the fetal lamb, pulmonary arterial blood has a PO_2 of approximately 18 mm Hg and oxygen saturation of 50%.[4] Because of high PVR, only about 16% of the combined ventricular output is directed to the lungs; the majority of right ventricular output passes through the ductus arteriosus to the descending aorta. The blood is then oxygenated by the placenta and returns to the body through the umbilical vein, with a PO_2 of ~32 to 35 mm Hg in lambs.[4] Based on the oxygen saturation difference between the umbilical vein (85%) and umbilical artery (52%), the fetus can achieve sufficient oxygen delivery at the low PO_2 levels needed for normal lung development.

In human fetuses, Doppler studies demonstrate that pulmonary blood flow is only 13% of combined ventricular output at 20 weeks of gestation (canalicular stage), representing a nadir during lung development (Fig. 3.1).[5] This finding is largely secondary to the lower cross-sectional area of the very immature pulmonary vascular bed. Furthermore, in fetal lambs at an equivalent point in gestation (~65% gestation), pulmonary blood flow does not increase in response to hyperoxia and PVR does not increase in response to hypoxia.[6,7] Similarly, in human pregnancies, maternal hyperoxygenation with face mask oxygen at 20 to 26 weeks of gestation does not result in pulmonary vasodilation.[8] Birth at this gestational age (23–26 weeks) is associated with a 2% risk of acute PH,[9,10] which perhaps explains the high rates of inhaled nitric oxide (iNO) therapy (6–8%) in extremely premature infants.[11-13]

As the lung develops through the early saccular stage, a rapid proliferation of pulmonary vessels and a marked increase in cross-sectional area of the pulmonary vascular bed occur, which decreases fetal PVR. At the same time, pulmonary vessels become more reactive to vasoconstrictors, such as hypoxia and endothelin, and vasodilators, such as oxygen. The net result is higher PVR and increased reactivity of the pulmonary vasculature. For instance, maternal hyperoxygenation testing (60% oxygen by face mask) is used to measure the reactivity of the fetal pulmonary vasculature in response to oxygen in late gestation and to predict postnatal survival in congenital diaphragmatic hernia.[14] Later in fetal life, studies in nonhuman primate and sheep models have shown that PVR is very sensitive to maternal hypoxemia (by administration of 12% oxygen) and hyperoxemia (by administration of 100% oxygen), independent of changes in umbilical flow.[15,16] These changes in PVR in turn determine the distribution of fetal cardiac output and oxygen delivery to the brain and heart. For instance, in pathologic conditions such as congenital diaphragmatic hernia, reduced pulmonary venous return and left ventricular filling may contribute to left ventricular hypoplasia.[17,18]

Pulmonary veins were originally regarded as passive conduit vessels, but they are now recognized to be reactive vessels that contribute to the overall regulation of PVR.[19] In the fetus, pulmonary veins contribute a significant fraction to total PVR and may play a more important role in regulating the fetal and newborn

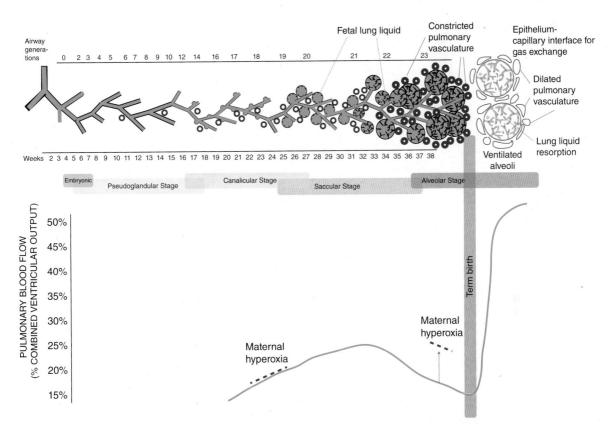

Fig. 3.1 Stages of lung development. Changes in airway morphology and pulmonary vasculature during various stages of lung development and at birth. The cross-sectional area of pulmonary vasculature increases with gestation. However, pulmonary vasculature develops sensitivity to oxygen during later gestation leading to hypoxic pulmonary vasoconstriction *(thick red vessels).* Pulmonary vasodilation secondary to ventilation and oxygenation at birth increased pulmonary blood flow. Changes in pulmonary blood flow (as a percentage of combined ventricular output) during the last half of human pregnancy and immediate postnatal life are shown in the bottom graph as a blue line. During early second trimester, pulmonary vasculature does not respond to changes in oxygen tension induced by maternal hyperoxia *(hyphenated red line).* During the third trimester, pulmonary blood flow increases with changes in oxygen tension *(hyphenated red line and red arrow).* After birth, following normal transition, the entire right ventricular output and left-to-right ductal shunt perfuses the lung establishing this organ as the site of gas exchange during postnatal period. (Copyright Satyan Lakshminrusimha and Robin H. Steinhorn.)

pulmonary circulation than in adults (Fig. 3.2). In perinatal sheep, NO stimulated endogenously by acetylcholine or given exogenously causes greater relaxation and accumulation of cGMP in pulmonary veins than in arteries.[20] At birth, the veins, as well as the arteries, relax in response to NO and dilator prostaglandins, thereby assisting in the fall in PVR (Fig. 3.3). These effects are oxygen-dependent and modulated by protein kinase G.[21] In a number of species, including the human, pulmonary veins are also the primary sites of action of certain vasoconstrictors, such as endothelin and thromboxane (Figs. 3.2 and 3.3).

Mediators of Fetal Pulmonary Vascular Development

The hypoxic conditions of fetal life support the tremendous lung vascular growth that occurs before birth. Hypoxia inducible factors (HIFs) are regarded as the "master regulators" of the transcriptional response to hypoxia and are involved in angiogenesis, survival, and metabolic pathways (Fig. 3.4). HIFs are heterodimers consisting of oxygen-sensitive α-subunits (HIF-1α, HIF-2α) and constitutively expressed β-subunits. Hypoxia stabilizes the α-subunit

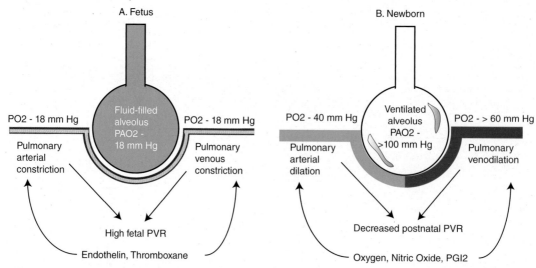

Fig. 3.2 Changes in pulmonary arterial and venous resistance at birth. (A) Relative hypoxia (with PO_2 in the 15–20 mm Hg range) in the fluid-filled alveoli and pulmonary arterial and venous blood contributes to high fetal pulmonary vascular resistance *(PVR)*. The pulmonary veins are highly responsive to vasoconstrictors such as endothelin and thromboxane. (B) At birth, with ventilation of alveoli, PAO_2 increases resulting in marked elevation of pulmonary venous PO_2. Pulmonary arterial PO_2 increases to a lesser extent. These changes contribute to a precipitous decrease in PVR at birth. Pulmonary veins are exquisitely sensitive to vasodilators such as oxygen, nitric oxide, and prostacyclin (PGI_2). (Copyright Satyan Lakshminrusimha and Robin Steinhorn.)

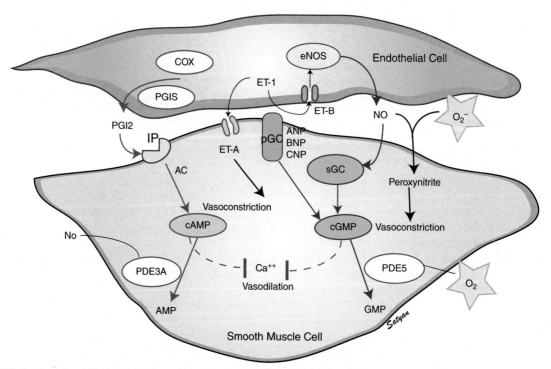

Fig. 3.3 Overview of endothelium-derived vasodilator (prostacyclin *[PGI$_2$]* and nitric oxide *[NO]*) and vasoconstrictor (endothelin *[ET-1]*) pathways. *AC*, Adenylate cyclase; *COX*, cyclooxygenase; *ET*, endothelin; *eNOS*, endothelial nitric oxide synthase; *PDE*, phosphodiesterase; *pGC*, particulate guanylate cyclase; *PGIS*, prostacyclin synthase; *sGC*, soluble guanylate cyclase.[71,169,170] (Copyright Satyan Lakshminrusimha and Robin H. Steinhorn.)

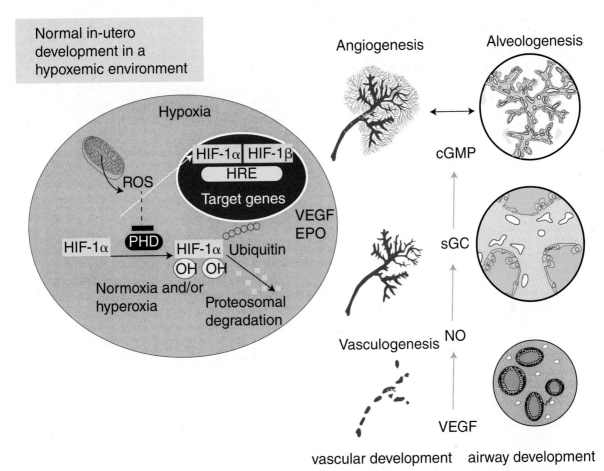

Fig. 3.4 Lung development occurs in utero in a relatively hypoxic environment. Under conditions of hypoxia, the hypoxia inducible factor *(HIF)* 1α is stabilized, dimerizes with HIF-1β, translocates to the nucleus, and binds to target genes that stimulate vascular endothelial growth factor *(VEGF)* production and angiogenesis. Under hyperoxic conditions, HIF is hydroxylated by prolyl hydroxylases *(PHD)* and ubiquinated for proteosomal degradation. Vascular and alveolar growth is mediated by VEGF through nitric oxide *(NO)* and soluble guanylate cyclase *(sGC)* pathways. Fetal or neonatal disruption of these pathways in animal models is associated with respiratory and vascular abnormalities. (Copyright Satyan Lakshminrusimha and Robin H. Steinhorn.)

leading to nuclear accumulation and activation of multiple target genes. HIF-1 regulates genes involved in angiogenesis (e.g., VEGF), oxygen transport (e.g., erythropoietin), and energy metabolism (e.g., glycolytic enzymes), among others.[22] The importance of HIFs in fetal lung development has been demonstrated by studies revealing that deletion of HIF-1 causes embryonic lethality, and deletion of HIF-2 reduces VEGF levels and leads to early death due to respiratory failure.[23] In the adult lung, hypoxia induces abnormal vascular remodeling, potentially by inducing HIF activity. However, hypoxia is the normal fetal condition and is a required environmental stimulus to sustain normal fetal lung and vascular development.

VEGF is a key regulator of lung vascular growth and development during fetal and postnatal life. VEGF transcription is regulated by HIF, and its signaling is transduced via two transmembrane tyrosine kinase receptors: VEGFR-2 and VEGFR-1. VEGF RNA and protein are localized to distal airway epithelial cells, while VEGFR-1 and VEGFR-2 mRNA expression is localized to the pulmonary endothelial cells closely approximated to the developing epithelium.[24] The importance of VEGF for vascular development has been demonstrated by a number of studies that inactivate or knock out VEGF or its receptors. Each of these will produce a lethal phenotype that is characterized by deficient organization of endothelial cells. Furthermore, VEGFR-1 and VEGFR-2 inhibitors (e.g., SU5416) impair alveolar development in fetal and newborn rodent models, producing pathologic findings similar to those seen in clinical bronchopulmonary dysplasia (BPD). Even in adult rats, chronic treatment with SU5416 causes PH and enlarges the air spaces, suggesting that normal VEGF function is required not only for the formation but also for the maintenance of the pulmonary vasculature and alveolar structures well after lung development is completed.[25]

VEGF-induced lung angiogenesis is in part mediated by NO. While NO is best known for its vasoactive properties, it also plays an important role in the structural development of the pulmonary vasculature. Lung endothelial NO synthase (eNOS) mRNA and protein are present in early fetal life in rats and sheep, and increase with advancing gestation in utero.[26,27] Lungs of fetal and neonatal mice deficient in eNOS have reduced alveolarization and vascularization and are more susceptible to the effects of hypoxia on vascular and alveolar growth.[28,29] VEGF inhibition is associated with decreased lung eNOS protein expression and NO production, and treatment with inhaled NO improves vascular and alveolar growth after VEGF inhibition. However, in neonatal mice that are eNOS deficient, recombinant human VEGF protein treatment restores lung structure after exposure to mild hyperoxia, suggesting that VEGF operates in part through mechanisms independent of eNOS.

Numerous transcription factors important to lung vascular development have been identified.[30] The Forkhead box (Fox) family of transcription factors regulate expression of genes involved in cellular proliferation and differentiation. Newborn mice with low Foxf1 levels die with defects in lung vascularization and alveolarization,[31] and endothelial-specific deletion of Foxf1 produces embryonic lethality, growth retardation, and vascular abnormalities in the lung, placenta, and retina.[32] These findings are directly relevant to human lung development, as, Foxf1 haploinsufficiency is found in 40% of infants with alveolar capillary dysplasia (ACD), a lethal disorder of lung vascular development.[33] NF-κB is a transcription factor traditionally associated with inflammation, but recent data suggest that it may play a very different, protective role in the neonatal lung. Blocking NF-κB activity during the alveolar stage of lung development in neonatal mice induced alveolar simplification and reduced pulmonary capillary density like that observed in BPD, effects that appear to be regulated by VEGFR-2.[34] Anecdotal reports of exacerbation of PH following intravitreal injection of VEGF inhibitors for retinopathy of prematurity suggest an ongoing role of VEGF in postnatal pulmonary vascular development in preterm infants.[35]

Lung endothelial progenitor cells (EPCs) have been recently identified as mediators of lung development, although their mechanistic role is not yet well understood. In rats, microvascular pulmonary endothelial cells proliferate twice as fast as endothelial cells isolated from large pulmonary arteries.[36] These highly proliferative cells express endothelial cell markers (CD31, CD144, eNOS, and von Willebrand factor) and progenitor cell antigens (CD34 and CD309). Thus, the pulmonary microcirculation seems to be enriched with EPCs that support vasculogenesis while maintaining endothelial microvascular functionality.[37]

Resident microvascular EPCs also share features of human cord blood–derived endothelial colony-forming cells (ECFCs). Developing human fetal and neonatal rat lungs contain ECFCs with robust proliferative and vasculogenic potential. The functionality of these cells can be disrupted during or after birth, potentially contributing to arrested alveolar growth after extremely preterm birth: for instance, human fetal lung ECFCs exposed to hyperoxia in vitro proliferate less and form fewer capillary-like networks. These findings also suggest a role for ECFCs in lung repair: in rodents, exogenous administration of human cord blood–derived ECFCs restored alveolar and lung vascular growth in hyperoxic rodents. Lung engraftment was low, suggesting that the ECFCs may support lung growth and repair through paracrine effects. Recent studies in a mouse model of ACD found that administration of EPCs stimulated neonatal lung angiogenesis through Foxf1-mediated signaling.[38] These findings suggest that pulmonary EPCs from patient-derived induced pluripotent stem cells could be a therapeutic avenue to restore vascular growth and function in the lungs of patients with pediatric pulmonary disorders such as ACD.[39]

Transitional Circulation and Postnatal Pulmonary Vascular Development

As gestation progresses, NO and cGMP become central to the emergence of pulmonary vascular reactivity. Inhibition of eNOS increases basal PVR as early as 0.75 gestation (112 days) in the fetal lamb, indicating that endogenous NOS activity contributes to vasoregulation during late gestation. Pulmonary vasodilation in response to NO (an endothelium-independent mediator) precedes the response to endothelium-dependent mediators such as acetylcholine and oxygen. The response to NO is dependent on expression and activity of soluble guanylate cyclase (sGC) in the smooth muscle cell (Fig. 3.3), which remains low through early preterm (126 days) gestation in fetal sheep and markedly increases toward the end of third trimester.[40] Intracellular cGMP levels are also tightly regulated by cGMP-specific phosphodiesterase (PDE5) activity, which increases during late gestation.

Pulmonary endothelial cells produce the prostaglandin molecules PGI_2 and PGE_2, which are both potent vasodilators. Prostacyclin (PGI_2) acts on its receptor in the smooth muscle cell to produce cyclic adenosine monophosphate (cAMP), which also mediates smooth muscle cell vasodilation (similar to cGMP, Fig. 3.3) and is inactivated by cAMP-specific phosphodiesterase 3A (PDE3A). While stimuli such as shear stress induce release of PGI_2, overall, prostaglandin release appears to play a less important role than NO in regulating fetal and transitional pulmonary vascular tone.

Constrictors also play a role in regulating the pulmonary vascular tone of the fetus. Endothelin-1 (ET-1) is produced by vascular endothelium and acts on the ET-A receptors in the smooth muscle cell to induce vasoconstriction by increasing ionic calcium concentrations. A second endothelial receptor, ET-B, on the endothelial cell stimulates NO release and vasodilation (Fig. 3.3). Although capable of both vasodilator and constrictor responses, ET-1 appears to primarily act as a pulmonary vasoconstrictor in the fetal pulmonary circulation and is elevated in infants with severe persistent pulmonary hypertension of the newborn (PPHN). Lipid mediators, such as thromboxane A_2, leukotrienes C_4 and D_4, and platelet-activating factor are potent pulmonary vasoconstrictors, but there is scant evidence that these agents influence PVR during fetal life and transition.

Endogenous serotonin (5-HT) production is another contributor to the high PVR of the fetus. Infusions of 5-HT increase PVR,[41,42] and infusions of ketanserin, a 5-HT 2A receptor antagonist, decrease fetal PVR in a dose-related fashion. Conversely, brief infusions of selective serotonin reuptake inhibitors (SSRIs), such as sertraline and fluoxetine, cause potent and sustained elevations of PVR. Together, these findings suggest that 5-HT causes pulmonary vasoconstriction and contributes to maintenance of high PVR in the normal fetus through stimulation of 5-HT 2A receptors and Rho kinase activation. These findings have important implications for SSRI treatment for maternal depression, as described below.

At birth, a rapid and dramatic series of circulatory events occur as the fetus transitions to extrauterine life. After birth and initiation of air breathing, several mechanisms operate simultaneously to rapidly reduce pulmonary arterial resistance and increase pulmonary blood flow. Of these, the most important stimuli are ventilation of the lungs and an increase in oxygen tension (Figs. 3.1 and 3.2).[43] Pulmonary blood flow increases by eightfold, resolving fetal PH.[44] Clamping of the umbilical cord removes the low-resistance placental circulation, increasing systemic arterial pressure as pulmonary arterial pressure falls. In some infants with in utero adverse events or with abnormalities of pulmonary transition at birth, PH persists into the newborn period, resulting in PPHN.

Pulmonary endothelial NO production increases markedly at the time of birth. NOS inhibitors (e.g., nitro-l-arginine) attenuate the decline in PVR after delivery of fetal lambs,[45,46] suggesting that the release of NO may be responsible for 50% of the rise in pulmonary blood flow at birth. Oxygen is an important catalyst for this increased NO production. In near-term fetal lambs, maternal hyperoxia induced by hyperbaric oxygenation increased pulmonary arterial PO_2 from 19 ± 1.5 to 48 ± 9 mm Hg, and pulmonary blood flow from 34 ± 3.3 to 298 ± 35 mL/kg/min, a 10-fold rise that nearly replicates the normal transition and is blocked by pretreatment with NOS inhibitors.[47] However, mice deficient in eNOS can successfully make the transition at birth without evidence of PPHN, suggesting the presence of alternate or compensatory vasodilator mechanisms, such as upregulation of other NOS isoforms or dilator prostaglandins.[48] Interestingly, eNOS-deficient mouse pups develop PH after relatively mild decreases in PaO_2 and have higher neonatal mortality when exposed to hypoxia after birth.[49] It is possible that eNOS deficiency alone may not be sufficient for the failure of postnatal adaptation, but that a decreased ability to produce NO during perinatal stressors such as hypoxia or inflammation may contribute to the development of postnatal PH. The similar timing of the peak in activity of pulmonary sGC and cGMP phosphodiesterase (PDE5) allows for fine regulation of vascular cGMP concentrations in the transitional and early neonatal period (Fig. 3.4).

The arachidonic acid-prostacyclin pathway also plays an important role in the transition at birth. Rhythmic lung distension and shear stress stimulate both PGI_2 and NO production in the late gestation fetus, although the effect of O_2 tension is predominantly on NO activity. PDE3A catalyzes the breakdown of cAMP (Fig. 3.3) and appears to create important crosstalk with the cGMP pathway.

Less is known about the pulmonary vascular transition after preterm birth, although similar mechanisms appear to be in effect.[50] In premature lambs at ~70% of gestation (112-115 days), the pulmonary vasodilator responses to rhythmic distension of the lung or increased PaO_2 are partly due to stimulation of NO release.[50] In human preterm infants, the decrease in PAP after birth is significantly slower compared to term infants, particularly if respiratory distress syndrome also exists.[51] Pulmonary arterial pressure elevations may persist for several days in extremely preterm infants.[52,53] Skimming et al. have questioned as to whether a "natural" increase in PVR affords benefit to the preterm infant by reducing the ductal steal and stabilizing systemic circulation.[54] However, recent prospective studies clearly indicate that early PH in extremely preterm babies is associated with BPD and late PH,[55] so it more likely indicates abnormal vascular development or function.

After birth, structural development of the lung and its vasculature continues. More than 90% of lung alveolarization occurs postnatally, with a prominent surge between birth and 6 months of age. Similarly, there is marked growth and development of the microvascular network during the alveolarization phase. A double capillary network is characteristic of the fetal and neonatal lung, but as alveolarization progresses, the interalveolar septae thin and the double capillary layer fuses into the single layer characteristic of the mature vasculature. The capillary network continues to expand its surface area through childhood by nearly 20-fold.[30]

Features of Abnormal Pulmonary Vascular Development

The histological features of early neonatal PPHN have been described in animal models and in fatal cases of PPHN in term infants.[56,57] In two autopsy series of infants with PPHN, vascular remodeling resulted in muscularization of the smallest arteries ($< 30\mu M$ external diameter) at the level of the alveolar duct and wall,[57,58] and a doubling of the medial wall thickness of the intra-acinar arteries (Fig. 3.5). These findings suggest that structural maldevelopment of the peripheral pulmonary arterial bed begins in utero and does not merely represent a failure of the fetal pattern to regress. Very similar patterns of remodeling are observed in animal models of PPHN, including the lamb model of antenatal ductal ligation.[59]

Thickening of the adventitia is observed in remodeled pulmonary vessels (Fig. 3.5)[59] and likely contributes to pulmonary artery stiffness.[60] Adventitial cells (including fibroblasts, pericytes, progenitor cells, etc.) also appear to be regulators of vascular wall function from the "outside in."[61,62] For example, NO is less potent when administered to the adventitial side of vessels. This may be partly due to the presence of constitutively active NADPH oxidase in adventitial cells, which generate superoxide anions that actively scavenge NO.

In contrast to PPHN, after very preterm birth, the developing lung is exposed to an extrauterine environment that disrupts the normal fetal vascular developmental patterns. On histology, the lungs of very preterm infants with BPD display evidence of arrested development, with reduced numbers of both alveoli and intra-acinar arteries. The pulmonary circulation in animal models and infants with BPD is characterized

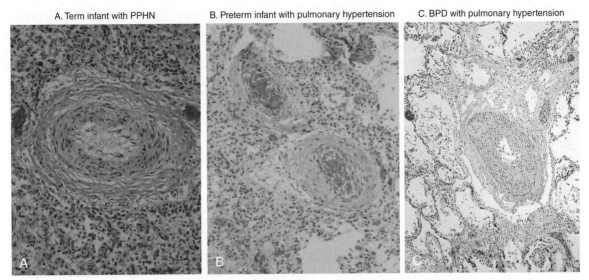

Fig. 3.5 Vascular remodeling in neonatal pulmonary hypertension. Histology of pulmonary arteries in the lung sections from three patients with pulmonary hypertension. (A) A 14-day-old, 37-week gestation infant with trisomy 21 (note the significant thickening of the medial and adventitial layers); (B) A 5-day-old, 25-week gestation preterm infant with pulmonary hypertension and severe hypoxemic respiratory failure; and (C) A 4-month-old, former 23-week gestation infant with bronchopulmonary dysplasia and pulmonary hypertension. *BPD*, Bronchopulmonary dysplasia; *PPHN*, persistent pulmonary hypertension of the newborn.

by vascular pruning, decreased vascular branching, and altered patterns of vascular distribution within the lung interstitium. Similar to early PPHN, smooth muscle proliferation also extends abnormally into the smaller peripheral arteries. In addition, intrapulmonary bronchopulmonary anastomoses have recently been identified that act as arteriovenous shunts that contribute to hypoxemia.[63] These anastomotic vessels may represent a compensatory mechanism to overcome the reduction in vascular surface area, or as a protective "pop-off" mechanism to reduce the severity of PH and protect the right ventricle.[64]

Signaling abnormalities in the remodeled vasculature include decreased expression of eNOS and reduced urinary levels of NO metabolites.[65,66] sGC expression and activity is also diminished in animal models of neonatal PH and congenital diaphragmatic hernia (CDH),[67,68] which is partly secondary to oxidation of sGC that renders it NO-insensitive.[69,70] Because NO and cGMP also inhibit vascular smooth muscle growth, it is likely that a combination of diminished eNOS expression, inactivation of sGC, and reduced cGMP levels also contribute to excessive muscularization of pulmonary vessels in PPHN and

BPD. Ventilation with high concentrations of inspired oxygen and exposure to reactive oxygen species (ROS) also decrease cGMP levels through increasing PDE5 activity, effects that appear to be mediated by ROS produced from the mitochondria (Fig. 3.3).[71] In fetal lambs with PPHN, pulmonary prostacyclin synthase (PGIS) and PGI_2 receptor (IP) protein levels in the lung are decreased, but levels of adenylate cyclase and PDE3A are not altered.[72]

Circulating levels of endothelin (ET-1), a potent vasoconstrictor and smooth muscle mitogen, are increased in human infants with PPHN,[73] and lung and vascular ET-1 levels are increased in fetal lambs with PPHN.[74,75] ET-1 appears also to be a marker for chronic PH, in that infants with congenital diaphragmatic hernia and poor outcomes have higher plasma ET-1 levels at 2 weeks of age and severity of PH than infants discharged on room air.[76] The constrictor effects of endothelin are mediated in part through activation of the RhoA-Rho kinase (ROCK) pathway.[75] Increased Rho kinase activity leads to phosphorylation of myosin light-chain kinase, which in turn increases intracellular calcium and causes vascular contraction. The ROCK pathway plays an important role in hypoxic pulmonary vasoconstriction,[77] and as a mediator of the impaired angiogenesis and increased contractility associated with chronic fetal PH (Fig. 3.3).[78]

Factors That Disrupt Fetal Pulmonary Vascular Development

GENETIC FACTORS

A number of gene mutations including mutations in the gene coding bone morphogenic protein receptor type 2 (BMPR2) and other genes (e.g., CAV1, KCNK3, EIF2AK4) have been identified in adults with PH. In contrast, PH is rarely familial in newborn infants and relatively few genetic mutations have been identified. Candidate gene analyses have not identified polymorphisms of the eNOS, VEGF, or other NO pathway genes in infants with PPHN.[79] However, polymorphisms have been identified in carbamoyl-phosphate synthetase 1, which catalyzes the first, rate-determining step of the urea cycle that leads to L-arginine synthesis, a key substrate required for NO generation.[66,80] In addition, higher rates of genetic variants for cortisol signaling (corticotropin releasing hormone receptor-1 [*CRHR1*] and CRH-binding protein) were observed in neonates with PPHN, as well as evidence for functional adrenal insufficiency.[79] More recently, variants in the T-box transcription factor 4 gene (TBX4) have been reported in infants with prolonged PH.[81] While the contribution of these novel variants to PPHN remains poorly characterized, whole genome sequencing should be considered in infants with atypical or prolonged PPHN.

Children with Down syndrome (trisomy 21) commonly develop PH in association with structural heart defects, but also have a 10-fold increased risk for idiopathic PPHN. In a Dutch cohort, PPHN was documented in 5.2% of Down syndrome infants without cardiac disease.[82] In addition, Down syndrome infants have worse pulmonary arterial hypertension in conjunction with anatomic cardiac disease than genetically normal infants with similar lesions and they are more likely to require ECMO support for PPHN.[83] One recent study showed that 85% of autopsy specimens from Down syndrome children displayed pulmonary vascular remodeling, suggesting that PH may occur even more commonly than clinically recognized.[84]

Dysregulation of angiogenic factors likely contributes to the pathogenesis of PH associated with Down syndrome. Chromosome 21 includes at least three genes with potent antiangiogenic properties which could affect fetal vascular development. One likely candidate, endostatin, is a known antiangiogenic factor that downregulates signaling of VEGF, which would be expected to impair angiogenesis and adversely affect lung structure. A threefold increase of endostatin mRNA expression has been reported in prenatal Down syndrome lungs, along with reduced microvascular density, thickened large and small pulmonary artery walls, and a persistent double capillary network.[85] More recent biomarker analysis of older children (ages 1–11 years) found elevated endostatin levels in the Down syndrome group relative to age-matched controls; levels were highest in those Down syndrome children with active or resolved PH.[86] On the other hand, Bush et al. reported elevated endostatin levels in Down syndrome children regardless of the presence of PH, raising questions about whether circulating endostatin levels are predictive of PH in this population.[87]

PLACENTAL INSUFFICIENCY AND MATERNAL VASCULAR UNDERPERFUSION

Epidemiology studies have reported an association between fetal growth restriction and the later development of PH in premature infants with BPD.[88,89] This association suggests that intrauterine stress could initiate the cascade that results in abnormal pulmonary vascular development and PH in preterm infants. Animal models have suggested that the pulmonary vascular maldevelopment underlying PH associated with chronic lung disease begins before birth in response to chronic fetal hypoxia.[90] Prospective cohort studies examining placental findings and cord blood biomarkers in preterm infants who develop acute PPHN or chronic PH associated with BPD showed a striking association with placental findings of maternal vascular underperfusion and decreased villous vascularity.[91-93] Moreover, cord blood angiogenic factors such as placental growth factor and VEGF-A were decreased in premature infants exposed to placental vascular underperfusion, and these fetal blood markers predicted the subsequent development of PH.[94] It is possible that disruption of placentation and placental vascular perfusion represents failed angiogenesis, as reflected by these biomarkers, and that this abnormal developmental angiogenesis may reflect global abnormalities of vascular signaling that contribute to postnatal vascular disease.[95] Additional preclinical studies suggest that disruption of angiogenesis because of adverse antenatal factors, such as chorioamnionitis, preeclampsia, or maternal smoking, can cause pulmonary vascular disease that not only leads to PH but also impairs lung growth and alveolarization.[64]

ANTENATAL DUCTAL CLOSURE

A patent ductus arteriosus (PDA) is critical for the normal fetal circulation. It not only directs right ventricular output to the aorta, but also protects the pulmonary circulation from volume overload and the right ventricle from pressure overload. Either partial or complete ductal ligation in the fetal lamb increases pulmonary arterial pressure without sustained elevation in pulmonary blood flow or in utero hypoxemia.[59,96,97] Endothelial dysfunction rapidly emerges and results in poor response to endothelium-dependent vasodilators such as oxygen and acetylcholine, along with decreased expression and activity of pulmonary eNOS.[98] There is also a strong constrictor "myogenic response" that may exist to protect the pulmonary capillary bed from high pulmonary blood flow and may be mediated by activation of the ROCK pathway.[99] Downstream signaling abnormalities emerge within days of ductal closure, including decreased activity and expression of sGC and increased activity of cGMP-phosphodiesterase (PDE5).[100] After birth, the newborns develop severe PH, a model that has been extensively utilized for preclinical studies to evaluate inhaled NO and other pulmonary vasodilators in PPHN.[101]

MATERNAL EXPOSURES

Two classes of medications, nonsteroidal antiinflammatory agents (NSAIDs) and SSRIs, have the most evidence to suggest a direct effect on pulmonary vascular development. Prostaglandins maintain ductal patency in utero and are important mediators of pulmonary vasodilation in response to ventilation at birth, and experimental closure or constriction of the ductus arteriosus in fetal lambs produces rapid development of pulmonary vascular remodeling and severe PPHN.[59] An association between PPHN and prostaglandin synthase

inhibitor use during late gestation was first reported 40 years ago, and indomethacin is avoided for tocolysis in the third trimester because of the risk of ductal closure.[102] Although early studies linked the presence of NSAIDs in meconium to risk for PPHN, a recent epidemiologic study suggests that an association with PPHN is only present for aspirin use during the third trimester and not for ibuprofen at any point in gestation.[103]

Exposure of pregnant rats to fluoxetine, an SSRI, produces PH, hypoxia, and increased mortality in the pups.[104,105] Large clinical meta-analyses have reported that the use of SSRIs after 20 weeks of gestation is associated with a twofold increase in the incidence of PPHN, with an estimated one additional PPHN case for every 285 to 5000 women treated.[106,107] However, the PPHN appears to be mild with lower need for mechanical ventilation and lower neonatal mortality rates in SSRI exposed versus nonexposed neonates with PPHN (3.4% vs. 8.3%, P = not significant).[108] The mechanism by which SSRIs induce PPHN remains poorly understood, although animal data indicate that SSRIs induce concentration-dependent constriction of the ductus arteriosus.[109]

Maternal medications also have the potential to reverse pathological fetal vascular development. In fetal lambs with PPHN induced by ductal ligation, maternal betamethasone reduced oxidative stress and improved the relaxation response to NO donors.[110] While not specifically examined, lower rates of PPHN could partially explain the benefit of antenatal steroids in late preterm infants.[111] In fetal rats with nitrofen-induced CDH, antenatal administration of sildenafil to the dam improved lung morphology and reduced pulmonary vascular remodeling and right ventricular hypertrophy.[112] However, in human clinical trials, maternal administration of sildenafil for severe fetal growth restriction did not improve perinatal morbidity or mortality, and in the Dutch cohort, PPHN was more common after antenatal sildenafil exposure.[113]

Clinical Implications and Controversies

PERSISTENT PULMONARY HYPERTENSION OF THE NEWBORN

PPHN is an acute, often life-threatening form of neonatal pulmonary hypertension (PH) caused by the failure of the normal pulmonary vascular transition at birth.

PPHN is not a single disease; rather, it refers to a syndrome characterized by sustained elevation of PVR and hypoxemia due to right-to-left extrapulmonary shunting of blood flow across the ductus arteriosus and/or foramen ovale. PPHN physiology occurs in term or preterm neonates with respiratory failure caused by multiple conditions, including meconium aspiration, sepsis, pneumonia, asphyxia, congenital diaphragmatic hernia, and respiratory distress syndrome. While the term hypoxemic respiratory failure is often used interchangeably with PPHN, many hypoxemic newborns lack echocardiographic findings of extrapulmonary shunting across the PDA or patent foramen ovale (PFO). Thus, PPHN specifically refers to hypoxemic newborns with evidence of extrapulmonary shunting. Its incidence is estimated at 0.4 to 6.8 per 1000 live births in term infants and 5.4 per 1000 live births in late preterm infants.[114,115] One-year mortality of all newborns with PPHN has been reported at 7.6%,[115] and surviving infants with PPHN are at increased risk of long-term morbidities, including ~25% neurodevelopmental impairment at 2 years.[116]

PERINATAL ASPHYXIA

Perinatal asphyxia interferes with the adaptation of the perinatal pulmonary vasculature by impeding the fall in PVR and increasing the risk for PPHN.[117] Multiple antenatal and postnatal mechanisms combine to cause respiratory failure and affect pulmonary circulation in asphyxia; for instance, fetal hypoxemia, ischemia, meconium aspiration, left ventricular dysfunction, and acidosis can all increase PVR.[117] Moreover, animal studies demonstrate exaggerated hypoxic pulmonary vasoconstriction with pH < 7.25.[118] Acute asphyxia is associated with reversible pulmonary vasoconstriction,[119] but chronic in utero asphyxia with or without meconium aspiration may be associated with vasoconstriction and vascular remodeling, and reduced responsiveness to pulmonary vasodilation.[58]

Given the above, it is not surprising that acute PPHN complicates the course of 25% of infants with perinatal asphyxia, which is an important consideration when providing therapeutic hypothermia for moderate-to-severe hypoxic ischemic encephalopathy (HIE). Deep hypothermia (temperature decreased to <32°C) increased mean pulmonary arterial pressure in neonatal lamb models,[120] and increased rates of

PPHN and ECMO in clinical trials,[121] and should be avoided. However, the effect of moderate hypothermia (33.5°C) on PVR appears to be modest, and randomized trials found that therapeutic hypothermia in that temperature range does not significantly increase the incidence of PPHN. In a secondary analysis of 280 infants enrolled in the hypothermia arm of one of the multicenter clinical trials of hypothermia for HIE, there was not a significant difference in death or moderate/severe disability among infants with HIE and PPHN versus those without PPHN (47% vs. 29%, respectively) after adjustment for severity of HIE, center and trial.[122]

CONGENITAL DIAPHRAGMATIC HERNIA

CDH occurs in approximately 1 in 2500 to 3000 pregnancies and represents ~8% of all major congenital anomalies. Approximately 30% of neonates with CDH fail medical management and require ECMO support for severe PPHN, and over the last decade, CDH has become the most common indication for neonatal ECMO.[123] Severe CDH develops early in the course of lung development: an incomplete closure of the diaphragm results in a diaphragm defect, herniation of the abdominal contents into the chest, and compression of the intrathoracic structures. An arrest in the normal pattern of airway branching occurs in both the lungs, resulting in pulmonary hypoplasia and impaired alveolarization. A similar developmental arrest occurs in pulmonary arterial branching, resulting in reduced cross-sectional area of the pulmonary vascular bed, thickened media and adventitia of small arterioles, and abnormal medial muscular hypertrophy extending distally to the level of the acinar arterioles.

Lung compression alone does not appear to fully explain the pulmonary vascular pruning, vascular remodeling, and refractory PH seen in CDH.[124] Additional evidence suggests that decreased pulmonary blood flow alone is sufficient to cause lung hypoplasia.[125] Histological findings of CDH show pulmonary vascular remodeling superimposed on pulmonary vascular bed hypoplasia,[126] and these are clinically associated with increased vascular tone and altered vasoreactivity after birth. High or suprasystemic PVR is commonly observed in the newborn with CDH, with elevated PA pressure in 94% of CDH cases in the first week of life, 43% in the third week, and 28% at the sixth week.[127] High PVR is caused by multiple factors, including the small cross-sectional area of pulmonary arteries, structural vascular remodeling, vasoconstriction with altered reactivity, and left ventricle (LV) dysfunction causing pulmonary venous hypertension. The mediators of altered pulmonary vascular reactivity in CDH remain under investigation, with substantial evidence for disruptions in NO-cGMP and endothelin signaling that persist in infants that develop chronic PH.[76]

Abnormalities of cardiac development and function are now recognized as key determinants of CDH pathophysiology.[128] The LV, left atrium, and intraventricular septum are hypoplastic in infants that die of CDH relative to age-matched controls, perhaps due to low fetal and postnatal pulmonary blood flow and/or compression by the hypertensive right ventricle. The degree of left ventricular dysfunction predicts the response to pulmonary vasodilators.[123] In infants with severe LV dysfunction, left atrial and pulmonary venous pressures increase, and the resulting pulmonary venous hypertension diminishes the clinical response to inhaled NO during the first few days of life. This likely explains why in the early clinical trials of iNO, infants with CDH did not experience a reduction in ECMO use or mortality. In one case series, CDH patients with PH and elevated pulmonary capillary wedge pressures identified by cardiac catheterization displayed worse pulmonary arterial hypertension severity, with prolonged need for invasive ventilation and hospital stays.[129] Some infants may have exceptionally severe left ventricular dysfunction that leads to dependence on the right ventricle for systemic perfusion[130]; this subset may depend on patency of the ductus arteriosus for survival in the early postnatal period. Determining the origins of these heart abnormalities will be key to understanding and treating these severely affected infants with CDH.

ALVEOLAR CAPILLARY DYSPLASIA

ACD, with or without misalignment of the pulmonary veins, is a rare form of vascular and parenchymal lung disease that presents as severe PH and refractory hypoxemia early in life.[33] The etiology of ACD is believed to be due to a genetic defect or early antenatal insult that prevents normal development of the pulmonary capillary bed. Findings include remodeling of the pulmonary arterioles, simplification of the alveolar architecture, and development of congested "misaligned pulmonary veins" residing in the same adventitial sheath. These so-called veins are actually bronchopulmonary anastomoses that link the systemic and pulmonary circulations and bypass the alveolar capillary bed.[131] Although ACD classically presents in the neonatal period, presentation occasionally occurs later, at several months of life.[132] While the disease is nearly universally lethal despite treatment with all known modalities, survival with medical therapy in one patient with confirmed ACD has been reported to 56 months and limited survival after lung transplantation has also been reported.[132,133]

FOXf1, a member of Fox family of transcription factors, is required for formation of pulmonary capillaries in mice and humans. Mutations or deletions in the FOXf1 transcription factor gene have been identified in up to 40% of infants with ACD and may eventually lead to therapeutic options via EPCs.[38,134] Other anomalies of the genitourinary, cardiovascular, and gastrointestinal systems are seen in up to half of infants with ACD and could also be explained by abnormal FOXf1 signaling.

ACUTE PULMONARY HYPERTENSION IN PRETERM INFANTS

Echocardiographic evidence of acute PH in the first 14 days of life is common in preterm infants (8–50% of infants born at ≤30 weeks of gestation), and at least one cohort study suggests the prevalence of the condition has increased.[135-138] The incidence of PH increases with lower gestational age and is a risk factor for mortality, BPD, and long-term cardiorespiratory morbidity.[89] Cohort studies indicate the presence of distinct phenotypes in this population: acute PPHN (right-to-left or bidirectional shunting across the PDA), flow-mediated PH (left-to-right nonrestrictive shunt across the PDA), and PH without an identifiable shunt.[135]

Some preterm infants develop severe early PH after prolonged rupture of membranes with oligohydramnios and some degree of pulmonary hypoplasia.[139,140] In animal studies, the pulmonary circulation of lambs with hypoplastic lungs created by a tracheoamniotic shunt had significantly increased PVR with high pulmonary artery pressure and reduced pulmonary blood flow.[141] Furthermore, changes in indices of lung ventilation were proportional to the changes in lung size, but accompanied by disproportionate changes in the pulmonary circulation associated with reduced density of pulmonary arterioles.[141] These findings suggest that oligohydramnios-induced pulmonary hypoplasia exerts a selective effect on lung vascular development and raises important questions about the role of the amniotic fluid in maintaining levels of lung vascular growth factors. Histologic changes of the pulmonary vasculature include reduced volume density of pulmonary arteries and increased acinar arterial wall muscle thickness.[142] In the clinical setting, mortality approaches 50% in preterm infants with prolonged rupture of membranes and PH.[143] One study documented low tracheal aspirate levels of nitrates/nitrites suggesting a specific deficiency of NO. While these infants responded promptly and dramatically to iNO, a survival benefit has not been found in larger matched cohort studies of preterm infants with pulmonary hypoplasia exposed versus not exposed to iNO.[10,143]

BRONCHOPULMONARY DYSPLASIA–ASSOCIATED PULMONARY HYPERTENSION

After birth, PVR decreases at a slower rate in very or extremely preterm compared to term neonates.[51] Echocardiographic markers of early pulmonary vascular dysfunction can be found in the first week of life in up to 50% of extremely preterm infants, and these findings are a strong risk factor for BPD and late PH.[137] In that same time frame, abnormalities of several circulating proteins related to extracellular matrix, growth factors, and angiogenesis are found.[144]

Preterm birth exposes the lung to ambient oxygen concentrations that are severalfold higher than fetal levels, and supplemental oxygen is frequently required to treat respiratory failure. The preterm lung is ill-equipped to cope with increased ambient oxygen concentrations, and exposure to hyperoxia during this developmentally sensitive period increases lipid and protein oxidation products, and disrupts normal parenchymal and vascular lung development.[145] In newborn rodents born at an immature saccular phase of lung development, short-term (24 hours) or chronic exposure to hyperoxia (7–21 days) causes PH and right ventricular hypertrophy that persists to day 14, which is associated with persistent diminished sGC

and increased cGMP phosphodiesterase activity.[146] In preterm lambs, early exposure to brief hyperoxic ventilation increases expression of prolyl hydroxylase (PHD2), which rapidly degrades HIF-1α and HIF-2α,[147] and disrupts expression of downstream targets such as VEGF (Fig. 3.4). Other stresses common to the sick preterm infant, such as nutritional deficiency, appear to amplify the effect of hyperoxia on the pulmonary vasculature, in part by reducing VEGF and NO synthase activity.[148]

Chronic PH complicates the course of 10% to 14% of extremely preterm infants at 36 weeks postmenstrual age and is even more common in infants with moderate-to-severe BPD. Not only severity of BPD, but also antenatal findings of fetal growth restriction and oligohydramnios are risk factors associated with development of PH.[88,135] BPD is associated with reduced cross-sectional perfusion area with decreased arterial density and abnormal muscularization of peripheral pulmonary arteries: the pathophysiology of PH in these infants is a combination of simplified lung parenchyma and impaired vascular development. Identifying PH in infants with BPD requires a high index of suspicion and longitudinal evaluation. Echocardiography remains the most practical screening tool and should be considered in all infants with risk factors, including BPD requiring oxygen supplementation at 36 weeks postmenstrual age. Cardiac catheterization may provide a more accurate quantification of the severity of disease, as well as support assessment of therapeutic responses via vasoreactivity testing.

PULMONARY VEIN STENOSIS

Pulmonary vein stenosis (PVS) most commonly presents as a complication of severe BPD that contributes to severe and progressive PH. The left-sided pulmonary veins (particularly the left upper vein) are most often affected, and severe PH can result after stenosis of only one vein. The mechanisms producing PVS are not yet known. A number of findings, including a median age of diagnosis of 6 months, a lack of concordance in twins, and association with necrotizing enterocolitis (NEC), suggest that the disease is postnatally acquired.[149,150] Fetal growth restriction, presence of a left-to-right shunt such as PDA, ASD, or ventricular septal defect (VSD), exposure to inflammatory cytokines from NEC, BPD, or maternal chorioamnionitis increase the risk of PVS (Fig 3.6). All infants screened for BPD-associated PH should have careful assessment of all four pulmonary veins by ultrasound; if the diagnosis is suspected, it is typically confirmed via CT angiography. Even with aggressive therapy, PVS tends to be progressive and is associated with high mortality (30%–50%) in the first two years after diagnosis.

Pulmonary Hypertension Treatment: Concepts and Controversies

OXYGEN TARGETS

Oxygen is a potent pulmonary vasodilator, and increased oxygen tension from fetal to ambient air levels is a key mediator of the fall in PVR at birth. The use of hyperoxia (100% oxygen) in the initial resuscitation of newborn lambs slightly enhances the rate of drop in PVR compared to normoxia,[151,152] although within minutes, PVR falls to similar levels in hyperoxic versus normoxic groups. After even brief hyperoxic ventilation, formation of ROS (e.g., hydrogen peroxide,

superoxide, and peroxynitrite) occurs due to immature or dysfunctional antioxidant defense mechanisms (e.g., superoxide dismutase, catalase) and/or increased activity of prooxidant enzymes such as NADPH oxidase.[153,154] These ROS can cause pulmonary vasoconstriction, impair relaxation to endogenous or inhaled NO, and cause vascular remodeling as seen in PPHN.[154,155] Considering that iNO is usually delivered with high concentrations of oxygen, these therapies could interact and lead to enhanced production of reactive oxygen and reactive nitrogen metabolites, which can further contribute to vasoconstriction and/or inadequate responses to iNO. A standardized weaning protocol that prioritizes initial weaning FiO$_2$ to 60%, followed by stepwise weaning of iNO and oxygen while maintaining SpO$_2$ >90% and/or PaO$_2$ >60 mm Hg achieved iNO weaning in 4.1 ± 3.4 days (Fig. 3.7).[156]

INHALED NITRIC OXIDE

Pulmonary vasodilator therapy in neonates is based on restoration of normal signaling pathways in the

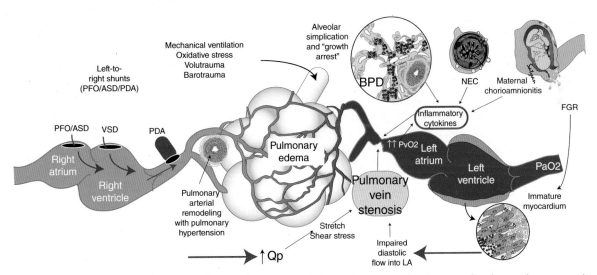

Fig. 3.6 Pathogenesis of pulmonary vein stenosis. Pulmonary vein stenosis is considered to be postinflammatory fibrosis secondary exposure to inflammatory cytokine release secondary to maternal chorioamnionitis, bronchopulmonary dysplasia *(BPD)*, necrotizing enterocolitis *(NEC)*, and oxidative stress due to high pulmonary venous PO$_2$ *(PvO$_2$)* compared to fetal levels. Fetal growth restriction *(FGR)* and prematurity contribute to immature myocardial function and impaired left atrial *(LA)* diastolic flow contributing to pulmonary venous hypertension. Increased pulmonary blood flow (compared to fetal levels) that is further exacerbated by left-to-right shunt (atrial septal defect *[ASD]*, patent ductus arteriosus *[PDA]*, and ventricular septal defect *[VSD]*), and pulmonary venous hypertension result in stretching of pulmonary veins increasing the risk of pulmonary vein stenosis. Pulmonary venous stenosis can lead to pulmonary edema and pulmonary arterial remodeling. (Based on Vyas-Read et al. Children. 2022. Copyright Satyan Lakshminrusimha.)

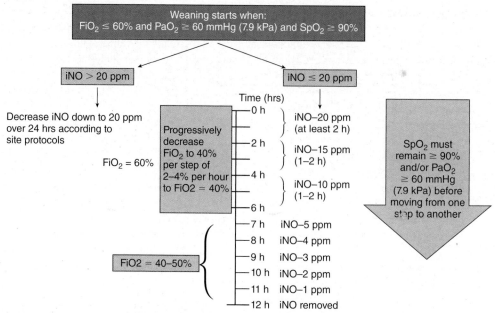

Fig. 3.7 Suggested weaning protocol from iNO, based on the protocol used in Pierce et al.[156] If an infant is receiving iNO at >20 ppm, the first step is to decrease iNO to 20 ppm. As oxygenation improves, FiO₂ should be decreased to 60%. Weaning of iNO can begin when the following conditions occur:

- iNO treatment is ≤20 ppm; AND
- FiO₂ ≤ 60%; AND
- PaO₂ ≥ 60 mm Hg and/or SpO₂ ≥90%.

During weaning, iNO should be decreased to 5 ppm by decrements of 5 ppm every 1 to 2 hours. At the same time, FiO₂ should be weaned by 2% to 4% per hour to 40%. After that, iNO should be weaned by 1 ppm every 1 to 2 hours down to 0 ppm. During this time, the infant's oxygen saturation should be monitored closely, and the FiO₂ may be increased as needed. PaO₂ must remain ≥60 mm Hg and/or SpO₂ ≥90% before moving from one step to the next. If the infant's oxygen saturation decreases at any time during weaning, iNO and FiO₂ should be increased as needed, and weaning should be attempted again when the infant is stable.

transitional pulmonary vascular circulation. NO was initially adapted for inhalational use by Warren Zapol, Claes Frostell, and Jay Roberts.[157] iNO was ultimately approved by the Food and Drug Administration (FDA) in 1999 after multiple placebo-controlled trials found improved oxygenation and decreased need for ECMO in neonates >34 weeks gestational age with moderate-to-severe hypoxemic respiratory failure (oxygenation index > 25). A starting dose of 20 ppm achieves the maximal benefit on oxygenation and avoids complications such as methemoglobinemia.

iNO has revolutionized the care of PPHN and has been widely adopted worldwide, although it is a relatively expensive therapy with limited use in low- and middle-income countries. iNO has not been shown to reduce mortality or length of hospitalization in any clinical trial, although in one retrospective cohort study, iNO responders had reduced ventilator

days (median 7 vs. 10 days, P = 0.02) and shorter hospitalization (median 22 vs. 30 days, P = 0.02) compared to nonresponders.[158] Treatment failure occurs in ~40% of infants in randomized trials and cohort studies. The failure to respond to iNO often indicates inadequate lung recruitment but may also be due to cardiac dysfunction or pulmonary vascular disease due to signaling abnormalities downstream of NO synthesis. Most infants recover and can be weaned from iNO within 4 to 5 days. Infants who remain hypoxemic with PH beyond that time are more likely to have an underlying developmental lung abnormality such as ACD, PVS, severe pulmonary hypoplasia, or progressive lung injury.

iNO is commonly used in infants with CDH. In one large US registry study, 57% of infants with CDH received iNO during their inpatient stay, although utilization varied substantially between centers

(34–92%). While the use of iNO increased between 2003 and 2011 across all registry centers, mortality rates did not change significantly during this time period or correlate with iNO therapy.

ADJUNCTIVE AND ALTERNATIVE THERAPIES

Several adjunctive therapies have been proposed to reduce the rate of treatment failure to iNO. While randomized, placebo-controlled trials have been undertaken for agents such as sildenafil, bosentan, and milrinone, meaningful endpoints have been difficult to develop, and most trials have been unable to complete their enrollment goals even after 18 to 64 months of recruitment.

PPHN and hyperoxia are associated with increased activity of cGMP-specific phosphodiesterase (PDE5), which would reduce the cGMP response to iNO. Pilot studies of enteral or intravenous sildenafil administered alone or in addition to iNO reported dramatic improvement in oxygenation and survival. Systemic hypotension was the most common adverse effect, particularly after rapid initiation of an intravenous loading dose. However, a recent multicenter trial incorporating a standardized iNO weaning protocol (Fig. 3.7) did not find any benefit from intravenous sildenafil on treatment failure or time on iNO.[156] Successful long-term use of enteral sildenafil has been reported in infants with chronic PH associated with congenital diaphragmatic hernia and BPD, although no randomized trials are available to confirm its safety and efficacy. Additional trials are underway to examine the effect of sildenafil on prevention of chronic BPD-associated PH.[159] Little information is available for other PDE5 inhibitors (e.g., tadalafil) for acute or chronic neonatal PH. Other promising approaches include agents that stimulate or enhance sGC activity such as riociguat. In one small high-risk cohort of infants with chronic PH, transitioning from sildenafil to riociguat therapy improved respiratory status and lowered pulmonary arterial pressure.[160]

The PGI$_2$-cAMP pathway has also been studied for acute and chronic PH treatment (Fig. 3.3). While intravenous PGI$_2$ is rarely used in neonates because of concerns about systemic hypotension and/or ventilation-perfusion mismatch, inhaled PGI$_2$ is commonly used for treatment of acute PH in adults and has been shown to produce transient pulmonary vasodilation and enhanced oxygenation in neonates. However, the alkaline solution needed to maintain drug stability could irritate the airway, and delivery of precise doses can be difficult because of loss of medication into the nebulization circuit. New, more stable preparations have emerged, such as treprostinil, which can be administered by the inhaled, intravenous, or subcutaneous route. A clinical trial studying the efficacy of treprostinil for PPHN was expected to complete enrollment in 2022 (NCT02261883).

In addition to administration of prostanoids, cAMP concentrations can be increased by inhibiting the activity of cAMP-specific phosphodiesterases (e.g., PDE3) with milrinone. Milrinone is an "inodilator" that improves right and left ventricular function and reduces pulmonary venous hypertension. Several clinical reports indicate that milrinone enhances pulmonary vasodilation and improves oxygenation in infants with PPHN refractory to iNO.

Plasma ET-1 levels are increased in infants with PPHN and in infants with severe CDH; these endothelin levels appear to correlate with the severity of illness. Bosentan, a nonspecific ET-1 receptor blocker, is an established treatment for PH in adults and is approved by the FDA for children over 3 years of age. Endothelin blockade enhances pulmonary vasodilation in experimental PPHN, and one single-center trial found that bosentan improved oxygenation in an iNO-naïve population of PPHN infants. In contrast, the FUTURE-4 multicenter trial found that bosentan as adjunctive therapy for iNO did not improve PPHN outcomes, time on iNO, or time to extubation, possibly in part due to inconsistent intestinal absorption.[161] There is little information on the efficacy of bosentan for chronic PH associated with BPD and CDH.

BLOOD PRESSURE MANAGEMENT

Systemic hypotension is common in neonates with acute PH, as pulmonary vasoconstriction decreases pulmonary venous return and left ventricular preload, which in turn reduces LV output and causes hypotension. Left ventricular dysfunction is observed in nearly 40% of infants with congenital diaphragmatic hernia and is associated with smaller LV volumes, left-to-right atrial shunting in the presence of suprasystemic pulmonary artery pressures, and worse outcomes.[162]

Dopamine is commonly used as the vasopressor of choice. When managing acute PH, many clinicians attempt to drive systemic blood pressure to higher "superphysiologic" levels to prevent right-to-left shunting across the PDA. This practice is not evidence based and is now under scrutiny, with attention directed toward better understanding of the underlying causes of systemic hypotension.[163] Dopamine can increase systemic vasoconstriction and LV afterload, which would potentially limit systemic perfusion and worsen acidosis. In addition, dopamine is a relatively nonspecific vasoconstrictor and may also exacerbate pulmonary vasoconstriction and right ventricular dysfunction (Fig 3.8). Thus, if titration of dopamine does not improve hemodynamic stability, evaluation of cardiac physiology by echocardiogram and use of inotropic agents that do not increase PVR (e.g., milrinone or dobutamine) should be considered. Milrinone may be especially useful in reversing left ventricular diastolic dysfunction in congenital diaphragmatic hernia; the benefit of milrinone for infants with CDH is currently under evaluation in a randomized clinical trial

(NCT02951130). However, systemic hypotension is a common side effect of milrinone therapy and may exacerbate right-to-left shunt. Additional cohort studies suggest that rescue therapy with arginine vasopressin can benefit infants with severe PH by raising systemic pressure via V_1 receptors and reducing pulmonary arterial pressure via activation of NO synthase.[164] Vasopressin is associated with oliguria and hyponatremia requiring close monitoring of urine output and serum electrolytes.

PULMONARY HYPERTENSION TREATMENT IN PRETERM INFANTS

While use of iNO is relatively common in preterm infants, the practice remains controversial. Prospective randomized trials with a primary outcome of death or BPD did not find enough benefit to recommend routine iNO use in this population. Several case series have reported that iNO rapidly improves oxygenation

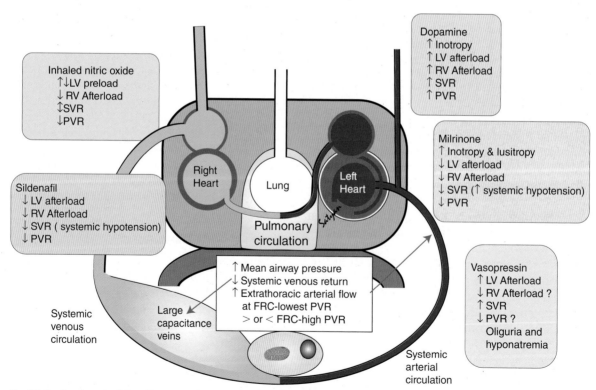

Fig. 3.8 Cardiopulmonary interactions secondary to mean airway pressure and vasoactive agents. *FRC,* Functional residual capacity; *LV,* left ventricle; *PVR,* pulmonary vascular resistance; *RV,* right ventricle; *SVR,* systemic vascular resistance. (Modified from Sehgal A, et al. *J Perinatol.* 2022. Copyright Satyan Lakshminrusimha.)

in preterm infants with PH, but there have not been randomized placebo-controlled trials assessing its effect on documented PPHN in this population, in part due to a lack of clinical equipoise. The multicenter PaTTerN registry compared iNO responses in the first week of life in a retrospective cohort of preterm (27–34 weeks of gestation, n = 55) versus term/near-term infants (≥34 weeks of gestation, n = 85) presenting with confirmed PPHN. The primary endpoint, a ≥25% reduction in oxygenation index at least 24 hours and up to 96 hours from baseline, was achieved in equivalent numbers of the preterm vs. term infants (90.9% vs. 88.2%).[165] However, the registry did not report on nonresponders that had iNO discontinued in the first 24 hours. Another retrospective cohort study evaluated in-hospital survival of infants with pulmonary hypoplasia and/or PPHN. Infants with PPHN who received iNO had a 33% reduced risk of in-hospital mortality compared with untreated infants, but this difference was not significant (HR, 0.67; 95% CI, 0.45–1.01).[143]

Even less is known about the benefit of adjunctive therapies in extremely preterm infants. One randomized trial of milrinone found the drug appeared safe but did not improve systemic blood flow in preterm infants without PH. Sildenafil is in early-phase testing for prevention of BPD in preterm infants, but it is not being tested in preterm infants with acute PH. It should also be noted that the use of sildenafil during pregnancy did not improve outcomes in fetuses affected by severe intrauterine growth restriction, and concerns were raised about possible harm. The international Sildenafil TheRapy In Dismal prognosis Early-onset intrauterine growth Restriction (STRIDER) consortium suspended their trial based on a 12% incidence of PH in the sildenafil arm of the Dutch cohort.[113] While increased PH was not observed in the UK or New Zealand/Australia STRIDER trial cohorts, the investigators did not find any benefit from maternal sildenafil therapy in this population.

Few studies are available to guide treatment of BPD-associated PH, although use of iNO, sildenafil, or a combination of the two is common in this population.[166] Cardiac catheterization is generally recommended in patients with PH who fail to respond or develop adverse responses such as pulmonary edema during empiric PH treatment.[167] In addition, clinical questions regarding the relative contributions of high flow through an unrestricted PDA, suspicion of LV dysfunction, and evaluation for PVS may warrant further assessment by cardiac catheterization. Empiric therapy with sildenafil is commonly initiated prior to cardiac catheterization in preterm infants. In a recent study using statistical decision modeling of a hypothetical cohort of BPD patients with PH identified by echo, Yang et al. estimated that initiating empiric oral sildenafil at 36 weeks postmenstrual age (PMA) after a positive echocardiography screen was more cost effective with equivalent long-term outcomes compared with mandatory invasive catheterization.[168]

Conclusions

In summary, lung vascular development is a dynamic process that begins in fetal life and continues through postnatal life. An increased understanding of the physiology of the fetal and neonatal pulmonary circulation has led to improved identification and management of acute and chronic PH in term and preterm infants. A number of open questions and controversies remain, including the role of cardiac dysfunction in PPHN (especially LV dysfunction in congenital diaphragmatic hernia), adjunctive and/or alternative therapies to iNO, and the causes and treatment of PH in the premature infant. Further research to overcome the challenges of conducting randomized trials and to develop strategies that prevent and ameliorate the long-term impact of pulmonary vascular disease is warranted.

REFERENCES

1. Thebaud B, Abman SH. Bronchopulmonary dysplasia: where have all the vessels gone? Roles of angiogenic growth factors in chronic lung disease. *Am J Respir Crit Care Med.* 2007;175(10):978-985.
2. Roth-Kleiner M, Post M. Similarities and dissimilarities of branching and septation during lung development. *Pediatr Pulmonol.* 2005;40(2):113-134.
3. Schwarz MA, Caldwell L, Cafasso D, et al. Emerging pulmonary vasculature lacks fate specification. *Am J Physiol Lung Cell Mol Physiol.* 2009;296(1):L71-L81.
4. Rudolph AM. Aortopulmonary transposition in the fetus: speculation on pathophysiology and therapy. *Pediatr Res.* 2007;61(3):375-380.
5. Rasanen J, Wood DC, Weiner S, et al. Role of the pulmonary circulation in the distribution of human fetal cardiac output during the second half of pregnancy. *Circulation.* 1996;94(5):1068-1073.

6. Morin FC III, Egan EA, Ferguson W, et al. Development of pulmonary vascular response to oxygen. *Am J Physiol*. 1988; 254(3 Pt 2):H542-H546.

7. Lewis AB, Heymann MA, Rudolph AM. Gestational changes in pulmonary vascular responses in fetal lambs in utero. *Circ Res*. 1976;39(4):536-541.

8. Rasanen J, Wood DC, Debbs RH, et al. Reactivity of the human fetal pulmonary circulation to maternal hyperoxygenation increases during the second half of pregnancy: a randomized study. *Circulation*. 1998;97(3):257-262.

9. Kumar VH, Hutchison AA, Lakshminrusimha S, et al. Characteristics of pulmonary hypertension in preterm neonates. *J Perinatol*. 2007;27(4):214-219.

10. Aikio O, Metsola J, Vuolteenaho R, et al. Transient defect in nitric oxide generation after rupture of fetal membranes and responsiveness to inhaled nitric oxide in very preterm infants with hypoxic respiratory failure. *J Pediatr*. 2012;161(3):397-403.e1.

11. Stenger MR, Slaughter JL, Kelleher K, et al. Hospital variation in nitric oxide use for premature infants. *Pediatrics*. 2012; 129(4):e945-e951.

12. Chow SSW, Le Marsney R, Haslam R, Lui K. *Report of the Australian and New Zealand Neonatal Network 2014*. Sydney: ANZNN; 2016. Available at: https://npesu.unsw.edu.au/sites/default/files/npesu/surveillances/Report%20of%20the%20Australian%20and%20New%20Zealand%20Neonatal%20Network%202014.pdf.

13. Handley SC, Steinhorn RH, Hopper AO, et al. Inhaled nitric oxide use in preterm infants in California neonatal intensive care units. *J Perinatol*. 2016;36(8):635-639.

14. Done E, Allegaert K, Lewi P, et al. Maternal hyperoxygenation test in fetuses undergoing FETO for severe isolated congenital diaphragmatic hernia. *Ultrasound Obstet Gynecol*. 2011;37(3):264-271.

15. Arraut AM, Frias AE, Hobbs TR, et al. Fetal pulmonary arterial vascular impedance reflects changes in fetal oxygenation at near-term gestation in a nonhuman primate model. *Reprod Sci*. 2013;20(1):33-38.

16. Konduri GG, Gervasio CT, Theodorou AA. Role of adenosine triphosphate and adenosine in oxygen-induced pulmonary vasodilation in fetal lambs. *Pediatr Res*. 1993;33(5):533-539.

17. Schwartz SM, Vermilion RP, Hirschl RB. Evaluation of left ventricular mass in children with left-sided congenital diaphragmatic hernia. *J Pediatr*. 1994;125(3):447-451.

18. Siebert JR, Haas JE, Beckwith JB. Left ventricular hypoplasia in congenital diaphragmatic hernia. *J Pediatr Surg*. 1984;19(5): 567-571.

19. Gao Y, Raj JU. Role of veins in regulation of pulmonary circulation. *Am J Physiol*. 2005;288(2):L213-L226.

20. Steinhorn RH, Morin FC III, Gugino SF, et al. Developmental differences in endothelium-dependent responses in isolated ovine pulmonary arteries and veins. *Am J Physiol*. 1993;264(6 Pt 2): H2162-H2167.

21. Gao Y, Dhanakoti S, Tolsa JF, et al. Role of protein kinase G in nitric oxide and cGMP induced relaxation of newborn ovine pulmonary veins. *J Appl Physiol*. 1999;87:993-998.

22. Semenza GL. Oxygen sensing, hypoxia-inducible factors, and disease pathophysiology. *Annu Rev Pathol*. 2014;9:47-71.

23. Compernolle V, Brusselmans K, Acker T, et al. Loss of HIF-2alpha and inhibition of VEGF impair fetal lung maturation, whereas treatment with VEGF prevents fatal respiratory distress in premature mice. *Nat Med*. 2002;8(7):702-710.

24. Ng YS, Rohan R, Sunday ME, et al. Differential expression of VEGF isoforms in mouse during development and in the adult. *Dev Dyn*. 2001;220(2):112-121.

25. Kasahara Y, Tuder RM, Taraseviciene-Stewart L, et al. Inhibition of VEGF receptors causes lung cell apoptosis and emphysema. *J Clin Invest*. 2000;106(11):1311-1319.

26. Parker TA, Le Cras TD, Kinsella JP, et al. Developmental changes in endothelial NO synthase expression in the ovine fetal lung. *Am J Physiol*. 2000;266:L202-L208.

27. North AJ, Star RA, Brannon TS, et al. NO synthase type I and type III gene expression are developmentally regulated in rat lung. *Am J Physiol*. 1994;266:L635-L641.

28. Han RN, Babaei S, Robb M, et al. Defective lung vascular development and fatal respiratory distress in endothelial NO synthase-deficient mice: a model of alveolar capillary dysplasia? *Circ Res*. 2004;94(8):1115-1123.

29. Balasubramaniam V, Tang JR, Maxey A, et al. Mild hypoxia impairs alveolarization in the endothelial nitric oxide synthase (eNOS) deficient mouse. *Am J Physiol*. 2003;284(6):L964-L971.

30. Gao Y, Cornfield DN, Stenmark KR, et al. Unique aspects of the developing lung circulation: structural development and regulation of vasomotor tone. *Pulm Circ*. 2016;6(4):407-425.

31. Kalinichenko VV, Lim L, Stolz DB, et al. Defects in pulmonary vasculature and perinatal lung hemorrhage in mice heterozygous null for the Forkhead Box f1 transcription factor. *Dev Biol*. 2001;235(2):489-506.

32. Ren X, Ustiyan V, Pradhan A, et al. FOXF1 transcription factor is required for formation of embryonic vasculature by regulating VEGF signaling in endothelial cells. *Circ Res*. 2014;115(8):709-720.

33. Bishop NB, Stankiewicz P, Steinhorn RH. Alveolar capillary dysplasia. *Am J Respir Crit Care Med*. 2011;184(2):172-179.

34. Iosef C, Alastalo TP, Hou Y, et al. Inhibiting NF-kappaB in the developing lung disrupts angiogenesis and alveolarization. *Am J Physiol Lung Cell Mol Physiol*. 2012;302(10):L1023-L1036.

35. Park L, Donohue L, Lakshminrusimha S, et al. Intravitreal bevacizumab injection for retinopathy of prematurity and pulmonary hypertension. *J Perinatol*. 2023;43(2):236-237.

36. Solodushko V, Fouty B. Proproliferative phenotype of pulmonary microvascular endothelial cells. *Am J Physiol Lung Cell Mol Physiol*. 2007;292(3):L671-L677.

37. Alvarez DF, Huang L, King JA, et al. Lung microvascular endothelium is enriched with progenitor cells that exhibit vasculogenic capacity. *Am J Physiol Lung Cell Mol Physiol*. 2008;294(3):L419-L430.

38. Wang G, Wen B, Deng Z, et al. Endothelial progenitor cells stimulate neonatal lung angiogenesis through FOXF1-mediated activation of BMP9/ACVRL1 signaling. *Nat Commun*. 2022; 13(1):2080.

39. Kolesnichenko OA, Whitsett JA, Kalin TV, et al. Therapeutic potential of endothelial progenitor cells in pulmonary diseases. *Am J Respir Cell Mol Biol*. 2021;65(5):473-488.

40. Mensah E, Morin FC III, Russell JA, et al. Soluble guanylate cyclase mRNA expression change during ovine lung development. *Pediatr Res*. 1998;43:290.

41. Delaney C, Gien J, Grover TR, et al. Pulmonary vascular effects of serotonin and selective serotonin reuptake inhibitors in the late-gestation ovine fetus. *Am J Physiol Lung Cell Mol Physiol*. 2011;301(6):L937-L944.

42. Delaney C, Gien J, Roe G, et al. Serotonin contributes to high pulmonary vascular tone in a sheep model of persistent pulmonary hypertension of the newborn. *Am J Physiol Lung Cell Mol Physiol*. 2013;304(12):L894-L901.

43. Teitel DF, Iwamoto HS, Rudolph AM. Changes in the pulmonary circulation during birth-related events. *Pediatr Res*. 1990; 27(4 Pt 1):372-378.

44. Lakshminrusimha S. The pulmonary circulation in neonatal respiratory failure. *Clin Perinatol*. 2012;39(3):655-683.

45. Abman SH, Chatfield BA, Hall SL, et al. Role of endothelium-derived relaxing factor during transition of pulmonary circulation at birth. *Am J Physiol.* 1990;259(6 Pt 2):H1921-H1927.

46. Fineman JR, Heymann MA, Soifer SJ. N omega-nitro-L-arginine attenuates endothelium-dependent pulmonary vasodilation in lambs. *Am J Physiol.* 1991;260(4 Pt 2):H1299-H1306.

47. Tiktinsky MH, Morin FC III. Increasing oxygen tension dilates fetal pulmonary circulation via endothelium-derived relaxing factor. *Am J Physiol Heart Circ Physiol.* 1993;265:H376-H380.

48. Fagan KA, Fouty BW, Tyler RC, et al. The pulmonary circulation of homozygous or heterozygous eNos-null mice is hyperresponsive to mild hypoxia. *J Clin Invest.* 1999;103:291-299.

49. Balasubramaniam V, Maxey AM, Morgan DB, et al. Inhaled NO restores lung structure in eNOS-deficient mice recovering from neonatal hypoxia. *Am J Physiol Lung Cell Mol Physiol.* 2006;291(1):L119-L127.

50. Kinsella JP, McQueston JA, Rosenberg AA, et al. Hemodynamic effects of exogenous nitric oxide in ovine transitional pulmonary circulation. *Am J Physiol.* 1992;263(3 Pt 2):H875-H880.

51. Randala M, Eronen M, Andersson S, et al. Pulmonary artery pressure in term and preterm neonates. *Acta Paediatr.* 1996;85(11):1344-1347.

52. Evans NJ, Archer LN. Doppler assessment of pulmonary artery pressure during recovery from hyaline membrane disease. *Arch Dis Child.* 1991;66(7 Spec No):802-804.

53. Evans NJ, Archer LN. Doppler assessment of pulmonary artery pressure and extrapulmonary shunting in the acute phase of hyaline membrane disease. *Arch Dis Child.* 1991;66(1 Spec No):6-11.

54. Skimming JW, Bender KA, Hutchison AA, et al. Nitric oxide inhalation in infants with respiratory distress syndrome. *J Pediatr.* 1997;130(2):225-230.

55. Mourani PM, Sontag MK, Younoszai A, et al. Early pulmonary vascular disease in preterm infants at risk for bronchopulmonary dysplasia. *Am J Respir Crit Care Med.* 2015;191(1):87-95.

56. Murphy JD, Rabinovitch M, Goldstein JD, et al. The structural basis of persistent pulmonary hypertension of the newborn infant. *J Pediatr.* 1981;98(6):962-967.

57. Ohara T, Ogata H, Tezuka F. Histological study of pulmonary vasculature in fatal cases of persistent pulmonary hypertension of the newborn. *Tohoku J Exp Med.* 1991;164(1):59-66.

58. Murphy JD, Vawter GF, Reid LM. Pulmonary vascular disease in fatal meconium aspiration. *J Pediatr.* 1984;104(5):758-762.

59. Wild LM, Nickerson PA, Morin FC III. Ligating the ductus arteriosus before birth remodels the pulmonary vasculature of the lamb. *Pediatr Res.* 1989;25(3):251-257.

60. Dodson RB, Morgan M, Galambos C, et al. Chronic intrauterine pulmonary hypertension increases main pulmonary artery stiffness and adventitial remodeling in fetal sheep. *Am J Physiol Lung Cell Mol Physiol.* 2014:307(11):L822-L828.

61. Stenmark KR, Davie N, Frid M, et al. Role of the adventitia in pulmonary vascular remodeling. *Physiology (Bethesda).* 2006;21:134-145.

62. Stenmark KR, Yeager ME, El Kasmi KC, et al. The adventitia: essential regulator of vascular wall structure and function. *Annu Rev Physiol.* 2013;75:23-47.

63. Galambos C, Sims-Lucas S, Abman SH. Histologic evidence of intrapulmonary anastomoses by three-dimensional reconstruction in severe bronchopulmonary dysplasia. *Ann Am Thorac Soc.* 2013;10(5):474-481.

64. Mourani PM, Abman SH. Pulmonary hypertension and vascular abnormalities in bronchopulmonary dysplasia. *Clin Perinatol.* 2015;42(4):839-855.

65. Villanueva ME, Zaher FM, Svinarich DM, et al. Decreased gene expression of endothelial nitric oxide synthase in newborns with persistent pulmonary hypertension. *Pediatr Res.* 1998;44(3):338-343.

66. Pearson DL, Dawling S, Walsh WF, et al. Neonatal pulmonary hypertension—urea-cycle intermediates, nitric oxide production, and carbamoyl-phosphate synthetase function. *N Engl J Med.* 2001;344(24):1832-1838.

67. Steinhorn RH, Russell JA, Morin FC III. Disruption of cGMP production in pulmonary arteries isolated from fetal lambs with pulmonary hypertension. *Am J Physiol.* 1995;268(4 Pt 2):H1483-H1489.

68. de Buys Roessingh A, Fouquet V, Aigrain Y, et al. Nitric oxide activity through guanylate cyclase and phosphodiesterase modulation is impaired in fetal lambs with congenital diaphragmatic hernia. *J Pediatr Surg.* 2011;46(8):1516-1522.

69. Chester M, Seedorf G, Tourneux P, et al. Cinaciguat, a soluble guanylate cyclase activator, augments cGMP after oxidative stress and causes pulmonary vasodilation in neonatal pulmonary hypertension. *Am J Physiol Lung Cell Mol Physiol.* 2011;301(5):L755-L764.

70. Farrow KN, Lakshminrusimha S, Czech L, et al. SOD and inhaled nitric oxide normalize phosphodiesterase 5 expression and activity in neonatal lambs with persistent pulmonary hypertension. *Am J Physiol Lung Cell Mol Physiol.* 2010;299(1):L109-L116.

71. Farrow KN, Groh BS, Schumacker PT, et al. Hyperoxia increases phosphodiesterase 5 expression and activity in ovine fetal pulmonary artery smooth muscle cells. *Circ Res.* 2008;102(2):226-233.

72. Lakshminrusimha S, Porta NF, Farrow KN, et al. Milrinone enhances relaxation to prostacyclin and iloprost in pulmonary arteries isolated from lambs with persistent pulmonary hypertension of the newborn. *Pediatr Crit Care Med.* 2009;10(1):106-112.

73. Christou H, Adatia I, Van Marter LJ, et al. Effect of inhaled nitric oxide on endothelin-1 and cyclic guanosine 5'-monophosphate plasma concentrations in newborn infants with persistent pulmonary hypertension. *J Pediatr.* 1997;130(4):603-611.

74. Ivy DD, Le Cras TD, Horan MP, et al. Chronic intrauterine pulmonary hypertension increases preproendothelin-1 and decreases endothelin B receptor mRNA expression in the ovine fetal lung. *Chest.* 1998;114(suppl 1):65S.

75. Gien J, Tseng N, Seedorf G, et al. Endothelin-1 impairs angiogenesis in vitro through Rho-kinase activation after chronic intrauterine pulmonary hypertension in fetal sheep. *Pediatr Res.* 2013;73(3):252-262.

76. Keller RL, Tacy TA, Hendricks-Munoz K, et al. Congenital diaphragmatic hernia: endothelin-1, pulmonary hypertension, and disease severity. *Am J Respir Crit Care Med.* 2010;182(4):555-561.

77. Fagan KA, Oka M, Bauer NR, et al. Attenuation of acute hypoxic pulmonary vasoconstriction and hypoxic pulmonary hypertension in mice by inhibition of Rho-kinase. *Am J Physiol Lung Cell Mol Physiol.* 2004;287(4):L656-L664.

78. Parker TA, Roe G, Grover TR, et al. Rho kinase activation maintains high pulmonary vascular resistance in the ovine fetal lung. *Am J Physiol Lung Cell Mol Physiol.* 2006;291(5):L976-L982.

79. Byers HM, Dagle JM, Klein JM, et al. Variations in CRHR1 are associated with persistent pulmonary hypertension of the newborn. *Pediatr Res.* 2012;71(2):162-167.

80. Kaluarachchi DC, Smith CJ, Klein JM, et al. Polymorphisms in urea cycle enzyme genes are associated with persistent pulmonary hypertension of the newborn. *Pediatr Res.* 2018;83(1-1):142-147.

81. Galambos C, Mullen MP, Shieh JT, et al. Phenotype characterisation of TBX4 mutation and deletion carriers with neonatal and paediatric pulmonary hypertension. *Eur Respir J.* 2019; 54(2):1801965.

82. Weijerman ME, van Furth AM, van der Mooren MD, et al. Prevalence of congenital heart defects and persistent pulmonary hypertension of the neonate with Down syndrome. *Eur J Pediatr.* 2010;169(10):1195-1199.

83. Southgate WM, Annibale DJ, Hulsey TC, et al. International experience with trisomy 21 infants placed on extracorporeal membrane oxygenation. *Pediatrics.* 2001;107(3):549-552.

84. Bush D, Abman SH, Galambos C. Prominent intrapulmonary bronchopulmonary anastomoses and abnormal lung development in infants and children with down syndrome. *J Pediatr.* 2017;180:156-162.e1.

85. Galambos C, Minic AD, Bush D, et al. Increased lung expression of anti-angiogenic factors in down syndrome: potential role in abnormal lung vascular growth and the risk for pulmonary hypertension. *PLoS One.* 2016;11(8):e0159005.

86. Griffiths M, Yang J, Vaidya D, et al. Biomarkers of pulmonary hypertension are altered in children with down syndrome and pulmonary hypertension. *J Pediatr.* 2022;241:68-76.e3.

87. Bush D, Wolter-Warmerdam K, Wagner BD, et al. EXPRESS: Angiogenic profile identifies pulmonary hypertension in children with down syndrome. *Pulm Circ.* 2019;9(3): 2045894019866549.

88. Check J, Gotteiner N, Liu X, et al. Fetal growth restriction and pulmonary hypertension in premature infants with bronchopulmonary dysplasia. *J Perinatol.* 2013;33(7):553-557.

89. Arjaans S, Zwart EAH, Ploegstra MJ, et al. Identification of gaps in the current knowledge on pulmonary hypertension in extremely preterm infants: a systematic review and meta-analysis. *Paediatr Perinat Epidemiol.* 2018;32(3):258-267.

90. Rozance PJ, Seedorf GJ, Brown A, et al. Intrauterine growth restriction decreases pulmonary alveolar and vessel growth and causes pulmonary artery endothelial cell dysfunction in vitro in fetal sheep. *Am J Physiol Lung Cell Mol Physiol.* 2011; 301(6):L860-L871.

91. Mestan, KK, Check J, Minturn L, et al. Placental pathologic changes of maternal vascular underperfusion in bronchopulmonary dysplasia and pulmonary hypertension. *Placenta.* 2014;35(8):570-574.

92. Yallapragada SG, Mestan KK, Palac H, et al. Placental villous vascularity is decreased in premature infants with bronchopulmonary dysplasia-associated pulmonary hypertension. *Pediatr Dev Pathol.* 2016;19(2):101-107.

93. Arjaans, S, Fries MWF, Schoots MH, et al. Clinical significance of early pulmonary hypertension in preterm infants. *J Pediatr.* 2022;251:74-81.e3.

94. Mestan KK, Gotteiner N, Porta N, et al. Cord blood biomarkers of placental maternal vascular underperfusion predict bronchopulmonary dysplasia-associated pulmonary hypertension. *J Pediatr.* 2017;185:33-41.

95. Mandell EW, Abman SH. Fetal vascular origins of bronchopulmonary dysplasia. *J Pediatr.* 2017;185:7-10.e1.

96. Abman SH, Accurso FJ. Acute effects of partial compression of ductus arteriosus on fetal pulmonary circulation. *Am J Physiol.* 1989;257(2 Pt 2):H626-H634.

97. Abman SH, Shanley PF, Accurso FJ. Failure of postnatal adaptation of the pulmonary circulation after chronic intrauterine pulmonary hypertension in fetal lambs. *J Clin Invest.* 1989; 83(6):1849-1858.

98. Shaul PW, Yuhanna IS, German Z, et al. Pulmonary endothelial NO synthase gene expression is decreased in fetal lambs with pulmonary hypertension. *Am J Physiol.* 1997;272(5 Pt 1): L1005-L1012.

99. Tourneux P, Chester M, Grover T, et al. Fasudil inhibits the myogenic response in the fetal pulmonary circulation. *Am J Physiol Heart Circ Physiol.* 2008;295(4):H1505-H1513.

100. Farrow KN, Wedgwood S, Lee KJ, et al. Mitochondrial oxidant stress increases PDE5 activity in persistent pulmonary hypertension of the newborn. *Respir Physiol Neurobiol.* 2010; 174(3):272-281.

101. Zayek M, Cleveland D, Morin FC III. Treatment of persistent pulmonary hypertension in the newborn lamb by inhaled nitric oxide. *J Pediatr.* 1993;122(5 Pt 1):743-750.

102. Talati AJ, Salim MA, Korones SB. Persistent pulmonary hypertension after maternal naproxen ingestion in a term newborn: a case report. *Am J Perinatol.* 2000;17(2):69-71.

103. Van Marter LJ, Hernandez-Diaz S, Werler MM, et al. Nonsteroidal antiinflammatory drugs in late pregnancy and persistent pulmonary hypertension of the newborn. *Pediatrics.* 2013; 131(1):79-87.

104. Belik J. Fetal and neonatal effects of maternal drug treatment for depression. *Semin Perinatol.* 2008;32(5):350-354.

105. Fornaro E, Li D, Pan J, et al. Prenatal exposure to fluoxetine induces fetal pulmonary hypertension in the rat. *Am J Respir Crit Care Med.* 2007;176(10):1035-1040.

106. Masarwa R, Bar-Oz B, Gorelik E, et al. Prenatal exposure to selective serotonin reuptake inhibitors and serotonin norepinephrine reuptake inhibitors and risk for persistent pulmonary hypertension of the newborn: a systematic review, meta-analysis, and network meta-analysis. *Am J Obstet Gynecol.* 2019; 220(1):57.e1-57.e13.

107. Munk-Olsen T, Bergink V, Rommel AS, et al. Association of persistent pulmonary hypertension in infants with the timing and type of antidepressants in utero. *JAMA Netw Open.* 2021;4(12):e2136639.

108. Norby U, Forsberg L, Wide K, et al. Neonatal morbidity after maternal use of antidepressant drugs during pregnancy. *Pediatrics.* 2016;138(5):e20160181.

109. Hooper CW, Delaney C, Streeter T, et al. Selective serotonin reuptake inhibitor exposure constricts the mouse ductus arteriosus in utero. *Am J Physiol Heart Circ Physiol.* 2016; 311(3):H572-H581.

110. Chandrasekar I, Eis A, Konduri GG. Betamethasone attenuates oxidant stress in endothelial cells from fetal lambs with persistent pulmonary hypertension. *Pediatr Res.* 2008; 63(1):67-72.

111. Gyamfi-Bannerman C, Thom EA, Blackwell SC, et al. Antenatal betamethasone for women at risk for late preterm delivery. *N Engl J Med.* 2016;374(14):1311-1320.

112. Luong C, Rey-Perra J, Vadivel A, et al. Antenatal sildenafil treatment attenuates pulmonary hypertension in experimental congenital diaphragmatic hernia. *Circulation.* 2011;123(19): 2120-2131.

113. Pels A, Onland W, Berger RMF, et al. Neonatal pulmonary hypertension after severe early-onset fetal growth restriction: post hoc reflections on the Dutch STRIDER study. *Eur J Pediatr.* 2022;181(4):1709-1718.

114. Walsh-Sukys MC, Tyson JE, Wright LL, et al. Persistent pulmonary hypertension of the newborn in the era before nitric oxide: practice variation and outcomes. *Pediatrics.* 2000;105(1 Pt 1):14-20.

115. Steurer MA, Jelliffe-Pawlowski LL, Baer RJ, et al. Persistent pulmonary hypertension of the newborn in late preterm and term infants in california. *Pediatrics.* 2017;139(1): CD000399.

116. Konduri GG, Vohr B, Robertson C, et al. Early inhaled nitric oxide therapy for term and near-term newborn infants with hypoxic respiratory failure: neurodevelopmental follow-up. *J Pediatr.* 2007;150(3):235-240.e1.

117. Lapointe A, Barrington KJ. Pulmonary hypertension and the asphyxiated newborn. *J Pediatr.* 2011;158(Suppl. 2):e19-e24.

118. Rudolph AM, Yuan S. Response of the pulmonary vasculature to hypoxia and H+ ion concentration changes. *J Clin Invest.* 1966;45(3):399-411.

119. Cornish JD, Dreyer GL, Snyder GE, et al. Failure of acute perinatal asphyxia or meconium aspiration to produce persistent pulmonary hypertension in a neonatal baboon model. *Am J Obstet Gynecol.* 1994;171(1):43-49.

120. Toubas PL, Hof RP, Heymann MA, et al. Effects of hypothermia and rewarming on the neonatal circulation. *Arch Fr Pediatr.* 1978;35(Suppl. 10):84-92.

121. Shankaran S, Laptook AR, Pappas A, et al. Effect of depth and duration of cooling on deaths in the NICU among neonates with hypoxic ischemic encephalopathy: a randomized clinical trial. *JAMA.* 2014;312(24):2629-2639.

122. Agarwal P, Shankaran S, Laptook AR, et al. Outcomes of infants with hypoxic ischemic encephalopathy and persistent pulmonary hypertension of the newborn: results from three NICHD studies. *J Perinatol.* 2021;41(3):502-511.

123. Bhombal S, Patel N. Diagnosis & management of pulmonary hypertension in congenital diaphragmatic hernia. *Semin Fetal Neonatal Med.* 2022;27(4):101383.

124. Derderian SC, Jayme CM, Cheng LS, et al. Mass effect alone may not explain pulmonary vascular pathology in severe congenital diaphragmatic hernia. *Fetal Diagn Ther.* 2016;39(2):117-124.

125. Tajchman UW, Tuder RM, Horan M, et al. Persistent eNOS in lung hypoplasia caused by left pulmonary artery ligation in the ovine fetus. *Am J Physiol.* 1997;272(5 Pt 1):L969-L978.

126. Pierro M, Thebaud B. Understanding and treating pulmonary hypertension in congenital diaphragmatic hernia. *Semin Fetal Neonatal Med.* 2014;19(6):357-363.

127. Lusk LA, Wai KC, Moon-Grady AJ, et al. Persistence of pulmonary hypertension by echocardiography predicts short-term outcomes in congenital diaphragmatic hernia. *J Pediatr.* 2015;166(2):251-266.e1.

128. Gien J, Kinsella JP. Management of pulmonary hypertension in infants with congenital diaphragmatic hernia. *J Perinatol.* 2016;36 Suppl 2:S28-S31.

129. Maia PD, Gien J, Kinsella JP, et al. Hemodynamic characterization of neonates with congenital diaphragmatic hernia-associated pulmonary hypertension by cardiac catheterization. *J Pediatr.* 2023;255:230-235.e2.

130. Altit S, Bhombal KP, Van Meurs K, et al. Ventricular performance is associated with need for ECMO in newborns with CDH. *J Pediatr.* 2017;191:28-34.e1.

131. Galambos C, Sims-Lucas S, Ali N, et al. Intrapulmonary vascular shunt pathways in alveolar capillary dysplasia with misalignment of pulmonary veins. *Thorax.* 2015;70(1):84-85.

132. Towe CT, White FV, Grady RM, et al. Clinical and histopathologic characterization of infants with atypical presentations of alveolar capillary dysplasia with misalignment of the pulmonary veins who underwent bilateral lung transplantation. *J Pediatr.* 2018;194:158-164.e1.

133. Yost CE, Putnam AR, Dishop MK, et al. A long-term survivor with alveolar capillary dysplasia. *JACC Case Rep.* 2020; 2(10):1492-1495.

134. Stankiewicz P, Sen P, Bhatt SS, et al. Genomic and genic deletions of the FOX gene cluster on 16q24.1 and inactivating mutations of FOXF1 cause alveolar capillary dysplasia and other malformations. *Am J Hum Genet.* 2009;84(6):780-791.

135. Arjaans S, Fries MWF, Schoots MH, et al. Clinical significance of early pulmonary hypertension in preterm infants. *J Pediatr.* 2022;251:74-81.e3.

136. Mirza H, Ziegler J, Ford S, et al. Pulmonary hypertension in preterm infants: prevalence and association with bronchopulmonary dysplasia. *J Pediatr.* 2014;165(5):909-914.e1.

137. Mourani PM, Sontag MK, Younoszai A, et al. Early pulmonary vascular disease in preterm infants at risk for bronchopulmonary dysplasia. *Am J Respir Crit Care Med.* 2015; 191(1):87-95.

138. Nakanishi H, Suenaga H, Uchiyama A, et al. Persistent pulmonary hypertension of the newborn in extremely preterm infants: a Japanese cohort study. *Arch Dis Child Fetal Neonatal Ed.* 2018;103(6):F554-F561.

139. Ball MK, Steinhorn RH. Inhaled nitric oxide for preterm infants: a Marksman's approach. *J Pediatr.* 2012;161(3):379-380.

140. de Waal K, Kluckow M. Prolonged rupture of membranes and pulmonary hypoplasia in very preterm infants: pathophysiology and guided treatment. *J Pediatr.* 2015;166(5):1113-1120.

141. Suzuki K, Hooper SB, Cock ML, et al. Effect of lung hypoplasia on birth-related changes in the pulmonary circulation in sheep. *Pediatr Res.* 2005;57(4):530-536.

142. Thibeault DW, Kilbride HK. Increased acinar arterial wall muscle in preterm infants with PROM and pulmonary hypoplasia. *Am J Perinatol.* 1997;14(8):457-460.

143. Ellsworth KR, Ellsworth MA, Weaver AL, et al. Association of early inhaled nitric oxide with the survival of preterm neonates with pulmonary hypoplasia. *JAMA Pediatr.* 2018; 172(7):e180761.

144. Wagner BD, Babinec AE, Carpenter C, et al. Proteomic profiles associated with early echocardiogram evidence of pulmonary vascular disease in preterm infants. *Am J Respir Crit Care Med.* 2018;197(3):394-397.

145. Saugstad OD. Oxygen and oxidative stress in bronchopulmonary dysplasia. *J Perinat Med.* 2010;38(6):571-577.

146. Lee, KJ, Berkelhamer SK, Kim GA, et al. Disrupted pulmonary artery cyclic guanosine monophosphate signaling in mice with hyperoxia-induced pulmonary hypertension. *Am J Respir Cell Mol Biol.* 2014;50(2):369-378.

147. Grover TR, Asikainen TM, Kinsella JP, et al. Hypoxia-inducible factors HIF-1alpha and HIF-2alpha are decreased in an experimental model of severe respiratory distress syndrome in preterm lambs. *Am J Physiol Lung Cell Mol Physiol.* 2007;292(6): L1345-L1351.

148. Wedgwood S, Warford C, Agvateesiri SC, et al. Postnatal growth restriction augments oxygen-induced pulmonary hypertension in a neonatal rat model of bronchopulmonary dysplasia. *Pediatr Res.* 2016;80(6):894-902.

149. Mahgoub, L, Kaddoura T, Kameny AR, et al. Pulmonary vein stenosis of ex-premature infants with pulmonary hypertension and bronchopulmonary dysplasia, epidemiology, and survival from a multicenter cohort. *Pediatr Pulmonol.* 2017; 52(8):1063-1070.

150. Heching HJ, Turner M, Farkouh-Karoleski C, et al. Pulmonary vein stenosis and necrotising enterocolitis: is there a possible link

with necrotising enterocolitis? *Arch Dis Child Fetal Neonatal Ed.* 2014;99(4):F282-F285.

151. Lakshminrusimha S, Russell JA, Steinhorn RH, et al. Pulmonary hemodynamics in neonatal lambs resuscitated with 21%, 50%, and 100% oxygen. *Pediatr Res.* 2007;62(3):313-318.

152. Lakshminrusimha S, Steinhorn RH, Wedgwood S, et al. Pulmonary hemodynamics and vascular reactivity in asphyxiated term lambs resuscitated with 21 and 100% oxygen. *J Appl Physiol (1985).* 2011;111(5):1441-1447.

153. Auten RL, Davis JM. Oxygen toxicity and reactive oxygen species: the devil is in the details. *Pediatr Res.* 2009;66(2):121-127.

154. Brennan LA, Steinhorn RH, Wedgwood S, et al. Increased superoxide generation is associated with pulmonary hypertension in fetal lambs: a role for NADPH oxidase. *Circ Res.* 2003;92(6):683-691.

155. Konduri GG, Bakhutashvili I, Eis A, et al. Oxidant stress from uncoupled nitric oxide synthase impairs vasodilation in fetal lambs with persistent pulmonary hypertension. *Am J Physiol Heart Circ Physiol.* 2007;292(4):H1812-H1820.

156. Pierce CM, Zhang MH, Jonsson B, et al. Efficacy and safety of IV sildenafil in the treatment of newborn infants with, or at risk of, Persistent Pulmonary Hypertension of the Newborn (PPHN): a multicenter, randomized, placebo-controlled trial. *J Pediatr.* 2021;237:154-161.e3.

157. Zapol WM. Nitric oxide story. *Anesthesiology.* 2019;130(3):435-440.

158. Dillard J, Pavlek LR, Korada S, et al. Worsened short-term clinical outcomes in a cohort of patients with iNO-unresponsive PPHN: a case for improving iNO responsiveness. *J Perinatol.* 2022;42(1):37-44.

159. Jackson W, Gonzalez D, Smith PB, et al. Safety of sildenafil in extremely premature infants: a phase I trial. *J Perinatol.* 2022;42(1):31-36.

160. Giesinger RE, Stanford AH, Thomas B, et al. Safety and feasibility of riociguat therapy for the treatment of chronic pulmonary arterial hypertension in infancy. *J Pediatr.* 2023;255:224-229.e1.

161. Steinhorn RH, Fineman J, Kusic-Pajic A, et al. Bosentan as adjunctive therapy for persistent pulmonary hypertension of the newborn: results of the FUTURE-4 study. *J Pediatr.* 2016;177:90-96.e3.

162. Wehrmann M, Patel SS, Haxel C, et al. Implications of atrial-level shunting by echocardiography in newborns with congenital diaphragmatic hernia. *J Pediatr.* 2020;219:43-47.

163. McNamara PJ, Giesinger RE, Lakshminrusimha S. Dopamine and neonatal pulmonary hypertension-pressing need for a better pressor? *J Pediatr.* 2022;246:242-250.

164. Shah S, Dhalait S, Fursule A, et al. Use of vasopressin as rescue therapy in refractory hypoxia and refractory systemic hypotension in term neonates with severe persistent pulmonary hypertension-a prospective observational Study. *Am J Perinatol.* 2022. doi:10.1055/a-1969-1119.

165. Nelin L, Kinsella JP, Courtney SE, et al. Use of inhaled nitric oxide in preterm vs term/near-term neonates with pulmonary hypertension: results of the PaTTerN registry study. *J Perinatol.* 2022;42(1):14-18.

166. Lagatta JM, Hysinger EB, Zaniletti I, et al. The impact of pulmonary hypertension in preterm infants with severe bronchopulmonary dysplasia through 1 year. *J Pediatr.* 2018;203:218-224.e3.

167. Abman SH, Hansmann G, Archer SL, et al. Pediatric pulmonary hypertension: guidelines from the American Heart Association and American Thoracic Society. *Circulation.* 2015;132(21):2037-2099.

168. Yang EL, Levy PT, Critser PJ, et al. The clinical and cost utility of cardiac catheterizations in infants with bronchopulmonary dysplasia. *J Pediatr.* 2022;246:56-63.e3.

169. Busch CJ, Graveline AR, Jiramongkolchai K, et al. Phosphodiesterase 3A expression is modulated by nitric oxide in rat pulmonary artery smooth muscle cells. *J Physiol Pharmacol.* 2010;61(6):663-669.

170. Chen B, Lakshminrusimha S, Czech L, et al. Regulation of phosphodiesterase 3 in the pulmonary arteries during the perinatal period in sheep. *Pediatr Res.* 2009;66(6):682-687.

Chapter 4

Airway Microbiome and Lung Injury

Rose M. Viscardi and Namasivayam Ambalavanan

Chapter Outline

Introduction

Newborn Lung Microbiome

Role of *Ureaplasma* Species in Intrauterine Infection and Neonatal Lung Injury

  Ureaplasma Species: Are There Species- or Serovar-Specific Virulence Factors?

  Potential Role of *Ureaplasma* Species in Preterm Birth and Intrauterine Inflammation

  Ureaplasma Spp. and Neonatal Lung Injury

Human and Experimental Evidence for Role of *Ureaplasma* Spp. in Bronchopulmonary Dysplasia

Developmental Deficiencies in Innate Immunity Contribute to Susceptibility to *Ureaplasma* Infection and Dysregulated Inflammation

Can Bronchopulmonary Dysplasia Be Prevented by *Ureaplasma* Eradication?

Summary

Key Points

- Contrary to conventional teaching, culture-independent molecular techniques have confirmed that the healthy lung is not sterile and the lung microbiome is likely established in early life, influences development of immune responses and pulmonary function, and is altered in disease states.

- Although the major pathway that microorganisms colonize the uterine cavity is vertical ascension from the vagina, there is emerging evidence suggesting transplacental transfer of microbiota as a route of infection.

- The airway microbiome of the newborn lung of term and preterm infants is similar in composition and diversity at birth, but the lung microbiome of bronchopulmonary dysplasia (BPD) infants differs in composition and is less diverse compared to term and non-BPD preterm infants.

- The genus *Lactobacillus* is decreased at birth in infants exposed to chorioamnionitis and in preterm infants who develop BPD.

- The mycoplasmas species *Ureaplasma parvum* and *Ureaplasma urealyticum* are commensals in the genital tract, but have been associated with intrauterine infection, preterm birth, and adverse neonatal outcomes including BPD. Current evidence indicates that these organisms modulate host immune responses.

Introduction

It has been determined that only 1% of all bacteria can be cultured[1] and many of the microbial species that normally (or abnormally) inhabit the human body are not identified by culture. Culture-independent molecular techniques have demonstrated that body sites, including the lung, are not sterile and are host to communities of microorganisms. The term *microbiota* refers specifically to the community of microorganisms living in a particular environment while the term *microbiome* refers to the communities of microorganisms and their encoded genes.[2] Microbial diversity measures how much variety exists in a microbial community and is characterized by richness (the number of different bacterial species present) and evenness (the relative abundance of the various species within the microbial community), while the term *dysbiosis* describes a microbial pattern associated with disease states.[3]

Culture-independent molecular methods show that the microbiota of humans is far greater than previously recognized.[4] The Human Microbiome Project focused particularly on the normal microbiome of the skin, mouth, nose, digestive tract, and vagina[5] and found that even healthy individuals differ remarkably in the diversity and abundance of the microbiome at the different sites. The relative abundance of members of a microbiome is most often determined by sequencing of the variables regions (V1–3 or V4–6) of the bacterial 16S ribosomal RNA (rRNA), but more extensive metagenomic and metatranscripomic sequencing provides more in-depth data on microbial gene function and possible host interactions.[6]

Due to the relative inaccessibility of the lower airways and the lungs, there has been less research on the airway and pulmonary microbiome as compared to the gastrointestinal or oral microbiome. Hilty et al.[7] found that lower airways of adults are not sterile, with approximately 2000 bacterial genomes per cm[2] surface sampled. They also found that the tracheobronchial tree contained a characteristic microbial flora that differs from the nares and oropharynx and between health and disease.[7,8] The major colonists in normal people are anaerobes such as *Bacteroidetes* (e.g., *Prevotella* spp.) grown with difficulty in culture while *Proteobacteria* (e.g., *Haemophilus*, *Moraxella*, *Neisseria* spp.) are strongly associated with airway disease in chronic obstructive pulmonary disease (COPD) and asthma.[7] It is possible that microbial immigration from the oral cavity contributes to the lung microbiome during health, although the lungs selectively eliminate *Prevotella* bacteria derived from the upper airways.[8] In healthy adult lungs, spatial variation in microbiota within an individual is significantly less than variation across individuals, and bronchoalveolar lavage (BAL) of a single lung segment is probably acceptable for sampling the healthy lung microbiome.[9] A limitation of bronchoscopic sampling of the airways is the possible contamination from the oral or nasal flora.[10] However, direct sampling of lung tissue derived from nonmalignant lung tissue samples from cancer patients determined that *Proteobacteria* is the dominant phylum, and other common phyla include *Firmicutes*, *Bacteroidetes*, and *Actinobacteria*.[11] Microbiota taxonomic alpha diversity increased with environmental exposures to air particulates, residency in high-density population areas, and smoking pack-years.[11]

Newborn Lung Microbiome

The newborn lung microbiome is even more technologically challenging to sample, since available sampling is limited to intubated infants with upper airways sampled by tracheal aspirates of the endotracheal tube and distal airways sampled by tracheal lavage. Despite this significant limitation, there have been some recent studies evaluating the airway microbiome in preterm infants, specifically in relation to development of bronchopulmonary dysplasia (BPD). Mourani et al.[12] evaluated serial tracheal aspirates (<72 hours, 7 days, 14 days, and 21 days) from 10 preterm infants who required mechanical ventilation for at least 21 days. Samples were analyzed by quantitative real-time polymerase chain reaction (PCR) assays for total bacterial load and by pyrosequencing for bacterial identification. Seventy-two organisms were observed in total. Seven organisms represented the dominant organism (>50% of total sequences) in 31 of the 32 samples with positive sequences. *Staphylococcus* and the genital mycoplasmas *Ureaplasma parvum* and *Ureaplasma urealyticum* were the most frequently identified dominant organisms, but *Pseudomonas*, *Enterococcus*, and *Escherichia* were also identified. Most infants in this series established either *Staphylococcus* spp. (*Firmicutes*) or *Ureaplasma* spp. (*Tenericutes*) as the predominant organism by 7 days of age. Lohmann et al.[13] evaluated tracheal aspirates of 25 preterm infants obtained at birth and on days 3, 7, and 28. Bacterial DNA was extracted, and 16S rRNA genes were amplified and sequenced. It was found that *Acinetobacter* was the predominant genus in the airways of all infants at birth. Infants who developed BPD had reduced bacterial diversity at birth.

Recently, we evaluated the airway microbiome of extremely preterm and term infants soon after birth and in preterm infants with established BPD.[14] Tracheal aspirates were collected from a discovery cohort of 23 extremely low-birth-weight (ELBW) infants and 10 full-term (FT) infants (with no respiratory disease) at birth or within 6 hours of birth at the time of intubation, as well as from 18 infants with established BPD in whom samples were obtained at 36 weeks postmenstrual age (PMA) at the time of endotracheal tube change.

A validation cohort was used consisting of tracheal aspirates from extremely preterm infants at a different institution. We were able to detect and characterize bacterial DNA by 16S rRNA sequencing in tracheal aspirates of all ELBW and FT infants soon after birth. The lung microbiome was similar at birth in ELBW and FT infants irrespective of gestational age. Both ELBW and FT infants had a predominance of *Firmicutes* and *Proteobacteria* on the first day of life, in addition to *Actinobacteria*, *Bacteroidetes*, *Tenericutes*, *Fusobacterium*, *Cyanobacteria*, and *Verrucomicrobia* (Fig. 4.1). The relative abundance of bacterial phyla and Shannon alpha diversity did not differ between ELBW and FT infants. Compared to newborn FT infants matched for PMA, the airway microbiome of infants after the diagnosis of BPD was characterized by increased phylum

Proteobacteria and decreased phyla *Firmicutes* and *Fusobacteria* (Fig. 4.2). At the genus level, the most abundant *Proteobacteria* in BPD patients were *Enterobacteriaceae*. To confirm the presence of *Proteobacteria* in the BPD patient samples, we also performed specific endotoxin assays. Endotoxin concentrations in the airway were similar between term and preterm infants at birth, but endotoxin levels were increased in infants with established BPD compared to concentrations at birth.[14] Serial samples in five ELBW infants who went on to develop BPD demonstrated a distinct temporal dysbiotic change with decreases in *Firmicutes* and increases in *Proteobacteria* over time. It was observed both in the discovery cohort and the validation cohort that genus *Lactobacillus* was less abundant even as early as birth in infants who later developed BPD, compared

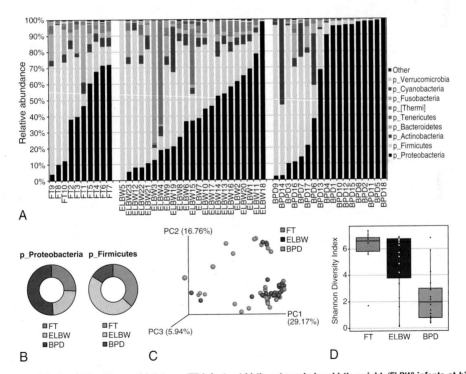

Fig. 4.1 Comparison of the lung microbiome of full-term *(FT)* **infants at birth, extremely low-birth-weight** *(ELBW)* **infants at birth, and ELBW patients with established bronchopulmonary dysplasia** *(BPD)*. **A,** Bar graph depicting the relative abundance of commonly encountered bacterial phyla between FT, ELBW, and BPD infants. **B,** Compared to newborn postmenstrual age-matched FT infants and ELBW infants, infants with BPD had increased *Proteobacteria* and decreased *Firmicutes* and *Fusobacteria*. **C,** Principal coordinates analysis "PCoA" plot (beta diversity) demonstrating unweighted UniFrac distance between samples with sample points colored for ELBW, FT, or BPD infants. Samples that are clustered closely together share a larger proportion of the phylogenetic tree in comparison to samples that are more separated. ELBW and FT infants have similar beta diversity, which is very different from the beta diversity of BPD infants. **D,** Shannon diversity index depicting decreased microbial alpha diversity in infants with BPD compared to FT and ELBW infants. (Figure taken from Lal CV et al. The Airway Microbiome at Birth. *Sci Rep.* 2016;6:31023.)

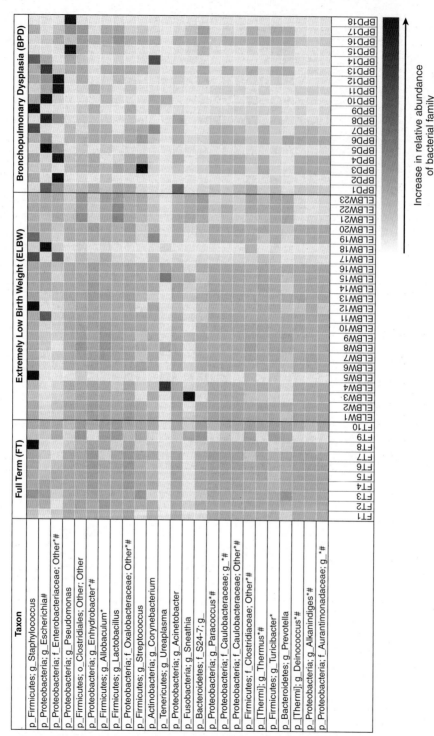

Fig. 4.2 Microbiome at genus level of extremely low-birth-weight (ELBW) infants, full-term (FT) infants, and patients with bronchopulmonary dysplasia (BPD). Heat map depicting the relative abundance of common bacterial families at the genus level. Statistically significant difference in microbial abundance is seen between lung microbiome of ELBW and BPD infants (*) and between FT and BPD infants (#). (Figure taken from Lal CV et al. The Airway Microbiome at Birth. *Sci Rep.* 2016;6:31023.)

to the infants who did not develop BPD (Fig. 4.2). Interestingly, preterm birth was associated with alterations in the vaginal microbial community with decreased relative abundance of *Lactobacillus*.[15]

Analyzing airway microbial community turnover in sequentially sampled tracheal aspirates from ventilated preterm infants, Wagner et al.[16] found that infants who eventually developed severe BPD had greater bacterial community turnover with age, acquired less *Staphylococcus* soon after birth, and had higher initial relative abundance of *Ureaplasma*.

As both extremely preterm and term infants had a similar diverse microbiome at birth, it is probable that the airway and lung microbiomes are established before birth, potentially through transplacental passage of bacterial products. This contention is supported by culture-independent studies of the uterine microbiome demonstrating the presence of bacteria in the placenta,[17] fetal membranes,[18] and amniotic fluid[19] of healthy pregnancies that have challenged the notion that the fetus develops in a sterile environment and have increased our understanding of infection-related preterm birth as a polymicrobial diease.[19] Using next-generation sequencing and metagenomic analyses, Aagaard et al.[17] identified a low abundance microbiota in the placenta of term and preterm placentas including *Escherichia coli*, *Prevotella tannerae*, *Bacteroides* species, and *Fusobacterium* species. Using 16S rDNA pyrosequencing to identify bacteria in placental membranes from term and preterm deliveries, Doyle et al.[18] found six genera (*Fusobacterium*, *Streptococcus*, *Mycoplasma*, *Aerococcus*, *Gardnerella*, and *Ureaplasma*) and one family (*Enterobacteriaceae*) that were more abundant in preterm membranes or absent in term membranes. There was reduced abundance of genus *Lactobacillus* and increased abundance of genera *Streptococcus*, *Aerococcus*, and *Ureaplasma* in membranes from preterm infants delivered by the vaginal route.[18] There is some evidence for a low biomass microbiome in both fetal lung and placenta even very early in gestation in the first trimester, which shows maturational changes with advancing gestational age.[20]

It is not currently known what proportion of the transferred bacterial DNA from the placenta are from live bacteria and what proportion is from "processed" bacterial products (DNA fragments, cell wall fragments, etc.). Our recent study indicated the presence of both bacterial DNA and bacterial lipopolysaccharide in neonatal airways at the time of birth.[14] Microbiome analysis evaluates bacterial DNA but does not indicate if the DNA is from live bacteria. It has been suggested that evaluation of susceptibility of the bacterial DNA to DNAse I may indicate the proportion of DNA from live bacteria, as live bacterial DNA is DNAse I resistant, but bacterial DNA from dead bacteria is DNAse I sensitive—63% of DNA in porcine BALF is DNAse I sensitive, suggesting the majority of airway bacterial DNA is from dead bacteria.[21]

It may be speculated that the establishment of the lung microbiome during fetal life enables the priming of the immune system in the fetus and later recognition of and response to bacterial flora encountered after birth. Alterations in the airway microbiome are associated with childhood pulmonary disorders such as asthma.[22,23] It is also likely that the lung microbiome contributes to normal alveolar development. Yun et al.[24] studied microbiota of sterilely excised lungs from mice of different origin including outbred wild mice caught in the natural environment or kept under non–specific pathogen-free (SPF) conditions as well as inbred mice maintained in non-SPF, SPF, or germ-free (GF) facilities. Metabolically active murine lung microbiota were found in all but GF mice.[24] Bacteria were detectable by fluorescent in situ hybridization (FISH) on alveolar epithelia in the absence of inflammation. A higher bacterial abundance in non-SPF mice correlated with more and smaller size alveolae (consistent with better alveolarization), which was corroborated by transplanting *Lactobacillus* spp. lung isolates into GF mice.[24] There is increasing evidence that lung and gut microbiota are altered by hyperoxia, with selective relative growth advantage of oxygen-tolerant microbes (e.g., *Staphylococcus aureus*), which may contribute to oxygen-induced lung injury in mice.[25] Willis et al.[26] have shown that perinatal maternal antibiotic exposure augments lung injury in newborn mice exposed to hyperoxia, while Dolma and colleagues[27] have shown that GF mice without a microbiome were protected from hyperoxia injury, showing improved lung structure and mechanics, and decreased inflammation compared to hyperoxia-exposed, non-GF mice. These studies indicate that dysbiosis is a contributor to lung injury and abnormal lung development in the BPD model.

There are many potential mechanisms by which the microbiome may modulate lung injury and repair. We have recently demonstrated that bacterial lipopolysaccharide (LPS) exposure alters exosomal microRNA in tracheal aspirates and reduces specific microRNA such as miR-876-3p that contributes to a BPD phenotype.[28] We have also shown that the early airway microbiome alters the metabolome, and that the airway metabolome of BPD-predisposed infants was enriched for metabolites involved in fatty acid activation and androgen and estrogen biosynthesis compared with BPD-resistant infants.[29] It is known that manipulation of the gut microbiota may influence lung pathology via the gut-lung axis,[30] but it is not clear if the manipulation of the gut microbiome also simultaneously alters the lung microbiome or if the effects in the lung can be due solely to alterations of the microbiome in the gut. It is possible that bacteria or bacterial products from the gut may be translocated to the systemic circulation and filtered from the pulmonary circulation into the lungs. It is known that the lung microbiome is enriched with gut bacteria in sepsis and the acute respiratory distress syndrome.[31]

In the next section, we will review the human and experimental evidence that the low-virulence pathogens *U. parvum* and *U. urealyticum* that are common members of the vaginal, amniotic fluid, placental, and preterm lung microbiota contribute to preterm birth and lung injury due to an augmented dysregulated inflammatory response that contributes to the development of BPD. Recent studies provide new insights into how these organisms evade the host immune response to establish colonization in the intrauterine cavity and fetal/newborn lung and identify these mechanisms as potential therapeutic targets.

Role of *Ureaplasma* Species in Intrauterine Infection and Neonatal Lung Injury

Ureaplasma is comprised of 2 species and 14 serovars. *U. parvum* contains serovars 1, 3, 6, and 14, and *U. urealyticum* contains the remaining serovars.[32] The *Ureaplasma* species are among the smallest self-replicating, free-living organisms with *U. parvum* serovar 3 genome containing the second smallest known genome with 751 Kbp.[33] Due to their small genome size, the *Ureaplasma* spp. have limited biosynthetic capacities,

requiring a parasitic relationship with a host. They lack a cell wall and generate ATP by hydrolyzing urea.[32] The following sections will focus on the evidence implicating the *Ureaplasma* species in preterm birth and neonatal lung disease.

UREAPLASMA SPECIES: ARE THERE SPECIES- OR SEROVAR-SPECIFIC VIRULENCE FACTORS?

U. parvum is more commonly isolated from clinical vaginal,[34] amniotic fluid,[35,36] and infant respiratory specimens,[37] and it is the predominant species in newborn serum and/or cerebrospinal fluid (CSF) samples detected by PCR.[38] It has been proposed that some serovars have greater association with adverse pregnancy outcomes than others.[34,39,40] Recently, Rittenschober-Bohm et al.[41] reported that vaginal colonization in early pregnancy with *U. parvum* serovar 3, but not other serovars, was associated with spontaneous preterm birth at very low (<32 weeks) and extremely low (<28 weeks) gestation. The risk for preterm birth was further increased in women with vaginal *U. parvum* serovar 3 and bacterial vaginosis or history of prior preterm birth. Payne et al.[42] identified a specific microbial DNA signature in vaginal swabs obtained mid-pregnancy that predicted pPROM and preterm birth risk, that consisted of DNA from *Gardnerella vaginalis* (clade 4), *Lactobacillis iners*, and *U. parvum* serovars 3 and 6. Utilizing 16S rRNA gene and whole genome sequencing of four *Ureaplasma* isolates from women with intraamniotic infection, Motomura et al.[36] found that *U. parvum* serovars were the most common, but that the isolates could not be differentiated by known virulence genes. Abele-Horn et al.[34] reported a higher rate of BPD in *U. urealyticum* respiratory tract–colonized infants. In contrast, Katz et al.[43] observed no difference in prevalence of either species detected by PCR between infants with and without BPD. In a prospective study of respiratory secretions in infants <33 weeks gestation, the distribution of *Ureaplasma* species and serovars was determined by real-time PCR using species and serovar-specific primers/probes.[37,44] *U. parvum* was the predominant species (63%), compared with *U. urealyticum* (33%). Serovars 3 and 6 alone and in combination accounted for 96% *U. parvum* isolates. *U. urealyticum* isolates were commonly a mixture of multiple serovars with serovar 11 alone or combined with other serovars (59%) as the most common serovar. No individual species/serovars or serovar mixtures were associated with moderate-to-severe BPD. This supports the contention that *Ureaplasma* virulence is species- and serovar-independent with regards to neonatal lung disease, but this needs to be confirmed. Recent research has shown that clinical isolates often have DNA hybrid genomes, proving that serovar-specific markers have been transferred horizontally.[45] These findings suggest that there could be innumerable serovars or strains based on different combinations of horizontally transferred genes. Thus, serotyping for diagnostic purposes or in an attempt to correlate pathogenicity at the serovar level is unlikely to be useful, and host factors likely contribute to different outcomes following *Ureaplasma* infection.[45]

Previously proposed ureaplasmal virulence factors include IgA protease, urease, phospholipases A and C, and production of hydrogen peroxide.[33] These factors may allow the organism to evade mucosal immune defenses by degrading IgA and injuring mucosal cells through the local generation of ammonia, membrane phospholipid degradation and prostaglandin synthesis, and membrane peroxidation, respectively. Although functionally active IgA protease and phospholipase A and C were found in *Ureaplasma* spp., the genes that code for these proteins have not been identified in the *U. parvum* serovar 3 genome.[33] The ureaplasmal enzymes may have unique sequences compared with analogous genes in other species.

The ureaplasmal MB antigen that contains both serovar-specific and cross-reactive epitopes is the predominant antigen recognized during ureaplasmal infections in humans. It exhibits highly variable size in vitro,[46] clinical isolates in vivo,[47] and in an experimental ovine intraamniotic infection model,[48] suggesting that antigen size variation may be another mechanism through which the organism evades host defenses. Ureaplasmas have multiple other host immune response avoidance mechanisms that facilitate establishing a chronic infection in the amniotic cavity and the neonatal respiratory tract. These include the ability to form biofilms,[49] presence of multiple nucleases that may degrade neutrophil extracellular traps that are formed when activated neutrophils release granule proteins and chromatin that kill bacteria,[50,51] and downregulation of various endogenous antimicrobial peptides by ureaplasmal-mediated chromatin modification alterations, including significantly decreased histone H3K9 acetylation.[52] Since neutrophil extracellular traps are abundant in chorioamniotic membranes with acute chorioamnionitis,[53] *Ureaplasma*-induced nuclease degradation may explain in part the prolonged subclinical intrauterine infection with these organisms. Further genetic studies of the ureaplasmal genome are likely to identify other virulence factors that may be novel therapeutic targets.

POTENTIAL ROLE OF *UREAPLASMA* SPECIES IN PRETERM BIRTH AND INTRAUTERINE INFLAMMATION

Because *Ureaplasma* is a commensal in the adult female genital tract, it has been considered of low virulence. However, it has been associated with multiple obstetrical complications including infertility, stillbirth, chorioamnionits,[36] and preterm delivery.[54] *Ureaplasma* spp. are the most common organisms isolated from amniotic fluid obtained from women who present with preterm onset of labor (POL) with intact membranes,[55] preterm premature rupture of membranes (pPROM),[56] short cervix associated with microbial invasion of the amniotic cavity,[57] and from infected placentas.[56] The prevalence of infected amniotic fluid with cultivated *Ureaplasma* as the only microbe ranges from 6% to 9% for pregnancies complicated by POL with intact membranes[55,58] to 22% for a cohort of women with POL or pPROM.[59] Detection of cultivated *Ureaplasma* in placental chorion in pregnancies producing very low birth weight (VLBW) infants ranges from 6% to 10% in homogenized frozen tissue[60,61] to 28% in fresh tissue and is inversely related to gestational age.[62] Recovery of *Ureaplasma* from the chorion increased with the duration of rupture membranes, suggesting an ascending route of infection.[62] However, *Ureaplasma* has also been detected in 31% of infected placentas with duration of rupture of membranes less than 1 hour,[63] suggesting the possibility of a preexisting infection. Indeed, *Ureaplasma* species have been detected in amniotic fluid as early as the time of genetic amniocentesis (16–20 weeks) in up to 13% asymptomatic women.[64,65] Placentas with the lowest rate of *Ureaplasma* recovery were from women delivered for preeclampsia or intrauterine growth restriction.[62]

The presence of *Ureaplasma* as the only identified microbial isolate in the upper genital tract is significantly associated with chorioamnionitis and adverse pregnancy outcomes, including premature delivery, neonatal morbidity, and perinatal death.[55,59,62,66] Placentas colonized with *Ureaplasma* exhibit a characteristic bistriate inflammatory pattern with maternal-derived neutrophils accumulating in the subchorion and amnion.[67] Experimental models of intrauterine *Ureaplasma* infection in mice,[36,68,69] sheep,[70-73] and nonhuman primates[74,75] have been described. Intraamniotic inoculation of *U. parvum* isolates stimulated POL in mice,[36,69] but not in sheep, and stimulated progressive uterine contractions and preterm delivery in rhesus macaques inoculated at 136 days gestation (80% term),[74] suggesting species differences in the host response or serovar differences in virulence. The rhesus macaque model is the first experimental model to definitely show a causal link between *Ureaplasma* intrauterine infection and POL.

In the presence of pPROM, cultivated *Ureaplasma* as the sole microbe was associated with increased leukocytes and proinflammatory cytokines (IL-6, IL-1β, and TNF-α) in amniotic fluid and increased cord blood IL-6 concentrations, indicating a robust inflammatory response to this infection.[76] However, amniotic fluid IL-8 levels were higher and amniocentesis-to-delivery interval was shorter when POL was caused by a combination of *Mycoplasma/Ureaplasma* and other bacteria than *Mycoplasma/Ureaplasma* alone.[77] Ureaplasmal bacterial load determined by quantitative PCR in amniotic fluid of women who delivered preterm was associated with histological chorioamnionitis, POL, PROM, and BPD.[35] The bacterial load correlated with amniotic fluid IL-8 concentrations. While the majority of women in whom subclinical *Ureaplasma* amniotic cavity infection is detected midtrimester deliver at term,[65] those with elevated amniotic fluid IL-6 levels have increased risk for adverse pregnancy outcome including fetal loss and preterm delivery.[78] In a mouse model, cervical injury facilitated ascending infection of vaginally inoculated *U. parvum*, followed by increase levels of proinflammatory cytokines and preterm birth.[69] In the rhesus monkey *U. parvum* intrauterine infection model, uterine activity was preceded by a rise in amniotic fluid leukocytes, inflammatory cytokines, prostaglandins PGE_2 and PGF_2 alpha, and matrix metalloproteinase (MMP) 9, demonstrating that *Ureaplasma* alone stimulates the mediators of POL.[74] Recently, Lal and coworkers[79] demonstrated that *Ureaplasma* spp. stimulate neutrophil MMP-9 release and serine protease prolyl endopeptidase expression that together induce collagen fragmentation, resulting in release of the tripeptide PGP (proline-glycine-proline), a neutrophil chemoattractant. These findings implicate *Ureaplasma* spp. in the causal pathway of preterm rupture of membranes and neutrophil influx causing chorioamnionitis.

In vitro studies have provided additional evidence supporting the contention that *Ureaplasma* spp. stimulate inflammation in the intrauterine compartment. Plasma from placental whole blood (source of maternal circulating leukocytes) that had been preincubated with *U. parvum* serovar 3 clinical isolate stimulated IL-1β and PGE_2 secretion by chorioamnion explants.[80] High inoculum (10^6 color changing units [CCU]/mL), but not low inoculum (10^2–10^4 CCU/mL) heat-killed *U. urealyticum* serotype 8 stimulated TNF-α, IL-10, and PGE_2 production by choriodecidual explants in vitro. In contrast, heat-killed *U. parvum* serovar 1 laboratory reference strain failed to stimulate a significant increase in cytokine and PGE_2 response in fetal membrane explants derived from term placentas. The apparent low virulence of *Ureaplasma* in these in vitro studies may be due, in part, to the use of a laboratory reference strain rather than more virulent clinical isolates or killed rather than live organisms. Alternatively, a decreased capacity to stimulate an inflammatory response in the intrauterine compartment may allow *Ureaplasma* infections to persist for long periods of time. In vitro exposure of pulmonary epithelial-like A549 cells to high inoculum ($\sim10^9$ CCU) ATCC reference *U. urealyticum* serovar 8 (ATCC27618) and *U. parvum* serovar 3 (ATCC27815) downregulated caspase 8 and 9 mRNA levels, but exposures of cultured human pulmonary microvascular endothelial cells to *Ureaplasma* spp. resulted in increased caspase 3, 8, and 9 protein expression and enzyme activity and cell death,[81] suggesting differential modulation of caspase expression by lung epithelial and endothelial cells with potential impact on lung inflammation and vascular development.

UREAPLASMA SPP. AND NEONATAL LUNG INJURY

Ureaplasma respiratory tract colonization has been associated with higher incidence of pneumonia[82] and BPD.[40,83-85] The rate of *Ureaplasma* respiratory tract colonization in infants <1500 g birth weight ranges from 20% to 47%, depending on study entry criteria, sampling source, frequency and timing of sampling, and detection methods.[86,87] In a recent cohort of infants <33 weeks gestation, *Ureaplasma* spp. were detected by combined culture/PCR during the first week of life in tracheal aspirates or nasopharyngeal specimens in 35% of infants.[38] *Ureaplasma*-colonized infants are more likely to be born extremely preterm (<28 weeks gestation) and to be delivered by spontaneous vaginal delivery following POL or pPROM.[88] Typically, they experience less respiratory distress in the first week of life with clinical deterioration in the second week, requiring increased oxygen and ventilatory support.[40,88] *Ureaplasma* respiratory tract colonization is associated with a peripheral blood leukocytosis [82,89] and early radiographic emphysematous changes of BPD.[88,90] These findings may be explained, in part, by an in utero onset of the inflammatory response and lung injury. Indeed, neonatal *Ureaplasma* respiratory colonization was associated with BPD in infants exposed to antenatal histological chorioamnionitis.[91] Clinical, radiographic, and laboratory characteristics of neonatal *Ureaplasma* respiratory tract colonization are summarized in Box 4.1.

The contribution of *Ureaplasma* respiratory tract colonization to the development of BPD has been debated; however, three meta-analyses of more than 40 studies over the past 30 years have confirmed that *Ureaplasma* respiratory colonization is an independent risk factor for BPD.[83,85,86] Overall, *Ureaplasma* respiratory tract colonization increased the risk for BPD at 28 days threefold and BPD at 36 weeks of PMA twofold.[85,92] Despite changes in neonatal care over the past three decades, this association has remained unchanged. In a prospective cohort[37] and in the recent azithromycin clinical trial,[93] we observed lower survival, higher rates of BPD, longer duration of hospitalization, mechanical ventilation and supplemental oxygen, and greater postnatal steroid exposure in infants with lower respiratory tract *Ureaplasma* infection than intubated infants without lower tract involvement or nonintubated infants. This suggests that lower tract infection, but not nasopharyngeal colonization, augments lung injury in mechanically ventilated infants.

HUMAN AND EXPERIMENTAL EVIDENCE FOR ROLE OF *UREAPLASMA* SPP. IN BRONCHOPULMONARY DYSPLASIA

Evidence from studies of human preterm infants[94-96] and intrauterine infection models in mice,[36,68,69] sheep,[70,71] and nonhuman primates[74,97] support that *Ureaplasma* infection is proinflammatory and profibrotic and results in a BPD phenotype. In a review of lung pathology of archived autopsy specimens from *Ureaplasma*-infected preterm infants, the most striking findings were (1) the presence of moderate-to-severe fibrosis, (2) increased myofibroblasts, (3) disordered elastin accumulation, and (4) increased numbers of TNF-α and transforming growth factor β_1 (TGFβ_1)-immunoreactive cells in all *Ureaplasma*-infected infants compared to gestational controls and infants who died with pneumonia from other causes.[94,95] The increase in fibrosis and elastic fiber accumulation in the distal lung correlated spatially and temporally with the presence of macrophages positive for TGFβ_1, suggesting that these are closely linked. Severity of fibrosis score and elastic fiber density exhibited strong correlation with duration of ventilation in *Ureaplasma*-positive infants, suggesting that *Ureaplasma* infection augments the inflammatory response to volutrauma.[94,95] Preterm infants with *Ureaplasma* respiratory colonization have elevated tracheal aspirate

---

BOX 4.1 CHARACTERISTIC CLINICAL AND LABORATORY FINDINGS IN *UREAPLASMA*-POSITIVE PRETERM INFANTS

Clinical Presentation	Laboratory/Radiographic Findings
• POL or pPROM[88,89]	• Bistriate inflammatory pattern chorioamnionitis[67]
• GA <28 weeks[37]	• Leukocytosis at birth[82,89,91]
• Mild RDS, but worsening gas exchange requiring increased respiratory support in second week of life[40,88]	• Early radiographic emphysematous changes[88,90] • Early lung fibrosis and disordered elastin[95]

POL, Preterm onset of labor; *pPROM*, preterm premature rupture of membranes.

IL-1β, TNF-α, IL-8, IL-17, and monocyte chemoattractant protein-1 (MCP-1) concentrations and neutrophil chemotactic activity but lower IL-10 during the first weeks of life compared to noncolonized infants.[96,98,99]

Experimental pneumonia models demonstrate the inflammatory response to Ureaplasma pulmonary infection. Intratracheal Ureaplasma inoculation caused an acute bronchiolitis in 140 days of preterm baboons,[100] and an acute interstitial pneumonia in newborn, but not 14 days of old mice.[101] Hyperoxia exposure increased mortality, lung inflammation, and delayed pathogen clearance in Ureaplasma-inoculated newborn mice,[102] consistent with the hypothesis that Ureaplasma augments the inflammatory response to secondary stimuli. In a mouse Ureaplasma pneumonia model, intratracheal inoculation with Ureaplasma induced a prolonged inflammatory response as indicated by a sustained recruitment of neutrophils and macrophages into the lung.[103]

Antenatal infection models provide insights into the effects of Ureaplasma on lung development. Intraamniotic inoculation with clinical U. parvum serovar 14 isolate induced proinflammatory cytokine increases in amniotic fluid, fetal membranes, and infected fetal organs including the fetal lung, spleen, and liver, but not maternal serum.[36] Experimental murine intrauterine U. parvum exposure stimulated fetal lung cytokine expression and augmented hyperoxia-induced lung injury.[68] Intraamniotic Ureaplasma (serovar 1) inoculation 2 days prior to delivery at 125 days (67% of term gestation) in the baboon caused an inflammatory response in the amniotic and fetal lung compartments and vertical transmission to the fetal lung that persisted for up to 2 weeks postnatally in half of the antenatal-exposed animals.[104] We observed extensive fibrosis, an increase in the myofibroblast phenotype, increased expression of proinflammatory (TNF-α, IL-1β) and profibrotic cytokines (TGFβ1; oncostatin M), and presence of macrophages as the predominant recruited leuokocyte in lungs of Ureaplasma-exposed immature baboons compared to gestational controls or noninfected ventilated animals.[97] After 14 days of ventilation, active TGFβ1 and TGFβ1-induced Smad signaling was increased in lung homogenates of Ureaplasma-infected animals compared to gestational and ventilated controls. Similarly, fetal sheep exposed to intraamniotic U. parvum

serovar 3 for 3 to 14 days prior to delivery at 124 days demonstrated increased fetal lung neutrophils after 3 days and decreased alveolar septa and elastin foci, and increased α-smooth muscle actin in arteries and bronchioli after 14 days exposure.[105] This demonstrated that short-term intrauterine exposure to Ureaplasma induces an inflammatory response and altered structural lung development. This may mimic the exposure with an ascending infection after rupture of membranes in the human condition.

Since subclinical Ureaplasma intrauterine infection has been detected early in human pregnancy, the effects of prolonged intrauterine exposure to this infection have been examined. In fetal sheep exposed to intraamniotic Ureaplasma for periods up to 10 weeks, long-term exposure was associated with improvement in lung function, but poor fetal growth, fetal acidemia, and evidence of fetal pulmonary inflammation.[70] Intraamniotic inoculation of U. parvum servovar 3 or 6 at midgestation in fetal sheep did not result in POL, but did cause placental and fetal pulmonary inflammation and altered lung development whether delivery occurred preterm or at term.[71] However, after intraamniotic inoculation of these serovars at 50 days gestation, there was evidence of persistent infection, lung inflammation, and increased surfactant and improved lung volumes, but no significant effects on indices of airspace and vascular morphology in fetuses delivered preterm at 125 days gestation.[106] With sequential exposure of pregnant sheep to 42 days U. parvum intraamniotic infection and LPS 7 days prior to delivery at 125 days (term 150 days), alveolar size increased with reduction in alveolar type II cells and Ki67+ proliferating cells and abnormal vascular development. In a nonhuman primate study of rhesus macaques, histologic changes in the fetal lungs depended on the duration of intrauterine exposure to U. parvum.[74] Infection exposure duration less than 136 hours resulted in neutrophil infiltration without epithelial injury. With progressive duration of exposure, there was an influx of neutrophils and macrophages, epithelial necrosis, and type II cell proliferation. For exposure duration >10 days, increased collagen and thickened alveolar walls were evident. These observations suggest that an early and prolonged exposure to Ureaplasma-mediated inflammation with or without secondary inflammatory stimulus may be necessary to adversely affect lung development. Discrepancies among the experimental models may be due to species differences as well as differences in *Ureaplasma* isolates used, inoculation timing, and route of administration. Overall, the experimental models confirm that intraamniotic *Ureaplasma* mimics many of the clinical features of the human disease.

The stimulatory effect of *Ureaplasma* on cytokine release has been confirmed in vitro. *Ureaplasma* stimulated TNF-α and IL-6 release by alveolar macrophages from preterm infant tracheal aspirates,[107] and cytokine, nitric oxide production, and upregulation of iNOS, nuclear factor-kappa B (NF-κB) activation, and VEGF and soluble and cell-associated ICAM-1 expression by human and murine-derived monocytic cells.[107-109] *Ureaplasma* induced apoptosis in A549 cells, a human type II cell line, and in THP-1 human monocytic cells.[110] These effects could be partially blocked by anti–TNF-α monoclonal antibody,[109,110] implicating TNF-α as a mediator of the host immune response to this infection that contributes to altered lung development. In cultured human monocytes, *Ureaplasma* stimulated release of TNF-α and IL-8.[111] Moreover, in the presence of bacterial endotoxic LPS, *Ureaplasma* greatly augmented monocyte production of proinflammatory cytokines while blocking expression of antiinflammatory cytokines (IL-6 and IL-10).

These data confirm that *Ureaplasma* infection contributes to chronic inflammation in the preterm lung. We propose that *Ureaplasma* infection initiated in utero and augmented postnatally by exposure to volutrauma and oxygen elicits a sustained, dysregulated inflammatory response in the immature lung that impairs alveolarization and vascular development, and stimulates myofibroblast proliferation and excessive collagen and elastin deposition.

Developmental Deficiencies in Innate Immunity Contribute to Susceptibility to *Ureaplasma* Infection and Dysregulated Inflammation

Immaturity of fetal host defense mechanisms may increase the susceptibility of the preterm lung to *Ureaplasma* infection and dysregulated inflammation. Surfactant protein A (SP-A), a product of the alveolar type II cell that is an important component of the lung's innate immune response, is deficient in the preterm lung. SP-A is critical for clearance of infection and limiting inflammation in the lung.[112] We have shown that SP-A binds to *Ureaplasma* isolates in a calcium-dependent manner and enhances phagocytosis and bacterial killing by RAW264.7 cells, a murine macrophage cell line.[113,114] Furthermore, bacterial clearance was delayed and inflammatory response exaggerated in SP-A–deficient mice compared to wild-type mice inoculated intratracheally with *U. parvum*.[113] Coadministration of purified human SP-A with the *Ureaplasma* inoculum to SP-A$^{-/-}$ mice reduced the inflammatory response to the infection but did not improve the rate of bacterial clearance. SP-A deficiency of the preterm lung may contribute to the prolonged inflammatory response, lung injury, and risk for fibrosis in *Ureaplasma*-infected infants contributing to the pathogenesis of BPD.

Other important components of the innate immune response are Toll-like receptors (TLRs) that respond to a broad range of pathogen-associated molecular patterns (PAMPs), including LPS, viral coat proteins, bacterial lipoproteins and glycolipids, viral RNA, and CpG-containing bacterial DNA.[115] Engagement of TLR proteins activates the expression of proinflammatory mediators by macrophages, neutrophils, dendritic cells, B cells, endothelial cells, and epithelial cells. TLR signaling activates the transcription factor NF-κB and subsequent upregulation of gene expression. Peltier et al.[116] and Shimizu et al.[117] demonstrated that Triton X-114 detergent extracted lipoproteins from *U. urealyticum* serovar 4 and *U. parvum* serovar 3 are responsible for NF-κB activation. Active lipoproteins identified for serovar 3 included the MB antigen.[117] The serovar 3 detergent extracts activated NF-κB through TLR2 cooperatively with TLR1 and TLR6,[117] while serovar 4 extracts activated both TLR2 and TLR4.[116] Further studies will need to determine if the different *Ureaplasma* species or serovars interact with different TLRs. If so, this could explain, in part, differences in host responses to the different serovars.

Little is known concerning TLR expression during human lung development. In mice, TLR2 and TLR4 mRNA levels were barely detectable early in gestation, increasing thereafter during late gestation and postnatally.[118] In fetal sheep lung, TLR2 and TLR4 mRNA levels increased throughout late gestation to reach half of adult levels at term, but were induced by intraamniotic LPS exposure.[119] In the immature baboon model, TLR2 and TLR4 mRNA and protein expressions were low in 125 days and 140 days nonventilated gestational controls, reached adult levels near term, and were increased in 125 days preterm baboons ventilated with oxygen for 21 days.[120] These data may explain, in part, the developmental susceptibility to *Ureaplasma* infection and interaction with other stimuli. Low TLR2 and TLR4 expression early in gestation may increase the susceptibility of the fetal lung to *Ureaplasma* infection and delay clearance, but postnatal exposures to mechanical ventilation, oxygen, and other infections may stimulate pulmonary TLR expression and enhance *Ureaplasma*-mediated inflammatory signaling. Single nucleotide polymorphisms in relevant TLRs may affect both the susceptibility to *Ureaplasma* respiratory infection and the risk of developing BPD in infected preterm infants.[121]

Can Bronchopulmonary Dysplasia Be Prevented by *Ureaplasma* Eradication?

Despite in vitro susceptibility of *Ureaplasma* to erythromycin,[122] trials of erythromycin therapy in the first few weeks of life in *Ureaplasma*-colonized preterm infants failed to demonstrate efficacy to prevent BPD[123,124] or eradicate respiratory tract colonization.[125] The failure to prevent BPD in these studies may have been due to the small sample size of each study, or to the initiation of erythromycin therapy too late to prevent the lung inflammation and injury that contribute to the pathogenesis of BPD.

The 14-membered macrolides that are derivatives of erythromycin and the related 15-member azalides have immunomodulatory effects, including effects on neutrophil function (e.g., chemotaxis, cell adhesion, oxidative burst, and phagocytosis), inhibition of cytokine release,[126] and nitric oxide production in vitro.[127] Macrolide antibiotics may exert immunomodulatory antiinflammatory effects in the setting of infection, and these may occur independently of a direct bactericidal effect.[128] Recently, Segal et al.[129] studied the effect of azithromycin on the lung microbiome and bacterial metabolites in adults with COPD in a placebo, double-blind, randomized trial. Although azithromycin did not alter bacterial abundance, it reduced alpha diversity and increased antiinflammatory bacterial metabolites glycolic acid and indol-3-acetate. In addition, azithromycin exhibits higher potency than erythromycin against clinical *Ureaplasma* isolates in vitro.[130] Pharmacokinetic studies in mice and humans have shown that azithromycin is preferentially concentrated in pulmonary epithelial lining fluid and alveolar macrophages.[131-133] Since neutrophil recruitment and activation has been implicated in BPD pathogenesis,[134] the experimental effects observed with azithromycin in vitro and in vivo indicate that this drug may be beneficial in the treatment of *Ureaplasma* infection and the prevention of BPD in preterm infants.

Since *Ureaplasma*-mediated lung injury may be initiated in utero and augmented postnatally by exposure to mechanical ventilation and hyperoxia, therapy to prevent BPD should be initiated antenatally or as soon as possible after birth in infants at risk. Treatment of intraamniotic *U. parvum*–infected pregnant mice with clarithromycin prevented preterm birth and neonatal mortality.[36] Walls et al.[135] demonstrated that azithromycin, but not erythromycin prophylaxis, improved outcomes and reduced inflammation in a murine neonatal *Ureaplasma* infection model. This suggests that azithromycin may be effective if administered immediately after birth. In a series of single-dose and multiple-dose intravenous azithromycin pharmacokinetic/pharmacodynamic studies in preterm infants, Viscardi and colleagues established that 20 mg/kg × 3 days was well tolerated, safe, and more effective than 10 mg/kg or 20 mg/kg single-dose regimens in eradicating *Ureaplasma* spp. from the preterm respiratory tract.[136-138] Based on these results, a randomized masked, multicenter, placebo-controlled phase IIb trial that enrolled 121 preterm infants 24 weeks 0 day to 28 weeks 6 days gestation (60 azithromycin, 61 placebo) was conducted.[93] In the study cohort, 36% of the infants were *Ureaplasma*-positive, and azithromycin effectively eradicated *Ureaplasma* in all treatment-assigned colonized infants. In the entire cohort, *Ureaplasma*-free survival was 92% (95% CI 82%–97%) for azithromycin versus 61% (95% CI 48%–73%) for placebo. Evaluation of this cohort at 2 years of age indicated that tracheal aspirate *Ureaplasma*-positive infants had a higher frequency of death or serious respiratory morbidity at 22 to

26 months corrected age (58%) than tracheal aspirate negative infants (34%) or nonintubated infants (21%) (p = 0.028), suggesting that infants with lower airway *Ureaplasma* should be targeted in future clinical trials.[139] No differences in longer-term pulmonary or neurodevelopmental outcomes were noted between azithromycin and placebo groups. A phase III randomized control trial (RCT) of a 10-day course of azithromycin (20 mg/kg × 3 days, followed by 10 mg/kg for a further 7 days) is currently enrolling ~800 preterm infants <30 weeks gestation in the United Kingdom (http://www.isrctn.com/ISRCTN11650227) to determine the safety and efficacy of this regimen to improve survival without BPD.[140]

Summary

Culture-independent techniques have provided insights into the microbial communities in the developing lung during health and disease. Future metagenomic and metabolomic studies will provide further information on microbial and lung cell gene expression and metabolic pathways that contribute to the balance of health versus disease states. Most studies of the genital mycoplasmas have focused on the host response to the single organism, but future studies including those involving therapeutic interventions should analyze the impact of the microbial communities in the placenta and fetal membranes and lungs on ureaplasmal gene expression, and host immune responses to identify approaches to better mitigate the risk for BPD.

REFERENCES

1. Staley JT, Konopka A. Measurement of in situ activities of nonphotosynthetic microorganisms in aquatic and terrestrial habitats. *Annu Rev Microbiol.* 1985;39:321-346.
2. Lynch SV. The Lung microbiome and airway disease. *Ann Am Thorac Soc.* 2016;13(suppl 5):S462-S465.
3. Gallacher DJ, Kotecha S. Respiratory microbiome of new-born infants. *Front Pediatr.* 2016;4:10.
4. Turnbaugh PJ, Ley RE, Hamady M, et al. The human microbiome project. *Nature.* 2007;449(7164):804-810.
5. Human Microbiome Project Consortium. Structure, function and diversity of the healthy human microbiome. *Nature.* 2012;486(7402):207-214.
6. Warner BB, Hamvas A. Lungs, microbes and the developing neonate. *Neonatology.* 2015;107(4):337-343.
7. Hilty M, Burke C, Pedro H, et al. Disordered microbial communities in asthmatic airways. *PLoS One.* 2010;5(1):e8578.
8. Bassis CM, Erb-Downward JR, Dickson RP, et al. Analysis of the upper respiratory tract microbiotas as the source of the lung and gastric microbiotas in healthy individuals. *mBio.* 2015;6(2):e00037.
9. Dickson RP, Erb-Downward JR, Freeman CM, et al. Spatial variation in the healthy human lung microbiome and the adapted island model of lung biogeography. *Ann Am Thorac Soc.* 2015;12(6):821-830.
10. Beck JM, Young VB, Huffnagle GB. The microbiome of the lung. *Transl Res.* 2012;160(4):258-266.
11. Yu G, Gail MH, Consonni D, et al. Characterizing human lung tissue microbiota and its relationship to epidemiological and clinical features. *Genome Biol.* 2016;17(1):163.
12. Mourani PM, Harris JK, Sontag MK, et al. Molecular identification of bacteria in tracheal aspirate fluid from mechanically ventilated preterm infants. *PLoS One.* 2011;6(10):e25959.
13. Lohmann P, Luna RA, Hollister EB, et al. The airway microbiome of intubated premature infants: characteristics and changes that predict the development of bronchopulmonary dysplasia. *Pediatr Res.* 2014;76(3):294-301.
14. Lal CV, Travers C, Aghai ZH, et al. The airway microbiome at birth. *Sci Rep.* 2016;6:31023.
15. DiGiulio DB, Callahan BJ, McMurdie PJ, et al. Temporal and spatial variation of the human microbiota during pregnancy. *Proc Natl Acad Sci U S A.* 2015;112(35):11060-11065.
16. Wagner BD, Sontag MK, Harris JK, et al. Airway microbial community turnover differs by BPD severity in ventilated preterm infants. *PLoS One.* 2017;12(1):e0170120.
17. Aagaard K, Ma J, Antony KM, et al. The placenta harbors a unique microbiome. *Sci Transl Med.* 2014;6(237):237ra265.
18. Doyle RM, Alber DG, Jones HE, et al. Term and preterm labour are associated with distinct microbial community structures in placental membranes which are independent of mode of delivery. *Placenta.* 2014;35(12):1099-1101.
19. Payne MS, Bayatibojakhi S. Exploring preterm birth as a polymicrobial disease: an overview of the uterine microbiome. *Front Immunol.* 2014;5:595. doi:10.3389/fimmu.2014.00595.
20. Al Alam D, Danopoulos S, Grubbs B, et al. Human fetal lungs harbor a microbiome signature. *Am J Respir Crit Care Med.* 2020;201(8):1002-1006.
21. Pezzulo AA, Kelly PH, Nassar BS, et al. Abundant DNase I-sensitive bacterial DNA in healthy porcine lungs and its implications for the lung microbiome. *Appl Environ Microbiol.* 2013;79(19):5936-5941.
22. Singanayagam A, Ritchie AI, Johnston SL. Role of microbiome in the pathophysiology and disease course of asthma. *Curr Opin Pulm Med.* 2017;23(1):41-47.
23. Huang YJ. The respiratory microbiome and innate immunity in asthma. *Curr Opin Pulm Med.* 2015;21(1):27-32.
24. Yun Y, Srinivas G, Kuenzel S, et al. Environmentally determined differences in the murine lung microbiota and their relation to alveolar architecture. *PLoS One.* 2014;9(12):e113466. doi:10.1371/journal.pone.0113466.
25. Ashley SL, Sjoding MW, Popova AP, et al. Lung and gut microbiota are altered by hyperoxia and contribute to oxygen-induced lung injury in mice. *Sci Transl Med.* 2020;12(556):eaau9959. doi:10.1126/scitranslmed.aau9959.
26. Willis KA, Siefker DT, Aziz MM, et al. Perinatal maternal antibiotic exposure augments lung injury in offspring in experimental bronchopulmonary dysplasia. *Am J Physiol Lung Cell Mol Physiol.* 2020;318(2):L407-L418.
27. Dolma K, Freeman AE, Rezonzew G, et al. Effects of hyperoxia on alveolar and pulmonary vascular development in germ-free

mice. *Am J Physiol Lung Cell Mol Physiol.* 2020;318(2):L421-L428.

28. Lal CV, Olave N, Travers C, et al. Exosomal microRNA predicts and protects against severe bronchopulmonary dysplasia in extremely premature infants. *JCI Insight.* 2018;3(5):e93994. doi:10.1172/jci.insight.93994.

29. Lal CV, Kandasamy J, Dolma K, et al. Early airway microbial metagenomic and metabolomic signatures are associated with development of severe bronchopulmonary dysplasia. *Am J Physiol Lung Cell Mol Physiol.* 2018;315(5):L810-L815.

30. Budden KF, Gellatly SL, Wood DL, et al. Emerging pathogenic links between microbiota and the gut-lung axis. *Nat Rev Microbiol.* 2017;15(1):55-63.

31. Dickson RP, Singer BH, Newstead MW, et al. Enrichment of the lung microbiome with gut bacteria in sepsis and the acute respiratory distress syndrome. *Nat Microbiol.* 2016;1(10):16113. doi:10.1038/nmicrobiol.2016.113.

32. Viscardi RM. Ureaplasma species: role in neonatal morbidities and outcomes. *Arch Dis Child Fetal Neonatal Ed.* 2014;99(1):F87-F92.

33. Glass JI, Lefkowitz EJ, Glass JS, Heiner CR, Chen EY, Cassell GH. The complete sequence of the mucosal pathogen *Ureaplasma urealyticum. Nature.* 2000;407(6805):757-762.

34. Abele-Horn M, Wolff C, Dressel P, Pfaff F, Zimmermann A. Association of *Ureaplasma urealyticum* biovars with clinical outcome for neonates, obstetric patients, and gynecological patients with pelvic inflammatory disease. *J Clin Microbiol.* 1997; 35:1199-1202.

35. Kasper DC, Mechtler TP, Reischer GH, et al. The bacterial load of *Ureaplasma parvum* in amniotic fluid is correlated with an increased intrauterine inflammatory response. *Diagn Microbiol Infect Dis.* 2010;67(2):117-121.

36. Motomura K, Romero R, Xu Y, et al. Intra-Amniotic Infection with *Ureaplasma parvum* causes preterm birth and neonatal mortality that are prevented by treatment with clarithromycin. *mBio.* 2020;11(3):e00797-20. doi:10.1128/mBio.00797-20.

37. Sung TJ, Xiao L, Duffy L, Waites KB, Chesko KL, Viscardi RM. Frequency of ureaplasma serovars in respiratory secretions of preterm infants at risk for bronchopulmonary dysplasia. *Pediatr Infect Dis J.* 2011;30(5):379-383.

38. Viscardi RM, Hashmi N, Gross GW, Sun CC, Rodriguez A, Fairchild KD. Incidence of invasive ureaplasma in VLBW infants: relationship to severe intraventricular hemorrhage. *J Perinatol.* 2008;28(11):759-765.

39. Grattard F, Soleihac B, De Barbeyrac B, Bebear C, Seffert P, Pozzetto B. Epidemiologic and molecular investigations of genital mycoplasmas from women and neonates at delivery. *Pediatr Infect Dis J.* 1995;14:853-858.

40. Hannaford K, Todd DA, Jeffrey H, John E, Byth K, Gilbert GL. Role of *Ureaplasma urealyticum* in lung disease of prematurity. *Arch Dis Child Fetal Neonatal Ed.* 1999;81:F162-F167.

41. Rittenschober-Bohm J, Waldhoer T, Schulz SM, et al. Vaginal *Ureaplasma parvum* serovars and spontaneous preterm birth. *Am J Obstet Gynecol.* 2019;220(6):594.e1-594.e9. doi:10.1016/j.ajog.2019.01.237.

42. Payne MS, Newnham JP, Doherty DA, et al. A specific bacterial DNA signature in the vagina of Australian women in midpregnancy predicts high risk of spontaneous preterm birth (the Predict1000 study). *Am J Obstet Gynecol.* 2021;224(6):635-636. doi:10.1016/j.ajog.2021.02.004.

43. Katz B, Patel P, Duffy L, Schelonka RL, Dimmitt RA, Waites KB. Characterization of ureaplasmas isolated from preterm infants with and without bronchopulmonary dysplasia. *J Clin Microbiol.* 2005;43(9):4852-4854.

44. Xiao L, Glass JI, Paralanov V, et al. Detection and characterization of human ureaplasma species and serovars by real-time PCR. *J Clin Microbiol.* 2010;48(8):2715-2723.

45. Xiao L, Paralanov V, Glass JI, et al. Extensive horizontal gene transfer in ureaplasmas from humans questions the utility of serotyping for diagnostic purposes. *J Clin Microbiol.* 2011;49(8): 2818-2826.

46. Zimmerman CU, Stiedl T, Rosengarten R, Spergser J. Alternate phase variation in expression of two major surface membrane proteins (MBA and UU376) of *Ureaplasma parvum* serovar 3. *FEMS Microbiol Lett.* 2009;292(2):187-193.

47. Zheng X, Watson HL, Waites KB, Cassell GH. Serotype diversity and antigen variation among invasive isolates of *Ureaplasma urealyticum* from neonates. *Infect Immun.* 1992;60:3472-3474.

48. Knox CL, Dando SJ, Nitsos I, et al. The severity of chorioamnionitis in pregnant sheep is associated with in vivo variation of the surface-exposed multiple-banded antigen/gene of *Ureaplasma parvum. Biol Reprod.* 2010;83(3):415-426.

49. Pandelidis K, McCarthy A, Chesko KL, Viscardi RM. Role of biofilm formation in Ureaplasma antibiotic susceptibility and development of bronchopulmonary dysplasia in preterm neonates. *Pediatr Infect Dis J.* 2013;32(4):394-398.

50. Paralanov V, Lu J, Duffy LB, et al. Comparative genome analysis of 19 *Ureaplasma urealyticum* and *Ureaplasma parvum* strains. *BMC Microbiol.* 2012;12:88. doi:10.1186/1471-2180-12-88.

51. Yamamoto T, Kida Y, Sakamoto Y, Kuwano K. Mpn491, a secreted nuclease of *Mycoplasma pneumoniae*, plays a critical role in evading killing by neutrophil extracellular traps. *Cell Microbiol.* 2016;19(3). doi:10.1111/cmi.12666.

52. Xiao L, Crabb DM, Dai Y, Chen Y, Waites KB, Atkinson TP. Suppression of antimicrobial peptide expression by ureaplasma species. *Infect Immun.* 2014;82(4):1657-1665.

53. Gomez-Lopez N, Romero R, Leng Y, et al. Neutrophil extracellular traps in acute chorioamnionitis: a mechanism of host defense. *Am J Reprod Immunol.* 2017;77(3):10.1111/aji.12617. doi:10.1111/aji.12617.

54. Van Mechelen K, Meeus M, Matheeussen V, Donders G, Jacquemyn Y, Mahieu L. Association between maternal cervicovaginal swab positivity for *Ureaplasma* spp. or other microorganisms and neonatal respiratory outcome and mortality. *J Perinatol.* 2021;41(6):1-11.

55. Yoon BH, Chang JW, Romero R. Isolation of *Ureaplasma urealyticum* from the amniotic cavity and adverse outcome in preterm labor. *Obstet Gynecol.* 1998;92:77-82.

56. Romero R, Yoon BH, Mazor M, et al. A comparative study of the diagnostic performance of amniotic fluid glucose, white blood cell count, interleukin-6, and Gram stain in the detection of microbial invasion in patients with preterm premature rupture of membranes. *Am J Obstet Gynecol.* 1993;169:839-851.

57. Hassan S, Romero R, Hendler I, et al. A sonographic short cervix as the only clinical manifestation of intra-amniotic infection. *J Perinat Med.* 2006;34(1):13-19.

58. Yoon BH, Romero R, Lim JH, et al. The clinical significance of detecting *Ureaplasma urealyticum* by the polymerase chain reaction in the amniotic fluid of patients with preterm labor. *Am J Obstet Gynecol.* 2003;189:919-924.

59. Kirchner L, Helmer H, Heinze G, et al. Amnionitis with *Ureaplasma urealyticum* or other microbes leads to increased morbidity and prolonged hospitalization in very low birth weight infants. *Eur J Obstet Gynecol Reprod Biol.* 2007;134(1):44-50.

60. Onderdonk AB, Delaney ML, DuBois AM, Allred EN, Leviton A. Detection of bacteria in placental tissues obtained from extremely low gestational age neonates. *Am J Obstet Gynecol.* 2008;198(1):110.e1-110.e7.

61. Olomu IN, Hecht JL, Onderdonk AO, Allred EN, Leviton A. Perinatal correlates of *Ureaplasma urealyticum* in placenta parenchyma of singleton pregnancies that end before 28 weeks of gestation. *Pediatrics.* 2009;123(5):1329-1336.

62. Kundsin RB, Leviton A, Allred EN, Poulin SA. *Ureaplasma urealyticum* infection of the placenta in pregnancies that ended prematurely. *Obstet Gynecol.* 1996;87:122-127.

63. Dammann O, Allred EN, Genest DR, Kundsin RB, Leviton A. Antenatal mycoplasma infection, the fetal inflammatory response and cerebral white matter damage in very-low-birth-weight infants. *Paediatr Perinat Epidemiol.* 2003;17(1):49-57.

64. Berg TG, Philpot KL, Welsh MS, Sanger WG, Smith CV. Ureaplasma/Mycoplasma-infected amniotic fluid: pregnancy outcome in treated and nontreated patients. *J Perinatol.* 1999; 19(4):275-277.

65. Perni SC, Vardhana S, Korneeva I, et al. *Mycoplasma hominis* and *Ureaplasma urealyticum* in midtrimester amniotic fluid: association with amniotic fluid cytokine levels and pregnancy outcome. *Am J Obstet Gynecol.* 2004;191(4):1382-1386.

66. Witt A, Berger A, Gruber CJ, et al. Increased intrauterine frequency of *Ureaplasma urealyticum* in women with preterm labor and preterm premature rupture of the membranes and subsequent cesarean delivery. *Am J Obstet Gynecol.* 2005; 193(5):1663-1669.

67. Namba F, Hasegawa T, Nakayama M, et al. Placental features of chorioamnionitis colonized with Ureaplasma species in preterm delivery. *Pediatr Res.* 2010;67(2):166-172.

68. Normann E, Lacaze-Masmonteil T, Eaton F, Schwendimann L, Gressens P, Thebaud B. A novel mouse model of Ureaplasma-induced perinatal inflammation: effects on lung and brain injury. *Pediatr Res.* 2009;65(4):430-436.

69. Pavlidis I, Spiller OB, Sammut Demarco G, et al. Cervical epithelial damage promotes *Ureaplasma parvum* ascending infection, intrauterine inflammation and preterm birth induction in mice. *Nat Commun.* 2020;11(1):199. doi:10.1038/s41467-019-14089-y.

70. Moss TJ, Nitsos I, Ikegami M, Jobe AH, Newnham JP. Experimental intrauterine *Ureaplasma* infection in sheep. *Am J Obstet Gynecol.* 2005;192(4):1179-1186.

71. Moss TJ, Knox CL, Kallapur SG, et al. Experimental amniotic fluid infection in sheep: effects of *Ureaplasma parvum* serovars 3 and 6 on preterm or term fetal sheep. *Am J Obstet Gynecol.* 2008;198(1):122.e1-122.e8.

72. Widowski H, Ophelders D, van Leeuwen A, et al. Chorioamnionitis induces changes in ovine pulmonary endogenous epithelial stem/progenitor cells in utero. *Pediatr Res.* 2021; 90(3):549-558.

73. Widowski H, Reynaert NL, Ophelders D, et al. Sequential exposure to antenatal microbial triggers attenuates alveolar growth and pulmonary vascular development and impacts pulmonary epithelial stem/progenitor cells. *Front Med (Lausanne).* 2021;8:614239. doi:10.3389/fmed.2021.614239.

74. Novy MJ, Duffy L, Axthelm MK, et al. *Ureaplasma parvum* or *Mycoplasma hominis* as sole pathogens cause chorioamnionitis, preterm delivery, and fetal pneumonia in rhesus macaques. *Reprod Sci.* 2009;16(1):56-70.

75. Kelleher MA, Liu Z, Wang X, et al. Beyond the uterine environment: a nonhuman primate model to investigate maternal-fetal and neonatal outcomes following chronic intrauterine infection. *Pediatr Res.* 2017;82(2):244-252.

76. Yoon BH, Romero R, Chang JW, et al. Microbial invasion of the amniotic cavity with *Ureaplasma urealyticum* is associated with a robust host response in fetal, amniotic, and maternal compartments. *Am J Obstet Gynecol.* 1998;179:1254-1260.

77. Yoneda N, Yoneda S, Niimi H, et al. Polymicrobial amniotic fluid infection with mycoplasma/ureaplasma and other bacteria induces severe intra-amniotic inflammation associated with poor perinatal prognosis in preterm labor. *Am J Reprod Immunol.* 2016;75(2):112-125.

78. Bashiri A, Horowitz S, Huleihel M, Hackmon R, Dukler D, Mazor M. Elevated concentrations of interleukin-6 in intra-amniotic infection with *Ureaplasma urealyticum* in asymptomatic women during genetic amniocentesis. *Acta Obstet Gynecol Scand.* 1999;78(5):379-382.

79. Lal CV, Xu X, Jackson P, et al. Ureaplasma infection-mediated release of matrix metalloproteinase-9 and PGP: a novel mechanism of preterm rupture of membranes and chorioamnionitis. *Pediatr Res.* 2017;81(1-1):75-79.

80. Estrada-Gutierrez G, Gomez-Lopez N, Zaga-Clavellina V, et al. Interaction between pathogenic bacteria and intrauterine leukocytes triggers alternative molecular signaling cascades leading to labor in women. *Infect Immun.* 2010;78(11):4792-4799.

81. Silwedel C, Fehrholz M, Speer CP, Ruf KC, Manig S, Glaser K. Differential modulation of pulmonary caspases: Is this the key to Ureaplasma-driven chronic inflammation? *PLoS One.* 2019; 14(5):e0216569. doi:10.1371/journal.pone.0216569.

82. Panero A, Pacifico L, Roggini M, Chiesa C. *Ureaplasma urealyticum* as a cause of pneumonia in preterm infants: analysis of the white cell response. *Arch Dis Child.* 1995;73:F37-F40.

83. Wang EL, Ohlsson A, Kellner JD. Association of *Ureaplasma urealyticum* colonization with chronic lung disease of prematurity: results of a metaanalysis. *J Pediatr.* 1995;127:640-644.

84. Castro-Alcaraz S, Greenberg EM, Bateman DA, Regan JA. Patterns of colonization with *Ureaplasma urealyticum* during neonatal intensive care unit hospitalizations of very low birth weight infants and the development of chronic lung disease. *Pediatrics.* 2002;110(4):E45-E45.

85. Lowe J, Watkins WJ, Edwards MO, et al. Association between pulmonary ureaplasma colonization and bronchopulmonary dysplasia in preterm infants: updated systematic review and meta-analysis. *Pediatr Infect Dis J.* 2014;33(7):697-702.

86. Schelonka RL, Katz B, Waites KB, Benjamin Jr DK. Critical appraisal of the role of Ureaplasma in the development of bronchopulmonary dysplasia with metaanalytic techniques. *Pediatr Infect Dis J.* 2005;24(12):1033-1039.

87. Brand MC, Mandy GT, Arora S, et al. Optimum Detection of Ureaplasma in Premature Infants. *Pediatr Infect Dis J.* 2018; 37(12):1294-1298.

88. Theilen U, Lyon AJ, Fitzgerald T, Hendry GM, Keeling JW. Infection with *Ureaplasma urealyticum*: is there a specific clinical and radiological course in the preterm infant? *Arch Dis Child Fetal Neonatal Ed.* 2004;89(2):F163-F167.

89. Sun T, Fu J. Analysis of the clinical features of intrauterine *Ureaplasma urealyticum* infection in preterm infants: a case-control study. *Front Pediatr.* 2021;9:774150. doi:10.3389/fped.2021.774150.

90. Pacifico L, Panero A, Roggini M, Rossi N, Bucci G, Chiesa C. *Ureaplasma urealyticum* and pulmonary outcome in a neonatal intensive care population. *Pediatr Infect Dis.* 1997;16:579-586.

91. Honma Y, Yada Y, Takahashi N, Momoi MY, Nakamura Y. Certain type of chronic lung disease of newborns is associated with *Ureaplasma urealyticum* infection in utero. *Pediatr Int.* 2007; 49(4):479-484.

92. Viscardi RM, Kallapur SG. Role of *Ureaplasma* respiratory tract colonization in bronchopulmonary dysplasia pathogenesis: current concepts and update. *Clin Perinatol.* 2015;42(4):719-738.

93. Viscardi RM, Terrin ML, Magder LS, et al. Randomised trial of azithromycin to eradicate Ureaplasma in preterm infants. *Arch Dis Child Fetal Neonatal Ed.* 2020;105(6):615-622.

94. Viscardi RM, Manimtim WM, Sun CCJ, Duffy L, Cassell GH. Lung pathology in premature infants with *Ureaplasma urealyticum* infection. *Pediatr Devel Pathol.* 2002;5:141-150.

95. Viscardi R, Manimtim W, He JR, et al. Disordered pulmonary myofibroblast distribution and elastin expression in preterm infants with *Ureaplasma urealyticum* pneumonitis. *Pediatr Dev Pathol.* 2006;9(2):143-151.

96. Glaser K, Gradzka-Luczewska A, Szymankiewicz-Breborowicz M, et al. Perinatal Ureaplasma exposure Is associated with increased risk of late onset sepsis and imbalanced inflammation in preterm infants and may add to lung injury. *Front Cell Infect Microbiol.* 2019;9:68. doi:10.3389/fcimb.2019.00068.

97. Viscardi RM, Atamas SP, Luzina IG, et al. Antenatal *Ureaplasma urealyticum* respiratory tract infection stimulates proinflammatory, profibrotic responses in the preterm baboon lung. *Pediatr Res.* 2006;60(2):141-146.

98. Groneck P, Goetze-Speer B, Speer CP. Inflammatory bronchopulmonary response of preterm infants with microbial colonisation of the airways at birth. *Arch Dis Child Fetal Neonatal Ed.* 1996;74:F51-F55.

99. Baier RJ, Loggins J, Kruger TE. Monocyte chemoattractant protein-1 and interleukin-8 are increased in bronchopulmonary dysplasia: relation to isolation of *Ureaplasma urealyticum*. *J Invest Med.* 2001;49(4):362-369.

100. Walsh WF, Butler J, Coalson J, Hensley D, Cassell GH, deLemos RA. A primate model of *Ureaplasma urealyticum* infection in the premature infant with hyaline membrane disease. *Clin Infect Dis.* 1993;17(suppl 1):S158-S162.

101. Rudd PT, Cassell GH, Waites KB, Davis JK, Duffy LB. *Ureaplasma urealyticum* pneumonia: experimental production and demonstration of age-related susceptibility. *Infect Immun.* 1989;57:918-925.

102. Crouse DT, Cassell GH, Waites KB, Foster JM, Cassady G. Hyeroxia potentiates *Ureaplasma urealyticum* pneumonia in newborn mice. *Infect Immun.* 1990;58:3487-3493.

103. Viscardi RM, Kaplan J, Lovchik JC, et al. Characterization of a murine model of *Ureaplasma urealyticum* pneumonia. *Infect Immun.* 2002;70:5721-5729.

104. Yoder BA, Coalson JJ, Winter VT, Siler-Khodr T, Duffy LB, Cassell GH. Effects of antenatal colonization with *Ureaplasma urealyticum* on pulmonary disease in the immature baboon. *Pediatr Res.* 2003;54:797-807.

105. Collins JJ, Kallapur SG, Knox CL, et al. Inflammation in fetal sheep from intra-amniotic injection of *Ureaplasma parvum*. *Am J Physiol Lung Cell Mol Physiol.* 2010;299(6):L852-L860.

106. Polglase GR, Dalton RG, Nitsos I, et al. Pulmonary vascular and alveolar development in preterm lambs chronically colonized with *Ureaplasma parvum*. *Am J Physiol Lung Cell Mol Physiol.* 2010;299(2):L232-L241.

107. Li YH, Brauner A, Jonsson B, et al. *Ureaplasma urealyticum*-induced production of proinflammatory cytokines by macrophages. *Pediatr Res.* 2000;48:114-119.

108. Li YH, Yan ZQ, Jensen JS, Tullus K, Brauner A. Activation of nuclear factor kappaB and induction of inducible nitric oxide synthase by *Ureaplasma urealyticum* in macrophages. *Infect Immun.* 2000;68(12):7087-7093.

109. Li YH, Brauner A, Jensen JS, Tullus K. Induction of human macrophage vascular endothelial growth factor and intercellular adhesion molecule-1 by *Ureaplasma urealyticum* and downregulation by steroids. *Biol Neonate.* 2002;82(1):22-28.

110. Li YH, Chen M, Brauner A, Zheng C, Skov Jensen J, Tullus K. *Ureaplasma urealyticum* induces apoptosis in human lung epithelial cells and macrophages. *Biol Neonate.* 2002;82(3): 166-173.

111. Manimtim WM, Hasday JD, Hester L, Fairchild KD, Lovchik JC, Viscardi RM. *Ureaplasma urealyticum* modulates endotoxin-induced cytokine release by human monocytes derived from preterm and term newborns and adults. *Infect Immun.* 2001; 69(6):3906-3915.

112. Depicolzuane L, Phelps DS, Floros J. Surfactant protein-A function: knowledge gained from SP-A knockout mice. *Front Pediatr.* 2021;9:799693. doi:10.3389/fped.2021.799693.

113. Famuyide ME, Hasday JD, Carter HC, Chesko KL, He JR, Viscardi RM. Surfactant protein-A limits Ureaplasma-mediated lung inflammation in a murine pneumonia model. *Pediatr Res.* 2009;66(2):162-167.

114. Okogbule-Wonodi AC, Chesko KL, Famuyide ME, Viscardi RM. Surfactant protein-A enhances ureaplasmacidal activity in Vitro. *Innate Immun.* 2011;17(2):145-151. doi:10.1177/1753425909360552.

115. Kaisho T, Akira S. Pleiotropic function of Toll-like receptors. *Microbes Infect.* 2004;6(15):1388-1394.

116. Peltier MR, Freeman AJ, Mu HH, Cole BC. Characterization of the macrophage-stimulating activity from *Ureaplasma urealyticum*. *Am J Reprod Immunol.* 2007;57(3):186-192.

117. Shimizu T, Kida Y, Kuwano K. *Ureaplasma parvum* lipoproteins, including MB antigen, activate NF-{kappa}B through TLR1, TLR2 and TLR6. *Microbiology.* 2008;154(Pt 5):1318-1325.

118. Harju K, Glumoff V, Hallman M. Ontogeny of Toll-like receptors Tlr2 and Tlr4 in mice. *Pediatr Res.* 2001;49(1):81-83.

119. Hillman NH, Moss TJ, Nitsos I, et al. Toll-like receptors and agonist responses in the developing fetal sheep lung. *Pediatr Res.* 2008;63(4):388-393.

120. Awasthi S, Cropper J, Brown KM. Developmental expression of Toll-like receptors-2 and -4 in preterm baboon lung. *Dev Comp Immunol.* 2008;32(9):1088-1098.

121. Winters AH, Levan TD, Vogel SN, Chesko KL, Pollin TI, Viscardi RM. Single nucleotide polymorphism in toll-like receptor 6 is associated with a decreased risk for ureaplasma respiratory tract colonization and bronchopulmonary dysplasia in preterm infants. *Pediatr Infect Dis J.* 2013;32(8):898-904.

122. Renaudin H, Bebear C. Comparative in vitro activity of azithromycin, clarithromycin, erythromycin and lomefloxacin against *Mycoplasma pneumoniae, Mycoplasma hominis* and *Ureaplasma urealyticum*. *Eur J Clin Microbiol Infect Dis.* 1990; 9(11):838-841.

123. Bowman ED, Dharmalingam A, Fan WQ, Brown F, Garland SM. Impact of erythromycin on respiratory colonization of *Ureaplasma urealyticum* and the development of chronic lung disease in extremely low birth weight infants. *Pediatr Infect Dis J.* 1998;17:615-620.

124. Jonsson B, Rylander M, Faxelius G. *Ureaplasma urealyticum*, erythromycin and respiratory morbidity in high-risk preterm neonates. *Acta Paediatr.* 1998;87:1079-1084.

125. Baier RJ, Loggins J, Kruger TE. Failure of erythromycin to eliminate airway colonization with *Ureaplasma urealyticum* in very low birth weight infants. *BMC Pediatr*. 2003;3:10. doi:10.1186/1471-2431-3-10.

126. Rubin BK. Macrolides as biologic response modifiers. *J Respir Dis*. 2002;23:S31-S38.

127. Ianaro A, Ialenti A, Maffia P, et al. Anti-inflammatory activity of macrolide antibiotics. *J Pharmacol Exp Ther*. 2000;292(1): 156-163.

128. Tsai WC, Standiford TJ. Immunomodulatory effects of macrolides in the lung: lessons from in-vitro and in-vivo models. *Curr Pharm Des*. 2004;10(25):3081-3093.

129. Segal LN, Clemente JC, Wu BG, et al. Randomised, double-blind, placebo-controlled trial with azithromycin selects for anti-inflammatory microbial metabolites in the emphysematous lung. *Thorax*. 2017;72(1):13-22.

130. Duffy LB, Crabb D, Searcey K, Kempf MC. Comparative potency of gemifloxacin, new quinolones, macrolides, tetracycline and clindamycin against Mycoplasma spp. *J Antimicrob Chemother*. 2000;45(suppl 1):29-33.

131. Girard AE, Cimochowski CR, Faiella JA. Correlation of increased azithromycin concentrations with phagocyte infiltration into sites of localized infection. *J Antimicrob Chemother*. 1996;37(suppl C):9-19.

132. Patel KB, Xuan D, Tessier PR, Russomanno JH, Quintiliani R, Nightingale CH. Comparison of bronchopulmonary pharmacokinetics of clarithromycin and azithromycin. *Antimicrob Agents Chemother*. 1996;40(10):2375-2379.

133. Capitano B, Mattoes HM, Shore E, et al. Steady-state intrapulmonary concentrations of moxifloxacin, levofloxacin, and azithromycin in older adults. *Chest*. 2004;125(3):965-973.

134. Liao L, Ning Q, Li Y, et al. CXCR2 blockade reduces radical formation in hyperoxia-exposed newborn rat lung. *Pediatr Res*. 2006;60(3):299-303.

135. Walls SA, Kong L, Leeming HA, Placencia FX, Popek EJ, Weisman LE. Antibiotic prophylaxis improves Ureaplasma-associated lung disease in suckling mice. *Pediatr Res*. 2009;66(2):197-202.

136. Hassan HE, Othman AA, Eddington ND, et al. Pharmacokinetics, safety, and biologic effects of azithromycin in extremely preterm infants at risk for ureaplasma colonization and bronchopulmonary dysplasia. *J Clin Pharmacol*. 2011;51(9): 1264-1275.

137. Viscardi RM, Othman AA, Hassan HE, et al. Azithromycin to prevent bronchopulmonary dysplasia in ureaplasma-infected preterm infants: pharmacokinetics, safety, microbial response, and clinical outcomes with a 20-milligram-per-kilogram single intravenous dose. *Antimicrob Agents Chemother*. 2013;57(5):2127-2133.

138. Merchan LM, Hassan HE, Terrin ML, et al. Pharmacokinetics, microbial response, and pulmonary outcomes of multidose intravenous azithromycin in preterm infants at risk for Ureaplasma respiratory colonization. *Antimicrob Agents Chemother*. 2015;59(1):570-578.

139. Viscardi RM, Terrin ML, Magder LS, et al. Randomized trial of azithromycin to eradicate Ureaplasma respiratory colonization in preterm infants: 2-year outcomes. *Pediatr Res*. 2022;91(1): 178-187. doi:10.1038/s41390-021-01437-2.

140. Lowe J, Gillespie D, Hubbard M, et al. Study protocol: azithromycin therapy for chronic lung disease of prematurity (AZTEC): a randomised, placebo-controlled trial of azithromycin for the prevention of chronic lung disease of prematurity in preterm infants. *BMJ Open*. 2020;10(10):e041528. doi:10.1136/bmjopen-2020-041528.

Chapter 5

Ventilator-Associated Pneumonia

Thomas Alexander Hooven and Richard A. Polin

Chapter Outline

Introduction

Definition

Epidemiology

Pathogenesis

Treatment

Prevention

Outcomes

Future Research Directions

Conclusion

Key Points

- Invasive mechanical ventilation of neonates increases their risk of developing bacterial infection of the lower airways and lung parenchyma, which is termed "ventilator-associated pneumonia" (VAP).
- VAP is diagnosed on the basis of defined clinical, radiographic, and laboratory criteria.
- Unlike other neonatal bacterial infections, culture isolation of a single, causative organism is unusual in VAP.
- Suspected VAP should initially be treated with broad-spectrum antibiotics covering both gram-negative and gram-positive microorganisms.
- Selection of antibiotics should depend on the antibiogram of organisms in the neonatal intensive care unit (NICU) or a given patient.
- As treatment progresses, empiric antibiotic coverage should be narrowed—as possible—based on available data.
- VAP is associated with prolonged hospitalization and poor clinical outcomes, including death.
- VAP "bundles," consisting of standard practices universally applied to prevent pneumonia among intubated patients, are accruing strong evidence and are now in widespread use.

Introduction

Infants in the neonatal intensive care unit (NICU) requiring mechanical ventilation (MV) can develop superimposed bacterial infection of the small airways and lung parenchyma, which is termed *ventilator-associated pneumonia* (VAP). VAP is classified as a type of health care–associated infection (also known as nosocomial infection). Health care–associated infections have come under increasing scrutiny as potentially preventable contributors to poor hospitalization outcomes and ballooning costs of inpatient care.

VAP is difficult to diagnose in the neonate and therefore requires a high index of suspicion. The concept of VAP first emerged in literature from adult ICUs, where a specific etiologic diagnosis can be aided by invasive airway sampling through bronchial brushings or lavage—techniques that are rarely used in the NICU. Adding further challenge to identifying VAP in the neonate is the fact that affected infants often have chronic pulmonary inflammation and dysfunction related to prematurity and respiratory support, which can complicate the diagnostic impression and make infection difficult to detect. Finally, as is the case with neonatal infection in general, infants with VAP show fewer localizing signs and symptoms than older children and adults, often presenting with general deterioration that may not immediately be attributed to VAP.

Nevertheless, with increasing awareness of VAP as a contributor to poor NICU outcomes, guidelines for diagnosis, management, and prevention have been developed and refined. This chapter reviews VAP epidemiology, pathogenesis, and the latest recommendations for limiting its impact on neonatal health.

Definition

The Centers for Disease Control and Prevention (CDC)/National Nosocomial Infections Surveillance (NNIS) define VAP as pneumonia occurring in the setting of at least 2 days of MV through an endotracheal tube (ETT). Noninvasive forms of ventilation such as nasal continuous positive airway pressure or intermittent positive pressure through nasal prongs do not qualify. Formal criteria for diagnosing pneumonia are based on a combination of radiographic, laboratory, and clinical findings.

When there is underlying respiratory or cardiac disease (such as respiratory distress syndrome, chronic lung disease, or a patent ductus arteriosus), at least two serial chest radiographs demonstrating a new or progressive focal infiltrate, consolidation, cavitation, or pneumatocele are required to meet the radiographic diagnostic criteria for pneumonia. For an infant with no preexisting pulmonary or cardiac disease, a single chest radiograph demonstrating one or more of the above features is sufficient.

The clinical and laboratory findings required to diagnose pneumonia in patients younger than 1 year of age include worsening gas exchange (manifesting as desaturations, need for increasing ventilator settings, and/or a rising fraction of inspired oxygen requirement) *and* at least three of the following:

- Temperature instability
- Leukopenia ($\leq$4000 white blood cells/mm^3) or leukocytosis ($\geq$15,000 white blood cells/mm^3) and left shift (>10% band forms)
- New onset of purulent sputum, change in character of sputum, or increased respiratory secretions requiring increased suctioning frequency
- Apnea, tachypnea, or retractions of the chest wall

- Wheezing, rales, or rhonchi
- Bradycardia (<100 beats/min) or tachycardia (>170 beats/min)

In studies of VAP that have reported on the frequency of different clinical signs in newborns, the need for increased ventilator settings, increased airway secretions, and a new radiographic infiltrate have been described as the most common.[1]

Some authors have argued for inclusion of microbiologic criteria in the definition of VAP, and positive culture results from suctioned sputum, bronchoscopy, blind bronchoalveolar lavage (BAL), or pleural fluid have sometimes been included as diagnostic criteria in clinical studies. However, there are several downsides to relying on microbiologic evidence of VAP in neonates. For example, suctioned secretion samples are frequently contaminated with bacteria colonizing the oropharynx and upper airway. The use of BAL may reduce this contamination. Comparisons between concurrent cultures of secretions suctioned from an ETT and BAL have shown that BAL samples are less likely to yield polymicrobial growth, suggesting less oropharyngeal and upper airway commensal contamination. However, BAL can be technically challenging in smaller patients and may not be feasible in an unstable infant. Bronchoscopy poses the same, if not greater, risks as BAL. Large infectious pleural effusions are unusual in neonatal VAP; therefore, pleurocentesis should be reserved for cases when an effusion is hindering respiratory mechanics. Blood cultures are not reliable for diagnosing VAP.

Although not required to diagnose VAP, gram stain and culture of a tracheal aspirate sample can provide valuable supplemental evidence. A gram stain of tracheal secretions that shows a significant leukocytic infiltrate and a high bacterial load is consistent with VAP, and the bacterial morphology can potentially help inform antibiotic selection (see "Treatment" section). Serial cultures and microscopic assessments of tracheal aspirate samples during treatment can be useful gauges of the patient's response to antibiotics. Results from tracheal suction samples should not be considered definitive, however, and the diagnosis of VAP can be made solely based on radiographic, clinical, and laboratory criteria described previously and summarized in Box 5.1.

BOX 5.1 CENTERS FOR DISEASE CONTROL AND PREVENTION/NATIONAL NOSOCOMIAL INFECTIONS SURVEILLANCE DEFINITION OF VAP[a]

Radiographic	Worsening Gas Exchange	Clinical/Laboratory Evidence
If there is an underlying pulmonary or cardiac disease, two serial x-rays demonstrating at least one of the following: • New or progressive infiltrate • Consolidation • Cavitation • Pneumatocele If there is no underlying pulmonary or cardiac disease, *one definitive imaging test result is acceptable.*	Any of the following: • Oxygen desaturation • Increased oxygen requirement • Increased ventilator demand	Must have *at least three* of the following: • Temperature instability • Leukopenia ($\leq$4000 WBC/mm^3) or leukocytosis ($\geq$15,000 WBC/mm^3) and left shift ($\geq$10% band forms) • New onset of purulent sputum or change in character of sputum, or increased respiratory secretions or increased suctioning requirements • Apnea, tachypnea, nasal flaring with retractions of the chest wall or nasal flaring with grunting • Wheezing, rales, or rhonchi • Cough • Bradycardia (<100 beats/min) or tachycardia (>170 beats/min)

VAP, Ventilator-associated pneumonia; *WBC*, white blood cell.
[a]Infants receiving mechanical ventilation through an endotracheal tube for at least 48 hours must meet criteria in *all three columns.*

Epidemiology

While the reported incidence of VAP varies depending on the source, neonatal VAP is common, accounting for 6.8% to 32.2% of health care–associated infections in level II and level III NICUs in the United States.[2] VAP rates appear to be decreasing. Sequential reports from the National Healthcare Safety Network, published in 2009 and 2013, showed a drop from 1.9 to 1.2 cases of VAP per 1000 ventilator days in level II and level III NICUs.[3,4] In 2021, the National Healthcare Safety Network chose to stop surveying and reporting neonatal VAP rates, electing instead to adopt a more broadly defined entity termed *ventilator-associated event* (VAE). A VAE consists of increased respiratory support requirements in a previously stable, mechanically ventilated patient. Radiographic and laboratory criteria are not part of the VAE definition. The reason for this change (which had already been implemented in adult populations) was the consensus that the CDC criteria for neonatal VAP diagnosis were too subjective for accurate inclusion in a surveillance algorithm. VAE is not intended as a clinical diagnosis and is meant for epidemiologic tracking only.

Prematurity, low birth weight, and duration of MV have all been identified as major risk factors for VAP in multiple studies. Since smaller, sicker patients tend to require longer treatment with MV, it is difficult to conclusively establish which of these variables are independent risks. Several authors have shown statistically significant differences in VAP incidence per 1000 ventilator days based on gestational age, but this analytical approach could be confounded by an uneven distribution of MV duration within preterm and term populations.

Cernada et al. published a prospective study of VAP in 198 neonates (gestational age range 27–37 weeks) intubated for more than 48 hours; VAP developed in 18 of the infants. In a multivariate regression model, only duration of MV emerged as an independent risk factor for VAP.[1] In contrast, Apisarnthanarak et al. performed logistical regression analysis on data from 19 extremely premature infants with VAP and found no significant independent risk from each additional week of MV.[5] Instead, that group identified prior bloodstream infection as an independent risk factor for preterm VAP, although there was no significant relationship between the organism causing the prior bloodstream infection and the isolate (if any) responsible for pneumonia. One possibility is that treatment of an earlier infection with antibiotics may alter the microbiome of the neonate and allow colonization with pathogens more likely to cause VAP.

The infection control infrastructure of the NICU may also significantly affect local rates of VAP. An observational study by Goldmann et al. reported a 16-fold decrease in VAP after relocation of their nursery to a new facility with 50% more staffing, improved isolation and cohorting capacity, more sinks, and better air filtration.[6] Other potential risk factors for VAP include administration of opiates for sedation during intubation, frequent suctioning (>8 times per day), and reintubation.[7]

Pathogenesis

The most common organisms cultured from respiratory cultures in the setting of neonatal VAP are *Pseudomonas aeruginosa*, *Enterobacter* spp., *Klebsiella* spp., and *Staphylococcus aureus* (Box 5.2). Tracheal aspirates from the ETT almost always yield polymicrobial growth owing to commensal contamination. BAL samples have a higher likelihood of growing a single isolate, but Cernada et al. still reported that 16% of BAL samples from neonates with VAP grew multiple organisms.[1] Therefore it is likely that VAP often results from polymicrobial overgrowth rather than a single pathogen.

Immature innate immunity in the neonate increases the risk of VAP. Low immunoglobin levels (particularly in the premature population) and functionally impaired alveolar neutrophils and macrophages limit

opsonization and phagocytosis of bacteria in the lower airways. Tissue damage from chronic inflammation, atelectasis, and pulmonary edema create potential niduses of infection and impede normal mucosal barrier functions and ciliary clearance of debris.

Although intubation can be lifesaving, the ETT itself contributes to VAP in multiple ways. It creates a physical barrier to ciliary action, prevents effective coughing, and provides a protected milieu for high-density bacterial colonization and biofilm formation. Zur et al. used electron microscopy to demonstrate progressive biofilm growth on the inner luminal and outer surfaces of ETTs from neonates intubated for at least 12 hours (Fig. 5.1).[8] Adair et al. performed within-patient comparisons of bacterial culture results from respiratory secretions and ETT biofilm swabs in 40 intubated patients and used genotyping to confirm clonal matches.[9] Patients with VAP showed high correlation between ETT and sputum isolates, whereas controls without VAP showed no statistical correlation, suggesting that the ETT serves as a reservoir for pathogenic organisms once infection is established.

VAP develops from overgrowth of bacteria colonizing the oropharynx, which may have been present before intubation or may become introduced afterward from contaminated oral or gastric secretions. Through alterations in the tracheobronchial milieu described earlier, MV leads to positive selection for these organisms, followed by tracheal colonization and population expansion in the lower airways (Fig. 5.2).

Patient positioning may influence pooling of orogastric secretions and the propensity of oropharyngeal commensals to be drawn into the trachea. Aly et al. performed a randomized controlled trial to test the hypothesis that gravity contributes to tracheal colonization, which may progress to VAP.[10] They compared tracheal cultures among 60 intubated infants who were maintained in either supine or side-lying positions and showed that after 5 days of intubation, there was significantly more tracheal colonization among the supine group, which also had higher tracheal bacterial density and greater introduction of new species over the observation period.

The contribution of gastric bacteria to VAP pathogenesis is uncertain. Some experimental evidence supports the hypothesis that the stomach serves as a

BOX 5.2 VAP PATHOGENS RANKED FROM MOST COMMON TO LEAST COMMON[a]

PATHOGEN

Pseudomonas aeruginosa
Enterobacter spp.
Klebsiella spp.
Staphylococcus aureus
Escherichia coli
Enterococcus spp.
Acinetobacter spp.
Proteus spp.
Citrobacter spp.
Stenotrophomonas maltophilia
Group B *Streptococcus*

[a]Based on multiple studies; exact order may vary depending on local factors.

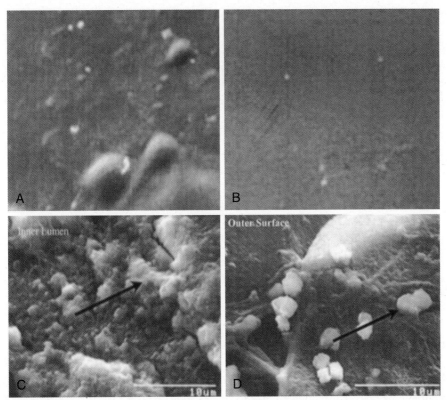

Fig. 5.1 Electron micrographs of the inner (A) and outer (B) surfaces of a sterile endotracheal tube before use and the inner (C) and outer (D) surfaces after 8 days of intubation. The 8-day micrographs demonstrate individual cocci *(arrows)* within a thick biofilm. (Adapted from Zur KB, Mandell DL, Gordon RE, et al. Electron microscopic analysis of biofilm on endotracheal tubes removed from intubated neonates. *Otolaryngol Head Neck Surg.* 2004;130(4):407-414. Reprinted with permission.)

reservoir for potential VAP pathogens. Gastric pepsin has been shown to be present in the lungs of intubated neonates, indicating that gastric secretions are commonly aspirated in this population. One study measured tracheal pepsin among intubated neonates and identified a reliable inverse relationship with the degree of head of bed elevation.[11] In a study of 19 intubated adults in a medical ICU, technetium labeling of gastric contents was followed by scintigraphy of endotracheal suctioning samples to assess for migration of gastric bacteria to the lungs. Radioactivity counts were compared between patients maintained in a supine versus a semirecumbent position. Migration occurred in both groups but happened more quickly among patients in the supine position, again indicating a role of patient positioning in the pathogenesis of VAP.[12]

Other studies have cast doubt on the theory that gastric bacteria are a major cause of VAP. Cardeñosa Cendrero et al. performed daily, simultaneous sampling of the trachea, pharynx, and stomach in 123 adults receiving MV to study temporal patterns of colonization and invasion. Nineteen patients in whom VAP developed subsequently underwent bronchoscopy with BAL and protected brush sampling. There was no evidence of primary gastric colonization for any of the VAP isolates, which generally matched preceding tracheal colonizers.[13] A smaller study by Feldman et al. with a similar design also did not reveal any evidence of primary gastric colonization with eventual VAP pathogens.[14]

Recent studies have begun to explore how early colonization events and subsequent evolution of airway colonizing bacteria affect neonatal health. Several

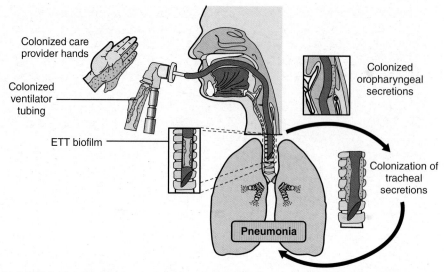

Fig. 5.2 Pathogenesis of ventilator-associated pneumonia. Colonization of the upper airway can originate from care provider hands, ventilator equipment, oropharyngeal secretions, or a biofilm within the endotracheal tube *(ETT)*. Ultimately, pathogenic organisms spread into the trachea, where the population expands and moves downward into the small airways and lung parenchyma, causing pneumonia. (Adapted from illustrations by Walter Earhart from Garland JS. Strategies to prevent ventilator-associated pneumonia in neonates. *Clin Perinatol.* 2010;37(3):629-643. Reprinted with permission.)

studies have shown that the newborn airway becomes colonized at the time of birth with a founder population of bacteria dominated by *Ureaplasma* and *Staphylococcus*.[15] With time, this early population gradually diversifies, eventually establishing "community states" characterized by temporally stable bacterial abundances.[16] While certain airway community states in low-birth-weight or premature infants may favor inflammatory immune activation and eventual development of pulmonary disease, such as bronchopulmonary dysplasia (BPD), it remains unclear whether there are identifiable airway microbiome patterns that predispose to neonatal VAP. Disruption of stable community states, such as through administration of broad-spectrum antibiotics, may allow expansion of virulent subpopulations. One longitudinal study of a cohort of preterm neonates showed increased abundance of *Pseudomonas aeruginosa* and a novel *Mycoplasma* species in one patient following antibiotic administration.[17] A very recent concept is the "gut-lung microbiome axis," which hypothesizes a dynamic interplay between evolving bacterial populations in the newborn intestine and airways—both influenced by and exerting influence over the infant's developing immune system.[16,18] Ongoing research in this field is revealing complex host-microbe interactions in the newborn lung that may eventually lead to greater insights about risk factors for VAP.

In summary, VAP pathogenesis data are limited and—in some regard—contradictory. The current model is also derived largely from adult research, which may limit its generalizability to the neonatal population. Based on the available evidence, the key steps of VAP pathogenesis seem to be initial tracheal colonization by one or more potentially virulent microorganisms, followed by progressive distal airway colonization and population expansion. This process is aided by the ETT itself, which offers a protected niche for potential pathogens, alterations in innate pulmonary immunity stemming from prematurity and chronic disease, abnormal establishment or disruption of commensal bacterial airway colonization, and possibly supine positioning, which favors bacterial spread from the upper airways into the lungs, may increase the risk of VAP.

Treatment

The central pillar of VAP treatment is an appropriate course of intravenous antibiotics. However, there are no consensus guidelines for specific antibiotics that should be used to treat VAP in the NICU. Instead, several general principles should guide therapy.

When VAP is suspected, empiric broad-spectrum antibiotics should be initiated promptly. The empiric regimen should be tailored, if possible, to antibiotic resistance patterns of pathogens commonly isolated in the unit and to any bacteria—particularly drug-resistant strains—previously cultured from the patient. Consideration should also be given to any prior courses of antibiotic therapy the patient has received, which might have been selected for drug-resistant organisms. In a recent report from the National Healthcare Safety Network of > 2500 health care facilities, NICUs had the lowest level of nonsusceptible pathogens compared with pediatric intensive care unit (PICU) and adult ICUs.[19] The consensus guidelines for the management of suspected VAP in adults differ between North American[20] and European experts.[21-23] Almost all the recommendations are based on low-quality or very low-quality evidence. Both guidelines agree on risk stratification of patients as low or high risk, but European and US experts define 'high risk' slightly differently (Fig. 5.3).[24] For low-risk patients, both guidelines recommend a single agent active against methicillin-sensitive *S. aureus* and nonresistant gram-negative pathogens or *Pseudomonas*.

Broader antimicrobial therapy is recommended for high-risk patients. Box 5.3 lists suggested empirical therapy for VAP in neonates. These recommendations are based on the degree of illness, likelihood of mortality,[25] and probability of colonization with a resistant pathogen.

Whenever possible, initial empiric therapy should subsequently be narrowed on the basis of culture results and sensitivity testing. Microbiologic data that can inform rational narrowing of empiric antibiotics can come from respiratory secretion cultures from the current illness and any prior cultures that revealed specific colonizers.

As noted earlier, methicillin-resistant *S. aureus* (MRSA) is a common cause of VAP. In a study on antibiotic resistance patterns in VAP isolates from adult patients, 62% of *S. aureus* recovered was methicillin resistant.[26] Prevalence rates of MRSA in the NICU differ between studies but are generally close to 2.0%.[27] Vancomycin or linezolid can be used to treat MRSA. Both drugs have been studied as monotherapy for nosocomial pneumonia (not necessarily ventilator-associated) caused by MRSA in adult and pediatric populations, although they have never been subject to head-to-head comparison in treatment of neonatal VAP. A recent network meta-analysis of randomized clinical trials comparing linezolid with

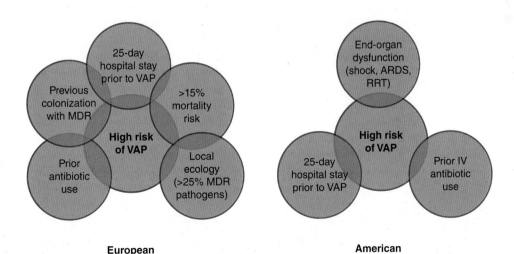

European   **American**

Fig. 5.3 Risk stratification models from European and American expert panels. Factors illustrated increase a patient's risk of developing ventilator-associated pneumonia *(VAP)*. (Adapted from Kelly DN, Martin-Loeches I. Comparing current US and European guidelines for nosocomial pneumonia. *Curr Opin Pulm Med.* 2019;25(3):263-270.)

BOX 5.3 EMPIRIC THERAPY OF SUSPECTED VAP IN THE NEONATAL ICU

1. Hemodynamically stable neonates *not known* to be colonized with MRSA or MDR gram-negative organisms and the prevalence of MRSA in the NICU < 10%
   a. Oxacillin and gentamicin
2. Hemodynamically stable neonates colonized with MRSA or ≥ 10% infants colonized with MRSA in the NICU
   a. Vancomycin and gentamicin
3. Hemodynamically stable neonates colonized with MDR gram-negative organism, but not MRSA and < 10% of infants positive for MRSA in the unit.
   a. Meropenem
4. Critically ill neonates with cardiopulmonary compromise and a high risk of mortality[a]
   a. Vancomycin and meropenem (or)
   b. Vancomycin and ceftazidime (if *Pseudomonas* is detected, add gentamicin)

MDR, Multiple drug resistant.
[a]nSOFA score can be used to estimate mortality.[25]

vancomycin concluded that cure rates were not significantly different.[28] Previous randomized trials and meta-analyses comparing the efficacy of linezolid with vancomycin reached varying conclusions.[29-33] In a prospective study of 39 children with nosocomial pneumonia treated with either linezolid or vancomycin, Jantausch et al. found no significant difference in overall cure rates.[34] However, the group treated with linezolid may have been more severely ill—with higher rates of multilobar pneumonia and longer duration of MV—at treatment initiation. Furthermore, the linezolid group experienced faster resolution of symptoms and shorter treatment durations compared with the vancomycin group.

While prompt initiation of broad-spectrum antibiotics to cover potential drug-resistant pathogens is important, prolonged or repeated treatment with empiric antibiotics increases the risk of a drug-resistant infection in the future and is associated with considerable cost. A Swiss study of antibiotic use among over 450 patients admitted to a combined PICU and NICU between 1998 and 1999 identified suspected pneumonia as the most common reason for initiation of antibiotics (probably reflecting the pediatric population more than the neonates, for whom rule-out sepsis episodes are more common). When the illnesses that prompted antibiotics were subjected to retrospective review, only 41% of

antibiotic courses corresponded to a proven bacterial infection.[35]

Given the challenges associated with isolating a VAP etiologic pathogen described earlier, rationally narrowing antibiotic coverage based on microbiologic evidence can be difficult. One approach is to wait 24 to 48 hours after starting empiric therapy before obtaining a suctioned ETT sample for culture. The rationale is that after exposure to a broad-spectrum regimen, much of the microbiome colonizing the airway will have been eliminated, increasing the chances of isolating any drug-resistant strains that might be causing disease. Obviously if the causative organism is actually sensitive to the empiric treatment, it will likely not be recovered, and—in this circumstance— any cultured organism is probably a nonpathogenic colonizer. In navigating these uncertainties, physicians are advised to incorporate multiple forms of evidence when planning therapy for suspected VAP. The patient's history and clinical response to empiric treatment, laboratory data, and caution regarding overuse of broad-spectrum antibiotics must all be included in the calculus.

There is no consensus on the best antibiotic course duration. One study in adults with VAP compared outcomes after either 8 or 15 days of therapy and found no overall difference in mortality or relapse rates. The subset of patients with VAP caused by gram-negative, nonfermenting bacilli (such as *P. aeruginosa*) did experience higher relapse rates when treated for only 8 days, suggesting that gram-negative infections may warrant a longer treatment course. On the other hand, patients in the 8-day treatment group were less likely to develop a multidrug-resistant infection in the future.[36]

Cantey et al. reported results of an extensive neonatal antibiotic stewardship program through which a "hard stop" for empiric antibiotics was introduced at 48 hours of treatment. At that point, antibiotic continuation required reordering, and the recommended treatment duration for pneumonia (ventilator-associated or otherwise) was 5 days total. The group assessed antibiotic usage and outcomes for 2502 patients: 1607 during a baseline period before the stewardship program began and 895 during the post-implementation period. There was no significant change in the percent of infants treated beyond

48 hours during the intervention period, but the proportion receiving 5 or fewer total days of antibiotics increased from 36% to 72%. Importantly, there was no corresponding increase in the number of patients treated for pneumonia requiring reinitiation of antibiotics within 14 days of the first course.[37]

When deciding on treatment duration for a neonate with suspected VAP, 7 days is a reasonable course, which can be adjusted based on clinical response. The guidelines from the United States and Europe each recommend treatment for 7 days. However, both guidelines acknowledge that the time frame may need to be altered based on the underlying clinical condition and resistance of the pathogen.

Goerens et al. proposed a three-pronged antibiotic stewardship program for infants with suspected VAP.[38] Following 24 to 36 hours of empiric antibiotic coverage, this group recommends deciding on treatment continuation based on reevaluation of (1) clinical status, (2) laboratory values, and (3) microbiologic data from cultures and a tracheal aspirate gram stain (Fig. 5.4).

Prevention

The Centers for Disease Control and Prevention and the American Thoracic Society have published guidelines for reducing the incidence of hospital-acquired pneumonia, including VAP.[39,40] Recommendations for preventing VAP are generally aimed at limiting opportunities for cross-contamination between caregivers and patients, decreasing tissue damage from prolonged or recurrent intubation, avoiding unnecessary medication that may promote infection and/or antibiotic resistance, and maximizing oral hygiene and pulmonary toilet.

The type of device used to suction ETTs (in-line or open) may also be an important variable. So-called in-line devices, which allow suctioning of the trachea and ETT lumen without disconnecting it from the ventilator, may prevent VAP in adults, but they are controversial. A Cochrane review of four studies in neonates concluded that in-line suctioning may yield improved short-term advantages—such as fewer desaturation events and improved ease of use by nursing staff—but there was no clear long-term benefit in terms of mortality or major morbidity. The included investigations did not allow strong conclusions about the effect on VAP rates.[41] A well-performed prospective study by Cordero and colleagues (not included in the Cochrane review) demonstrated no significant difference in infectious or noninfectious complications between in-line and open suctioning systems in 175 randomly assigned premature infants, but reported a nursing preference for the convenience and

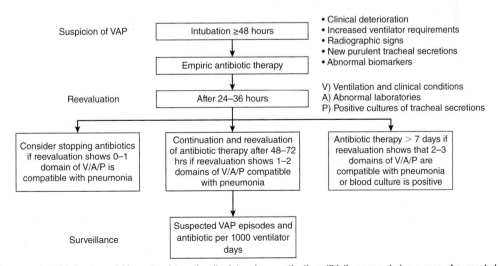

Fig. 5.4 A proposed antibiotic stewardship protocol to rationally determine a patient's antibiotic course during a case of suspected ventilator-associated pneumonia (VAP). (Adapted from Goerens A, Lehnick D, Büttcher M, et al. Neonatal Ventilator Associated Pneumonia: A Quality Improvement Initiative Focusing on Antimicrobial Stewardship. *Front Pediatr.* 2018;6:262.)

ease of the in-line system.[42] While the data are arguably too limited to draw definite conclusions about in-line suctioning and neonatal VAP, there is no strong evidence that one type of suctioning apparatus has marked advantages for infection prevention over the others. A semirecumbent position ($\geq 30°$) may reduce clinically suspected VAP compared to a 0 to 10 degrees supine position. However, the evidence is seriously limited with a high risk of bias.[43]

In the adult population, use of probiotics has been studied as a strategy to prevent VAP. Most of the trials have been small, single-center studies, and there was not consistent dosing or choice of probiotic. Systematic reviews have reached differing conclusions. In a review of five randomized clinical trials (n = 689), Siempos et al. concluded that the incidence of VAP was significantly lower in mechanically ventilated adults receiving probiotics (OR 0.61, CI 0.41–0.91).[44] Other meta-analyses by Petrof et al. (23 trials encompassing 2153 adults; RR 0.75, CI 0.59–0.97)[45] and Bo (8 RCTs with 1083 adults; OR 0.70, CI 0.62–0.95)[46] reached similar conclusions. In contrast, Wang et al. concluded in their meta-analysis (5 RCTs; n = 844 adults) that probiotics did not significantly reduce the incidence of VAP (RR 0.94, CI 0.85–1.04).[47] In the most recently published meta-analysis by Batra et al., which included 9 RCTs (n = 1127 adults), the incidence of VAP (RR 0.70, CI 0.56–0.88) and in-hospital mortality were both significantly reduced.[48] Although the adult data suggest that probiotics may be effective in reducing the incidence of VAP, randomized trials using pharmaceutical grade probiotics are still lacking. There have been a limited number of RCTs in neonates.[49,50] In a RCT by Xue Chao Li (n = 165), the probiotic group exhibited a lower bacterial strain colonization rate in the oropharynx than a control group.[49] In a very small study, Xiang-Lan Wu demonstrated that the incidence of VAP was reduced in infants receiving probiotics containing bifidobacteria (n = 81).[50]

Several studies have tested the hypothesis that neonatal oral care with human breast milk/colostrum—which is rich in antimicrobial substances—might decrease VAP rates. In a recent Cochrane review of early oropharyngeal colostrum, six studies were analyzed (n = 335 infants). There was no reduction in infectious complications, NEC, or pneumonia. However, the time taken to achieve full enteral feeds was shorter.[51] In a systematic review

published in 2020, Ma et al. identified eight randomized trials. Three studies used a double-blind controlled design and five trials were single blinded (n = 682).[52] Only three studies reported VAP as an outcome measure. In those studies, there was a significant reduction in VAP (OR 0.38, CI 0.17–0.88). There was a trend toward a reduction in mortality. The time to full enteral feedings was significantly shorter. In 2021, Aggarwal reported on a randomized clinical trial comparing oropharyngeal colostrum or donor breast milk with sterile water.[53] There were no significant differences in any primary or secondary outcome including VAP. Although use of oropharyngeal colostrum is considered safe, the efficacy of oropharyngeal colostrum as a VAP preventative has not been proven. Products containing chlorhexidine for mouth care are not recommended for infants under 2 months.

Some bundle components that are standard in adult units—such as using cuffed ETTs—are generally inapplicable to neonates, but other components are feasible in the NICU, and an emerging literature indicates that neonatal VAP bundles are also effective. The implementation of care bundles to prevent VAP has generally been effective, but none of them have been studied in randomized clinical trials.[54] In a recent meta-analysis of care bundles in PICU and NICU, the studies demonstrated a reduction in VAP in mechanically ventilated neonates and children (n = 3989). However, all of the studies were observational and nonrandomized. The validity of five of the studies was considered substandard, and there were variations in the care bundle components.[54] Furthermore, only two of the studies were conducted in NICUs. The main elements of the neonatal care bundles were head-of-bed elevation, oral care (saline, sterile water, or human milk every 3–4 hours), daily assessment for extubation readiness, hand hygiene, clean aseptic techniques when suctioning and handling of respiratory equipment, and limiting ventilator circuit breaks. In a recent prospective observational study from NICUs in Spain, implementation of a care bundle reduced the incidence of VAP episodes from 11.79 to 1.93 per 1000 ventilator days.[55] The components of that bundle were similar to those described earlier. Pepin et al. were also able to reduce the VAP rate in their 60-bed NICU through a bundle-based quality improvement effort.[56]

Proper hand hygiene is likely the single most important defense against VAP. Potential pathogens on caregivers' hands can be passed to patients during examination, routine care, or through contamination of medical equipment. An observational study of nosocomial infection rates before and after an intensive hospital-wide hand hygiene improvement initiative documented a decrease in neonatal VAP rates from 16.9 to 6.4 per 1000 ventilator days.[57] A similar Taiwanese study performed during hospital quality reforms that nearly doubled local handwashing rates documented a simultaneous threefold decrease in neonatal respiratory infections.[58]

Several studies have investigated possible approaches to limiting introduction of VAP pathogens from contaminated equipment. One well-examined strategy involves scheduled exchanges of ventilators, tubing, and suctioning equipment. The rationale for this approach is that regular substitution of sterilized equipment might decrease accumulation of bacterial contamination. This hypothesis, however, has not been borne out in clinical trials. Routine disconnection and replacement of ventilator circuits probably actually creates unnecessary opportunities for contamination. The consensus of multiple agencies, therefore, is that ventilator equipment—including tubing and suctioning apparatuses—should be replaced only when visibly soiled or malfunctioning.

Other neonatal VAP bundle components intended to prevent infection from equipment contamination include ensuring that at least two people are present during ETT retaping or repositioning; draining ventilator condensate away from the patient every 2 to 4 hours; clearing secretions before ETT retaping or repositioning, patient repositioning, or extubation; and using only sterilized laryngoscopes and newly opened ETTs that have not touched any environmental surfaces.

As discussed previously, there is some evidence that patient positioning can affect the likelihood of tracheal contamination from gastric secretions, but this is controversial. Some investigators have suggested that intubated infants should be kept in a side-lying position as tolerated, with the head of the bed elevated 15 to 30 degrees, but this is not evidence-based. Other measures that can prevent gastric reflux from contributing to VAP include minimizing large gastric residuals by monitoring gastric aspirates every 4 hours and adjusting enteral feed volume and duration as needed. Although not well studied in neonatal populations, gastric antacid medications and histamine-2 receptor blockers have been shown to promote bacterial growth in the stomach and secondary tracheal colonization. These medications should be avoided in the NICU unless there is a clear indication that outweighs potential risks.

In general, excess oral secretions should be removed because pooling of saliva may create a niche for colonization by potential pathogens. The evidence for a strong effect of oral hygiene is weaker in neonates, who are less susceptible to cavities and bacterial gingivitis. One small study of intubated preterm infants investigated routine oral swabbing with a pharmacologic gel containing several potentially antimicrobial compounds (e.g., lactoperoxidase, lysozyme, lactoferrin) or sterile water as a control. The authors reported a statistically nonsignificant drop in VAP rates among the experimental group, who also had lower neutrophil density in tracheal aspirates relative to controls, possibly suggesting decreased airway inflammation. The safety profile of the gel was acceptable, with no significant differences in noninfectious morbidities between the two groups.[59]

Box 5.4 summarizes VAP bundle elements that are generally believed to help prevent neonatal VAP.

Outcomes

Outcomes for VAP in neonates are difficult to determine because of imprecision in diagnostic criteria. VAP undoubtedly increases mortality and morbidity (including BPD), although the precise degree of risk for neonates has so far not been determined. In a prospective observational study in an academic NICU in France, Dell'Orto et al. demonstrated that BPD was significantly higher in infants with VAP (75%) than unexposed infants (26.8%).[60] However, this difference was of borderline significance when adjusted for confounders ($P = 0.049$). The combined outcome of BPD and mortality was not significantly different. Infants with VAP needed ventilation for a longer period of time than those without. Multiple other neonatal studies have demonstrated that VAP increases hospital length of stay and duration of ventilation, but sample sizes have not been sufficient to draw firm conclusions about the degree of increased mortality risk attributable to

BOX 5.4 POSSIBLE COMPONENTS OF A NEONATAL VAP PREVENTION BUNDLE[a]

HAND HYGIENE

Meticulous hand hygiene before and after patient contact and handling respiratory equipment.

Wear gloves when handling ventilator condensate and other respiratory/oral secretions.

INTUBATION

Use a new, sterile ETT for each intubation attempt.

Ensure that the ETT does not contact environmental surfaces before insertion.

Use a sterilized laryngoscope.

Have at least two NICU staff members present for ETT retaping or repositioning.

SUCTIONING PRACTICES

Clear secretions from the posterior oropharynx before:
- ETT manipulation
- Patient repositioning
- Extubation
- Reintubation

FEEDING

Prevent gastric distention.

Monitor gastric residuals.

Adjust feeding to prevent large residuals and/or distention.

POSITIONING

Use side-lying position as tolerated.

Keep the head of bed elevated 15 to 30 degrees as tolerated.

Use left lateral positioning after feedings as tolerated.

ORAL CARE

Provide oral care:
- Within 24 hours after intubation
- Every 3 to 4 hours
- Before reintubation as time allows
- Before orogastric tube insertion

Use sterile water, breast milk, or approved pharmaceutical oral care solution.

RESPIRATORY EQUIPMENT

Use a separate suction catheter, connection tubing, and canister for oral and tracheal suction.

Drain ventilator condensate away from the patient every 2 to 4 hours and before repositioning.

Avoid unnecessary disconnection of the ventilator circuit.

Change ventilator equipment when visibly soiled or mechanically malfunctioning.

Use heated ventilator circuits.

ETT, Endotracheal tube; *NICU*, neonatal intensive care unit.
[a]Elements have been adapted from the adult literature, and there is no consensus on a universal bundle.

neonatal VAP.[5,7] Long-term functional respiratory outcomes have not been assessed in infants with VAP. Implementation of VAP prevention bundles has inconsistently reduced mortality[54] and BPD.[55]

Future Research Directions

Accurate diagnostic tests that allow discrimination between normal oropharyngeal colonization and true infection are needed, and work in this direction is underway. Several laboratories have investigated individual or grouped biomarkers as indicators of VAP. Harwood et al. investigated the potential of glutathione sulfonamide (GSA), a by-product of neutrophil-mediated oxidation, to detect the presence of infectious airway inflammation. They measured GSA concentrations in tracheal aspirates from intubated preterm neonates and correlated levels with culture results. GSA concentration was significantly correlated with the presence of potential pathogenic bacteria and—importantly—did not increase in the presence of likely commensals such

as *Staphylococcus epidermidis*. The study was not powered to identify a significant relationship between GSA concentration and diagnosed VAP.[61]

Conclusion

Recognition of neonatal VAP as a disease with potentially serious consequences is a relatively recent development. VAP, which has been better studied in adult populations, is inherently difficult to diagnose with certainty—even more so in the NICU, where invasive airway testing is rarely feasible. Bacterial contamination of the airway is a significant challenge, which currently can be surmounted only by using multimodal clinical, laboratory, and radiographic diagnostic criteria.

Nevertheless, prompt diagnosis and evidence-based antibiotic treatment of VAP can speed extubation, decrease NICU admission duration, and save lives. Several important questions about the best approach to VAP diagnosis and management remain unanswered, making VAP an inviting topic for impactful scientific research.

REFERENCES

1. Cernada M, Aguar M, Brugada M, et al. Ventilator-associated pneumonia in newborn infants diagnosed with an invasive bronchoalveolar lavage technique. *Pediatr Crit Care Med.* 2013;14(1):55-61.
2. Dudeck MA, Edwards JR, Allen-Bridson K, et al. National Healthcare Safety Network report, data summary for 2013, Device-associated Module. *Am J Infect Control.* 2015;43(3):206-221.
3. Edwards JR, Peterson KD, Mu Y, et al. National Healthcare Safety Network (NHSN) report: data summary for 2006 through 2008, issued December 2009. *Am J Infect Control.* 2009;37(10):783-805.
4. Dudeck MA, Horan TC, Peterson KD, et al. National Healthcare Safety Network report, data summary for 2011, device-associated module. *Am J Infect Control.* 2013;41(4):286-300.
5. Apisarnthanarak A, Holzmann-Pazgal G, Hamvas A, et al. Ventilator-associated pneumonia in extremely preterm neonates in a neonatal intensive care unit: characteristics, risk factors, and outcomes. *Pediatrics.* 2003;112:1283-1289.
6. Goldmann DA, Freeman J, Durbin JWA. Nosocomial infection and death in a neonatal intensive care unit. *J Infect Dis.* 1983;147(4):635-641.
7. Singh-Naz N, Yuan TM, Chen LH, et al. Risk factors and outcomes for ventilator-associated pneumonia in neonatal intensive care unit patients. *J Perinat Med.* 2007;35(4):334-338.
8. Zur KB, Mandell DL, Gordon RE, Holzman I, Rothschild MA. Electron microscopic analysis of biofilm on endotracheal tubes removed from intubated neonates. *Otolaryngol Head Neck Surg.* 2004;130:407-414.
9. Adair CG, Gorman SP, Feron BM, et al. Implications of endotracheal tube biofilm for ventilator-associated pneumonia. *Intensive Care Med.* 1999;25:1072-1076.
10. Aly H, Badawy M, El-Kholy A, Nabil R, Mohamed A. Randomized, controlled trial on tracheal colonization of ventilated infants: can gravity prevent ventilator-associated pneumonia? *Pediatrics.* 2008;122:770-774.
11. Garland JS, Alex CP, Johnston N, Yan JC, Werlin SL. Association between tracheal pepsin, a reliable marker of gastric aspiration, and head of bed elevation among ventilated neonates. *J Neonatal Perinatal Med.* 2014;7:185-192.
12. Torres A, Serra-Batlles J, Ros E, et al. Pulmonary aspiration of gastric contents in patients receiving mechanical ventilation: the effect of body position. *Ann Intern Med.* 1992;116:540-543.
13. Cendrero JAC, Solé-Violán J, Benítez AB, et al. Role of different routes of tracheal colonization in the development of pneumonia in patients receiving mechanical ventilation. *Chest.* 1999;116:462-470.
14. Feldman C, Kassel M, Cantrell J, et al. The presence and sequence of endotracheal tube colonization in patients undergoing mechanical ventilation. *Eur Respir J.* 1999;13:546-551.
15. Payne MS, Goss KCW, Connett GJ, et al. Molecular microbiological characterization of preterm neonates at risk of bronchopulmonary dysplasia. *Pediatr Res.* 2010;67:412-418.
16. Grier A, McDavid A, Wang B, et al. Neonatal gut and respiratory microbiota: coordinated development through time and space. *Microbiome.* 2018;6:193.
17. Costello EK, Carlisle EM, Bik EM, Morowitz MJ, Relman DA. Microbiome assembly across multiple body sites in low-birth-weight infants. *MBio.* 2013;4:e00782-13.
18. Tirone C, Pezza L, Paladini A, et al. Gut and lung microbiota in preterm infants: immunological modulation and implication in neonatal outcomes. *Front Immunol.* 2019;10:2910.
19. Weiner-Lastinger LM, Abner S, Edwards JR, et al. Antimicrobial-resistant pathogens associated with adult healthcare-associated infections: summary of data reported to the National Healthcare Safety Network, 2015–2017. *Infect Control Hosp Epidemiol.* 2020;41:1-18.
20. Kalil AC, Metersky ML, Klompas M, et al. Management of adults with hospital-acquired and ventilator-associated pneumonia: 2016 clinical practice guidelines by the Infectious Diseases Society of America and the American Thoracic Society. *Clin Infect Dis.* 2016;63:e61-e111.
21. Zaragoza R, Vidal-Cortés P, Aguilar G, et al. Update of the treatment of nosocomial pneumonia in the ICU. *Crit Care.* 2020;24:383.
22. Torres A, Niederman MS, Chastre J, et al. International ERS/ESICM/ESCMID/ALAT guidelines for the management of hospital-acquired pneumonia and ventilator-associated pneumonia. *Eur Respir J.* 2017;50:1700582.
23. Martin-Loeches I, Rodriguez AH, Torres A. New guidelines for hospital-acquired pneumonia/ventilator-associated pneumonia. *Curr Opin Crit Care.* 2018;24:347-352.
24. Kelly DN, Martin-Loeches I. Comparing current US and European guidelines for nosocomial pneumonia. *Curr Opin Pulm Med.* 2019;25:263-270.
25. Fleiss N, Coggins SA, Lewis AN, et al. Evaluation of the neonatal sequential organ failure assessment and mortality risk in preterm infants with late-onset infection. *JAMA Netw Open.* 2020;4:e2036518.
26. Trouillet JL, Chastre J, Vuagnat A, et al. Ventilator-associated pneumonia caused by potentially drug-resistant bacteria. *Am J Resp Crit Care.* 1998;157:531-539.
27. Grohs E, Hill-Ricciuti A, Kelly N, et al. Spa typing of staphylococcus aureus in a neonatal intensive care unit during routine surveillance. *J Pediatric Infect Dis Soc.* 2021;10:766-773.
28. Zhang Y, Wang Y, Driel ML, et al. Network meta-analysis and pharmacoeconomic evaluation of antibiotics for the treatment of patients infected with complicated skin and soft structure infection and hospital-acquired or ventilator-associated pneumonia. *Antimicrob Resist Infect Control.* 2019;8:72.
29. Bally M, Dendukuri N, Sinclair A, et al. A network meta-analysis of antibiotics for treatment of hospitalised patients with suspected or proven methicillin-resistant staphylococcus aureus infection. *Int J Antimicrob Agents.* 2012;40:479-495.
30. Wunderink RG, Niederman MS, Kollef MH, et al. Linezolid in methicillin-resistant staphylococcus aureus nosocomial pneumonia: a randomized, controlled study. *Clin Infect Dis.* 2012;54:621-629.
31. Falagas ME, Siempos II, Vardakas KZ. Linezolid versus glycopeptide or β-lactam for treatment of gram-positive bacterial infections: meta-analysis of randomised controlled trials. *Lancet Infect Dis.* 2008;8:53-66.
32. Walkey AJ, O'Donnell MR, Wiener RS. Linezolid vs Glycopeptide antibiotics for the treatment of suspected methicillin-resistant staphylococcus aureus nosocomial pneumonia a meta-analysis of randomized controlled trials. *Chest.* 2011;139:1148-1155.
33. Wang Y, Zou Y, Xie J, et al. Linezolid versus vancomycin for the treatment of suspected methicillin-resistant staphylococcus aureus nosocomial pneumonia: a systematic review employing meta-analysis. *Eur J Clin Pharmacol.* 2015;71:107-115.
34. Jantausch BA, Deville J, Adler S, et al. Linezolid for the treatment of children with bacteremia or nosocomial pneumonia caused by resistant gram-positive bacterial pathogens. *Pediatric Infect Dis J.* 2003;22:S164-S171.

35. Fischer JE, Ramser M, Fanconi S. Use of antibiotics in pediatric intensive care and potential savings. *Intensive Care Med.* 2000; 26:959-966.

36. Chastre J, Wolff M, Fagon JY, et al. Comparison of 8 vs 15 days of antibiotic therapy for ventilator-associated pneumonia in adults: a randomized trial. *JAMA.* 2003;290:2588-2598.

37. Cantey JB, Wozniak PS, Pruszynski JE, Sánchez PJ. Reducing unnecessary antibiotic use in the neonatal intensive care unit (SCOUT): a prospective interrupted time-series study. *Lancet Infect Dis.* 2016;16:1178-1184.

38. Goerens A, Lehnick D, Büttcher M, et al. Neonatal ventilator associated pneumonia: a quality improvement initiative focusing on antimicrobial stewardship. *Front Pediatr.* 2018;6:262.

39. American Thoracic Society, Infectious Diseases Society of America. Guidelines for the management of adults with hospital-acquired, ventilator-associated, and healthcare-associated pneumonia. *Am J Respir Crit Care Med.* 2005;171(4):388-416.

40. Tablan OC, Anderson LJ, Besser R, Bridges C. Guidelines for preventing healthcare-associated pneumonia, 2003. *MMWR.* 2004. Available at: https://www.cdc.gov/mmwr/preview/mmwrhtml/rr5303a1.htm.

41. Taylor JE, Hawley G, Flenady V, Woodgate PG. Tracheal suctioning without disconnection in intubated ventilated neonates. *Cochrane Database Syst Rev.* 2011;2011(12):CD003065. doi:10.1002/14651858.cd003065.pub2.

42. Cordero L, Sananes M, Ayers LW. Comparison of a closed (Trach Care MAC) with an open endotracheal suction system in small premature infants. *J Perinatol.* 2000;20:151-156.

43. Wang L, Li X, Yang Z, et al. Semi-recumbent position versus supine position for the prevention of ventilator-associated pneumonia in adults requiring mechanical ventilation. *Cochrane Database Syst Rev.* 2016;2016:CD009946.

44. Siempos II, Ntaidou TK, Falagas ME. Impact of the administration of probiotics on the incidence of ventilator-associated pneumonia: a meta-analysis of randomized controlled trials. *Crit Care Med.* 2010;38:954-962.

45. Petrof EO, Dhaliwal R, Manzanares W, Johnstone J, Cook D, Heyland DK. Probiotics in the critically ill. *Crit Care Med.* 2012; 40:3290-3302.

46. Bo L, Li J, Tao T, et al. Probiotics for preventing ventilator-associated pneumonia. *Cochrane Database Syst Rev.* 2014;10:CD009066.

47. Wang J, Liu K, Ariani F, Tao L, Zhang J, Qu JM. Probiotics for preventing ventilator-associated pneumonia: a systematic review and meta-analysis of high-quality randomized controlled trials. *PLoS One.* 2013;8:e83934.

48. Batra P, Soni KD, Mathur P. Efficacy of probiotics in the prevention of VAP in critically ill ICU patients: an updated systematic review and meta-analysis of randomized control trials. *J Intensive Care.* 2020;8:81.

49. Li XC, Wang JZ, Liu YH. Effect of probiotics on respiratory tract pathogen colonization in neonates undergoing mechanical ventilation. *Zhongguo Dang Dai Er Ke Za Zhi.* 2012;14:406-408.

50. Wu XL, Li YF, Zhou BY, Wu LJ, Wu ZJ. Effects of bifidobacteria on respiratory and gastrointestinal tracts in neonates receiving mechanical ventilation. *Zhongguo Dang Dai Er Ke Za Zhi.* 2011; 13:704-707.

51. Nasuf AWA, Ojha S, Dorling J. Oropharyngeal colostrum in preventing mortality and morbidity in preterm infants. *Cochrane Database Syst Rev.* 2018;9(9):CD011921.

52. Ma A, Yang J, Li Y, Zhang X, Kang, Y. Oropharyngeal colostrum therapy reduces the incidence of ventilator-associated pneumonia in very low birth weight infants: a systematic review and meta-analysis. *Pediatr Res.* 2020;89:1-9.

53. Aggarwal R, Plakkal N, Bhat V. Does oropharyngeal administration of colostrum reduce morbidity and mortality in very preterm infants? A randomised parallel-group controlled trial. *J Paediatr Child Health.* 2021;57:1467-1472.

54. Niedzwiecka T, Patton D, Walsh S, Moore Z, O'Connor T, Nugent L. What are the effects of care bundles on the incidence of ventilator-associated pneumonia in paediatric and neonatal intensive care units? A systematic review. *J Spec Pediatr Nurs.* 2019;24:e12264.

55. Pinilla-González A, Solaz-García Á, Parra-Llorca A, et al. Preventive bundle approach decreases the incidence of ventilator-associated pneumonia in newborn infants. *J Perinatol.* 2021;41:1-7.

56. Pepin BJ, Lesslie D, Berg W, Spaulding AB, Pokora T. ZAP-VAP: A Quality Improvement Initiative to Decrease Ventilator-Associated Pneumonia in the Neonatal Intensive Care Unit, 2012-2016. *Adv Neonat Care.* 2019;19(4):253-261.

57. Lam BCC, Lee J, Lau YL. Hand hygiene practices in a neonatal intensive care unit: a multimodal intervention and impact on nosocomial infection. *Pediatrics.* 2004;114:e565-e571.

58. Won SP, Chou HC, Hsieh WS, et al. Handwashing program for the prevention of nosocomial infections in a neonatal intensive care unit. *Infect Control Hosp Epidemiol.* 2004;25:742-746.

59. Stefanescu BM, Hétu C, Slaughter JC, O'Shea TM, Shetty AK. A pilot study of Biotene OralBalance® gel for oral care in mechanically ventilated preterm neonates. *Contemp Clin Trials.* 2013;35:33-39.

60. Dell'Orto V, Raschetti R, Centorrino R, et al. Short- and long-term respiratory outcomes in neonates with ventilator-associated pneumonia. *Pediatr Pulmonol.* 2019;54:1982-1988.

61. Harwood DT, Darlow BA, Cheah FC, McNeill N, Graham P, Winterbourn CC. Biomarkers of neutrophil-mediated glutathione and protein oxidation in tracheal aspirates from preterm infants: association with bacterial infection. *Pediatr Res.* 2011; 69:28-33.

Chapter 6

Noninvasive Respiratory Support for Preterm Infants: An Alternative to Mechanical Ventilation

Brett J. Manley, Kate A. Hodgson, Amit Mukerji, and Peter G. Davis

Chapter Outline

Introduction

Why Do Preterm Infants Experience Respiratory Failure and How Can Noninvasive Respiratory Support Help?

Respiratory Distress Syndrome

Apnea of Prematurity

The Role of Continuous Positive Airway Pressure

A Brief History of Neonatal Mechanical Ventilation and Noninvasive Respiratory Support

Nasal Continuous Positive Airway Pressure

Nasal Continuous Positive Airway Pressure Interfaces

Nasal Continuous Positive Airway Pressure Devices

How Much Pressure Should Be Used?

Nasal CPAP for Babies With RDS or at Risk of Developing RDS

CPAP in the "Surfactant Era"

Is CPAP a Suitable Alternative to Routine Intubation of Very Preterm Infants at Birth?

Is CPAP With Early Intubation for Surfactant and Brief Mechanical Ventilation Better Than CPAP Alone?

Less Invasive or Minimally Invasive Surfactant Administration

Nasal Continuous Positive Airway Pressure for Postextubation Support

CPAP "Failure": When Should Preterm Infants Be Intubated?

Complications of Nasal CPAP

Weaning From CPAP

Nasal Intermittent Positive-Pressure Ventilation

Mechanisms of Nasal Intermittent Positive-Pressure Ventilation

Synchronized Versus Unsynchronized Nasal Intermittent Positive-Pressure Ventilation

Clinical Evidence on Use of Nasal Intermittent Positive-Pressure Ventilation for Primary Respiratory Support

Clinical Evidence on Use of Nasal Intermittent Positive-Pressure Ventilation as a Postextubation Mode

Nasal Intermittent Positive-Pressure Ventilation for Apnea of Prematurity

Nasal Intermittent Positive-Pressure Ventilation Settings

Summary and Recommendations

Noninvasive High-Frequency Ventilation

Mechanisms of Action of Noninvasive High-Frequency Ventilation

Clinical Studies of Noninvasive High-Frequency Ventilation

Settings During Noninvasive High-Frequency Ventilation

Summary And Recommendations for Noninvasive High-Frequency Ventilation Use

Nasal High Flow

How Does Nasal High Flow Work?

Evidence From Randomized Trials in Preterm Infants

Safety of Nasal High Flow

Potential Concerns With Use of Nasal High Flow in Neonates

Should Nasal High Flow Be Used to Treat Preterm Infants?

Future Directions

Key Points

- Continuous positive airway pressure (CPAP) provides effective respiratory support for preterm infants for a range of indications, especially when delivered via binasal prongs or nasal masks at set pressures equal to or greater than 5 cm H_2O.

- Extremely preterm infants may be managed with CPAP from the delivery room onward as an alternative to routine intubation and mechanical ventilation.

- Nasal intermittent positive-pressure ventilation is a useful method for augmenting the benefits of CPAP, especially when synchronized with the infant's breathing.

- Noninvasive high-frequency ventilation is a promising modality that requires further study in randomized trials.

- Nasal high flow is an alternative to CPAP for postextubation support for preterm infants and as primary support if CPAP is available as backup.

Introduction

The primary concern of the clinician making choices about treatment is whether one therapy leads to better outcomes than the alternatives. This chapter focuses on current modes of noninvasive respiratory support in clinical use or under investigation in clinical trials: nasal continuous positive airway pressure (CPAP), nasal intermittent positive-pressure ventilation (NIPPV), noninvasive high-frequency ventilation (NIHFV), and nasal high flow (nHF). It draws heavily on evidence from randomized controlled trials (RCTs) and reviews found in the neonatal module of the Cochrane Library (https://neonatal.cochrane.org).

Why Do Preterm Infants Experience Respiratory Failure and How Can Noninvasive Respiratory Support Help?

RESPIRATORY DISTRESS SYNDROME

Respiratory distress syndrome (RDS) is a disease of newborn infants, increasing in prevalence with decreasing gestational age. It is characterized by immature lung development and inadequate surfactant production. The lungs of affected infants may not expand normally immediately after birth, do not easily maintain a residual volume, and are at risk of atelectasis. Other factors also contribute to a loss of lung volume, including muscle hypotonia, a compliant chest wall, and slow clearance of fetal lung liquid. Repeated lung expansion, followed by atelectasis during expiration, leads to shearing forces and stretch injury that damage the airway and saccular alveolar epithelium and cause leakage of protein-rich fluid from the pulmonary capillaries. This leakage in turn inhibits any endogenous surfactant present.[1] Damage to the lungs is exacerbated by mechanical ventilation (MV), high oxygen concentrations, and infection.[2]

APNEA OF PREMATURITY

The pharyngeal airway of the preterm newborn is very compliant. The cartilaginous components are more flexible, and the fat-laden superficial fascia of the neck that stabilizes the upper airway of term infants is not well developed. The intrathoracic airways, including trachea, bronchi, and small airways, are similarly compliant and prone to collapse during expiration. The breathing patterns of very premature infants are frequently erratic and at times inadequate to maintain oxygenation (see Chapter 8). The causes of apnea of prematurity include hypoxia due to a reduced functional residual capacity, particularly in active sleep. Upper airway obstruction, alone or in combination with a central respiratory pause, accompanies most apneic events.[3]

THE ROLE OF CONTINUOUS POSITIVE AIRWAY PRESSURE

CPAP effectively supports the breathing of preterm infants through several mechanisms. It mechanically splints the upper airway, thereby minimizing obstruction and reducing apnea.[4] Distension of the airways reduces resistance to air flow and so diminishes work of breathing.[5] CPAP aids lung expansion and therefore reduces ventilation-perfusion mismatch and improves oxygenation. By preventing repeated alveolar collapse and reexpansion, CPAP reduces protein leak and helps conserve surfactant.

MV via an endotracheal tube (ETT) has been the mainstay of neonatal intensive care almost since its inception. Many lives have been saved by this technique, but its adverse effects are well documented. These include cardiovascular and cerebrovascular instability during intubation; complications of the ETT, including subglottic stenosis and tracheal lesions; infections, both pulmonary and systemic; and acute and chronic lung damage, primarily related to stretch mediated effects of nonhomogeneous tidal volume delivery at the cellular level. By avoiding the local mechanical problems of an ETT as well as those of volutrauma, the use of CPAP has been shown to improve outcomes for preterm infants.[6,7]

A Brief History of Neonatal Mechanical Ventilation and Noninvasive Respiratory Support

The first form of assisted ventilation for neonates was MV provided via an ETT, which became widespread in the late 1960s and early 1970s. George Gregory and associates[8] were the first to describe the use of CPAP in neonates in 1971, a therapy they developed because of the high mortality observed in infants weighing less than 1500 g, particularly those requiring assisted ventilation in the first 24 hours of life. The first series of 20 "severely ill" infants with RDS were treated with CPAP delivered predominantly via an ETT. In an attempt to avoid the complications of endotracheal intubation, other interfaces were developed, including a pressurized plastic bag[9] and a tight-fitting face mask.[10] Two infants in the initial Gregory series were managed in a pressure chamber around the infant's head.[8] In 1976, Ahlström and colleagues[11] described the use of a face chamber providing pressures up to 15 cm of water (H_2O). Rhodes and Hall[12] conducted a controlled trial involving alternate allocation of subjects to CPAP via a tight-fitting face mask or to conventional therapy consisting of warmed humidified oxygen. A trend toward increased survival was noted in the CPAP group, which was statistically significant in the subgroup of infants weighing more than 1500 g.

The local pressure effects of these devices, combined with the problems of accessibility, particularly for suctioning and feeding, led to the development of alternative interfaces for the delivery of CPAP. Novogroder and coworkers[13] described a device composed of two ETTs inserted through the nose and then positioned under direct laryngoscopy in the posterior pharynx, joined by a Y-connector, and attached to a pressure source. Others described

shorter binasal devices that were simpler to manufacture and insert.[14,15] An even simpler single nasal prong, made by cutting down an ETT, became widely used.[16] These were followed by development of a variable flow device that used jet nozzles to assist inspiratory flow while diverting flow away from the patient in expiration.[17] This design was claimed to be superior to "conventional" CPAP in reducing work of breathing.[18]

It should be noted that of all these trials, only the one conducted by Rhodes and Hall[12] used a control group. Novogroder and coworkers[13] had plans to subject their device to a randomized trial but abandoned them when "the dramatic effect of CPAP (was) observed after a brief period of treatment in all patients." It is likely that other researchers were so convinced of the virtues of endotracheal intubation that trials comparing MV with CPAP were considered inappropriate. In an accompanying commentary to the study by Rhodes and Hall, Chernick[19] congratulated the investigators on conducting a "daring controlled study" and suggested that although one or two such studies of CPAP would be welcome, many more "would be foolish." With some notable exceptions, it seems researchers heeded his advice. The following sections describe these exceptions.

Nasal Continuous Positive Airway Pressure

NASAL CONTINUOUS POSITIVE AIRWAY PRESSURE INTERFACES

Several interfaces have been developed for delivering nasal CPAP (Fig. 6.1). Nasal prongs may be short, lying 1 to 2 cm inside the nose, or long, with the tip in the nasopharynx. They may be single or binasal. Both are associated with a leak around the prongs and nasal trauma. Nasal masks have been developed as an alternative interface to ameliorate these problems. An important determinant of effectiveness of nasal CPAP devices is their ability to transmit the pressure to the airways. This ability depends on the resistance to flow of the device, which in turn depends on the length and diameter of the prongs. In an in vitro comparison of popular devices, nasal mask interfaces had lower resistance than short binasal prongs, which in turn had lower resistance than single or long nasopharyngeal prongs.[20]

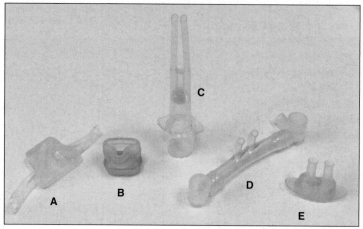

Fig. 6.1 Examples of noninvasive nasal CPAP interfaces—nasal masks (A: Nasal Mask, Medical Innovations GmbH, Puchheim, Germany, B: Nasal Mask, Fisher & Paykel Healthcare, Auckland, New Zealand), nasopharyngeal prongs (C: Binasal Airway, Neotech Products Inc., Valencia, CA, USA), and short binasal prongs (D: Hudson Prongs, Teleflex Medical, North Carolina, Durham, USA, and E: Infant Flow System Nasal Prongs, Viasys Healthcare, Palm Springs, CA, USA). (With permission from Dr Louise Owen, The Royal Women's Hospital, Melbourne, Australia.)

The highest resistance was seen with the "RAM" nasal cannula,[20] which has been an increasingly popular interface in recent years, particularly in North America. Several bench studies suggest significant limitations in the ability of the RAM nasal cannula to provide ventilator set peak or distending pressure during CPAP or NIPPV support.[21-23] These studies show that only 60% to 70% of the set pressure is delivered to the proximal airway resulting in only minimal delivery of tidal volume. Two small RCTs have compared the RAM cannula to alternate interfaces for the delivery of NIPPV to preterm infants with RDS. Gokce et al. randomized 126 infants to receive NIPPV via RAM cannula or Hudson prongs.[24] Infants in the RAM cannula group were more likely to require invasive ventilation (32.8% vs. 9.6%) and surfactant therapy (42.1% vs. 19.3%). In a noninferiority trial, Hochwald et al. randomized 166 preterm infants to receive NIPPV via short binasal prongs or mask, or via RAM cannula.[25] In contrast to the advice from most nasal cannula manufacturers, the RAM cannula were fitted snuggly, aiming to fill about 80% of the nares. Surfactant administration was allowed in both groups and was not considered a NIPPV treatment failure. They found no difference in rates of endotracheal intubation but less nasal trauma in infants managed with RAM cannula.

Two recent meta-analyses have compared mask CPAP with prong CPAP.[26,27] The findings of both are consistent with the benchtop studies showing that the lower resistance of the mask interface delivers more effective CPAP levels to the infant. King et al. noted that while the quality of the evidence included in the review was low, the use of a nasal mask decreased the rate of nasal CPAP failure compared with nasal prongs.[26] Likewise, Jasani and colleagues reported in a pooled analysis that treating nine infants with nasal mask rather than prongs would prevent one intubation.[27] These authors noted that the mask was also associated with a reduction in the rate of nasal injury.

NASAL CONTINUOUS POSITIVE AIRWAY PRESSURE DEVICES

There are several ways to deliver CPAP. The most common method is "bubble" CPAP, which uses a continuous gas flow that is directed past, and into, the infant's nose, and an underwater seal at the distal end of the expiratory limb of the breathing circuit to generate circuit pressure. Tubing is inserted to a specific underwater depth to obtain the desired circuit pressure. The other type of continuous flow CPAP is ventilator-generated CPAP, where the ventilator expiratory assembly employs various methods to maintain a set pressure within the circuit that is applied to the infant.

The alternative to continuous flow CPAP is variable flow CPAP, where alterations to the gas flow result in changes in the delivered pressure. Since its description by Moa and colleagues[17] in 1988, the variable flow nasal CPAP device—Aladdin nasal CPAP Infant Flow System (now called the Arabella; Hamilton Medical AG, Reno, NV), EME Infant Flow Nasal CPAP (CareFusion, San Francisco), or Infant Flow Driver (Electro Medical Equipment Ltd, Brighton, Sussex, UK)—has become widely used around the world. In vitro studies using models of neonatal ventilation have demonstrated less pressure variation and work of breathing with the variable flow device. Pandit and colleagues[28] measured work of breathing in preterm infants with the use of respiratory inductance plethysmography and esophageal pressure monitoring. They demonstrated less work of breathing with variable flow CPAP than with continuous flow CPAP. The same group showed, in a crossover study, that the variable flow device led to better lung recruitment than either nasal cannula or continuous flow CPAP.[29]

There are no large-scale RCTs investigating differences between CPAP devices. Several small studies exist, but there is little convincing evidence to support one form over another.[30] A recent systematic review of bubble CPAP versus other CPAP delivery modes included 19 studies. The authors report that there was no difference in mortality or bronchopulmonary dysplasia (BPD) between modes, but there was less CPAP failure within seven days with bubble CPAP (risk ratio [RR] 0.75, 95% confidence interval [CI] 0.57–0.98). However, more nasal injury was observed with bubble CPAP than other modes (RR 2.04, 95% CI 1.33–3.14).[31]

HOW MUCH PRESSURE SHOULD BE USED?

The purpose of nasal CPAP is to deliver a set pressure to the airways and lungs. If sufficient pressure is consistently achieved, the choice of device may not be important. A pressure of 5 cm H_2O is a traditional starting point. Some neonatal intensive care units (NICUs) hardly vary this pressure and claim good results.[32] There is some evidence from the *Cochrane Review* of postextubation nasal CPAP that pressures <5 cm H_2O are ineffective in this setting.[33] In their landmark publication on CPAP, Gregory and associates used pressures up to 15 mm Hg.[8] A study of

infants with mild RDS showed the highest end-expiratory lung volume and tidal volume, the lowest respiratory rate, and the least thoracoabdominal asynchrony occurred at a pressure of 8 cm H_2O, when compared with 0, 2, 4, and 6 cm H_2O.[34] It is uncertain whether these results apply to more immature infants with more severe lung disease.

A study from Buzzella and colleagues[35] suggests that CPAP pressures of 8 cm H_2O compared to 5 cm H_2O may be more effective at preventing extubation failure in extremely low birth weight infants. Additionally, the higher pressure seems to be well tolerated from a cardiovascular standpoint. Comparisons of cardiac output, cerebral circulation, and venous return suggest the higher pressure does not compromise cerebral circulation or venous return but may reduce pulmonary shunting across the ductus arteriosus.[36] The choice of CPAP pressure should be tailored to the infant's clinical condition. A baby with RDS, relatively stiff lungs, a high fraction of inspired oxygen (FiO_2), and a chest X-ray showing opaque lungs may need a higher pressure to support lung volume than a baby with a low FiO_2 being treated for apneic episodes. If CPAP is to be effective in infants with very low lung compliance, the pressure may need to be increased to 8 to 10 cm H_2O in increments of 1 cm H_2O and the effect observed. It is important to note, however, that high distending pressures, if used in a baby with compliant lungs, can interfere with pulmonary blood flow and cause overdistention, leading to carbon dioxide retention.

The optimal CPAP pressure is likely to vary between infants and over time as an individual infant's pulmonary mechanics change. In the absence of evidence-based guidelines, we typically use CPAP pressures in the range 5 to 8 cm H_2O, adjusting them on the basis of FiO_2 and clinical progress.

NASAL CPAP FOR BABIES WITH RDS OR AT RISK OF DEVELOPING RDS

The focus of studies on the use of nasal CPAP in infants who have, or are at risk for, RDS has changed over the decades. From a clinical perspective, studies conducted before the availability of surfactant are of limited relevance in the modern neonatal intensive care era. In general, presurfactant trials comparing the risk and benefit of prophylactic CPAP versus no continuous distending pressure (i.e., oxygen by hood or standard nasal cannula therapy) showed that CPAP was associated with lower risk of treatment failure (RR 0.64, 95% CI 0.50–0.82), lower use of ventilatory assistance (RR 0.72, 95% CI 0.54–0.96), and lower overall mortality (RR 0.53, 95% CI 0.34–0.83). However, CPAP was associated with increased risk of pneumothorax (typical RR 2.48, 95% CI 1.16–5.30).[37]

CPAP IN THE "SURFACTANT ERA"

Surfactant is the most comprehensively evaluated treatment in neonatology. Initial randomized trials of surfactant were done nearly 30 years ago, when early CPAP was not commonly used for very preterm infants, antenatal corticosteroids were given to only 10% of eligible mothers, and rates of neonatal mortality and morbidity were much higher than at present. Surfactant therapy was provided via an ETT, and whether given prophylactically or as treatment, surfactant reduced mortality and the combined outcome of death or chronic lung disease.[38,39] Surfactant therapy appeared more beneficial when given early in the course of RDS.[40] It became common practice for all very preterm infants to be intubated in the delivery room for surfactant administration. In the past few years, a number of randomized trials have evaluated "less invasive" approaches to surfactant administration in conjunction with CPAP support.

IS CPAP A SUITABLE ALTERNATIVE TO ROUTINE INTUBATION OF VERY PRETERM INFANTS AT BIRTH?

More than a decade ago, several groups reported their experience following policy change from early intubation to early nasal CPAP,[41,42] describing lower mortality and morbidity in the CPAP-treated group. Since then, several RCTs have compared intubation in the delivery room with early nasal CPAP. The "COIN" trial[43] randomly assigned 610 breathing infants at 25 to 29 weeks' gestation to CPAP or intubation and ventilation if they manifested signs of respiratory distress at 5 minutes after birth. Surfactant was administered to intubated infants at the discretion of the treating clinician. There were no important differences in the rates of death or BPD between the groups. CPAP halved the intubation rate, decreased the risk of the combined outcome of death or the

need for oxygen therapy at 28 days, and resulted in fewer days of MV. However, the CPAP group had a higher rate of pneumothorax (9% vs. 3% in the intubated group).

The "SUPPORT" trial[44] enrolled 1316 infants between 24 and 27 weeks' gestation who were randomly allocated before birth to immediate CPAP or intubation in the delivery room. Intubated infants were also treated with surfactant within 1 hour after birth. The rates of death or BPD did not differ significantly between the groups after adjustment for gestational age, center, and familial clustering. Although more than 80% of infants in the CPAP group ultimately required intubation and MV, only about one-third were intubated in the delivery room. Overall, infants randomly assigned to CPAP were less likely to be intubated, less likely to receive postnatal corticosteroids, had fewer days of MV, and were more likely to be alive without MV by day 7.

A Vermont Oxford Network trial[45] compared three approaches to initial respiratory management in 648 very preterm infants born at 26 to 29 completed weeks' gestation: (1) prophylactic surfactant followed by a period of MV, (2) prophylactic surfactant with rapid extubation to CPAP, or (3) initial management with CPAP and selective surfactant treatment. The primary outcome was the incidence of death or BPD at 36 weeks' postmenstrual age. Both prophylactic surfactant with rapid extubation to CPAP and initial management with CPAP reduced the RR of death or BPD compared with prophylactic surfactant followed by a period of MV. About half the infants managed with initial CPAP avoided MV and surfactant. Mortality and other adverse outcomes were similar between the groups.

A meta-analysis including these RCTs and a fourth trial[46] found a significant reduction in the combined outcome of death or BPD, at 36 weeks' corrected gestation for infants treated with early CPAP: RR 0.91 (95% CI 0.84–0.99); number needed to treat: 25 infants. The trials show that nasal CPAP can be safely used from birth in very preterm infants and that nearly half of such infants may not need ventilation or surfactant treatment. Current evidence supports the use of early nasal CPAP as the initial respiratory mode for most extremely preterm infants in an effort to prevent intubation/MV and subsequent BPD.

IS CPAP WITH EARLY INTUBATION FOR SURFACTANT AND BRIEF MECHANICAL VENTILATION BETTER THAN CPAP ALONE?

A systematic review has investigated whether early, brief intubation for surfactant administration (the Intubation, SURfactant, Extubation, or 'INSURE' procedure) followed by extubation to nasal CPAP was better than nasal CPAP and selective intubation, surfactant, and continued MV.[47] Meta-analysis of the six studies identified showed that intubation, ventilation, and early surfactant therapy followed by extubation to nasal CPAP ventilation was associated with lower rates of later MV (RR 0.67, 95% CI 0.57–0.79), air leak syndromes (RR 0.52, 95% CI 0.28–0.96), and supplemental oxygen requirement at 28 days of age (RR 0.51, 95% CI 0.26–0.99). There was no difference in supplemental oxygen requirement at 36 weeks' postmenstrual age. The early surfactant group received about 60% more surfactant than the selective intubation group. Stratified analysis of FiO_2 at study entry suggested that a lower treatment threshold (FiO_2 <0.45) reduced air leaks and oxygen requirement at 28 days of age compared with a higher threshold (FiO_2 ≥0.45).

Further studies have been published since this review. The Colombian Neonatal Network enrolled infants of 27 to 31 weeks' gestation, who were receiving oxygen and had increased work of breathing, at 15 to 60 minutes after birth.[48] The infants were treated with bubble nasal CPAP 6 cm H_2O and then randomly allocated to either nasal CPAP plus surfactant (n = 141) or nasal CPAP alone (n = 137). The primary outcome was the need for MV started because either the FiO_2 was > 0.75 or the partial pressure of carbon dioxide ($PaCO_2$) was > 65 mm Hg. The nasal CPAP plus surfactant group received two doses of surfactant (Survanta™, Abbott Nutrition, Abbott Park, IL, USA), 2 minutes apart, and were then extubated, if possible, to nasal CPAP 6 cm H_2O. The need for MV was significantly lower in the nasal CPAP plus surfactant group (26% vs. 39%, RR 0.69 [95% CI 0.49–0.97]), although all babies who had received surfactant had been temporarily intubated and ventilated. Mortality, BPD, duration of MV, and oxygen therapy did not differ between the groups. There were fewer air leaks in the group receiving surfactant.

The "CURPAP" trial randomly assigned 208 infants born at 25 to 28 weeks' gestation who were not intubated within 30 minutes of birth to either (1) intubation, surfactant (Curosurf™, Cornerstone Therapeutics, Inc., Cary NC, USA) and extubation within an hour (if possible) to nasal CPAP or (2) nasal CPAP with early selective surfactant.[46] Infants were intubated for MV when the FiO_2 exceeded 0.40, the infant had four episodes of apnea per hour, or for $PaCO_2$ >65 mm Hg. There were no significant differences between the groups in the need for MV at 5 days of life, death or BPD, or the rate of pneumothorax.

These trials show that outcomes in infants stabilized in the delivery room with either nasal CPAP or prophylactic surfactant and extubation to nasal CPAP appear to be similar to those in infants managed with surfactant followed by MV.

LESS INVASIVE OR MINIMALLY INVASIVE SURFACTANT ADMINISTRATION

Over the last decade, various techniques of administering surfactant to spontaneously breathing preterm infants on noninvasive respiratory support without using an ETT, known as less invasive surfactant administration (LISA) or minimally invasive surfactant therapy (MIST), have been described and studied (Fig. 6.2). RCTs of LISA are heterogeneous, with differences in method of delivering the intervention, the mode of noninvasive respiratory support used, and the study population. Pooled analyses of these RCTs[49-51] found that LISA reduced rates of MV, the composite outcome of death or BPD at 36 weeks, and BPD in survivors.

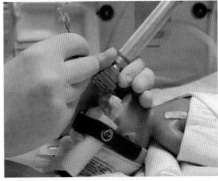

Fig. 6.2 Minimally invasive surfactant therapy. (Photo provided by Professor Peter Dargaville, Hobart, Australia.)

The recent Cochrane Review included 2164 preterm infants in 16 studies and compared LISA techniques with endotracheal intubation and surfactant.[52] The management of infants in the control group varied between studies: either early extubation after surfactant, delayed extubation after surfactant, or continuation of nasal CPAP and rescue surfactant administration only when prespecified criteria were met. Pooled analysis showed that LISA decreased the risk of the composite outcome of death or BPD: RR 0.59 (95% CI 0.48–0.73); the need for intubation within 72 hours: RR 0.63 (95% CI 0.54–0.74); severe intraventricular hemorrhage: RR 0.63 (95% CI 0.42–0.96); death during first hospitalization: RR 0.63 (95% CI 0.47–0.84); and BPD among survivors: RR 0.57 (95% CI 0.45–0.74). There was no significant difference in risk of air leak requiring drainage. Only two of the included RCTs have reported longer-term outcomes at 2 years,[53,54] and more evidence of longer-term effects is required. Herting et al.[55] found no statistically significant differences in weight, length, or neurodevelopmental outcome. However, Mehler and colleagues[56] reported lower incidences of a psychomotor development index <70 in infants receiving LISA and a lower incidence of mental developmental index <70 in the subgroup of more mature infants born 25 to 26 weeks' gestation who received LISA.

Since that Cochrane Review, Dargaville and colleagues have completed the largest RCT of the "MIST" technique[57] to date: the "OptiMIST-A" trial.[58] The trial enrolled preterm infants 25 to 28 weeks' gestation supported with nasal CPAP and receiving an $FiO_2 \geq$ 0.30 within 6 hours of birth. Infants were randomized to either receive surfactant (200 mg/kg of *poractant alfa*) via a 16-gauge vascular catheter under direct vision of the vocal cords or to continue CPAP without routine surfactant. Nasal CPAP was continued thereafter in both groups unless specified intubation criteria were met. OptiMIST-A was unique in that the control group underwent a sham procedure so that caregivers and outcome assessors were blinded to treatment allocation. The planned sample size was 606 infants. Ultimately, the trial, conducted at 33 centers around the world, enrolled 485 preterm infants.

In the OptiMIST-A trial, the primary outcome of death or BPD occurred in 43.6% of the MIST group and 49.6% of the control group: RR 0.87 (95%

CI 0.74–1.03), $P = 0.10$.[58] The overall incidence of death before 36 weeks' postmenstrual age did not differ significantly between the groups. However, there was an interaction between death and gestational age: the more immature subgroup of infants born 25 to 26 weeks' gestational age who received LISA seemed to have a higher rate of death. BPD was lower in the MIST group: RR 0.83 (95% CI 0.70–0.98). The incidence of other adverse events was similar between groups. There were some additional apparent benefits of MIST, including reductions in the incidence of intubation within 72 hours of birth and at any time, pneumothorax requiring drainage, patent ductus arteriosus requiring medical therapy, and the need for oxygen at home after discharge. The requirement for surfactant therapy via ETT was halved after treatment with MIST (32.8% vs. 68.4%), and MIST reduced the duration of MV (1 vs. 4 days), CPAP (17 vs. 22 days), and all forms of mechanical respiratory support (40 vs. 45 days).

The results of the OptiMIST-A trial, combined with evidence from earlier meta-analyses of RCTs, suggest important benefits from LISA/MIST. However, some caution is warranted in the most immature infants born 25 to 26 weeks' gestation given the signal for higher mortality. Overall, the evidence suggests that LISA/MIST may be preferable to routine endotracheal intubation for surfactant therapy in infants born $\geq$25 weeks' gestation. Of course, this procedure still requires skill with laryngoscopy. These findings are now being incorporated into clinical practice.[59]

NASAL CONTINUOUS POSITIVE AIRWAY PRESSURE FOR POSTEXTUBATION SUPPORT

It is generally accepted that early extubation of preterm infants is desirable. The benefits include reducing the risks of infection, local tissue damage, and BPD. On the other hand, failure of extubation and the need for reintubation are associated with instability and local trauma. The Cochrane Review on the topic[33] identified nine randomized trials of varying methodologic quality and using different CPAP pressures and devices.[60-68] Pooled analysis showed that in preterm infants, nasal CPAP after extubation was associated with a lower rate of respiratory failure (apnea, respiratory acidosis, or increased oxygen requirements) than management in an oxygen hood (RR 0.62 [95% CI 0.51–0.76]). Four of the studies allowed rescue nasal CPAP for infants in whom the oxygen hood failed. Because rescue treatment with nasal CPAP was frequently successful, there was no significant difference in the rate of reintubation between the groups: RR 0.93 (95% CI 0.72–1.19). A study that directly compared elective with rescue nasal CPAP ventilation after extubation found no differences in reintubation rates.[69]

Therefore, it can reasonably be concluded that nasal CPAP should be used when a very preterm infant is extubated, to prevent the instability associated with possible subsequent respiratory failure and reintubation.

CPAP "FAILURE": WHEN SHOULD PRETERM INFANTS BE INTUBATED?

There is no universally accepted definition of CPAP "failure." Polin and Sahni[70] suggested that "an infant with ventilation that is not improving or inadequate oxygenation with $FiO_2 > 0.60$" should be intubated and given surfactant. Others recommend intubation when the FiO_2 exceeds 0.35 to 0.40.[71] Studies suggest that lower gestational age (<26–27 weeks), more severe radiographic disease, and evidence of escalating FiO_2 are risk factors for nasal CPAP failure in preterm infants, although not necessarily strong predictors.[72,73] The following failure criteria were set for infants randomly allocated to nasal CPAP in the COIN trial of CPAP in the delivery room: $FiO_2 > 0.60$ or pH <7.25 with a $PaCO_2 > 60$ mm Hg, or more than one apneic episode per hour requiring stimulation.[43] More recently, a lower threshold of $FiO_2 > 0.30$ has been recommended in international guidelines as an indication for surfactant administration.[74] Whatever threshold is applied, it is important that remediable causes of CPAP failure are sought and treated before intubation. They include airway obstruction with secretions, inappropriate (too small) prong size, and inadequate distending pressure. Treating a large mouth leak and raising the applied pressure may be useful strategies before CPAP is deemed to have failed.

COMPLICATIONS OF NASAL CPAP

Nasal CPAP ventilation is a comparatively simple form of respiratory support, yet it is not without complications. The major problems during the early days of CPAP, i.e., intracerebellar hemorrhages[75] and hydrocephalus,[76] were solved by alterations in delivery technique. However, nasal trauma may still occur with prongs, ranging in severity from redness and excoriation of the nares to necrosis of the columella and nasal septum requiring surgery. Observational studies suggest that all nasal CPAP devices may cause trauma.[77] Robertson and coworkers[78] reported a complication rate of 20%, including necrosis or nasal deformities, in a series of very low birth weight babies managed with the Infant Flow Driver. To minimize the incidence of nasal trauma, we try to select a prong with a diameter that is sufficient to snugly fit the infant's nostril (avoiding excessive leak around the device), but which does not cause blanching of the nares. Positioning of the binasal prongs so that there is no pressure on the columella may sometimes be difficult to achieve, but this is critical. We have observed that supervision by skilled nurses experienced in the technique of securing nasal CPAP prongs reduces rates of nasal trauma.

Pneumothoraces may occur in preterm infants treated with CPAP. In the COIN trial,[43] there were significantly more pneumothoraces in the CPAP group than in the ventilated group (9% vs. 3%, respectively), raising concerns in some quarters about the use of early nasal CPAP. In the Colombian Neonatal Network study, the group managed with early surfactant therapy had fewer pneumothoraces compared with the group managed with nasal CPAP alone (2% vs. 9%).[48] The SUPPORT trial found no difference in the rate of pneumothoraces between early CPAP and early MV groups.[44] An RCT of early CPAP compared with headbox oxygen therapy after birth for newborn infants with respiratory distress born in Australian nontertiary centers by Buckmaster and colleagues found an almost threefold increase in pneumothorax rate in the CPAP-treated group (9% vs. 3%).[79] The benefits of CPAP are clear, but clinicians caring for infants receiving CPAP (particularly those infants with RDS who have not received surfactant therapy) must be aware of the risk of pneumothoraces and be able to diagnose and treat them.

WEANING FROM CPAP

The optimal method of weaning a baby from nasal CPAP remains uncertain, and practices vary among units. An RCT comparing a strategy of weaning through reducing pressure with one of increasing time "off" nasal CPAP showed a significantly shorter duration of weaning with the "pressure" strategy.[80] Another trial determined that weaning directly off nasal CPAP, rather than gradual titration over increasing time intervals, resulted in discontinuing nasal CPAP earlier.[81] Follow-up from that study suggests that utilizing a standardized approach to weaning from nasal CPAP in very preterm infants born <30 weeks' gestation is associated with improved outcomes, including decreased rates of BPD.[82] A multicenter trial by Jensen and colleagues[83] included 372 very preterm infants and compared "sudden" CPAP discontinuation with a gradual CPAP pressure wean prior to the discontinuation of CPAP. They found no difference in the primary outcome of weight gain velocity. However, among infants born before 28 weeks' gestation, infants in the gradual pressure wean group were more often successfully weaned from CPAP during the first attempt, without a longer duration of CPAP treatment.

Five RCTs have assessed the role of nHF in weaning from nasal CPAP. Trials by Tang et al.[84] and Soonsawad et al.[85] found nHF contributed to shorter time receiving nasal CPAP, but the overall duration of noninvasive respiratory support was reduced. In the study by Abdel-Hady et al.,[86] the use of nHF with gas flow 2 L/min to wean from CPAP resulted in more days on oxygen and respiratory support, with no difference in success of CPAP weaning. In contrast, Badiee[87] found that nHF 2 L/min significantly reduced the duration of supplemental oxygen and hospital stay, without increasing successful weaning from CPAP. Clements et al. recently found that weaning using nHF was noninferior to discontinuing CPAP from 5 cm H_2O in very preterm infants.[88]

The use of nHF to facilitate weaning from CPAP ventilation requires further investigation. In the absence of clear evidence, our practice is to incrementally wean infants to nasal CPAP 5 cm H_2O and discontinue CPAP when the infant is stable with FiO_2 <0.30 and recommence it if the oxygen requirement or frequency of apnea increases. We do not recommend the use of nHF as a routine weaning method.

Nasal Intermittent Positive-Pressure Ventilation

Despite the advantages of CPAP, many preterm infants experience treatment failure with CPAP and require additional support.[73] This led to clinicians applying ventilator-derived inflations via nasal interfaces as early as 1970.[89,90] NIPPV delivers an intermittent increase in pressure level, referred to as the peak inspiratory pressure (PIP), superimposed on a baseline positive end-expiratory pressure, which is similar to CPAP. The level and duration of set PIPs have varied across clinical studies. Some ventilators are capable of delivering inflations in synchrony with the infant's spontaneous breathing efforts. NIPPV may be used for primary support for infants with respiratory distress and in the postextubation setting.[91,92] Most forms of NIPPV aim to mimic normal tidal ventilation with relatively short inspiratory times and PIPs set similar to those on invasive ventilation. Biphasic CPAP is a form of noninvasive support where relatively longer inspiratory times and lower peak pressures are utilized.[93]

MECHANISMS OF NASAL INTERMITTENT POSITIVE-PRESSURE VENTILATION

Increased tidal volume delivery to the lungs was originally thought to be the primary mechanism of action of NIPPV. While some studies have demonstrated that NIPPV may improve tidal volume and minute ventilation,[94] others have shown that the pressure transmission to the lung is variable,[95] and the delivered tidal volume is low.[96] Studies assessing CO_2 clearance have shown inconsistent results.[94,97-99] Other proposed mechanisms include reducing airway resistance, improving the respiratory drive, and inducing paradoxical Head's reflex.[100] Finally, part of the mechanism of action may relate simply to the fact that the mean airway pressure (MAP) during NIPPV is generally higher than during CPAP. A few studies have evaluated short-term physiological impact of CPAP and NIPPV when used at equivalent MAP and have found no differences.[101,102] Further studies comparing CPAP and NIPPV at equivalent MAP are warranted to fully understand whether there are any independent mechanisms of action of NIPPV, and if there are any differences in clinical outcomes.

SYNCHRONIZED VERSUS UNSYNCHRONIZED NASAL INTERMITTENT POSITIVE-PRESSURE VENTILATION

NIPPV can be broadly classified into synchronized and nonsynchronized with the infant's spontaneous respiratory efforts. Asynchronous breaths (delivered late in the inspiratory phase or during patients' expiratory phase) may alter the spontaneous breathing pattern and may even lead to closure of the glottis, which in turn may potentially divert gas flow to the stomach.[103-106] It has been shown that majority of delivered breaths during nonsynchronized NIPPV (nsNIPPV) are asynchronous with patients' efforts and result in minimal tidal volume delivery.[107]

The two most common means of achieving synchronization are flow sensors and pneumatic capsules such as the Graseby capsule (Graseby Medical, Watford, United Kingdom). Synchronization using flow sensors in a system with a substantial and variable leak is challenging. Some have reliably achieved synchronization using flow sensors during NIPPV,[94] while others have reported lack of success.[108] Similarly, the accuracy of a pneumatic capsule may be affected by positioning and movement. However, there are some data reporting that the Graseby capsule correctly detected onset of inspiration about 90% of the time.[107] Many devices that performed synchronized NIPPV (sNIPPV) are no longer commercially available (e.g., Infant Star ventilator). Surveys show most centers using NIPPV employ the nonsynchronized mode.[100]

There are very limited clinical data on direct comparison of sNIPPV versus nsNIPPV. Some studies have reported physiological benefits of sNIPPV over nsNIPPV,[99,107,109] but important clinical outcomes are lacking.

A relatively new form of synchronization, neurally adjusted ventilator assist (NAVA), uses electrical diaphragmatic signals detected by a catheter which also functions as a feeding tube. This technology can be applied to both invasive and noninvasive respiratory support (NIV-NAVA). The signal is used to deliver ventilation in synchrony with and in proportion to the infant's breathing efforts. While early data show promise, a recent Cochrane Review identified only two small crossover trials.[110] More studies are required before this technique is adopted into routine clinical practice.

CLINICAL EVIDENCE ON USE OF NASAL INTERMITTENT POSITIVE-PRESSURE VENTILATION FOR PRIMARY RESPIRATORY SUPPORT

A Cochrane Review published in 2016 evaluated outcomes from RCTs comparing NIPPV and CPAP and demonstrated a lower risk of respiratory failure within the first week and a lower risk of intubation with the use of NIPPV.[91] There were no differences in rates of important morbidities between groups. However, none of the included studies attempted to match the MAP between NIPPV and CPAP groups. A more recent review[93] included eight new trials representing an additional 850 infants. The results were largely concordant with the Cochrane Review with one notable exception—the pooled estimate of the risk of developing BPD was lower in the NIPPV group: RR 0.72 (95% CI 0.56–0.93). The authors noted that the overall difference was fully attributable to the reduction in BPD seen in studies using ventilator-generated sNIPPV.

CLINICAL EVIDENCE ON USE OF NASAL INTERMITTENT POSITIVE-PRESSURE VENTILATION AS A POSTEXTUBATION MODE

A Cochrane Review assessing outcomes with the use of NIPPV (including bilevel CPAP, nsNIPPV, and sNIPPV) versus CPAP for preterm infants following extubation was published in 2017.[92] Ten trials comprising 1431 infants were included. There was a significantly lower risk of respiratory failure in the first week postextubation with use of NIPPV compared with CPAP (RR 0.70 [95% CI 0.60–0.80]) as well as a lower risk of reintubation (RR 0.76 [95% CI 0.65–0.88]). Subgroup analyses showed benefits were confined to studies evaluating traditional NIPPV, rather than bilevel CPAP. There were no differences in mortality, BPD, or necrotizing enterocolitis. Pulmonary air leaks were lower with use of NIPPV: RR 0.48 (95% CI 0.28–0.82). BPD rates were lower for traditional NIPPV but not bilevel CPAP. Subgroup analyses by presence or absence of synchronization found a lower risk of extubation failure with both sNIPPV and ns-NIPPV. The pooled estimate of risk of developing BPD was also lower where sNIPPV was used, based on limited data from three trials representing 181 infants. Similar to the limitations of the meta-analysis of pre-extubation NIPPV use, none of the included studies matched the MAP between the intervention and control arms, and data to conduct subgroup analyses for the smallest infants (<28 weeks' gestational age or <1000 g) were not available.

A more recent review included an additional five trials (total of 1013 infants).[93] Extubation failure was again noted to be lower with NIPPV, and the greatest benefit was noted with sNIPPV based on data from six trials totaling 352 infants: RR 0.24 (95% CI 0.15–0.39). Similar to the Cochrane Review, the overall risk of BPD was not lower with NIPPV, but when limited to studies that used traditional sNIPPV, the pooled estimate was lower (4 trials, 289 infants).

NASAL INTERMITTENT POSITIVE-PRESSURE VENTILATION FOR APNEA OF PREMATURITY

A recent meta-analysis comparing NIPPV and CPAP for apnea of prematurity found that apnea frequency was similar between the groups.[111] However, in a post hoc analysis, there was a lower risk of occurrence of any apnea. None of the studies compared the modes at equivalent MAPs. The limited quality of the included studies precluded firm conclusions.

NASAL INTERMITTENT POSITIVE-PRESSURE VENTILATION SETTINGS

There are limited data informing the choice of pressure, rate, and inspiratory time settings to use during NIPPV. Traditional forms of NIPPV use similar settings to those used during conventional MV. The PEEPs utilized in RCTs have ranged from 3 to 8 cm H_2O, while set PIPs have ranged from 15 to 24 cm H_2O.[91,92] The inspiratory time is generally ≤0.5 seconds, although occasionally higher inspiratory times may be used. Rates are set typically between 20 and 40 per minute. On the other hand, during bilevel CPAP, the two levels of PEEP are generally no more than 3 to 5 cm H_2O apart. Lower PEEP levels are set similar to the levels used in traditional NIPPV. During bilevel CPAP, the time spent on the higher CPAP level is often longer, typically 1 second. While guidelines for settings to be used during NIPPV have been published,[112] it is recognized that these are based on expert opinion and NIPPV settings in published trials, rather than rigorous studies comparing settings.

Summary and Recommendations

NIPPV is a mode of noninvasive respiratory support that superimposes intermittent higher pressures on a background PEEP level, the duration and frequency of which can be set by the clinician. There are several devices available to provide NIPPV. These include traditional NIPPV typically provided by a ventilator which aims to mimic tidal ventilation (higher peak pressures and shorter inspiratory times) and bilevel CPAP (lower peak pressure and longer inspiratory times). NIPPV may be synchronized or nonsynchronized with patient efforts. NIPPV appears to be superior to CPAP both as a primary and as a postextubation support mode. Subgroup analyses suggest that sNIPPV using higher pressures may be the most effective. NIV-NAVA is promising but has yet to be studied in large RCTs.

Noninvasive High-Frequency Ventilation

Recently, NIHFV has been employed in some NICUs, seeking to combine the advantages of noninvasive respiratory support with the efficacy of invasive high-frequency ventilation delivered via an ETT.[113,114] Although its first clinical use in neonates was described as far back as 1998,[115] evidence regarding safety and efficacy of NIHFV is limited.

MECHANISMS OF ACTION OF NONINVASIVE HIGH-FREQUENCY VENTILATION

The MAP is primarily responsible for the maintenance of functional residual capacity. Similar to CPAP, some loss of pressure is expected with NIHFV. This has been demonstrated in bench models.[116,117] Gas exchange during high-frequency ventilation via an ETT is due to a variety of mechanisms. These include Taylor dispersion, Pendelluft, and asymmetric gas velocity profiles, in addition to the bulk flow and molecular diffusion that occur during conventional ventilation.[118,119] The same mechanisms may be involved during NIHFV. A number of bench and in vivo studies have demonstrated that oscillatory pressures and volumes can be delivered to the airways and distal lung parenchyma.[117,120-122]

A variety of interfaces have been used during NIHFV. While initial studies of NIHFV used a single nasopharyngeal tube, the presence of higher resistance, secretions, and leak via the contralateral nostril led to a shift toward short binasal prongs and/or nasal masks, based on experience with CPAP.[27,123] Bench models suggest that while both short binasal prongs and masks can deliver oscillatory pressure and volume, larger prong diameters may be more efficient,[117,124] and nasal masks may lead to lower transmission compared with prongs.[116]

The presence of leak during NIHFV may also be important. One bench model suggested that ventilation may remain effective during NIHFV even in the presence of a leak.[125] Another reported that NIHFV with a moderate level of leak provided more effective CO_2 elimination than that without any leak.[126] These findings raise the possibility of dead-space washout as an important mechanism of NIHFV.

CLINICAL STUDIES OF NONINVASIVE HIGH-FREQUENCY VENTILATION

Observational and Crossover Studies

Initial studies of NIHFV focused on its use as a rescue mode following failure of other noninvasive respiratory support modes or as postextubation "prophylaxis" in a group of high-risk infants. Van der Hoeven et al. described the use of NIHFV in 21 preterm and term infants with CO_2 retention and/or increasing FiO_2 requirements, of whom only 5 ultimately required intubation.[115] Czernik et al. reported its use in 20 infants deemed to be at high risk of extubation failure, of whom 14 avoided reintubation.[127] Mukerji et al. reported both rescue and prophylactic use of NIHFV in a cohort of 52 preterm infants and noted that NIHFV prevented intubation in the majority of these infants; these latter findings were replicated in another cohort.[128,129] Recently, two observational studies with control groups have been reported, one of which reported a lower incidence of failure with NIHFV versus bilevel CPAP.[130] The other study reported no differences in reintubation rates between NIHFV and CPAP.[131]

Other studies have focused on physiological outcomes, chiefly CO_2 elimination. Colaizy et al. noted a decline in CO_2 from 50($\pm$6) to 45($\pm$9) mm Hg in 14 neonates transferred from CPAP to NIHFV.[132] Bottino et al. conducted a crossover trial with 30 neonates placed on either CPAP or NIHFV for two 1-hour periods on each mode. The transcutaneous CO_2 fell during NIHFV (47.5 $\pm$ 7.6 mm Hg) compared with CPAP (49.9 $\pm$ 7.2 mm Hg).[133] Two other crossover trials did not find any significant change in CO_2 levels.[134,135] The reasons for these contrasting findings are unclear.

Randomized Controlled Trials

There have been 10 parallel RCTs of NIHFV recruiting a total of 2530 infants evaluating clinical outcomes.[136-144] Sample sizes in individual trials ranged from 39 to 1440 participants. While most trials have assessed the use of NIHFV as a primary mode, the largest is a three-arm trial assessing its use post-extubation.[145] Many of these trials have been included in systematic and narrative reviews.[146-148] Despite heterogeneity within their populations and design, the trials have generally favored NIHFV. Treatment failure and/or need for intubation were reported to be lower in the NIHFV group in five studies,[136-138,141,143,145] whereas three did not detect any important differences.[139,140,142] Duration of respiratory support was noted to be shorter with NIHFV in three studies.[138,140,141] Li et al.[138] reported a reduction in rates of BPD with the use of NIHFV; however, this effect was not seen in other studies reporting the outcome. Summary of key findings from the RCTs is depicted in Table 6.1.

These studies have important limitations. The populations studied and the indications for use are heterogeneous. Studies of NIHFV as the primary mode of support included both infants who had received surfactant and those who had not, and they had differing inclusion criteria with respect to gestational age. Finally, none of the caregivers were blinded to treatment allocation. Pooled analyses show a lower incidence of intubation when NIHFV was used as primary support (RR 0.44 [95% CI 0.29–0.67]); lower incidence of intubation across all indications (RR 0.50 [95% CI 0.36–0.70]); and reduction in $PaCO_2$.[146,147] The most recent meta-analysis, restricted to use of NIHFV as primary support, did not find any significant differences in BPD, mortality, necrotizing enterocolitis, or air leak syndromes.[147]

SETTINGS DURING NONINVASIVE HIGH-FREQUENCY VENTILATION

There are no clinical studies that have compared the effectiveness of different settings during NIHFV. Many trials comparing NIHFV to other modes have either used a higher initial MAP or allowed for a higher range with NIHFV. This leads to uncertainty as to whether differences in outcomes are related to the use of higher distending pressures or the mechanisms of NIHFV itself. While some advocate for a higher MAP during use of NIHFV,[148] there are no data to refute the hypothesis that similar benefits in clinical outcomes could be achieved by simply raising the CPAP pressure. The

TABLE 6.1 Characteristics and Key Findings from Randomized Controlled Trials of NIHFV Assessing Clinical Outcomes

Author, Year	Population	NIHFV and Comparator: Initial (Range) of MAP	Key Outcomes With NIHFV	Comments
Dumas De La Roque, 2011	N = 46 with TTN (primary use) GA: NIHFV arm: 38 ± 0.5 weeks CPAP arm: 37 ± 0.4 weeks	NIHFV: 5 cm H_2O CPAP: 5 cm H_2O	Lower respiratory distress duration[a] Lower duration of oxygen supplementation	
Mukerji, 2017	N = 39 with CPAP failure GA: NIHFV arm: 26.1 (1.3) weeks CPAP arm: 26.5 (1.6) weeks	NIHFV: 8 (maximum 10) cm H_2O Biphasic CPAP: PIP 8/ PEEP 5 (maximum 10/7) cm H_2O	Treatment failure: ND Need for MV <72 hours and <7 days: ND BPD: ND $PaCO_2$ gradient: ND	Pilot feasibility trial
Zhu, 2017	N = 76 with RDS (primary use) GA: NIHFV arm: 31.7 ± 1.7 weeks CPAP arm: 32.0 ± 1.9 weeks	NIHFV: 6 (up to 10) cm H_2O CPAP: 6 (up to 10) cm H_2O	Less need for MV[a] BPD: ND IVH: ND	Patients had received surfactant prior to randomization
Iranpour, 2019	N = 68 with RDS (primary use) GA: NIHFV arm: 33 (31–35) weeks CPAP arm: 33 (30–34) weeks	NIHFV: 8 cm H_2O CPAP: 6–7 cm H_2O	Lower noninvasive respiratory support duration[a] Less need for MV Less IVH BPD: ND $PaCO_2$[b]: ND	
Malakian, 2019	N = 124 with RDS (primary use) GA: NIHFV arm: 31.08 ± 2.9 weeks CPAP arm: 31.07 ± 2.8 weeks	NIHFV: 4 (maximum 8) cm H_2O CPAP: 4 (maximum 8) cm H_2O	Intubation within 72 hours[a]: ND Lower duration of respiratory support IVH: ND	None of the included patients developed BPD
Chen, 2019	N = 206 post-extubation GA: NIHFV arm: 226.8 ± 16.9 days CPAP arm: 229.5 ± 16.8 days	NIHFV: 10 (5–16) cm H_2O CPAP: 6 (4–8) cm H_2O	Less reintubation[a] Lower $PaCO_2$ BPD: ND IVH: ND	
Li, 2021	N = 149 post-extubation GA: NIHFV arm: 29.0 ± 1.9 weeks NIPPV arm: 28.9 ± 2.0 weeks CPAP arm: 29.0 ± 1.7 weeks	NIHFV: 10 (6–12) cm H_2O NIPPV: PIP 15/PEEP 4 (15–25/4–8) cm H_2O CPAP: 5 (3–8) cm H_2O	Less reintubation within 7 days[a] (vs. both CPAP and NIPPV) Lower $PaCO_2$ (vs. both CPAP and NIPPV) Lower noninvasive respiratory support duration (vs. CPAP only) Less BPD (vs. CPAP only) IVH: ND	Three-arm trial
Wu, 2021	N = 80 post-extubation after cardiac surgery Age: NIHFV arm: 2.2 (0.4) months CPAP arm: 2.3 (0.4) months	NIHFV: 5–10 cm H_2O CPAP: 3–8 cm H_2O	Postextubation failure[a]: ND Lower $PaCO_2$ Noninvasive respiratory support duration: ND	

TABLE 6.1 Characteristics and Key Findings from Randomized Controlled Trials of NIHFV Assessing Clinical Outcomes (Continued)

Author, Year	Population	NIHFV and Comparator: Initial (Range) of MAP	Key Outcomes With NIHFV	Comments
Zhu, 2021	N = 302 with RDS (primary use) GA: NIHFV arm: 30.6 (1.7) weeks CPAP arm: 30.9 (1.8) weeks	NIHFV: 6 (6–10) cm H_2O CPAP: 6 (6–8) cm H_2O	Need for MV <7 days[a]: ND Noninvasive respiratory support duration: ND BPD: ND Severe IVH: ND	Need for MV/treatment failure was lower in a lower GA subgroup (26–29 weeks)
Zhu, 2022	N = 1440 post-extubation GA: NIHFV arm: 29.4 (1.8) weeks NIPPV arm: 29.4 (1.8) weeks CPAP arm: 29.5 (1.7) weeks	NIHFV: 10 (maximum 16) cm H_2O NIPPV: PIP 15/PEEP 5 (maximum 25/8) cm H_2O CPAP: 5 (maximum 8) cm H_2O	Lower duration of MV (vs. CPAP and NIPPV) Lower risk of reintubation (vs. CPAP) BPD: ND Air leaks: ND	

[a]Primary outcome.
[b]Post-hoc outcome.

BPD, Bronchopulmonary dysplasia; *CPAP*, continuous positive airway pressure; *cm H_2O*, centimeters of water; *GA*, gestational age; *IVH*, intraventricular hemorrhage; *MV*, mechanical ventilation; *ND*, no difference; *NIHFV*, noninvasive high-frequency ventilation; *NIPPV*, nasal intermittent positive-pressure ventilation; *PaCO₂*, partial pressure of carbon dioxide; *PEEP*, positive end-expiratory pressure; *PIP*, positive inflation pressure; *RDS*, respiratory distress syndrome; *TTN*, transient tachypnea of the newborn.

concern of CO_2 retention when using high MAPs without oscillations (e.g., high pressures on CPAP) raised by some authors[148] remain speculative.

Frequencies used in NIFHV trials have mostly been around 10 Hz. Some bench models have demonstrated that lower frequencies improve ventilation,[149] similar to invasive high-frequency ventilation. It is unclear whether different frequencies should be applied in different lung conditions (i.e., higher frequencies for lung conditions with lower time constants such as RDS and lower frequencies for conditions with higher time constants such as BPD).[150] At present, the choice of 10 Hz as a starting point appears reasonable with adjustments made to achieve the desired ventilation goals. Most studies report setting the amplitude to achieve a visible or palpable chest shake, which seems appropriate.

SUMMARY AND RECOMMENDATIONS FOR NONINVASIVE HIGH-FREQUENCY VENTILATION USE

NIHFV remains a relatively untested form of noninvasive respiratory support for preterm neonates. Bench models and in vivo studies suggest NIHFV may retain the ventilation properties seen during high-frequency ventilation via an ETT. While a number of studies suggest that CO_2 removal is improved compared with CPAP, this has not been consistently described. Many studies suggest favorable clinical outcomes with the use of NIHFV, but heterogeneity in study designs and inconsistencies in the outcomes preclude firm conclusions. The optimal indications remain unclear, and the currently available data do not justify its routine widespread use outside of rigorously designed clinical trials.

Nasal High Flow

Nasal high flow (nHF) (Fig. 6.3) is an increasingly popular mode of noninvasive respiratory support for newborn infants, particularly preterm infants. nHF provides heated, humidified, blended air and oxygen at high gas flows, usually set at 2 to 8 L/min.[151,152] The prongs should not occlude the nares in order to avoid excessive pressure generation.[151] The perceived benefits of nHF over CPAP include the simpler interface, ease of application, and infant comfort.[153] nHF is preferred by parents[154] and nurses.[155] Rates of nasal trauma are lower with the use of nHF, compared with CPAP.[151,156]

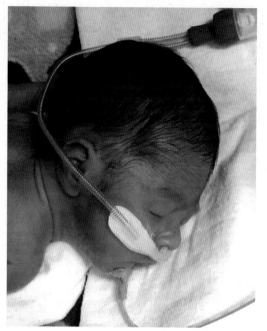

Fig. 6.3 A very preterm infant treated with nasal high-flow therapy. (Fisher & Paykel Optiflow Junior, Fisher & Paykel Healthcare, Auckland, New Zealand).

The use of nHF as an alternative to CPAP for preterm infants in developed countries has dramatically increased over the past decade. For example, the Australian and New Zealand Neonatal Network has reported a fourfold increase in nHF exposure of included infants from 2009 to 2019.[157] Surveys have demonstrated that 89% of Canadian tertiary centers[158] and 95% of responding units in a UK survey[159] use nHF in some capacity. In NICUs, nHF is used as an alternative to nasal CPAP for preterm infants for several indications: primary respiratory support soon after birth for prophylaxis or treatment of RDS; postextubation support following a period of MV; to treat apnea of prematurity; to reduce nasal trauma; and as a weaning mode from nasal CPAP.[160-163]

The two most widely used commercially available neonatal nHF systems are Vapotherm Precision Flow (Vapotherm Inc., Exeter, NH) and Optiflow Junior (Fisher & Paykel Healthcare, Auckland, NZ). These systems include a range of infant nasal prong sizes with varying outer diameters and septum widths. The Fisher & Paykel system includes a pressure relief valve

in the circuit, whereas Vapotherm does not. Only one small trial comparing older versions of the devices has been published.[164] Hence, there is no evidence that one device is superior to the other.

HOW DOES NASAL HIGH FLOW WORK?

nHF provides respiratory support through a number of mechanisms. There is probably some overlap between the mechanisms of action of nHF and CPAP. nHF delivers heated and humidified gases, which can help improve mucociliary function and pulmonary compliance.[165] There is some reported variation in temperature and humidity of gas between devices and at different gas flows.[165-167] nHF produces a distending airway pressure, which unlike CPAP, is not routinely set. In vivo and in vitro studies with different methodologies have attempted to measure the distending airway pressure produced by nHF devices. In these studies, pharyngeal pressures were similar to, or less than, those commonly achieved with CPAP, provided a leak in the circuit was maintained.[168-172] Pressures increase with increasing gas flow but vary considerably between infants. Higher pressures are measured in smaller infants at the same gas flow.[165,168-178]

Another mechanism of gas exchange during nHF is washout of the nasopharyngeal dead space.[179,180] This improves carbon dioxide clearance, with a greater effect observed when higher gas flows are applied.[181,182] An animal study showed that the effect of increasing gas flow on carbon dioxide removal and oxygenation was independent of the pressures generated, and that both ventilation and oxygenation improved in a flow-dependent manner.[175] A high-leak interface produced better ventilation than a low-leak interface until flow rates were high. nHF may also minimize the resistance to gas flow in the nasopharynx by providing a gas flow matching or exceeding the peak inspiratory flow of the patient, thus reducing the work of breathing.[183-187]

EVIDENCE FROM RANDOMIZED TRIALS IN PRETERM INFANTS

Stabilization in the Delivery Room

There are no published randomized trials of nHF use in the delivery room; however, Siva and Reynolds published a single-center 5-year retrospective cohort study of 292 preterm infants born before 32 weeks' gestation.[188] Delivery room stabilization of the infants involved delayed cord clamping, followed by nHF at 7 to 8 L/min if infants were spontaneously breathing. If infants were not spontaneously breathing, they received inflation breaths, followed by consideration of nHF if breathing was subsequently established. Of the total 491 infants born <32 weeks' gestation, 292 (59%) were stabilized on nHF in the delivery room and the median FiO_2 on NICU admission was 0.25. Infants managed with nHF had a higher median gestational age and birth weight than those who required intubation in the delivery room. Of infants commenced on nHF, 78% of infants remained on this therapy at 72 hours of age and overall, about half of the infants required surfactant treatment. RCTs are required before the use of nHF for delivery room stabilization can be recommended.

Nasal High Flow as Primary Respiratory Support for Preterm Infants With Respiratory Distress

Nasal High Flow Versus Continuous Positive Airway Pressure

Eleven RCTs[189-199] enrolling a total of more than 2100 preterm infants have compared nHF with CPAP for primary respiratory support soon after birth. These trials vary in the gestational ages and birth weights of the infants enrolled and included very few extremely preterm infants. The studies also differ in the use of CPAP to treat infants in the nHF group before inclusion, the nHF and CPAP devices studied, the starting and maximal gas flows (for nHF) and pressures (for CPAP) studied, the administration of surfactant before the primary outcome was determined, and the use of "rescue" modes of noninvasive respiratory support once treatment failure occurred.

Pooled analyses of nine studies found a higher incidence of treatment failure within 72 hours of trial entry in infants treated with nHF for primary respiratory support after birth, compared with CPAP (RR 1.70 [95% CI 1.41–2.06]) (Fig. 6.4). However, there was no difference between groups for the outcome of MV within 72 hours of trial entry: RR 1.04 (95% CI 0.82–1.31) (Fig. 6.5). This is likely due to the use of second-line CPAP prior to intubation, which was permitted in some trials for infants who met treatment failure criteria on nHF.

Nasal High Flow Versus Nasal Intermittent Positive-Pressure Ventilation

Four studies enrolling a total of 343 infants have compared nHF with NIPPV for primary respiratory support soon after birth.[194,197,200,201] There was no difference in the incidence of treatment failure (based on trial criteria) when nHF was compared with NIPPV: RR 1.27 (95% CI 0.90–1.79). Similarly, there was no difference in the incidence of MV: RR 0.90 (95% CI 0.55–1.46).

Nasal High Flow to Prevent Extubation Failure in Preterm Infants

Several meta-analyses have compared nHF with CPAP for postextubation support after a period of MV or after intubation for surfactant provision (INtubation, SURfactant, Extubation, or INSURE) in preterm infants.

Since publication of a 2016 Cochrane Review[202] that included six trials,[189,203-207] three further systematic reviews have evaluated the efficacy of nHF to prevent extubation failure in preterm infants.[208-210] Five additional studies were included in these new reviews.[211-214] All reviews concluded that there was no significant difference in the rate of treatment failure or reintubation when nHF was compared with CPAP for postextubation support of preterm infants. In two of the reviews,[209,210] nHF was associated with a lower incidence of air leak (pneumothorax) and nasal trauma. In contrast to the findings of these meta-analyses, a recent Japanese RCT found a higher rate of treatment failure with nHF than CPAP in preterm infants born <34 weeks' gestation, although it must be noted that infants in the CPAP group could also receive NIPPV. Ramaswamy et al. also performed a sensitivity analysis comparing different devices to deliver nHF, concluding that further studies comparing devices were required.[209]

Overall, the evidence suggests that nHF is a suitable alternative to nasal CPAP for postextubation support of preterm infants, and may have some benefits, but caution is recommended for extremely preterm infants born <28 weeks' gestation. Few trials have enrolled these high-risk infants, and gestational age subgroup data are not available from all trials.

SAFETY OF NASAL HIGH FLOW

Adverse events, including death, BPD, and pneumothorax, were included outcomes in the Cochrane

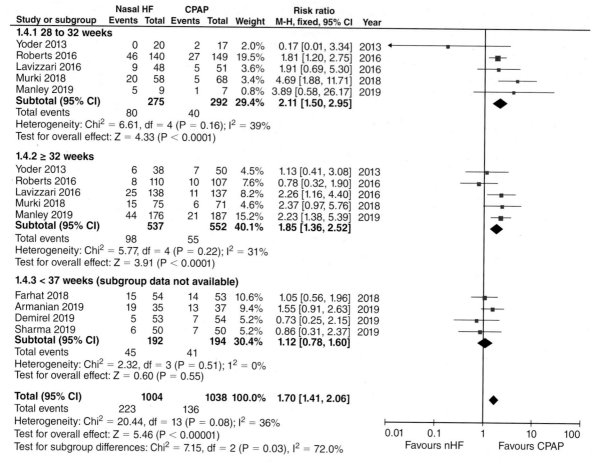

Study or subgroup	Nasal HF Events	Total	CPAP Events	Total	Weight	Risk ratio M-H, fixed, 95% CI	Year
1.4.1 28 to 32 weeks							
Yoder 2013	0	20	2	17	2.0%	0.17 [0.01, 3.34]	2013
Roberts 2016	46	140	27	149	19.5%	1.81 [1.20, 2.75]	2016
Lavizzari 2016	9	48	5	51	3.6%	1.91 [0.69, 5.30]	2016
Murki 2018	20	58	5	68	3.4%	4.69 [1.88, 11.71]	2018
Manley 2019	5	9	1	7	0.8%	3.89 [0.58, 26.17]	2019
Subtotal (95% CI)		**275**		**292**	**29.4%**	**2.11 [1.50, 2.95]**	
Total events	80		40				
Heterogeneity: Chi^2 = 6.61, df = 4 (P = 0.16); I^2 = 39%							
Test for overall effect: Z = 4.33 (P < 0.0001)							
1.4.2 ≥ 32 weeks							
Yoder 2013	6	38	7	50	4.5%	1.13 [0.41, 3.08]	2013
Roberts 2016	8	110	10	107	7.6%	0.78 [0.32, 1.90]	2016
Lavizzari 2016	25	138	11	137	8.2%	2.26 [1.16, 4.40]	2016
Murki 2018	15	75	6	71	4.6%	2.37 [0.97, 5.76]	2018
Manley 2019	44	176	21	187	15.2%	2.23 [1.38, 5.39]	2019
Subtotal (95% CI)		**537**		**552**	**40.1%**	**1.85 [1.36, 2.52]**	
Total events	98		55				
Heterogeneity: Chi^2 = 5.77, df = 4 (P = 0.22); I^2 = 31%							
Test for overall effect: Z = 3.91 (P < 0.0001)							
1.4.3 < 37 weeks (subgroup data not available)							
Farhat 2018	15	54	14	53	10.6%	1.05 [0.56, 1.96]	2018
Armanian 2019	19	35	13	37	9.4%	1.55 [0.91, 2.63]	2019
Demirel 2019	5	53	7	54	5.2%	0.73 [0.25, 2.15]	2019
Sharma 2019	6	50	7	50	5.2%	0.86 [0.31, 2.37]	2019
Subtotal (95% CI)		**192**		**194**	**30.4%**	**1.12 [0.78, 1.60]**	
Total events	45		41				
Heterogeneity: Chi^2 = 2.32, df = 3 (P = 0.51); I^2 = 0%							
Test for overall effect: Z = 0.60 (P = 0.55)							
Total (95% CI)		**1004**		**1038**	**100.0%**	**1.70 [1.41, 2.06]**	
Total events	223		136				
Heterogeneity: Chi^2 = 20.44, df = 13 (P = 0.08); I^2 = 36%							
Test for overall effect: Z = 5.46 (P < 0.00001)							
Test for subgroup differences: Chi^2 = 7.15, df = 2 (P = 0.03), I^2 = 72.0%							

0.01   0.1   1   10   100
Favours nHF   Favours CPAP

Fig. 6.4 Nasal high flow *(HF)* versus continuous positive airway pressure *(CPAP)* as primary support for preterm infants: treatment failure (study definition, 9 studies).

Review.[202] No differences were demonstrated in the rates of death or BPD between nHF and CPAP/NIPPV for any of the studied clinical indications. Trials published since this have similarly found no difference in rates of death or BPD.[190-194] Despite early concerns that unregulated distending pressure generation in the lung with nHF might increase the risk of air leaks from the lung,[215] pneumothorax rates were low in all randomized trials and there was no difference in rates of pneumothorax between nHF and CPAP on pooled analysis.[202,210,216] In fact, the risk of pneumothorax may actually be lower with the use of nHF, compared with CPAP.[209] While trials have consistently reported lower rates of nasal trauma with nHF compared with CPAP, and this

reduction is confirmed with pooled analysis in the Cochrane Review,[202] none of the studies included blinded assessment of this outcome. It should also be noted that individual studies were not powered to detect differences in the rates of most secondary outcomes.

POTENTIAL CONCERNS WITH USE OF NASAL HIGH FLOW IN NEONATES

While the results of clinical trials are generally reassuring, there are several factors that warrant caution and further investigation. Though no differences in rates of BPD have been described with nHF use compared to CPAP/NIPPV, trials have used varying definitions of BPD. No nHF trials have been powered sufficiently to

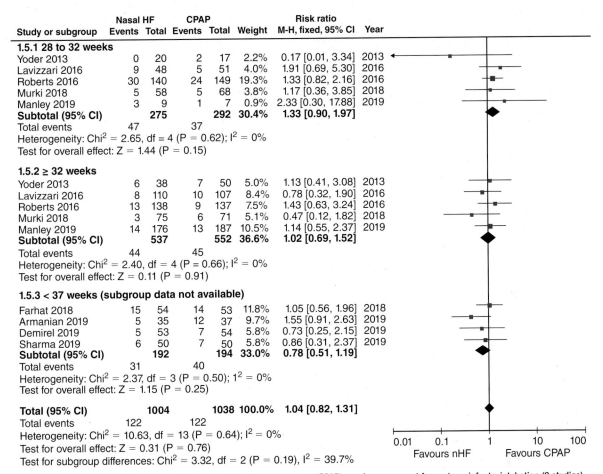

Study or subgroup	Nasal HF Events	Total	CPAP Events	Total	Weight	Risk ratio M-H, fixed, 95% CI	Year
1.5.1 28 to 32 weeks							
Yoder 2013	0	20	2	17	2.2%	0.17 [0.01, 3.34]	2013
Lavizzari 2016	9	48	5	51	4.0%	1.91 [0.69, 5.30]	2016
Roberts 2016	30	140	24	149	19.3%	1.33 [0.82, 2.16]	2016
Murki 2018	5	58	5	68	3.8%	1.17 [0.36, 3.85]	2018
Manley 2019	3	9	1	7	0.9%	2.33 [0.30, 17.88]	2019
Subtotal (95% CI)		**275**		**292**	**30.4%**	**1.33 [0.90, 1.97]**	
Total events	47		37				
Heterogeneity: Chi^2 = 2.65, df = 4 (P = 0.62); I^2 = 0%							
Test for overall effect: Z = 1.44 (P = 0.15)							
1.5.2 ≥ 32 weeks							
Yoder 2013	6	38	7	50	5.0%	1.13 [0.41, 3.08]	2013
Lavizzari 2016	8	110	10	107	8.4%	0.78 [0.32, 1.90]	2016
Roberts 2016	13	138	9	137	7.5%	1.43 [0.63, 3.24]	2016
Murki 2018	3	75	6	71	5.1%	0.47 [0.12, 1.82]	2018
Manley 2019	14	176	13	187	10.5%	1.14 [0.55, 2.37]	2019
Subtotal (95% CI)		**537**		**552**	**36.6%**	**1.02 [0.69, 1.52]**	
Total events	44		45				
Heterogeneity: Chi^2 = 2.40, df = 4 (P = 0.66); I^2 = 0%							
Test for overall effect: Z = 0.11 (P = 0.91)							
1.5.3 < 37 weeks (subgroup data not available)							
Farhat 2018	15	54	14	53	11.8%	1.05 [0.56, 1.96]	2018
Armanian 2019	5	35	12	37	9.7%	1.55 [0.91, 2.63]	2019
Demirel 2019	5	53	7	54	5.8%	0.73 [0.25, 2.15]	2019
Sharma 2019	6	50	7	50	5.8%	0.86 [0.31, 2.37]	2019
Subtotal (95% CI)		**192**		**194**	**33.0%**	**0.78 [0.51, 1.19]**	
Total events	31		40				
Heterogeneity: Chi^2 = 2.37, df = 3 (P = 0.50); I^2 = 0%							
Test for overall effect: Z = 1.15 (P = 0.25)							
Total (95% CI)		**1004**		**1038**	**100.0%**	**1.04 [0.82, 1.31]**	
Total events	122		122				
Heterogeneity: Chi^2 = 10.63, df = 13 (P = 0.64); I^2 = 0%							
Test for overall effect: Z = 0.31 (P = 0.76)							
Test for subgroup differences: Chi^2 = 3.32, df = 2 (P = 0.19), I^2 = 39.7%							

0.01 0.1 1 10 100
Favours nHF   Favours CPAP

Fig. 6.5 Nasal high flow *(HF)* versus continuous positive airway pressure *(CPAP)* as primary support for preterm infants: intubation (9 studies).

demonstrate a difference in BPD rates, and none have reported using an oxygen reduction test or grading the severity of BPD. Several studies have however reported a longer duration of weaning from respiratory support or oxygen with nHF use compared with CPAP,[189,190,200,205,217] which may be influenced by weaning practices.

Some infants initially managed with nHF develop respiratory failure but may be successfully "rescued" with CPAP and avoid MV. Hence, availability of CPAP is an important consideration if nHF is used as first-line therapy. Finally, relatively few extremely preterm infants born before 28 weeks' gestation, the population at highest risk of BPD, have been included in randomized trials, and caution is recommended when using nHF in this population.

SHOULD NASAL HIGH FLOW BE USED TO TREAT PRETERM INFANTS?

There is evidence that nHF may be used as an alternative to nasal CPAP for postextubation support in preterm infants ≥ 28 weeks' gestation. In contrast, CPAP is a superior therapy to nHF for primary support of RDS. In this setting, nHF is associated with a higher rate of treatment failure, but no difference in the rate of MV, where surfactant and/or CPAP are available to escalate therapy. Due to the perceived benefits of nHF, some clinicians may still choose to use nHF as first-line therapy for this indication, keeping CPAP in reserve for infants who require more support. nHF may be a good option for stable preterm infants with (or at risk of) CPAP-related nasal trauma or other pressure injuries. Until further data are available, we do not recommend the use of nHF for the stabilization of newborn infants in the delivery room.

In the absence of an evidence-based nHF weaning guideline, it is important to be diligent in weaning the gas flow as clinically indicated to avoid unnecessarily prolonging exposure to respiratory support. It is not recommended to prescribe gas flows higher than 8 L/min for preterm infants unless in a clinical trial setting. When using nHF to treat preterm infants, units should determine clear, objective criteria to expedite escalation of therapy when nHF is failing.

Future Directions

Opportunities to advance knowledge in the field of noninvasive respiratory support include studies of:

- Alternative techniques of surfactant administration in spontaneously breathing infants receiving noninvasive respiratory support
- Methods available at the bedside to judge optimal levels of nasal CPAP and to predict which preterm infants will require intubation and surfactant
- NIPPV, to determine the best settings in terms of pressures, rates, and synchronization
- NIHFV, to identify optimal approach(es), including comparison of devices and settings, and to assess systemic effects as well as the effects on lung injury and developmental lung biology
- nHF, to compare devices, assess efficacy and safety in extremely preterm infants, assess optimal gas flows and how best to increase and wean them, and whether nHF may be used for stabilization of newborn infants in the delivery room.

Acknowledgments

The authors thank Professor Colin Morley and Professor Bradley Yoder for their work on the previous versions of this chapter. BJM is supported by a NHRCM Investigator Grant (No. 2016662). PGD is supported by an NHMRC Practitioner Fellowship (No. 1059111). AM is supported by a Research Early Career Award from Hamilton Health Sciences Foundation (2019–2022).

REFERENCES

1. Ikegami M, Jacobs H, Jobe A. Surfactant function in respiratory distress syndrome. *J Pediatr.* 1983;102(3):443-447.
2. deLemos RA, Coalson JJ. The contribution of experimental models to our understanding of the pathogenesis and treatment of bronchopulmonary dysplasia. *Clin Perinatol.* 1992;19(3):521-539.
3. Di Fiore JM, Martin RJ, Gauda EB. Apnea of prematurity: perfect storm. *Respir Physiol Neurobiol.* 2013;189(2):213-222.
4. Alex CG, Aronson RM, Onal E, et al. Effects of continuous positive airway pressure on upper airway and respiratory muscle activity. *J Appl Physiol (1985).* 1987;62(5):2026-2030.
5. Saunders RA, Milner AD, Hopkin IE. The effects of continuous positive airway pressure on lung mechanics and lung volumes in the neonate. *Biol Neonate.* 1976;29(3-4):178-186.
6. Schmolzer GM, Kumar M, Pichler G, et al. Non-invasive versus invasive respiratory support in preterm infants at birth: systematic review and meta-analysis. *BMJ.* 2013;347:f5980.
7. Subramaniam P, Ho JJ, Davis PG. Prophylactic nasal continuous positive airway pressure for preventing morbidity and mortality in very preterm infants. *Cochrane Database Syst Rev.* 2016;(6):CD001243.
8. Gregory GA, Kitterman JA, Phibbs RH, et al. Treatment of the idiopathic respiratory-distress syndrome with continuous positive airway pressure. *N Engl J Med.* 1971;284:1333-1340.
9. Barrie H. Simple method of applying continuous airway pressure in respiratory-distress syndrome. *Lancet.* 1972;1(7754):776-777.
10. Ackerman BD, Stein MP, Sommer JS, et al. Continuous positive airway pressure applied by means of a tight-fitting face-mask. *J Pediatr.* 1974;85:408-411.
11. Ahlström H, Jonson B, Svenningsen NW. Continuous positive airways pressure treatment by a face chamber in idiopathic respiratory distress syndrome. *Arch Dis Child.* 1976;51:13-21.
12. Rhodes PG, Hall RT. Continuous positive airway pressure delivered by face mask in infants with the idiopathic respiratory distress syndrome: a controlled study. *Pediatrics.* 1973;52(1):1-5.
13. Novogroder M, MacKuanying N, Eidelman AI, et al. Nasopharyngeal ventilation in respiratory distress syndrome: a simple and efficient method of delivering continuous positive airway pressure. *J Pediatr.* 1973;82(6):1059-1062.
14. Wung JT, Driscoll Jr JM, Epstein RA, et al. A new device for CPAP by nasal route. *Crit Care Med.* 1975;3(2):76-78.
15. Caliumi-Pellegrini G, Agostino R, Orzalesi M, et al. Twin nasal cannula for administration of continuous positive airway pressure to newborn infants. *Arch Dis Child.* 1974;49(3):228-230.
16. Field D, Vyas H, Milner AD, et al. Continuous positive airway pressure via a single nasal catheter in preterm infants. *Early Hum Dev.* 1985;11(3-4):275-280.
17. Moa G, Nilsson K, Zetterstrom H, Jonsson LO. A new device for administration of nasal continuous positive airway pressure in the newborn: an experimental study. *Crit Care Med.* 1988;16(12):1238-1242.
18. Courtney SE, Aghai ZH, Saslow JG, Pyon KH, Habib RH. Changes in lung volume and work of breathing: a comparison of two variable-flow nasal continuous positive airway pressure devices in very low birth weight infants. *Pediatr Pulmonol.* 2003;36(3):248-252.
19. Chernick V. Continuous distending pressure in hyaline membrane disease: of devices, disadvantages, and a daring study. *Pediatrics.* 1973;52(1):114-115.

20. Green EA, Dawson JA, Davis PG, De Paoli AG, Roberts CT. Assessment of resistance of nasal continuous positive airway pressure interfaces. *Arch Dis Child Fetal Neonatal Ed.* 2019; 104(5):F535-F539.

21. Iyer NP, Chatburn R. Evaluation of a nasal cannula in noninvasive ventilation using a lung simulator. *Respir Care.* 2015;60(4): 508-512.

22. Mukerji A, Belik J. Neonatal nasal intermittent positive pressure ventilation efficacy and lung pressure transmission. *J Perinatol.* 2015;35(9):716-719.

23. Gerdes JS, Sivieri EM, Abbasi S. Factors influencing delivered mean airway pressure during nasal CPAP with the RAM cannula. *Pediatr Pulmonol.* 2016;51(1):60-69.

24. Gokce IK, Kaya H, Ozdemir R. A randomized trial comparing the short binasal prong to the RAM cannula for noninvasive ventilation support of preterm infants with respiratory distress syndrome. *J Matern Fetal Neonatal Med.* 2021;34(12):1868-1874.

25. Hochwald O, Riskin A, Borenstein-Levin L, et al. Cannula with long and narrow tubing vs short binasal prongs for noninvasive ventilation in preterm infants: noninferiority randomized clinical trial. *JAMA Pediatr.* 2021;175(1):36-43.

26. King BC, Gandhi BB, Jackson A, et al. Mask versus prongs for nasal continuous positive airway pressure in preterm infants: a systematic review and meta-analysis. *Neonatology.* 2019;116(2): 100-114.

27. Jasani B, Ismail A, Rao S, et al. Effectiveness and safety of nasal mask versus binasal prongs for providing continuous positive airway pressure in preterm infants: a systematic review and meta-analysis. *Pediatr Pulmonol.* 2018;53(7):987-992.

28. Pandit PB, Courtney SE, Pyon KH, et al. Work of breathing during constant- and variable-flow nasal continuous positive airway pressure in preterm neonates. *Pediatrics.* 2001;108(3): 682-685.

29. Courtney SEM. Lung recruitment and breathing pattern during variable versus continuous flow nasal continuous positive airway pressure in premature infants: an evaluation of three devices. *Pediatrics.* 2001;107(2):304-308.

30. De Paoli AG, Davis PG, Faber B, et al. Devices and pressure sources for administration of nasal continuous positive airway pressure (NCPAP) in preterm neonates. *Cochrane Database Syst Rev.* 2008;(1):CD002977.

31. Bharadwaj SK, Alonazi A, Banfield L, et al. Bubble versus other continuous positive airway pressure forms: a systematic review and meta-analysis. *Arch Dis Child Fetal Neonatal Ed.* 2020; 105(5):526-531.

32. De Klerk AM, De Klerk RK. Nasal continuous positive airway pressure and outcomes of preterm infants. *J Paediatr Child Health.* 2001;37(2):161-167.

33. Davis PG, Henderson-Smart DJ. Nasal continuous positive airways pressure immediately after extubation for preventing morbidity in preterm infants. *Cochrane Database Syst Rev.* 2003;(2):CD000143.

34. Elgellab A, Riou Y, Abbazine A, et al. Effects of nasal continuous positive airway pressure (NCPAP) on breathing pattern in spontaneously breathing premature newborn infants. *Intensive Care Med.* 2001;27(11):1782-1787.

35. Buzzella B, Claure N, D'Ugard C, et al. A randomized controlled trial of two nasal continuous positive airway pressure levels after extubation in preterm infants. *J Pediatr.* 2014; 164(1):46-51.

36. Fajardo MF, Claure N, Swaminathan S, et al. Effect of positive end-expiratory pressure on ductal shunting and systemic blood flow in preterm infants with patent ductus arteriosus. *Neonatology.* 2014;105(1):9-13.

37. Ho JJ, Subramaniam P, Davis PG. Continuous positive airway pressure (CPAP) for respiratory distress in preterm infants. *Cochrane Database Syst Rev.* 2020;10:CD002271.

38. Soll RF. Prophylactic synthetic surfactant for preventing morbidity and mortality in preterm infants. *Cochrane Database Syst Rev.* 2000;(2):CD001079.

39. Soll RF. Prophylactic natural surfactant extract for preventing morbidity and mortality in preterm infants. *Cochrane Database Syst Rev.* 2000;(2):CD000511.

40. Yost CC, Soll RF. Early versus delayed selective surfactant treatment for neonatal respiratory distress syndrome. *Cochrane Database Syst Rev.* 2000;(2):CD001456.

41. Lindner W, Vossbeck S, Hummler H, et al. Delivery room management of extremely low birth weight infants: spontaneous breathing or intubation? *Pediatrics.* 1999;103:961-967.

42. Aly H, Massaro AN, Patel K, et al. Is it safer to intubate premature infants in the delivery room? *Pediatrics.* 2005;115(6): 1660-1665.

43. Morley CJ, Davis PG, Doyle LW, Brion LP, Hascoet JM, Carlin JB. Nasal CPAP or intubation at birth for very preterm infants. *N Engl J Med.* 2008;358(7):700-708.

44. Finer NN, Carlo WA, Walsh MC, et al. Early CPAP versus surfactant in extremely preterm infants. *N Engl J Med.* 2010; 362(21):1970-1979.

45. Dunn MS, Kaempf J, de Klerk A, et al. Randomized trial comparing 3 approaches to the initial respiratory management of preterm neonates. *Pediatrics.* 2011;128(5):e1069-e1076.

46. Sandri F, Plavka R, Ancora G, et al. Prophylactic or early selective surfactant combined with nCPAP in very preterm infants. *Pediatrics.* 2010;125(6):e1402-e1409.

47. Stevens TP, Harrington EW, Blennow M, Soll RF. Early surfactant administration with brief ventilation vs. selective surfactant and continued mechanical ventilation for preterm infants with or at risk for respiratory distress syndrome. *Cochrane Database Syst Rev.* 2007;(4):CD003063.

48. Rojas MA, Lozano JM, Rojas MX, et al. Very early surfactant without mandatory ventilation in premature infants treated with early continuous positive airway pressure: a randomized, controlled trial. *Pediatrics.* 2009;123(1):137-142.

49. Aldana-Aguirre JC, Pinto M, Featherstone RM, Kumar M. Less invasive surfactant administration versus intubation for surfactant delivery in preterm infants with respiratory distress syndrome: a systematic review and meta-analysis. *Arch Dis Child Fetal Neonatal Ed.* 2017;102(1):F17-F23.

50. Rigo V, Lefebvre C, Broux I. Surfactant instillation in spontaneously breathing preterm infants: a systematic review and meta-analysis. *Eur J Pediatr.* 2016;175(12):1933-1942.

51. Isayama T, Iwami H, McDonald S, et al. Association of noninvasive ventilation strategies with mortality and bronchopulmonary dysplasia among preterm infants: a systematic review and meta-analysis. *JAMA.* 2016;316(6):611-624.

52. Abdel-Latif ME, Davis PG, Wheeler KI, et al. Surfactant therapy via thin catheter in preterm infants with or at risk of respiratory distress syndrome. *Cochrane Database Syst Rev.* 2021;5:CD011672.

53. Gopel W, Kribs A, Ziegler A, et al. Avoidance of mechanical ventilation by surfactant treatment of spontaneously breathing preterm infants (AMV): an open-label, randomised, controlled trial. *Lancet.* 2011;378(9803):1627-1634.

54. Kribs A, Roll C, Gopel W, et al. Nonintubated surfactant application vs conventional therapy in extremely preterm

infants: a randomized clinical trial. *JAMA Pediatr.* 2015; 169(8):723-730.

55. Herting E, Kribs A, Hartel C, et al. Two-year outcome data suggest that less invasive surfactant administration (LISA) is safe: results from the follow-up of the randomized controlled AMV (avoid mechanical ventilation) study. *Eur J Pediatr.* 2020;179(8): 1309-1313.

56. Mehler K, Broer A, Roll C, et al. Developmental outcome of extremely preterm infants is improved after less invasive surfactant application: developmental outcome after LISA. *Acta Paediatr.* 2021;110(3):818-825.

57. Dargaville PA, Aiyappan A, Cornelius A, et al. Preliminary evaluation of a new technique of minimally invasive surfactant therapy. *Arch Dis Child Fetal Neonatal Ed.* 2011;96(4):F243-F248.

58. Dargaville PA, Kamlin COF, Orsini F, et al. Effect of minimally invasive surfactant therapy vs sham treatment on death or bronchopulmonary dysplasia in preterm infants with respiratory distress syndrome: the OPTIMIST-A Randomized Clinical Trial. *JAMA.* 2021;326(24):2478-2487.

59. Roberts CT, Halibullah I, Bhatia R, et al. Outcomes after introduction of minimally invasive surfactant therapy in two Australian tertiary neonatal units. *J Pediatr.* 2021;229:141-146.

60. Annibale DJ, Hulsey TC, Engstrom PC, Wallin LA, Ohning BL. Randomized, controlled trial of nasopharyngeal continuous positive airway pressure in the extubation of very low birth weight infants. *J Pediatr.* 1994;124:455-460.

61. Davis P, Jankov R, Doyle L, Henschke P. Randomised, controlled trial of nasal continuous positive airway pressure in the extubation of infants weighing 600 to 1250 g. *Arch Dis Child Fetal Neonatal Ed.* 1998;79(1):F54-F57.

62. Dimitriou G, Greenough A, Kavvadia V, et al. Elective use of nasal continuous positive airways pressure following extubation of preterm infants. *Eur J Pediatr.* 2000;159(6):434-439.

63. Tapia JL, Bancalari A, Gonzalez A, Mercado ME. Does continuous positive airway pressure (CPAP) during weaning from intermittent mandatory ventilation in very low birth weight infants have risks or benefits? A controlled trial. *Pediatr Pulmonol.* 1995;19(5):269-274.

64. Engelke SC, Roloff DW, Kuhns LR. Postextubation nasal continuous positive airway pressure: a prospective controlled study. *Am J Dis Child.* 1982;136(4):359-361.

65. Higgins RD, Richter SE, Davis JM. Nasal continuous positive airway pressure facilitates extubation of very low birth weight neonates. *Pediatrics.* 1991;88(5):999-1003.

66. So BH, Tamura M, Mishina J, Watanabe T, Kamoshita S. Application of nasal continuous positive airway pressure to early extubation in very low birthweight infants. *Arch Dis Child Fetal Neonatal Ed.* 1995;72(3):F191-F193.

67. Chan V, Greenough A. Randomised trial of methods of extubation in acute and chronic respiratory distress. *Arch Dis Child.* 1993;68:570-572.

68. Peake M, Dillon P, Shaw NJ. Randomized trial of continuous positive airways pressure to prevent reventilation in preterm infants. *Pediatr Pulmonol.* 2005;39(3):247-250.

69. Robertson NJ, Hamilton PA. Randomised trial of elective continuous positive airway pressure (CPAP) compared with rescue CPAP after extubation. *Arch Dis Child Fetal Neonatal Ed.* 1998;79(1):F58-F60.

70. Polin RA, Sahni R. Newer experience with CPAP. *Semin Neonatol.* 2002;7(5):379-389.

71. Goldbart AD, Gozal D. Non-invasive ventilation in preterm infants. *Pediatr Pulmonol Suppl.* 2004;26:158-161.

72. Ammari A, Suri M, Milisavljevic V, et al. Variables associated with the early failure of nasal CPAP in very low birth weight infants. *J Pediatr.* 2005;147(3):341-347.

73. Dargaville PA, Aiyappan A, De Paoli AG, et al. Continuous positive airway pressure failure in preterm infants: incidence, predictors and consequences. *Neonatology.* 2013;104(1):8-14.

74. Sweet DG, Carnielli V, Greisen G, et al. European consensus guidelines on the management of respiratory distress syndrome: 2019 update. *Neonatology.* 2019;115(4):432-450.

75. Pape KE, Armstrong DL, Fitzhardinge PM. Central nervous system patholgoy associated with mask ventilation in the very low birthweight infant: a new etiology for intracerebellar hemorrhages. *Pediatrics.* 1976;58(4):473-483.

76. Vert P, Andre M, Sibout M. Continuous positive airway pressure and hydrocephalus. *Lancet.* 1973;2(7824):319.

77. Buettiker V, Hug MI, Baenziger O, Meyer C, Frey B. Advantages and disadvantages of different nasal CPAP systems in newborns. *Intensive Care Med.* 2004;30(5):926-930.

78. Robertson NJ, McCarthy LS, Hamilton PA, Moss AL. Nasal deformities resulting from flow driver continuous positive airway pressure. *Arch Dis Child Fetal Neonatal Ed.* 1996;75(3):F209-F212.

79. Buckmaster AG, Arnolda G, Wright IM, Foster JP, Henderson-Smart DJ. Continuous positive airway pressure therapy for infants with respiratory distress in non tertiary care centers: a randomized, controlled trial. *Pediatrics.* 2007;120(3):509-518.

80. Bowe L, Smith J, Clarke P, Glover K, Pasquill A, Robinson M. NasalCPAP weaning of VLBW infants: Is decreasing CPAP pressure or increasing time off the better strategy - results of a randomised controlled trial. *Pediatric Academic Society Meeting, San Francisco (Abstract).* 2006.

81. Todd DA, Wright A, Broom M, et al. Methods of weaning preterm babies <30 weeks gestation off CPAP: a multicentre randomised controlled trial. *Arch Dis Child Fetal Neonatal Ed.* 2012;97(4):F236-F240.

82. Heath Jeffery RC, Broom M, Shadbolt B, Todd DA. CeasIng Cpap At standarD criteriA (CICADA): implementation improves neonatal outcomes. *J Paediatr Child Health.* 2016;52(3): 321-326.

83. Jensen CF, Sellmer A, Ebbesen F, et al. Sudden vs pressure wean from nasal continuous positive airway pressure in infants born before 32 weeks of gestation: a randomized clinical trial. *JAMA Pediatr.* 2018;172(9):824-831.

84. Tang J, Reid S, Lutz T, Malcolm G, Oliver S, Osborn DA. Randomised controlled trial of weaning strategies for preterm infants on nasal continuous positive airway pressure. *BMC Pediatr.* 2015;15:147.

85. Soonsawad S, Tongsawang N, Nuntnarumit P. Heated humidified high-flow nasal cannula for weaning from continuous positive airway pressure in preterm infants: a randomized controlled trial. *Neonatology.* 2016;110(3):204-209.

86. Abdel-Hady H, Shouman B, Aly H. Early weaning from CPAP to high flow nasal cannula in preterm infants is associated with prolonged oxygen requirement: a randomized controlled trial. *Early Hum Dev.* 2011;87(3):205-208.

87. Badiee Z, Eshghi A, Mohammadizadeh M. High flow nasal cannula as a method for rapid weaning from nasal continuous positive airway pressure. *Int J Prev Med.* 2015;6:33.

88. Clements J, Christensen PM, Meyer M. A randomised trial comparing weaning from CPAP alone with weaning using heated humidified high flow nasal cannula in very preterm infants: the CHiPS study. *Arch Dis Child Fetal Neonatal Ed.* 2022. doi:10.1136/archdischild-2021-323636.

89. Helmrath TA, Hodson WA, Oliver Jr TK. Positive pressure ventilation in the newborn infant: the use of a face mask. *J Pediatr.* 1970;76(2):202-207.

90. Llewellyn MA, Tilak KS, Swyer PR. A controlled trial of assisted ventilation using an oro-nasal mask. *Arch Dis Child.* 1970; 45(242):453-459.

91. Lemyre B, Laughon M, Bose C, Davis PG. Early nasal intermittent positive pressure ventilation (NIPPV) versus early nasal continuous positive airway pressure (NCPAP) for preterm infants. *Cochrane Database Syst Rev.* 2016;12(12):CD005384.

92. Lemyre B, Davis PG, De Paoli AG, Kirpalani H. Nasal intermittent positive pressure ventilation (NIPPV) versus nasal continuous positive airway pressure (NCPAP) for preterm neonates after extubation. *Cochrane Database Syst Rev.* 2017;2(2): CD003212.

93. Rüegger CM, Owen LS, Davis PG. Nasal intermittent positive pressure ventilation for neonatal respiratory distress syndrome. *Clin Perinatol.* 2021;48(4):725-744.

94. Moretti C, Gizzi C, Papoff P, et al. Comparing the effects of nasal synchronized intermittent positive pressure ventilation (nSIPPV) and nasal continuous positive airway pressure (nCPAP) after extubation in very low birth weight infants. *Early Hum Dev.* 1999;56(2-3):167-177.

95. Owen LS, Morley CJ, Davis PG. Pressure variation during ventilator generated nasal intermittent positive pressure ventilation in preterm infants. *Arch Dis Child Fetal Neonatal Ed.* 2010; 95(5):F359-F364.

96. Owen LS, Morley CJ, Dawson JA, Davis PG. Effects of non-synchronised nasal intermittent positive pressure ventilation on spontaneous breathing in preterm infants. *Arch Dis Child Fetal Neonatal Ed.* 2011;96(6):F422-F428.

97. Bisceglia M, Belcastro A, Poerio V, et al. A comparison of nasal intermittent versus continuous positive pressure delivery for the treatment of moderate respiratory syndrome in preterm infants. *Minerva Pediatr.* 2007;59(2):91-95.

98. Ali N, Claure N, Alegria X, D'Ugard C, Organero R, Bancalari E. Effects of non-invasive pressure support ventilation (NI-PSV) on ventilation and respiratory effort in very low birth weight infants. *Pediatr Pulmonol.* 2007;42(8):704-710.

99. Gizzi C, Montecchia F, Panetta V, et al. Is synchronised NIPPV more effective than NIPPV and NCPAP in treating apnoea of prematurity (AOP)? A randomised cross-over trial. *Arch Dis Child Fetal Neonatal Ed.* 2015;100(1):F17-F23.

100. Owen LS, Manley BJ. Nasal intermittent positive pressure ventilation in preterm infants: equipment, evidence, and synchronization. *Semin Fetal Neonatal Med.* 2016;21(3):146-153.

101. Mukerji A, Abdul Wahab MG, Razak A, et al. High CPAP vs. NIPPV in preterm neonates - A physiological cross-over study. *J Perinatol.* 2021;41(7):1690-1696.

102. Owen LS, Morley CJ, Davis PG. Do the pressure changes of Neonatal Non-Synchronised NIPPV (NS Nasal Intermittent Positive Pressure Ventilation) confer advantages over cpap, or are high CPAP pressures as effective? *Pediatr Res.* 2011;70(5):16.

103. Moretti C, Gizzi C. Synchronized nasal intermittent positive pressure ventilation. *Clin Perinatol.* 2021;48(4):745-759.

104. Praud JP, Samson N, Moreau-Bussière F. Laryngeal function and nasal ventilatory support in the neonatal period. *Paediatr Respir Rev.* 2006;7(suppl 1):S180-S182.

105. Roy B, Samson N, Moreau-Bussiere F, et al. Mechanisms of active laryngeal closure during noninvasive intermittent positive pressure ventilation in nonsedated lambs. *J Appl Physiol (1985).* 2008;105(5):1406-1412.

106. Jounieaux V, Aubert G, Dury M, Delguste P, Rodenstein DO. Effects of nasal positive-pressure hyperventilation on the glottis in normal sleeping subjects. *J Appl Physiol (1985).* 1995;79(1): 186-193.

107. Chang HY, Claure N, D'Ugard C, Torres J, Nwajei P, Bancalari E. Effects of synchronization during nasal ventilation in clinically stable preterm infants. *Pediatr Res.* 2011;69(1):84-89.

108. Courtney SE, Barrington KJ. Continuous positive airway pressure and noninvasive ventilation. *Clin Perinatol.* 2007;34(1): 73-92, vi.

109. Huang L, Mendler MR, Waitz M, Schmid M, Hassan MA, Hummler HD. Effects of synchronization during noninvasive intermittent mandatory ventilation in preterm infants with respiratory distress syndrome immediately after extubation. *Neonatology.* 2015;108(2):108-114.

110. Goel D, Oei JL, Smyth J, Schindler T. Diaphragm-triggered non-invasive respiratory support in preterm infants. *Cochrane Database Syst Rev.* 2020;3(3):CD012935.

111. Sabsabi B, Harrison A, Banfield L, Mukerji A. Nasal intermittent positive pressure ventilation versus continuous positive airway pressure and apnea of prematurity: a systematic review and meta-analysis. *Am J Perinatol.* 2021. doi:10.1055/s-0040-1722337.

112. Bhandari V. Nasal intermittent positive pressure ventilation in the newborn: review of literature and evidence-based guidelines. *J Perinatol.* 2010;30(8):505-512.

113. Mukerji A, Shah PS, Shivananda S, et al. Survey of noninvasive respiratory support practices in Canadian neonatal intensive care units. *Acta Paediatr.* 2017;106(3):387-393.

114. Fischer HS, Bohlin K, Buhrer C, et al. Nasal high-frequency oscillation ventilation in neonates: a survey in five European countries. *Eur J Pediatr.* 2015;174(4):465-471.

115. van der Hoeven M, Brouwer E, Blanco CE. Nasal high frequency ventilation in neonates with moderate respiratory insufficiency. *Arch Dis Child Fetal Neonatal Ed.* 1998;79(1):F61-F63.

116. Centorrino R, Dell'Orto V, Gitto E, Conti G, De Luca D. Mechanics of nasal mask-delivered HFOV in neonates: a physiologic study. *Pediatr Pulmonol.* 2019;54(8):1304-1310.

117. De Luca D, Carnielli VP, Conti G, Piastra M. Noninvasive high frequency oscillatory ventilation through nasal prongs: bench evaluation of efficacy and mechanics. *Intensive Care Med.* 2010;36(12):2094-2100.

118. Chang HK. Mechanisms of gas transport during ventilation by high-frequency oscillation. *J Appl Physiol Respir Environ Exerc Physiol.* 1984;56(3):553-563.

119. Muhlethaler V, Malcolm G. Mechanical ventilation in the newborn; a simplified approach. Part 2: high-frequency ventilation. *J Paediatr Child Health.* 2014;50(10):E10-E13.

120. Gaertner VD, Waldmann AD, Davis PG, et al. Transmission of oscillatory volumes into the preterm lung during noninvasive high-frequency ventilation. *Am J Respir Crit Care Med.* 2021; 203(8):998-1005.

121. Gaertner VD, Waldmann AD, Davis PG, et al. Lung volume distribution in preterm infants on non-invasive high-frequency ventilation. *Arch Dis Child Fetal Neonatal Ed.* 2022;107(5): 551-557. doi:10.1136/archdischild-2021-322990.

122. De Luca D, Costa R, Visconti F, Piastra M, Conti G. Oscillation transmission and volume delivery during face mask-delivered HFOV in infants: Bench and in vivo study. *Pediatr Pulmonol.* 2016;51(7):705-712.

123. De Paoli AG, Davis PG, Faber B, Morley CJ. Devices and pressure sources for administration of nasal continuous positive

airway pressure (NCPAP) in preterm neonates. *Cochrane Database Syst Rev.* 2008;2008(1):CD002977. doi:10.1002/14651858.CD002977.pub2.

124. De Luca D, Piastra M, Pietrini D, Conti G. Effect of amplitude and inspiratory time in a bench model of non-invasive HFOV through nasal prongs. *Pediatr Pulmonol.* 2012;47(10):1012-1018.

125. Schäfer C, Schumann S, Fuchs H, Klotz D. Carbon dioxide diffusion coefficient in noninvasive high-frequency oscillatory ventilation. *Pediatr Pulmonol.* 2019;54(6):759-764.

126. Klotz D, Schaefer C, Stavropoulou D, et al. Leakage in nasal high-frequency oscillatory ventilation improves carbon dioxide clearance-A bench study. *Pediatr Pulmonol.* 2017;52(3):367-372.

127. Czernik C, Schmalisch G, Buhrer C, et al. Weaning of neonates from mechanical ventilation by use of nasopharyngeal high-frequency oscillatory ventilation: a preliminary study. *J Matern Fetal Neonatal Med.* 2012;25(4):374-378.

128. Mukerji A, Singh B, Helou SE, et al. Use of noninvasive high-frequency ventilation in the neonatal intensive care unit: a retrospective review. *Am J Perinatol.* 2015;30(2):171-176.

129. Ali YAH, Seshia MM, Ali E, Alvaro R. Noninvasive high-frequency oscillatory ventilation: a retrospective chart review. *Am J Perinatol.* 2022;39(6):666-670. doi:10.1055/s-0040-1718738.

130. Lai SH, Xie YL, Chen ZQ, et al. Non-invasive high-frequency oscillatory ventilation as initial respiratory support for preterm infants with respiratory distress syndrome. *Front Pediatr.* 2021;9:792160. doi:10.3389/fped.2021.792160.

131. Thatrimontrichai A, Sirianansopa K, Janjindamai W, Dissanevate S, Maneenil G. Comparison of endotracheal reintubation between nasal high-frequency oscillation and continuous positive airway pressure in neonates. *Am J Perinatol.* 2020;37(4):409-414.

132. Colaizy TT, Younis UM, Bell EF, Klein JM. Nasal high-frequency ventilation for premature infants. *Acta Paediatr.* 2008;97(11):1518-1522. doi:10.1111/j.1651-2227.2008.00900.x.

133. Bottino R, Pontiggia F, Ricci C, et al. Nasal high-frequency oscillatory ventilation and CO_2 removal: a randomized controlled crossover trial. *Pediatr Pulmonol.* 2018;53(9):1245-1251. doi:10.1002/ppul.24120.

134. Klotz D, Schneider H, Schumann S, Mayer B, Fuchs H. Non-invasive high-frequency oscillatory ventilation in preterm infants: a randomised controlled cross-over trial. *Arch Dis Child Fetal Neonatal Ed.* 2018;103(4):F1-F5. doi:10.1136/archdischild-2017-313190.

135. Rüegger CM, Lorenz L, Kamlin COF, et al. The effect of noninvasive high-frequency oscillatory ventilation on desaturations and bradycardia in very preterm infants: a randomized cross-over trial. *J Pediatr.* 2018;201:269-273.e2. doi:10.1016/j.jpeds.2018.05.029.

136. Zhu XW, Zhao JN, Tang SF, Yan J, Shi Y. Noninvasive high-frequency oscillatory ventilation versus nasal continuous positive airway pressure in preterm infants with moderate-severe respiratory distress syndrome: a preliminary report. *Pediatr Pulmonol.* 2017;52(8):1038-1042. doi:10.1002/ppul.23755.

137. Zhu X, Feng Z, Liu C, Shi L, Shi Y, Ramanathan R. Nasal high-frequency oscillatory ventilation in preterm infants with moderate respiratory distress syndrome: a multicenter randomized clinical trial. *Neonatology.* 2021;118(3):325-331. doi:10.1159/000515226.

138. Li Y, Wei Q, Zhao D, et al. Non-invasive high-frequency oscillatory ventilation in preterm infants after extubation:

a randomized, controlled trial. *J Int Med Res.* 2021;49(2):300060520984915. doi:10.1177/0300060520984915.

139. Wu HL, Lei YQ, Xie WP, Chen Q, Zheng YR. Nasal high-frequency oscillatory ventilation vs. nasal continuous positive airway pressure as therapy for postextubation respiratory failure in infants after congenital heart surgery. *Front Pediatr.* 2021;9:700632. doi:10.3389/fped.2021.700632.

140. Malakian A, Bashirnezhadkhabaz S, Aramesh MR, Dehdashtian M. Noninvasive high-frequency oscillatory ventilation versus nasal continuous positive airway pressure in preterm infants with respiratory distress syndrome: a randomized controlled trial. *J Matern Fetal Neonatal Med.* 2020;33(15):2601-2607. doi:10.1080/14767058.2018.1555810.

141. Iranpour R, Armanian AM, Abedi AR, Farajzadegan Z. Nasal high-frequency oscillatory ventilation (nHFOV) versus nasal continuous positive airway pressure (NCPAP) as an initial therapy for respiratory distress syndrome (RDS) in preterm and near-term infants. *BMJ Paediatr Open.* 2019;3(1):e000443. doi:10.1136/bmjpo-2019-000443.

142. Mukerji A, Sarmiento K, Lee B, Hassall K, Shah V. Non-invasive high-frequency ventilation versus bi-phasic continuous positive airway pressure (BP-CPAP) following CPAP failure in infants <1250 g: a pilot randomized controlled trial. *J Perinatol.* 2017;37(1):49-53.

143. Chen L, Wang L, Ma J, Feng Z, Li J, Shi Y. Nasal high-frequency oscillatory ventilation in preterm infants with respiratory distress syndrome and ARDS after extubation: a randomized controlled trial. *Chest.* 2019;155(4):740-748.

144. Dumas De La Roque E, Bertrand C, Tandonnet O, et al. Nasal high frequency percussive ventilation versus nasal continuous positive airway pressure in transient tachypnea of the newborn: a pilot randomized controlled trial (NCT00556738). *Pediatr Pulmonol.* 2011;46(3):218-223. doi:10.1002/ppul.21354.

145. Zhu X, Qi H, Feng Z, Shi Y, De Luca D, Nasal Oscillation Post-Extubation Study Group. Noninvasive high-frequency oscillatory ventilation vs nasal continuous positive airway pressure vs nasal intermittent positive pressure ventilation as postextubation support for preterm neonates in china: a randomized clinical trial. *JAMA Pediatr.* 2022;176(6):551-559. doi:10.1001/jamapediatrics.2022.0710.

146. Li J, Li X, Huang X, Zhang Z. Noninvasive high-frequency oscillatory ventilation as respiratory support in preterm infants: a meta-analysis of randomized controlled trials. *Respir Res.* 2019;20(1):58. doi:10.1186/s12931-019-1023-0.

147. Li J, Chen L, Shi Y. Nasal high-frequency oscillatory ventilation versus nasal continuous positive airway pressure as primary respiratory support strategies for respiratory distress syndrome in preterm infants: a systematic review and meta-analysis. *Eur J Pediatr.* 2022;181(1):215-223. doi:10.1007/s00431-021-04190-0.

148. De Luca D, Centorrino R. Nasal high-frequency ventilation. *Clin Perinatol.* 2021;48(4):761-782.

149. Mukerji A, Finelli M, Belik J. Nasal high-frequency oscillation for lung carbon dioxide clearance in the newborn. *Neonatology.* 2013;103(3):161-165.

150. Keszler M. Mechanical ventilation strategies. *Semin Fetal Neonatal Med.* 2017;22(4):267-274. doi:10.1016/j.siny.2017.06.003.

151. Wilkinson D, Andersen C, O'Donnell CP, De Paoli AG, Manley BJ. High flow nasal cannula for respiratory support in preterm infants. *Cochrane Database Syst Rev.* 2016;2:CD006405. doi:10.1002/14651858.CD006405.pub3.

152. Yoder BA, Manley B, Collins C, et al. Consensus approach to nasal high-flow therapy in neonates. *J Perinatol.* 2017;37(7):809-813.

153. Osman M, Elsharkawy A, Abdel-Hady H. Assessment of pain during application of nasal-continuous positive airway pressure and heated, humidified high-flow nasal cannulae in preterm infants. *J Perinatol.* 2015;35(4):263-267.

154. Klingenberg C, Pettersen M, Hansen EA, et al. Patient comfort during treatment with heated humidified high flow nasal cannulae versus nasal continuous positive airway pressure: a randomised cross-over trial. *Arch Dis Child Fetal Neonatal Ed.* 2014;99(2):F134-F137. doi:10.1136/archdischild-2013-304525.

155. Roberts CT, Manley BJ, Dawson JA, Davis PG. Nursing perceptions of high-flow nasal cannulae treatment for very preterm infants. *J Paediatr Child Health.* 2014;50(10):806-810. doi:10.1111/jpc.12636.

156. Imbulana DI, Manley BJ, Dawson JA, Davis PG, Owen LS. Nasal injury in preterm infants receiving non-invasive respiratory support: a systematic review. *Arch Dis Child Fetal Neonatal Ed.* 2018;103(1):F29-F35. doi:10.1136/archdischild-2017-313418.

157. Chow SSW, Creighton P, Chambers GM, Lui K. *Report of the Australian and New Zealand Neonatal Network 2019.* Sydney, Australia: ANZNN; 2021.

158. Mukerji A, Shah PS, Shivananda S, et al. Survey of noninvasive respiratory support practices in Canadian neonatal intensive care units. *Acta Paediatr.* 2017;106(3):387-393. doi:10.1111/apa.13644.

159. Naples R, Harigopal S. Nasal high flow in extremely preterm infants: current evidence and practice in the United Kingdom. *Acta Paediatr.* 2022;111(2):302-304.

160. Hough JL, Shearman AD, Jardine LA, Davies MW. Humidified high flow nasal cannulae: current practice in Australasian nurseries, a survey. *J Paediatr Child Health.* 2012;48(2):106-113.

161. Motojima Y, Ito M, Oka S, Uchiyama A, Tamura M, Namba F. Use of high-flow nasal cannula in neonates: nationwide survey in Japan. *Pediatr Int.* 2016;58(4):308-310.

162. Ojha S, Gridley E, Dorling J. Use of heated humidified high-flow nasal cannula oxygen in neonates: a UK wide survey. *Acta Paediatr.* 2013;102(3):249-253.

163. Shetty S, Sundaresan A, Hunt K, et al. Changes in the use of humidified high flow nasal cannula oxygen. *Arch Dis Child Fetal Neonatal Ed.* 2016;101(4):F371-F372.

164. Miller SM, Dowd SA. High-flow nasal cannula and extubation success in the premature infant: a comparison of two modalities. *J Perinatol.* 2010;30(12):805-808.

165. Chang GY, Cox CA, Shaffer TH. Nasal cannula, CPAP, and high-flow nasal cannula: effect of flow on temperature, humidity, pressure, and resistance. *Biomed Instrum Technol.* 2011;45(1):69-74.

166. Waugh JB, Granger WM. An evaluation of 2 new devices for nasal high-flow gas therapy. *Respir Care.* 2004;49(8):902-906.

167. Roberts CT, Kortekaas R, Dawson JA, Manley BJ, Owen LS, Davis PG. The effects of non-invasive respiratory support on oropharyngeal temperature and humidity: a neonatal manikin study. *Arch Dis Child Fetal Neonatal Ed.* 2016;101(3):F248-F252. doi:10.1136/archdischild-2015-308991.

168. Spence KL, Murphy D, Kilian C, McGonigle R, Kilani RA. High-flow nasal cannula as a device to provide continuous positive airway pressure in infants. *J Perinatol.* 2007;27(12):772-775.

169. Kubicka ZJ, Limauro J, Darnall RA. Heated, humidified high-flow nasal cannula therapy: yet another way to deliver continuous positive airway pressure? *Pediatrics.* 2008;121(1):82-88.

170. Wilkinson DJ, Andersen CC, Smith K, Holberton J. Pharyngeal pressure with high-flow nasal cannulae in premature infants. *J Perinatol.* 2008;28(1):42-47.

171. Volsko TA, Fedor K, Amadei J, Chatburn RL. High flow through a nasal cannula and CPAP effect in a simulated infant model. *Respir Care.* 2011;56(12):1893-1900. doi:10.4187/respcare.01204.

172. Lampland AL, Plumm B, Meyers PA, Worwa CT, Mammel MC. Observational study of humidified high-flow nasal cannula compared with nasal continuous positive airway pressure. *J Pediatr.* 2009;154(2):177-182.

173. Collins CL, Holberton JR, Konig K. Comparison of the pharyngeal pressure provided by two heated, humidified high-flow nasal cannulae devices in premature infants. *J Paediatr Child Health.* 2013;49(7):554-556.

174. Hasan RA, Habib RH. Effects of flow rate and airleak at the nares and mouth opening on positive distending pressure delivery using commercially available high-flow nasal cannula systems: a lung model study. *Pediatr Crit Care Med.* 2011;12(1):e29-e33.

175. Frizzola M, Miller TL, Rodriguez ME, et al. High-flow nasal cannula: impact on oxygenation and ventilation in an acute lung injury model. *Pediatr Pulmonol.* 2011;46(1):67-74.

176. Iyer NP, Mhanna MJ. Association between high-flow nasal cannula and end-expiratory esophageal pressures in premature infants. *Respir Care.* 2016;61(3):285-290.

177. Sivieri EM, Gerdes JS, Abbasi S. Effect of HFNC flow rate, cannula size, and nares diameter on generated airway pressures: an in vitro study. *Pediatr Pulmonol.* 2013;48(5):506-514.

178. Moore C, Rebstock D, Katz IM, et al. The influence of flowrate and gas density on positive airway pressure for high flow nasal cannula applied to infant airway replicas. *J Biomech.* 2020;112:110022.

179. Dysart K, Miller TL, Wolfson MR, Shaffer TH. Research in high flow therapy: mechanisms of action. *Respir Med.* 2009;103(10):1400-1405.

180. Shaffer TH, Alapati D, Greenspan JS, Wolfson MR. Neonatal non-invasive respiratory support: physiological implications. *Pediatr Pulmonol.* 2012;47(9):837-847.

181. Sivieri EM, Foglia EE, Abbasi S. Carbon dioxide washout during high flow nasal cannula versus nasal CPAP support: an in vitro study. *Pediatr Pulmonol.* 2017;52(6):792-798.

182. Van Hove SC, Storey J, Adams C, et al. An experimental and numerical investigation of CO_2 distribution in the upper airways during nasal high flow therapy. *Ann Biomed Eng.* 2016;44(10):3007-3019.

183. Saslow JG, Aghai ZH, Nakhla TA, et al. Work of breathing using high-flow nasal cannula in preterm infants. *J Perinatol.* 2006;26(8):476-480.

184. de Jongh BE, Locke R, Mackley A, et al. Work of breathing indices in infants with respiratory insufficiency receiving high-flow nasal cannula and nasal continuous positive airway pressure. *J Perinatol.* 2014;34(1):27-32.

185. Shetty S, Hickey A, Rafferty GF, Peacock JL, Greenough A. Work of breathing during CPAP and heated humidified high-flow nasal cannula. *Arch Dis Child Fetal Neonatal Ed.* 2016;101(5):F404-F407.

186. Boumecid H, Rakza T, Abazine A, Klosowski S, Matran R, Storme L. Influence of three nasal continuous positive airway pressure devices on breathing pattern in preterm infants. *Arch Dis Child Fetal Neonatal Ed.* 2007;92(4):F298-F300.

187. Lavizzari A, Veneroni C, Colnaghi M, et al. Respiratory mechanics during NCPAP and HHHFNC at equal distending pressures. *Arch Dis Child Fetal Neonatal Ed.* 2014;99(4):F315-F320.

188. Siva NV, Reynolds PR. Stabilisation of the preterm infant in the delivery room using nasal high flow: a 5-year retrospective analysis. *Acta Paediatr.* 2021;110(7):2065-2071. doi:10.1111/apa.15824.

189. Yoder BA, Stoddard RA, Li M, King J, Dirnberger DR, Abbasi S. Heated, humidified high-flow nasal cannula versus nasal CPAP for respiratory support in neonates. *Pediatrics.* 2013;131(5):e1482-e1490.

190. Roberts CT, Owen LS, Manley BJ, et al. Nasal high-flow therapy for primary respiratory support in preterm infants. *N Engl J Med.* 2016;375(12):1142-1151.

191. Lavizzari A, Colnaghi M, Ciuffini F, et al. Heated, humidified high-flow nasal cannula vs nasal continuous positive airway pressure for respiratory distress syndrome of prematurity: a randomized clinical noninferiority trial. *JAMA Pediatr.* 2016. doi:10.1001/jamapediatrics.2016.1243.

192. Murki S, Singh J, Khant C, et al. High-flow nasal cannula versus CPAP for primary respiratory support in preterm infants with respiratory distress: a randomized controlled trial. *Neonatology.* 2018;113(3):235-241.

193. Manley BJ, Arnolda GRB, Wright IMR, et al. Nasal high-flow therapy for newborn infants in special care nurseries. *N Engl J Med.* 2019;380(21):2031-2040.

194. Farhat AS, Mohammadzadeh A, Mamuri GA, et al. Comparison of nasal non-invasive ventilation methods in preterm neonates with respiratory distress syndrome. *Iran J Neonatol.* 2018;9(4):53-60.

195. Demirel G, Vatansever B, Tastekin A. High flow nasal cannula versus nasal continuous positive airway pressure for primary respiratory support in preterm infants: a prospective randomized study. *Am J Perinatol.* 2021;38(3):237-241.

196. Poonia A, Sharma P, Bansal R. Comparison of efficacy of nasal continuous positive airway pressure and heated humidified high-flow nasal cannula as a primary respiratory support in preterm infants. *J Clin Neonatol.* 2019;8(2):102.

197. Armanian A-M, Iranpour R, Parvaneh M, et al. Heated Humidified High Flow Nasal Cannula (HHHFNC) is not an effective method for initial treatment of Respiratory Distress Syndrome (RDS) versus nasal intermittent mandatory ventilation (NIMV) and nasal continuous positive airway pressure (NCPAP). *J Res Med Sci.* 2019;24(1):265625.

198. Shin J, Park K, Lee EH, et al. Humidified high flow nasal cannula versus CPAP as initial respiratory support in preterm infants. *J Korean Med Sci.* 2017;32(4):650-655.

199. Nair G, Karna P. *Comparison of the effects of Vapotherm and nasal CPAP in respiratory distress.* Washington DC: Pediatric Academic Societies Meeting USA; 2005.

200. Kugelman A, Riskin A, Said W, Shoris I, Mor F, Bader D. A randomized pilot study comparing heated humidified high-flow nasal cannulae with NIPPV for RDS. *Pediatr Pulmonol.* 2015;50(6):576-583.

201. Wang Z, Xiang JW, Gao WW, et al. Comparison of clinical efficacy of two noninvasive respiratory support therapies for respiratory distress syndrome in very low birth weight preterm infants. *Zhongguo Dang Dai Er Ke Za Zhi.* 2018;20(8):603-607.

202. Wilkinson D, Andersen C, O'Donnell CPF, et al. High flow nasal cannula for respiratory support in preterm infants. *Cochrane Database Syst Rev.* 2016;2(2):CD006405.

203. Campbell DM, Shah PS, Shah V, et al. Nasal continuous positive airway pressure from high flow cannula versus Infant Flow for Preterm infants. *J Perinatol.* 2006;26(9):546-549.

204. Collins CL, Holberton JR, Barfield C, et al. A randomized controlled trial to compare heated humidified high-flow nasal cannulae with nasal continuous positive airway pressure postextubation in premature infants. *J Pediatr.* 2013;162(5):949.

205. Manley BJ, Owen LS, Doyle LW, et al. High-flow nasal cannulae in very preterm infants after extubation. *N Engl J Med.* 2013;369(15):1425-1433.

206. [Efficacy and safety of heated humidified high-flow nasal cannula for prevention of extubation failure in neonates]. *Zhonghua Er Ke Za Zhi.* 2014;52(4):271-276.

207. Mostafa-Gharehbaghi M, Mojabi H. Comparing the effectiveness of Nasal Continuous Positive Airway Pressure (NCPAP) and High Flow Nasal Cannula (HFNC) in prevention of post extubation assisted ventilation. *Zahedan J Res Med Sci.* 2015;17(6):e984. doi:10.17795/zjrms984.

208. Colleti Junior J, Azevedo R, Araujo O, Carvalho WB. High-flow nasal cannula as a post-extubation respiratory support strategy in preterm infants: a systematic review and meta-analysis [Canula nasal de alto fluxo como estrategia de suporte respiratorio pos-extubacao em recem-nascidos prematuros: uma revisao sistematica e metanalise]. *J Pediatr (Rio J).* 2020;96(4):422-431. Available at: http://dx.doi.org/10.1016/j.jped.2019.11.004.

209. Ramaswamy VV, Oommen VI, Gupta A, et al. Efficacy of noninvasive respiratory support modes as postextubation respiratory support in preterm neonates: a systematic review and network meta-analysis. *Pediatr Pulmonol.* 2020;55(11):2924-2939.

210. Fleeman N, Dundar Y, Shah PS, Shaw BNJ. Heated humidified high-flow nasal cannula for preterm infants: an updated systematic review and meta-analysis. *Int J Technol Assess Health Care.* 2019;35(4):298-306.

211. Soonsawad S, Swatesutipun B, Limrungsikul A, Nuntnarumit P. Heated humidified high-flow nasal cannula for prevention of extubation failure in preterm infants. *Indian J Pediatr.* 2017;84(4):262-266.

212. Kadivar M, Mosayebi Z, Razi N, Nariman S, Sangsari R. High flow nasal cannulae versus nasal continuous positive airway pressure in neonates with respiratory distress syndrome managed with INSURE method: a randomized clinical trial. *Iranian J Med Sci.* 2016;41(6):494-500.

213. Kang WQ, Xu BL, Liu DP, et al. Efficacy of heated humidified high-flow nasal cannula in preterm infants aged less than 32 weeks after ventilator weaning. *Zhongguo Dang Dai Er Ke Za Zhi.* 2016;18(6):488-491. doi:10.7499/j.issn.1008-8830.2016.06.004.

214. Elkhwad M, Dako JA, Jennifer G, Harriet F, Anand K. Randomized control trial: heated humidity high flow nasal cannula in comparison with NCPAP in the management of RDS in extreme low birth infants in immediate post extubation period. *Neonatal Pediatr Med.* 2017;3:121. doi:10.4172/2572-4983.1000121.

215. Jasin LR, Kern S, Thompson S, Walter C, Rone JM, Yohannan MD. Subcutaneous scalp emphysema, pneumo-orbitis and pneumocephalus in a neonate on high humidity high flow nasal cannula. *J Perinatol.* 2008;28(11):779-781.

216. Kotecha SJ, Adappa R, Gupta N, Watkins WJ, Kotecha S, Chakraborty M. Safety and efficacy of high-flow nasal cannula therapy in preterm infants: a meta-analysis. *Pediatrics.* 2015;136(3):542-553.

217. Abdel-Hady H, Shouman B, Nasef N. Weaning preterm infants from continuous positive airway pressure: evidence for best practice. *World J Pediatr.* 2015;11(3):212-218.

Chapter 7

Newer Strategies for Surfactant Delivery

Peter A. Dargaville

Chapter Outline

Introduction
   Administration of Surfactant to Infants on CPAP
Techniques of Surfactant Administration Without an Endotracheal Tube
   Aerosolization
   Pharyngeal Instillation of Surfactant
   Delivery of Surfactant by Laryngeal Mask Airway
   Delivery of Surfactant Via a Thin Catheter
Surfactant Administration Via Brief Tracheal Catheterization
   Methods of Surfactant Delivery Via Thin Catheter
   Depth of Catheter Insertion
   Observational and Cohort Studies of Surfactant Delivery
   Clinical Trials of Surfactant Administration Via Tracheal Catheterization
   Summation of the Clinical Trials, and Findings of Meta-Analysis
Surfactant Administration Via Brief Tracheal Catheterization—Scientific and Practical Considerations
   Effectiveness of Surfactant Delivery and Distribution

   Laboratory Studies of Surfactant Distribution
   Use of Premedication for Tracheal Catheterization
   Procedural Complications
Surfactant Administration Via Brief Tracheal Catheterization—Recommendations
   Selection of Infants
Surfactant Administration Via Brief Tracheal Catheterization—Future Research Directions
   Longer-Term Outcomes After Surfactant Delivery Via Thin Catheter
   The Role of Spontaneous Breathing in Surfactant Distribution
   Optimal Premedication for Babies at Different Gestation Ranges
   Methods for Determining that the Catheter is Correctly Positioned in the Trachea
   Role of Videolaryngoscopy

Key Points

- As fewer preterm infants are managed with an endotracheal tube (ETT) in early life, the usual conduit for surfactant delivery is lacking. With this approach has come a dilemma regarding how and when to deliver surfactant to those showing features of surfactant-deficient respiratory distress syndrome (RDS).

- Brief intubation solely for surfactant delivery has been widely practiced, but has disadvantages, not the least of which is difficulty with extubation.

- Several less invasive approaches to delivering surfactant have been applied to preterm infants with RDS, including aerosolization, pharyngeal instillation, laryngeal mask administration, and brief tracheal catheterization.

- Recent experience has been gained with the approach of surfactant delivery using a thin catheter briefly inserted through the vocal cords, and this method has found its way into clinical practice.

- Numerous randomized controlled trials of surfactant administration via thin catheter have now been conducted, with heterogeneity in the settings in which the studies were conducted, and many aspects of trial design.

- Pooled data from these trials suggest that surfactant delivery via thin catheter has advantages over delivery via ETT, with improvement in survival free of bronchopulmonary dysplasia and reduction in the need for mechanical ventilation in the first 72 hours of life.

- A recent clinical trial also suggests that surfactant administration via thin catheter in the first 6 hours of life in infants with moderate RDS has advantages over continuation of noninvasive respiratory support without surfactant.

- Circumstantial evidence suggests that delivery of surfactant to a spontaneously breathing infant on continuous positive airway pressure leads to better surfactant distribution within the lung than when an equivalent dose is given via an ETT with the aid of positive pressure ventilation. Further laboratory and clinical studies are needed to confirm this.

- Application of surfactant therapy via thin catheter needs to be considered as part of a less-invasive approach to respiratory support in preterm infants, taking account of gestation, age, and apparent severity of RDS.

Introduction

Since its introduction into clinical practice more than four decades ago, exogenous surfactant therapy has become a universal standard, used early, repeatedly, and certainly to good effect in dealing with the scourge of respiratory distress syndrome (RDS) and its complications in the preterm infant.[1,2] Now, in the wake of the findings of large clinical trials suggesting a benefit of early continuous positive airway pressure (CPAP) rather than intubation,[3-5] the practice of routine endotracheal intubation at the beginning of life for preterm infants is being questioned,[6] and in many centers this approach has been superseded by an intent to apply CPAP at the outset for respiratory support.[7,8] The avoidance of endotracheal tube (ETT) placement has many ramifications, not the least of which is the lack of the usual conduit for the administration of surfactant, heretofore our enduring security blanket in treating RDS. As

frequency of routine intubation has gradually diminished, it has become clear on the one hand that many infants with RDS can be successfully supported without a dose of surfactant, particularly at gestations beyond 28 weeks.[7,9] On the other hand, however, there is now firm evidence that for some preterm infants with RDS, primary CPAP alone fails to provide enough support, prompting a resort to intubation followed by a dose of surfactant given at a later than ideal time.[10-16] This pathway is known from both cohort[10-15,17] and population-based[16] studies to be associated with adverse outcomes, including a higher incidence of pneumothorax, bronchopulmonary dysplasia (BPD), and severe intraventricular hemorrhage (IVH). A dilemma thus exists in the management of preterm infants with RDS—should they be intubated early in life to be given a dose of surfactant, or managed on CPAP to avoid the pitfalls of ventilation and the risk of ventilator-induced lung injury?[18,19]

ADMINISTRATION OF SURFACTANT TO INFANTS ON CONTINUOUS POSITIVE AIRWAY PRESSURE

A first attempt at overcoming the CPAP-surfactant dilemma was in the form of the technique of intubation, surfactant administration, and extubation (INSURE).[20] This method has been widely practiced, but its advantages over continuation of CPAP have more recently come into question. While some clinical trials have found a reduced need for mechanical ventilation with INSURE,[21,22] others have not, mostly attributable to difficulty with extubation after the procedure.[5,23] This limitation, and the difficulty of the intubation itself,[24] has deterred many clinicians from using INSURE in clinical practice.

In view of the difficulties and limitations of the INSURE technique, a number of less invasive means of delivering surfactant to the preterm infant with RDS have been developed and pursued. These newer strategies for surfactant delivery are the subject of this chapter, which will draw upon the published evidence from nonrandomized and randomized studies, as well as reviews[18,19,25-34] and meta-analyses,[35-45] to portray the current state of knowledge and bounds of accepted practice, and to highlight the areas of uncertainty in this rapidly changing field.

TABLE 7.1 Techniques for Surfactant Delivery without Intubation

Technique	First Report(s)	Equipment Used
Aerosolization	Robillard et al. 1964[46], Chu et al. 1967[47]	Variety of aerosolization devices
Pharyngeal instillation	Ten Centre Study Group 1987[48]	Instillation catheter
Laryngeal mask administration	Brimacombe 2004[49]	Laryngeal mask airway, sizes 0.5–1
Tracheal catheterization	Verder et al. 1992[50]	Laryngoscope, variety of thin catheters, Magill forceps (some cases), other devices for directing catheter (some cases)

Techniques of Surfactant Administration Without an Endotracheal Tube

The long-standing ingenuity of neonatologists has led to a multiplicity of methods for delivery of exogenous surfactant to the lung without using an ETT.[27,28,46-50] In some cases, these methods are far from new, but have been rediscovered and reapplied as more infants avoid intubation in early life. The full gamut of reported techniques is documented in Table 7.1 and described in further detail below.

AEROSOLIZATION

While aerosolization is currently used infrequently to deliver medications of any sort to the neonatal lung, it has the attraction of being potentially the least invasive approach to surfactant administration, involving no direct instrumentation of the airway.[28] It is little known that aerosolization was the first method of surfactant therapy in newborn infants with RDS, being first described in 1964.[46] The clinical effects in this and another pioneering clinical study[47] were modest, a testament to the difficulties in effective surfactant delivery and distribution using aerosolized surfactant, but also attributable in these early studies to the surfactant preparation used (pure DPPC with no spreading agents). Even with the advent of third-generation surfactant preparations with enhanced biophysical properties, and the development of sophisticated nebulization devices capable of dispersion of surfactant into droplets <5 μm, surfactant aerosolization for infants with RDS remains in the province of research.

Following on from observational studies[51-53] and a small clinical trial[54] have come the results of two recent randomized controlled trials (RCTs) in preterm infants with mild-to-moderate RDS.[55,56] Minocchieri and coworkers investigated the use of a vibrating membrane nebulizer for aerosolization of poractant alfa in infants 29 to 33 weeks' gestation (n = 64) and reported a clinical benefit in relation to need for subsequent intubation (odds ratio [OR] 0.56, 95% confidence interval [CI] 0.34–0.93).[55] However, the proportion of infants requiring intubation and surfactant therapy in the control group was considerably higher than that usually reported at this gestation. Moreover the degree of RDS as indicated by oxygen requirement at study entry was relatively mild (FiO_2 0.22–0.30 at age <4 hours).

More recently, a large multicentre RCT with pragmatic design (the Aero-O2 study) has examined whether, in infants of median gestation 33 weeks (n = 457) with mild-to-moderate RDS, aerosolization of calfactant at a dose of 210 mg/kg phospholipid could reduce the need for intubation for standard surfactant instillation compared with a control group receiving expectant management.[56] Infants were eligible if they had suspected or confirmed RDS and were receiving noninvasive respiratory support. Initially the FiO_2 entry threshold was set between 0.25 and 0.40 at age 1 to 12 hours, but soon after the start of the trial the lower FiO_2 limit was altered to room air. Surfactant dosing via aerosolization could be repeated up to a total of three doses (minimum interval 4 hours) as long as there was a positive response to the previous dose. Aerosolization of the surfactant took on average 68 minutes (~30 minutes per kg body weight), and one-third of infants received two or more doses. The primary outcome of need for intubation followed by liquid surfactant instillation occurred in 26% of the aerosolization group and 50% of the control group (relative risk [RR] 0.48; 95% CI 0.36–0.62; P <0.001). The risk reduction was most apparent at gestations beyond 30 weeks. No difference was noted between groups in secondary outcomes, including pneumothorax and mode of respiratory support on days 3, 7, and 28. The authors concluded that surfactant aerosolization may expand the opportunities for surfactant therapy while avoiding intubation.

Interpretation and translation of the findings of the Aero-O2 study are hampered to a considerable degree by several elements of the study design. The removal of the lower limit on FiO_2 at study entry meant that many infants with minimal or mild RDS were included. The mean FiO_2 for the two groups at study entry was relatively low (0.30 and 0.32 in the active treatment and control groups, respectively), especially when considered alongside the median gestation of 33 weeks. Furthermore, the study was not blinded, and no criteria for intubation were imposed on treating clinicians in either group. The study investigators provided an analysis indicating that the lack of intubation criteria had not contributed to treatment bias. It was stated that the intubation rate of 50% in the control group was lower than expected, but no evidence in support of this was provided.

Further well-designed studies of surfactant aerosolization will be needed for this therapy to become accepted as an alternative to more selective intubation for surfactant administration.[57] Ultimately head-to-head trials comparing this technique with other less invasive forms of surfactant therapy will be necessary. Given the relatively low proportional deposition of surfactant within the lung with any form of aerosolization, it is likely that this mode of surfactant administration could only find a place in the management of mild RDS occurring in infants ≥28 weeks' gestation.[57]

PHARYNGEAL INSTILLATION OF SURFACTANT

Although used several decades ago for initial surfactant delivery,[48] the method of pharyngeal surfactant instillation shortly after birth was largely forgotten until rediscovery by Kattwinkel and coworkers, who applied the technique in preterm infants of gestational age 27 to 30 weeks, with some suggestion of

an oxygenation response.[58] The approach has also been explored in extremely preterm infants <25 weeks' gestation, with suggestion of a better transition and lesser need for intubation compared with nonrandomized controls.[59]

More recently, a multicentre RCT focusing on the efficacy of delivery room pharyngeal surfactant administration has been completed in 251 preterm infants ≤28 weeks' gestation (POPART trial, EudraCT 2016-004198-41).[60] Randomization occurred prenatally, and infants were assigned to receive either oropharyngeal surfactant before cord clamping or standard care. The surfactant dose was 120 mg poractant alfa for infants <26 weeks' gestation and 240 mg for those at 26 to 28 weeks' gestation. The primary outcome for the study was the need for intubation in the first 5 days, and clinicians were required to adhere to prespecified criteria regarding intubation in all enrolled infants. Preliminary results indicate that the need for intubation did not differ between groups (oropharyngeal surfactant 63%; control group 65%; P = 0.79).[61] Among secondary outcomes, there was a higher incidence of pneumothorax in infants receiving oropharyngeal surfactant compared to controls (17% vs 7%, P = 0.031) but no other discernible differences in relevant in-hospital outcomes.

The results of the POPART study dampen enthusiasm for oropharyngeal surfactant administration soon after delivery in extremely preterm infants. For more mature infants at gestations beyond 28 weeks, any form of surfactant delivery used unselectively in the delivery room is unlikely to offer an advantage over early rescue therapy in those exhibiting features of RDS not manageable by CPAP alone.[62]

DELIVERY OF SURFACTANT BY LARYNGEAL MASK AIRWAY

The laryngeal mask airway (LMA) is designed to enclose the larynx in a cuffed seal and is increasingly promoted as a tool for facilitating neonatal resuscitation.[63,64] After initial reports of its use as a conduit for the administration of exogenous surfactant,[49,65] further studies including a number of clinical trials have been conducted in preterm infants.[66-72] Interest in surfactant delivery by LMA has been stimulated by the difficulties encountered with airway instrumentation and procedural tolerance associated with other less invasive techniques, especially at more mature gestations.[33] A total of six RCTs have explored surfactant delivery via LMA (reviewed in Roberts et al.[33]); in four cases this mode of delivery was compared to surfactant therapy after intubation,[68-71] and in two others LMA surfactant administration was compared to expectant management including continuation of CPAP.[67,72] All studies have concentrated on infants at 28 weeks' gestation and above, this being the lower limit of gestation at which the smallest LMA (size 0.5 or 1) can be reliably positioned. Surfactant delivery via LMA has been noted to be relatively easy to perform, with placement achievable in almost all cases. Two of the studies used post-procedure gastric aspiration as a way of confirming surfactant delivery to the lung, although the validity of this method has been questioned.[73] The rate of surfactant redosing has also been rather high after LMA administration (~38% in two studies combined[69,70]). A figure of around 20% might be expected in infants of gestation ≥28 weeks, both with ETT administration and by thin catheter.[74] For the outcome of avoidance of mechanical ventilation, overall the studies have shown a benefit of LMA surfactant administration compared to either continued CPAP (RR 0.57, 95% CI 0.38–0.85) or surfactant administration via ETT (RR 0.43, 95% CI 0.31–0.61).[75] An advantage of LMA surfactant has not been apparent for other outcomes.

Ultimately the role and uptake of the LMA as a conduit for surfactant therapy in preterm infants will depend on the results of further and larger well-designed RCTs comparing LMA surfactant delivery to other forms of less invasive surfactant administration. One such study (SURFSUP trial, ACTRN12620001184965) is now underway and aims to recruit 1000 preterm infants >1250 g with RDS, comparing surfactant delivery via LMA with that via thin catheter placed in the trachea, with a primary outcome of treatment failure, indicated by need for repeat surfactant therapy or need for mechanical ventilation.

DELIVERY OF SURFACTANT VIA A THIN CATHETER

The alternative of using a thin catheter to deliver surfactant to the trachea rather than an ETT was first reported by Verder et al., with an unstated number of preterm infants treated by this method among 34 preterm infants on CPAP given surfactant therapy in a pilot study.[50] The method was rediscovered and championed by Kribs and colleagues in Cologne,[76] and enthusiasm for tracheal catheterization as a means of surfactant delivery has burgeoned since. Given the wide experience and clinical applicability of this technique, the remainder of this chapter will focus on this approach to surfactant delivery.

Surfactant Administration Via Brief Tracheal Catheterization

METHODS OF SURFACTANT DELIVERY VIA THIN CATHETER

Reported techniques for surfactant delivery via thin catheter are shown in Table 7.2.[76-80] Some of them involve the use of instrumentation to aid passage of the catheter tip through the vocal cords (e.g., Magill's forceps); yet others use no internal guide and rely on the skill of the proceduralist to direct the catheter into the trachea. A semi-rigid rather than flexible catheter has generally been used for this latter approach, with the exception of the RCT of Kanmaz et al.,[77] in which the trachea was catheterized with a flexible catheter without use of Magill's forceps.

TABLE 7.2 Published Methods of Tracheal Catheterization		
Method, Reference	**Catheter Type**	**Guidance Through Vocal Cords**
Cologne method (LISA)[76]	Flexible nasogastric tube	Magill's forceps
Take Care method[77]	Flexible nasogastric tube	No forceps
Hobart method[78]	Semi-rigid vascular catheter	No forceps
SONSURE[79]	Flexible nasogastric tube	Magill's forceps
QuickSF[80]	Soft catheter	Intrapharyngeal guide

Beyond these original reports, a wide range of different catheters have now been used for surfactant delivery, including umbilical, suction, and urethral catheters, inserted by both oral and nasal routes.[81-83]

DEPTH OF CATHETER INSERTION

As with surfactant instillation via an ETT, the position of the catheter tip in the trachea is critically important, with surfactant reflux into the pharynx, or surfactant delivery preferentially into the right lung, being the potential consequences of an overly shallow or deep tip position, respectively. Reported catheter insertion depth has been 1 to 2 cm beyond vocal cords, depending on gestation. Based on information from a postmortem study of tracheal dimensions,[84] a recommended catheter tip position of 1.5 cm beyond cords at <27 weeks' gestation, and 2 cm for more mature infants, has been made.[85] Optimal insertion depth for the catheter tip has also been estimated using radiological measurements of carina position, with the following recommendations: <750 g: 1.5 cm; 750–1499 g: 2 cm; 1500–2499 g: 2.5 cm; 2500–3500 g: 3 cm.[86] Note that for many catheters (vascular catheter, feeding tube), a mark has to be drawn near the tip to indicate the required depth; a wax pencil is most suitable for this purpose.[87]

OBSERVATIONAL AND COHORT STUDIES OF SURFACTANT DELIVERY

Beyond the first descriptions of tracheal catheterization techniques, numerous single and multicentre experiences with this approach to surfactant delivery have now been reported. The experience of surfactant delivery via thin catheter runs to many thousands of infants.[88] Readers are referred to recent reviews and meta-analyses for discussion of individual studies.[31,32,34,42,45,89]

CLINICAL TRIALS OF SURFACTANT ADMINISTRATION VIA TRACHEAL CATHETERIZATION

There are now at least 20 RCTs in which surfactant delivery via thin catheter has been evaluated in preterm infants with RDS. Commentary on the most influential RCTs[87,90,91] is found hereunder, followed by a summary of the findings of a recent meta-analysis.[45]

AMV Trial[90]

The AMV trial was the first reported RCT of surfactant administration via tracheal catheterization, conducted in 12 tertiary level NICUs in Germany. Enrolled infants (n = 220) were of gestational age 26 to 28 weeks and being managed on CPAP with features of RDS. An FiO_2 threshold of >0.30 in the first 12 hours of life was set for inclusion. Randomization was to receive either surfactant via thin catheter using the Cologne method or continue on CPAP. All infants were thereafter managed with CPAP unless intubation criteria were reached, including an FiO_2 threshold that varied from 0.30 to 0.60 between participating centers. Primary outcome for the study was need for intubation on day 2 or 3 of life, and infants in the intervention group had a lower rate of this outcome. There was no difference in the rate of pneumothorax or other adverse events. The intervention group had a lower requirement for oxygen at 28 days, but not at 36 weeks' gestation.

Interpretation of the results of the AMV trial is hampered by several limitations of design[25]: (1) only 65 of the 108 infants randomized to the intervention actually received surfactant via thin catheter, (2) both groups included infants intubated at the outset, and (3) postintervention management differed considerably between centers. Nevertheless, the finding of a reduction in the need for mechanical ventilation after surfactant administration via thin catheter in this first clinical trial was important and led the authors to speculate that this approach may be included in a bundle of gentler respiratory care for preterm infants in the years to come.[90]

NINSAPP Trial[87]

Kribs and coworkers conducted a further RCT of the Cologne method of surfactant administration in 13 tertiary level NICUs in Germany. The study was notable for the enrollment of extremely preterm infants <27 weeks' gestation (n = 211) and is the only RCT of surfactant delivery via thin catheter to focus on this vulnerable group. Control infants received surfactant via ETT and remained intubated and ventilated until extubation criteria were met. Enrollment was in the first 2 hours of life and could occur after 10 minutes if FiO_2 was ≥0.30 and/or Silverman score reached 5. Caffeine was administered prior to surfactant delivery in the group receiving it via thin catheter but was delayed in the intubated group.

The primary outcome for the NINSAPP trial (survival without BPD) did not differ in incidence between the study groups, but there were some significant differences in secondary outcomes suggesting a benefit of surfactant delivery via thin catheter. More infants in this group survived without major complications (50% vs. 36%), and the rate of severe IVH was reduced (10% vs. 22%), as was the pneumothorax rate, and the overall duration of mechanical ventilation. The incidence of BPD was not significantly different between groups.

The intervention in the NINSAPP trial was applied as part of a less invasive bundle of respiratory management for extremely preterm infants, with avoidance of intubation in the delivery room even at 23 and 24 weeks' gestation. This is a substantial departure from what would be considered standard practice for most neonatologists in the most immature infants. It is noteworthy that the improvement in survival free of major complications in the group receiving surfactant via thin catheter occurred despite nearly half of the infants in this group requiring intubation in the first 72 hours of life, with almost all infants at 23 and 24 weeks being intubated at some time. The implication is that even a day or a few days during which the extremely preterm infant is spontaneously breathing on CPAP (facilitated by less invasive surfactant administration) may be to their advantage in early life.

OPTIMIST-A Trial[91]

The OPTIMIST-A trial was a multicentre RCT examining the efficacy of administration of surfactant via a thin catheter using the Hobart method (minimally invasive surfactant therapy, MIST). It is, to date, the largest study evaluating any of the less invasive forms of surfactant delivery, including a total of 485 infants in the gestation range 25 to 28 weeks. The comparison group in this trial was continued on CPAP, and the one-time intervention (MIST or sham treatment) was blinded from treating clinicians. Infants were eligible for enrollment if of age <6 hours, requiring respiratory support with CPAP and exhibiting an oxygen requirement of at least 30%. After intervention, criteria for intubation were imposed for all infants, including an FiO_2 ≥0.45, with discretion above 0.40. For the primary outcome of death or BPD, there was not a significant difference between groups (MIST 43.6%, sham treatment 49.6%; RR 0.87; 95% CI 0.74–1.03; $P = 0.10$). There was stronger evidence for a benefit of MIST in relation to BPD in survivors to 36 postmenstrual weeks (MIST 37.3%, sham 45.3%; RR 0.83; 95% CI, 0.70–0.98; $P = 0.03$). Among secondary outcomes, the need for intubation <72 hours was substantially reduced in the MIST group (MIST 36.5%, sham 72.1%; RR 0.50; 95% CI 0.40–0.64; $P < 0.001$), and the risk of pneumothorax was more than halved (MIST 4.6%, sham 10.2%; RR 0.44; 95% CI 0.25–0.78; $P = 0.005$). There were reductions in the duration of mechanical ventilation (median difference −1.96 days; 95% CI −3.19 to −0.73 days) and in all forms of respiratory support (median difference −6.42 days; 95% CI −11.95 to −0.89 days). The technique of MIST was widely applicable, requiring only one attempt in 76% of cases, and appeared to be well tolerated.

Prespecified sub-group analyses, although underpowered, noted an interaction between gestation stratum and treatment allocation in relation to mortality, such that infants in the 25 to 26 weeks' stratum who received MIST had a higher mortality than those receiving sham treatment. No single cause for this effect on mortality was identifiable.

A key strength of the design of the OPTIMIST-A trial was the blinding of the procedural invention (MIST or sham treatment) from the treating clinicians. This involved the assembly of a study team not involved in clinical management to perform the randomization and intervention. Furthermore, the success of blinding was measured (and confirmed) using a questionnaire for clinicians. An important weakness of the study was that enrollment ceased prior to reaching the prespecified sample size (606 infants), meaning that there was less statistical power than planned for the detection of small but meaningful differences in the primary and other outcomes.

SUMMATION OF THE CLINICAL TRIALS, AND FINDINGS OF META-ANALYSIS

The RCTs of surfactant delivery via tracheal catheterization are heterogeneous in many aspects of design, including gestation range, thresholds for study entry, surfactant administration technique, comparator group, and postintervention management. Moreover, some are conducted in established centers of excellence with low rates of mortality and morbidity even at extremely low gestation,[87] whereas others are conducted in NICUs in low- or middle-income countries with a developing experience of neonatal intensive care, in some cases hampered by lack of resources (e.g., nurse-patient ratio of 1 to 10).[92] Higher rates of mortality and morbidity are thus inevitable in studies from these centers, and these outcomes may be affected by a simple one-time intervention, such as less invasive surfactant delivery, in a way that cannot be replicated in more sophisticated NICUs. Caution is thus required in the interpretation of the pooled findings of the RCTs, and of the published meta-analyses, in relation to the applicability of the findings to NICUs with different resourcing and clinical expertise.

A further note of caution comes in relation to the gestation range studies in the RCTs to date, with an overrepresentation of infants between 26 and 28 weeks' gestation, in whom the combination of effective surfactant delivery and avoidance of intubation is most likely to have sustained effects, including the possibility of an effect on BPD. Infants beyond 28 weeks' gestation have been less completely studied in RCTs. Such infants are unlikely to gain a lasting benefit from less invasive surfactant delivery in an advanced NICU setting, in which rates of BPD, other complications, and mortality should already be very low in infants starting life on CPAP.[9] Conversely, for infants <26 weeks' gestation (only ~230 randomized in RCTs to date), any advantage of surfactant via thin catheter on lung injury may be obscured or negated by the influence of a large number of other factors contributing to the development of BPD. The possibility that even brief avoidance of ventilation in the first days of life could have lasting effects on nonpulmonary morbidities such as IVH in the most immature infants is raised by the result of the NINSAPP trial,[87] but requires confirmation.

A recent Cochrane review examined the findings of RCTs in which surfactant administration via thin catheter was compared with INSURE (12 studies) or with surfactant therapy via ETT with delayed extubation (2 studies).[45] The certainty of evidence was low-moderate, with only one study in which the intervention was reported to be blinded.[93] Meta-analyses of these 14 studies showed a significant decrease in the

risk of death or BPD (RR 0.59; 95% CI 0.48–0.73; number needed to benefit 9; 1324 infants) (Fig. 7.1), and a benefit of the thin catheter method in relation to need for intubation <72 hours (RR 0.63; 95% CI 0.54–0.74; number needed to benefit 8; 1422 infants) (Fig. 7.2). Surfactant administration via thin catheter was also noted to have advantages in relation to severe IVH, death during first hospitalization, and BPD in survivors to 36 weeks postmenstrual age.

Meta-analyses of RCTs[40-43] and of RCTs along with nonrandomized studies[38,43] published as the evidence emerged have in large part shown similar findings to the Cochrane review. Network meta-analysis, which allows the incorporation of evidence from multiple RCTs of respiratory interventions in preterm infants, has shown surfactant administration via thin catheter to be the most effective among strategies of less-invasive respiratory support in reducing the composite outcome of death or BPD.[39] A further network meta-analysis compared surfactant administration via thin catheter, laryngeal mask, nebulization, pharyngeal instillation, INSURE, as well as no surfactant administration in the management of preterm infants with RDS, and found surfactant delivery via thin catheter to be associated with a lower incidence of mortality, BPD, and need for mechanical ventilation compared with the INSURE approach.[44]

Surfactant Administration Via Brief Tracheal Catheterization—Scientific and Practical Considerations

EFFECTIVENESS OF SURFACTANT DELIVERY AND DISTRIBUTION

The clinical experience of surfactant therapy via thin catheter in spontaneously breathing preterm infants on CPAP is of a rapid, profound, and sustained improvement in oxygenation, equivalent or better than that seen after administration via an ETT (Fig. 7.3). Several lines of inquiry have been pursued to more fully understand how spontaneous breathing and an active glottis may help to optimize the distribution of surfactant delivered into the trachea with these techniques.

LABORATORY STUDIES OF SURFACTANT DISTRIBUTION

Exogenous surfactant distribution after administration by ETT has long been studied in animal models of lung

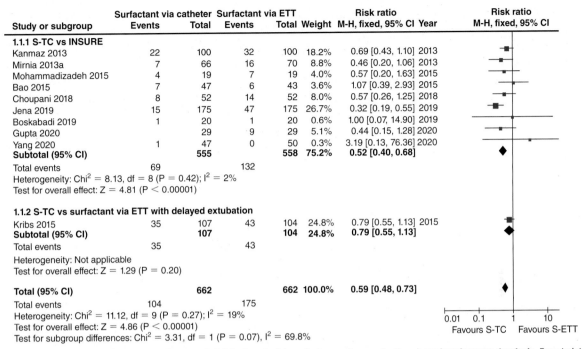

Study or subgroup	Surfactant via catheter Events	Total	Surfactant via ETT Events	Total	Weight	Risk ratio M-H, fixed, 95% CI	Year	Risk ratio M-H, fixed, 95% CI
1.1.1 S-TC vs INSURE								
Kanmaz 2013	22	100	32	100	18.2%	0.69 [0.43, 1.10]	2013	
Mirnia 2013a	7	66	16	70	8.8%	0.46 [0.20, 1.06]	2013	
Mohammadizadeh 2015	4	19	7	19	4.0%	0.57 [0.20, 1.63]	2015	
Bao 2015	7	47	6	43	3.6%	1.07 [0.39, 2.93]	2015	
Choupani 2018	8	52	14	52	8.0%	0.57 [0.26, 1.25]	2018	
Jena 2019	15	175	47	175	26.7%	0.32 [0.19, 0.55]	2019	
Boskabadi 2019	1	20	1	20	0.6%	1.00 [0.07, 14.90]	2019	
Gupta 2020		29	9	29	5.1%	0.44 [0.15, 1.28]	2020	
Yang 2020	1	47	0	50	0.3%	3.19 [0.13, 76.36]	2020	
Subtotal (95% CI)		**555**		**558**	**75.2%**	**0.52 [0.40, 0.68]**		
Total events	69		132					

Heterogeneity: Chi² = 8.13, df = 8 (P = 0.42); I² = 2%
Test for overall effect: Z = 4.81 (P < 0.00001)

1.1.2 S-TC vs surfactant via ETT with delayed extubation								
Kribs 2015	35	107	43	104	24.8%	0.79 [0.55, 1.13]	2015	
Subtotal (95% CI)		**107**		**104**	**24.8%**	**0.79 [0.55, 1.13]**		
Total events	35		43					

Heterogeneity: Not applicable
Test for overall effect: Z = 1.29 (P = 0.20)

Total (95% CI)		**662**		**662**	**100.0%**	**0.59 [0.48, 0.73]**		
Total events	104		175					

Heterogeneity: Chi² = 11.12, df = 9 (P = 0.27); I² = 19%
Test for overall effect: Z = 4.86 (P < 0.00001)
Test for subgroup differences: Chi² = 3.31, df = 1 (P = 0.07), I² = 69.8%

0.01 0.1 1 10
Favours S-TC   Favours S-ETT

Fig. 7.1 Meta-analysis of studies of surfactant administration via thin catheter—outcome: death or bronchopulmonary dysplasia. Forest plot for composite outcome of death or bronchopulmonary dysplasia including data from RCTs comparing surfactant administration via thin catheter *(S-TC)* to delivery via endotracheal tube *(ETT)*. This analysis shows data for those studies in which surfactant via ETT was given using the intubate-surfactant-extubate *(INSURE)* approach and those in which there was the intent of delayed extubation; results for all studies combined are shown at the bottom. (Reproduced from Abdel-Latif ME, Davis PG, Wheeler KI, et al. Surfactant therapy via thin catheter in preterm infants with or at risk of respiratory distress syndrome. *Cochrane Database Syst Rev.* 2021;5:CD011672.)

disease, with evidence for a benefit of higher surfactant concentration, larger surfactant volume, and more rapid instillation time.[94] On the other hand, given the recent emergence of less-invasive approaches to surfactant therapy, the laboratory evidence is currently lagging behind clinical practice. Two published studies have examined the impact of spontaneous breathing (as compared to positive pressure ventilation [PPV]) *during*[95] or *after*[96] surfactant administration, with somewhat conflicting and inconclusive results. Niemarkt and coworkers compared the effect on surfactant distribution of spontaneous breathing or PPV during surfactant administration in preterm lambs (n = 4 per group).[95] Lobar distribution of surfactant was *less homogeneous* after spontaneous breathing, with a reduction in delivery to the right upper lobe. The small number of animals in each group limits the interpretation of this finding, which clearly should be verified in

further studies. Bohlin and coworkers found spontaneous breathing *after* surfactant administration to lead to greater tissue incorporation of labeled exogenous surfactant in preterm rabbits (n = 8–15 per group), and along with it improved dynamic compliance. The conclusion drawn was the mechanical ventilation impaired or delayed tissue incorporation of surfactant and reinforced the notion that surfactant delivery in the clinical setting should be followed by spontaneous breathing wherever possible.

The advent of surfactant administration via thin catheter now requires some further laboratory studies to reexamine questions previously investigated in the era of surfactant delivery by PPV in intubated subjects. Factors influencing surfactant distribution, including the optimal rate of administration of surfactant, need to be reexplored. Clinical studies report a wide range of different approaches to deliver the surfactant dose,

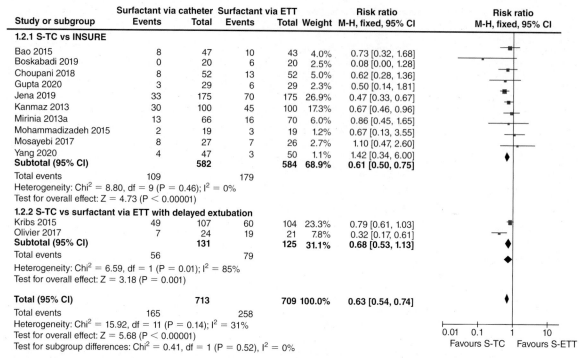

Study or subgroup	Surfactant via catheter Events	Total	Surfactant via ETT Events	Total	Weight	Risk ratio M-H, fixed, 95% CI	Risk ratio M-H, fixed, 95% CI
1.2.1 S-TC vs INSURE							
Bao 2015	8	47	10	43	4.0%	0.73 [0.32, 1.68]	
Boskabadi 2019	0	20	6	20	2.5%	0.08 [0.00, 1.28]	
Choupani 2018	8	52	13	52	5.0%	0.62 [0.28, 1.36]	
Gupta 2020	3	29	6	29	2.3%	0.50 [0.14, 1.81]	
Jena 2019	33	175	70	175	26.9%	0.47 [0.33, 0.67]	
Kanmaz 2013	30	100	45	100	17.3%	0.67 [0.46, 0.96]	
Mirinia 2013a	13	66	16	70	6.0%	0.86 [0.45, 1.65]	
Mohammadizadeh 2015	2	19	3	19	1.2%	0.67 [0.13, 3.55]	
Mosayebi 2017	8	27	7	26	2.7%	1.10 [0.47, 2.60]	
Yang 2020	4	47	3	50	1.1%	1.42 [0.34, 6.00]	
Subtotal (95% CI)		**582**		**584**	**68.9%**	**0.61 [0.50, 0.75]**	
Total events	109		179				

Heterogeneity: $Chi^2 = 8.80$, $df = 9$ ($P = 0.46$); $I^2 = 0\%$
Test for overall effect: $Z = 4.73$ ($P < 0.00001$)

1.2.2 S-TC vs surfactant via ETT with delayed extubation							
Kribs 2015	49	107	60	104	23.3%	0.79 [0.61, 1.03]	
Olivier 2017	7	24	19	21	7.8%	0.32 [0.17, 0.61]	
Subtotal (95% CI)		**131**		**125**	**31.1%**	**0.68 [0.53, 1.13]**	
Total events	56		79				

Heterogeneity: $Chi^2 = 6.59$, $df = 1$ ($P = 0.01$); $I^2 = 85\%$
Test for overall effect: $Z = 3.18$ ($P = 0.001$)

Total (95% CI)		**713**		**709**	**100.0%**	**0.63 [0.54, 0.74]**	
Total events	165		258				

Heterogeneity: $Chi^2 = 15.92$, $df = 11$ ($P = 0.14$); $I^2 = 31\%$
Test for overall effect: $Z = 5.68$ ($P < 0.00001$)
Test for subgroup differences: $Chi^2 = 0.41$, $df = 1$ ($P = 0.52$), $I^2 = 0\%$

Fig. 7.2 Meta-analysis of studies of surfactant administration via thin catheter—outcome: intubation < 72 hours. Forest plot for the outcome of intubation < 72 hours, including data from RCTs comparing surfactant administration via thin catheter *(S-TC)* to delivery via endotracheal tube *(ETT)*. (Reproduced from Abdel-Latif ME, Davis PG, Wheeler KI, et al. Surfactant therapy via thin catheter in preterm infants with or at risk of respiratory distress syndrome. *Cochrane Database Syst Rev.* 2021;5:CD011672.)

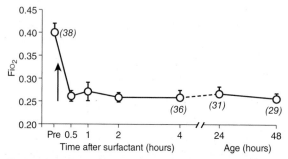

Fig. 7.3 Oxygen requirement after surfactant administration via thin catheter. Fraction of inspired oxygen *(FiO₂)* in the first 4 hours after surfactant delivery, and at 24 and 48 hours of life, in 38 preterm infants of median gestation 27 weeks and birth weight 880 g. Mean and standard error. *Black arrow* indicates the timing of surfactant administration, which was performed at a median age of 3.1 hours. All postsurfactant FiO_2 values differ from that presurfactant, **P <0.01,** paired t-test. (Redrawn from Dargaville PA, Aiyappan A, De Paoli AG, et al. Minimally-invasive surfactant therapy in preterm infants on continuous positive airway pressure. *Arch Dis Child Fetal Neonatal Ed.* 2013;98:F122-F126.)

including as three boluses over around 30 seconds, or as an infusion over 3 to 5 minutes. This latter approach requires careful appraisal—past studies of surfactant delivery by intratracheal infusion found this method to be inferior to bolus therapy in terms of surfactant distribution[97] and postsurfactant lung function.[97,98]

Some clinical evidence regarding surfactant distribution has been gained from two studies that have examined the effect of surfactant administration on regional lung aeration measured using electrical impedance tomography (EIT) in preterm infants with RDS.[99,100] Combined data from these studies, which were done several years apart in the same NICU, suggest that the aeration changes after intratracheal surfactant administration were more evenly distributed if surfactant was given via thin catheter and under conditions of spontaneous breathing,[100] rather than via ETT with PPV.[99] The gravity-dependent regions were seen to increase in aeration immediately after

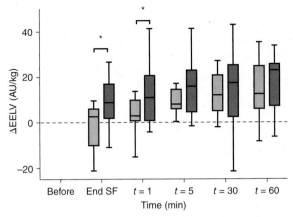

Fig. 7.4 Alteration in end-expiratory lung volume *(ΔEELV)* after surfactant administration by thin catheter. EELV changes in ventral *(gray boxes)* and dorsal *(carmine boxes)* lung regions directly after surfactant administration *(End SF)*, and at time points 1, 5, 30, and 60 minutes after the end of surfactant administration, relative to post-surfactant. Data from 15 preterm infants of median gestation 29 weeks and birth weight 1385 g. ΔEELV measured by electrical impedance tomography and expressed as arbitrary units *(AU)* per kg body weight. Box: median and interquartile range; whiskers: minimum and maximum values. *P < .05 versus before surfactant. (From van der Burg PS, de Jongh FH, Miedema M, et al. Effect of minimally invasive surfactant therapy on lung volume and ventilation in preterm infants. *J Pediatr.* 2016;170:67-72.)

surfactant instillation with both delivery methods, but a delayed increase in aeration in the nondependent lung regions was then noted preferentially in the group receiving surfactant via thin catheter (Fig. 7.4). The authors concluded that surfactant distribution may have been optimized by spontaneous breathing, but acknowledged that the evidence is circumstantial and needs further verification by a direct comparison between methods. Another study using EIT found that surfactant administration via thin catheter led to resolution of pendelluft and synchronous filling of nondependent and dependent regions during tidal ventilation.[101]

USE OF PREMEDICATION FOR TRACHEAL CATHETERIZATION

Minimization of Discomfort

Tracheal catheterization is currently performed under direct vision using a standard laryngoscope and in some cases instrumentation with Magill's forceps, followed by insertion of a catheter through the glottis. These maneuvers, although brief, are likely to be uncomfortable and may induce apnea and/or bradycardia. For this reason, due consideration has been given to methods of maintaining comfort and enhancing tolerability during the procedure. Evidence concerning the safety and tolerability of tracheal catheterization is far from complete and at present consists of nonrandomized observational studies,[102] surveys of practice,[81,82] and one small single-center RCT.[103] Premedication with narcotic or anesthetic agents appears more common in Nordic countries[82] than elsewhere.[74,77,104,105] A retrospective study of discretionary use of propofol (1 mg/kg) prior to tracheal catheterization indicated that this agent relieved discomfort during the procedure but led to a higher need for PPV.[102] An RCT performed in the same center compared 1 mg/kg propofol to no premedication in preterm infants 26 to 36 weeks' gestation (n = 78).[103] The proportion of infants with satisfactory pain scores was higher in the propofol group (76% vs. 22%, p <0.001). However, the incidence of hypoxia (SpO$_2$ <85%) during the procedure and need for noninvasive positive pressure ventilation were considerably higher after propofol premedication. No clear effects were seen in relation to other clinical outcomes.

Nonpharmacologic means of enhancing tolerance of the tracheal catheterization procedure include swaddling, tactile stimulation, and administration of 25% sucrose. The individual or combined benefit of these measures has not been formally evaluated.

The issue of sedation for surfactant delivery via thin catheter remains unresolved and requires further research.[83,89] At present it seems reasonable to individualize preintervention therapy (pharmacologic and nonpharmacologic) based on factors such as severity of RDS, gestational age, and unit experience.[106]

Maintenance of Respiratory Effort and Avoidance of Bradycardia

It is widely accepted that premedication with caffeine should be a prerequisite to surfactant delivery via thin catheter for infants <30 weeks' gestation, with selective use of caffeine in more mature infants. Beyond this, respiratory effort during the procedure is promoted by maintenance of CPAP wherever possible, cutaneous stimulation in the event of apnea, and PPV if absolutely necessary.

Bradycardia during brief tracheal catheterization most usually occurs during the direct laryngoscopy, sometimes requiring easing of blade pressure on the anterior hypopharyngeal wall, or even temporary cessation of laryngoscopy to resolve. Premedication with atropine in doses of 5 to 20 μg/kg has been used sporadically, and in one observational study appeared to contribute to a reduction in the incidence of bradycardia from 53% to 8.6%. Some centers report routine use of atropine prior to surfactant administration via thin catheter,[107,108] and surveys suggest it to be part of premedication in around 30% to 40% of neonatal units. Atropine was used as premedication in only 3% of infants prior to MIST in the OPTIMIST-A trial, in which the incidence of transient bradycardia was relatively high (~30%).[91] Further evidence will be required to make a firm recommendation on the use of atropine in this context.

PROCEDURAL COMPLICATIONS
Repeated Catheterization Attempts

Most studies of tracheal catheterization for surfactant delivery report high rates of catheterization of the trachea on the first attempt (first introduction of the laryngoscope), with a second or subsequent attempt required in around 20% to 30% (24% in the OPTIMIST-A trial).[91] Failure of catheterization on repeated attempts occurs with a frequency of <5%.

Hypoxia and Bradycardia

Not surprisingly, hypoxic and bradycardic episodes are commonly reported during tracheal catheterization for surfactant delivery, with the occurrence of hypoxia (SpO_2 <80%) being around 40% to 60% and of bradycardia (heart rate <100 bpm) being 10% to 40%. Need for PPV to aid recovery from these events remains relatively low and can mostly be avoided by skilled proceduralists. Intubation during or after the procedure is rarely needed.

Surfactant Reflux

Appearance of some surfactant in the mouth during instillation via the catheter is noted in around one-third of reported cases and does not appear to correlate with a lesser surfactant response. Closure of the mouth and promotion of spontaneous breathing may aid in returning the surfactant to the lung. PPV and suction are rarely needed in this circumstance.

Surfactant Administration Via Brief Tracheal Catheterization— Recommendations

Notwithstanding the gaps in the evidence, and with the recognition of relatively widespread uptake of brief tracheal catheterization as an alternative to standard intubation for surfactant delivery,[81-83,87,109] some recommendations regarding application of this approach in a specific NICU environment are put forward below and are summarized in Table 7.3.

SELECTION OF INFANTS
Gestational Age Range

In choosing the gestation range at which to apply a less invasive approach to surfactant delivery, it is apparent that NICUs will need to examine their local profile of prematurity-related complications, along with the Unit philosophy in relation to use of CPAP from the outset. The thresholds at which infants on noninvasive support would be considered eligible are also gestation-specific and should be selected based on local experience.

Inclusion Criteria

It is clear from observational and interventional studies that not all preterm infants managed on noninvasive respiratory support will gain a benefit from surfactant delivery via thin catheter. Particularly at more mature gestations, where surfactant deficiency may be less pronounced, many infants with RDS will have sufficient respiratory resilience to be sustained by CPAP alone, without surfactant therapy. The thresholds for treatment used in previous studies, and those proposed below, aim to identify in a pragmatic way those infants with RDS of at least moderate severity, for whom surfactant therapy is likely to provide benefit, and without it, CPAP failure is more likely to occur. Previous studies of CPAP failure provide examples of how local data can help to identify a suitable

TABLE 7.3	Examples of Inclusion and Exclusion Criteria for Surfactant Delivery Via Thin Catheter

Inclusion Criteria

All Gestations:
- Respiratory insufficiency thought related to RDS and managed with noninvasive respiratory support.

23–25 Weeks' Gestation:[a]
- CPAP level ≥6 cm H_2O.
- Any requirement for oxygen to maintain SpO_2 in the local target range.
- Age <6 hours, and preferably <2 hours.

26–28 Weeks' Gestation:
- CPAP level ≥6 cm H_2O, or nasal HF with flow ≥7 L/min.
- FiO_2 ≥0.30 to maintain SpO_2 in the local target range.
- Age <24 hours, with an emphasis on early recognition and treatment at an age < 6–12 hours.

Beyond 28 Weeks' Gestation:
- CPAP level ≥6 cm H_2O, or HF with flow ≥7 L/min.
- FiO_2 ≥0.30 to 0.35[b] to maintain SpO_2 in the local target range.
- Age <24 hours.

Exclusion Criteria

Absolute Contraindications:
- Severe RDS with high oxygen requirements and/or severe respiratory acidosis with prominent atelectasis radiologically, such that ongoing ventilatory support will be necessary after surfactant therapy.
- Suggested FiO_2 threshold at which intubation for surfactant should be considered:
- FiO_2 >0.40–0.50 (lower gestations); FiO_2 >0.60 (more mature infants).
- Maxillofacial, tracheal, or known pulmonary malformations.
- An alternative cause for respiratory distress (e.g., congenital pneumonia or pulmonary hypoplasia).
- No experienced personnel available to perform the tracheal catheterization.

Relative Contraindications:
- Infant <26 weeks' gestation—procedure can be technically challenging and destabilizing in inexperienced hands.
- Pneumothorax requiring drainage.
- Prominent apnea despite caffeine administration.

CPAP, Continuous positive airway pressure; *HF*, high flow; *RDS*, respiratory distress syndrome.
[a]Delivery room therapy remains controversial.
[b]For infants >28 weeks' gestation, the lower FiO_2 threshold (FiO_2 ≥0.30) may be preferable (i) at an age <6 hours, (ii) at higher CPAP levels (7 cm H_2O or more), and (iii) for less mature or growth-restricted infants.
Adapted from Vento M, Bohlin K, Herting E, et al. Surfactant administration via thin catheter: A practical guide. *Neonatology*. 2019;116:211-226.

threshold (Fig. 7.5).[14] Such analysis should take into account the Unit approach to CPAP (conservative vs. aggressive titration), the use (if any) of nasal high flow as primary therapy, and the uptake of adjuncts such as nasal intermittent positive-pressure ventilation (NIPPV). A lower FiO_2 threshold would be appropriate where high CPAP levels or NIPPV are commonly used at an early stage. Silverman scores and scoring of radiological appearances could also contribute to the inclusion criteria if familiar to local clinicians. Similarly a functional surfactant assay may identify infants with more serious RDS at an early stage,[110] but such tests are not commonly used outside the province of research.

Exclusion Criteria

Some infants surpassing the treatment threshold have factors that may limit the effectiveness of surfactant delivery via a thin catheter indicating that surfactant alone may be insufficient to overcome the degree of respiratory compromise. Examples include the infant with severe or very severe RDS or a comorbidity such as pneumothorax or recurrent apnea. Adoption of locally agreed exclusion criteria will thus also be

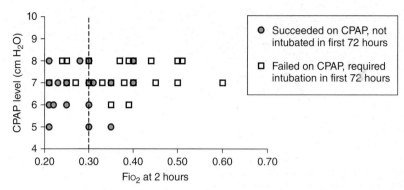

Fig. 7.5 Prediction of CPAP failure in preterm infants on CPAP. This shows individual data points for highest CPAP level and appropriate FiO_2 in the first 2 hours in preterm infants 25 to 28 weeks' gestation who commenced life on CPAP (n = 66), including those succeeding on CPAP (n = 36), and those requiring intubation <72 hours (n = 30). *Dashed line* at FiO_2 = 0.30 indicates predictive cut point. Odds ratio for CPAP failure in infants above and below this FiO_2 threshold: 5.6 (95% CI 1.7–18). *CPAP*, Continuous positive airway pressure. (Data derived from Dargaville PA, Aiyappan A, De Paoli AG, et al. Continuous positive airway pressure failure in preterm infants: incidence, predictors and consequences. *Neonatology.* 2013;104:8-14.)

essential, acknowledging that surfactant therapy by standard intubation will remain the best option in some circumstances, including the lack of a proceduralist sufficiently skilled and experienced in the method.

Surfactant Administration Via Brief Tracheal Catheterization—Future Research Directions

LONGER-TERM OUTCOMES AFTER SURFACTANT DELIVERY VIA THIN CATHETER

While there do appear to be clinical advantages of delivering surfactant via tracheal catheterization, information is only just emerging from RCTs regarding any effect on longer-term outcomes. Herting and coworkers reported the 2-year follow data after the AMV trial,[90] finding the motor and cognitive performance to be similar in the two groups.[111] Conversely, outcomes at 2 years postmenstrual age following randomization into the NINSAPP trial[87] were seen to be superior in the group receiving surfactant via thin catheter compared to that receiving surfactant via ETT (psychomotor development index 22% vs. 42%, $P = 0.012$).[112] In both cases, the number of infants initially recruited meant that the follow-up studies were underpowered to detect more subtle differences in incidence of cerebral palsy and cognitive impairments. Further follow-up data are needed to examine any lasting benefits or

ill-effects following surfactant delivery by this and other less invasive methods.

THE ROLE OF SPONTANEOUS BREATHING IN SURFACTANT DISTRIBUTION

The studies showing benefits of surfactant via thin catheter over INSURE in delivery of surfactant (as shown in Figs. 7.1 and 7.2) raise the possibility that spontaneous breathing is more effective for dispersion and distribution of surfactant from the trachea than positive pressure ventilation. Experimental studies in which surfactant distribution has been directly measured during spontaneous breathing are few, and the results are thus far contradictory. Further laboratory and clinical studies are needed to completely understand the influence of an infant's respiratory effort on surfactant distribution.

OPTIMAL PREMEDICATION FOR BABIES AT DIFFERENT GESTATION RANGES

Opinions range widely on the use of premedication for tracheal catheterization. Further studies will be needed to fully understand the risk/benefit ratio associated with the use of agents which have the potential to cause respiratory depression.

METHODS FOR DETERMINING THAT THE CATHETER IS CORRECTLY POSITIONED IN THE TRACHEA

The role of CO_2 measurement or another means of identifying catheter tip position in confirming correct placement of the surfactant delivery catheter has yet to be definitively explored.

ROLE OF VIDEOLARYNGOSCOPY

Beyond its use as a training tool, videolaryngoscopy may be of benefit in confirming catheter placement and in minimizing the discomfort associated with standard laryngoscopy.

Conflict of interest: As Chief Investigator of the OPTIMIST-A trial, the author has received support from the Royal Hobart Hospital Research Foundation, the Australian National Health and Medical Research Council (grant #1049114), and in-kind support from Chiesi Farmaceutici.

REFERENCES

1. Jobe AH. Pulmonary surfactant therapy. *N Engl J Med.* 1993; 328:861-868.
2. Suresh GK, Soll RF. Overview of surfactant replacement trials. *J Perinatol.* 2005;25(suppl 2):S40-S44.
3. Morley CJ, Davis PG, Doyle LW, et al. Nasal CPAP or intubation at birth for very preterm infants. *N Engl J Med.* 2008;358:700-708.
4. Finer NN, Carlo WA, Walsh MC, et al. Early CPAP versus surfactant in extremely preterm infants. *N Engl J Med.* 2010; 362:1970-1979.
5. Dunn MS, Kaempf J, de KA, et al. Randomized trial comparing 3 approaches to the initial respiratory management of preterm neonates. *Pediatrics.* 2011;128:e1069-e1076.
6. Jobe AH. Transition/adaptation in the delivery room and less RDS: "Don't just do something, stand there!". *J Pediatr.* 2005; 147:284-286.
7. Hatch LD III, Clark RH, Carlo WA, et al. Changes in use of respiratory support for preterm infants in the US, 2008-2018. *JAMA Pediatr.* 2021;175:1017-1024.
8. Sweet DG, Carnielli V, Greisen G, et al. European Consensus Guidelines on the Management of Respiratory Distress Syndrome - 2019 Update. *Neonatology.* 2019;115:432-450.
9. Dargaville PA, Ali SKM, Jackson HD, et al. Impact of minimally invasive surfactant therapy in preterm infants at 29-32 weeks gestation. *Neonatology.* 2018;113:7-14.
10. Ammari A, Suri M, Milisavljevic V, et al. Variables associated with the early failure of nasal CPAP in very low birth weight infants. *J Pediatr.* 2005;147:341-347.
11. Aly H, Massaro AN, Patel K, et al. Is it safer to intubate premature infants in the delivery room? *Pediatrics.* 2005;115: 1660-1665.
12. Fuchs H, Lindner W, Leiprecht A, et al. Predictors of early nasal CPAP failure and effects of various intubation criteria on the rate of mechanical ventilation in preterm infants of <29 weeks gestational age. *Arch Dis Child Fetal Neonatal Ed.* 2011;96: F343-F347.
13. De Jaegere AP, van der Lee JH, Cante C, et al. Early prediction of nasal continuous positive airway pressure failure in preterm infants less than 30 weeks gestation. *Acta Paediatr.* 2011;101:374-379.
14. Dargaville PA, Aiyappan A, De Paoli AG, et al. Continuous positive airway pressure failure in preterm infants: incidence, predictors and consequences. *Neonatology.* 2013;104:8-14.
15. Tagliaferro T, Bateman D, Ruzal-Shapiro C, et al. Early radiologic evidence of severe respiratory distress syndrome as a predictor of nasal continuous positive airway pressure failure in extremely low birth weight newborns. *J Perinatol.* 2015;35:99-103.
16. Dargaville PA, Gerber A, Johansson S, et al. Incidence and outcome of CPAP failure in preterm infants. *Pediatrics.* 2016;138: e20153985.
17. Gulczynska E, Szczapa T, Hozejowski R, et al. Fraction of inspired oxygen as a predictor of CPAP failure in preterm infants with respiratory distress syndrome: a prospective multicenter study. *Neonatology.* 2019;116:171-178.
18. Bohlin K. RDS—CPAP or surfactant or both. *Acta Paediatr Suppl.* 2012;101:24-28.
19. Dargaville PA. CPAP, surfactant or both for the preterm infant. Resolving the dilemma. *JAMA Pediatrics.* 2015;169:715-717.
20. Verder H, Robertson B, Greisen G, et al. Surfactant therapy and nasal continuous positive airway pressure for newborns with respiratory distress syndrome. Danish-Swedish Multicenter Study Group. *N Engl J Med.* 1994;331:1051-1055.
21. Escobedo MB, Gunkel JH, Kennedy KA, et al. Early surfactant for neonates with mild to moderate respiratory distress syndrome: a multicenter, randomized trial. *J Pediatr.* 2004;144:804-808.
22. Reininger A, Khalak R, Kendig JW, et al. Surfactant administration by transient intubation in infants 29 to 35 weeks' gestation with respiratory distress syndrome decreases the likelihood of later mechanical ventilation: a randomized controlled trial. *J Perinatol.* 2005;25:703-708.
23. Sandri F, Plavka R, Ancora G, et al. Prophylactic or early selective surfactant combined with nCPAP in very preterm infants. *Pediatrics.* 2010;125:e1402-e1409.
24. O'Donnell CP, Kamlin CO, Davis PG, Morley CJ. Endotracheal intubation attempts during neonatal resuscitation: success rates, duration, and adverse effects. *Pediatrics.* 2006;117:e16-e21.
25. Cools F. A new method of surfactant administration in preterm infants. *Lancet.* 2011;378:1607-1608.
26. Kribs A. How best to administer surfactant to VLBW infants? *Arch Dis Child Fetal Neonatal Ed.* 2011;96:F238-F240.
27. Dargaville PA. Innovation in surfactant therapy I: surfactant lavage and surfactant administration by fluid bolus using minimally invasive techniques. *Neonatology.* 2012;101:326-336.
28. Pillow JJ, Minocchieri S. Innovation in surfactant therapy II: surfactant administration by aerosolization. *Neonatology.* 2012; 101:337-344.
29. Blennow M, Bohlin K. Surfactant and noninvasive ventilation. *Neonatology.* 2015;107:330-336.
30. Aguar M, Vento M, Dargaville PA. Minimally-invasive surfactant therapy - an update. *Neoreviews.* 2014;15:e275.
31. Kribs A. Minimally invasive surfactant therapy and noninvasive respiratory support. *Clin Perinatol.* 2016;43:755-771.
32. Shim GH. Update of minimally invasive surfactant therapy. *Korean J Pediatr.* 2017;60:273-281.
33. Roberts CT, Manley BJ, O'Shea JE, et al. Supraglottic airway devices for administration of surfactant to newborn infants with respiratory distress syndrome: a narrative review. *Arch Dis Child Fetal Neonatal Ed.* 2021;106:336-341.
34. Kakkilaya V, Gautham KS. Should less invasive surfactant administration (LISA) become routine practice in US neonatal units? *Pediatr Res.* 2023;93:1188-1198. doi:10.1038/s41390-022-02265-8.

35. Abdel-Latif ME, Osborn DA. Nebulised surfactant in preterm infants with or at risk of respiratory distress syndrome. *Cochrane Database Syst Rev.* 2012;10:CD008310.

36. Abdel-Latif ME, Osborn DA. Pharyngeal instillation of surfactant before the first breath for prevention of morbidity and mortality in preterm infants at risk of respiratory distress syndrome. *Cochrane Database Syst Rev.* 2011;3:CD008311.

37. Abdel-Latif ME, Osborn DA. Laryngeal mask airway surfactant administration for prevention of morbidity and mortality in preterm infants with or at risk of respiratory distress syndrome. *Cochrane Database Syst Rev.* 2011;CD008309.

38. More K, Sakhuja P, Shah PS. Minimally invasive surfactant administration in preterm infants: a meta-narrative review. *JAMA Pediatr.* 2014;168:901-908.

39. Isayama T, Iwami H, McDonald S, Beyene J. Association of noninvasive ventilation strategies with mortality and bronchopulmonary dysplasia among preterm infants: a systematic review and meta-analysis. *JAMA.* 2016;316:611-624.

40. Ali E, Abdel WM, Alsalami Z, et al. New modalities to deliver surfactant in premature infants: a systematic review and meta-analysis. *J Matern Fetal Neonatal Med.* 2016;29:3519-3524.

41. Aldana-Aguirre JC, Pinto M, Featherstone RM, Kumar M. Less invasive surfactant administration versus intubation for surfactant delivery in preterm infants with respiratory distress syndrome: a systematic review and meta-analysis. *Arch Dis Child Fetal Neonatal Ed.* 2017;102:F17-F23.

42. Rigo V, Lefebvre C, Broux I. Surfactant instillation in spontaneously breathing preterm infants: a systematic review and meta-analysis. *Eur J Pediatr.* 2016;175:1933-1942.

43. Wu W, Shi Y, Li F, Wen Z, Liu H. Surfactant administration via a thin endotracheal catheter during spontaneous breathing in preterm infants. *Pediatr Pulmonol.* 2017;52:844-854.

44. Bellos I, Fitrou G, Panza R, Pandita A. Comparative efficacy of methods for surfactant administration: a network meta-analysis. *Arch Dis Child Fetal Neonatal Ed.* 2021;106:474-487.

45. Abdel-Latif ME, Davis PG, Wheeler KI, et al. Surfactant therapy via thin catheter in preterm infants with or at risk of respiratory distress syndrome. *Cochrane Database Syst Rev.* 2021;5:CD011672.

46. Robillard E, Alarie Y, Dagenais-Perusse P, et al. Microaerosol administration of synthetic beta-gamma-dipalmitoyl-l-alpha-lecithin in the respiratory distress syndome: a preliminary report. *Can Med Assoc J.* 1964;90:55-57.

47. Chu J, Clements JA, Cotton EK, et al. Neonatal pulmonary ischemia. I. Clinical and physiological studies. *Pediatrics.* 1967;40(suppl):709-782.

48. Ten Centre Study Group. Ten centre trial of artificial surfactant (artificial lung expanding compound) in very premature babies. Ten Centre Study Group. *British Medical Journal.* 1987;294:991-996.

49. Brimacombe J, Gandini D, Keller C. The laryngeal mask airway for administration of surfactant in two neonates with respiratory distress syndrome. *Paediatr Anaesth.* 2004;14:188-190.

50. Verder H, Agertoft L, Albertsen P, et al. Surfactant treatment of newborn infants with respiratory distress syndrome primarily treated with nasal continuous positive air pressure. A pilot study. *Ugeskr Laeger.* 1992;154:2136-2139.

51. Jorch G, Hartl H, Roth B, et al. Surfactant aerosol treatment of respiratory distress syndrome in spontaneously breathing premature infants. *Pediatr Pulmonol.* 1997;24:222-224.

52. Arroe M, Pedersen-Bjergaard L, Albertsen P, Bode S, Griesen G, Jonsbo F. Inhalation of aerosolized surfactant (exosurf) to neonates treated with nasal continuous positive airway pressure. *Prenat Neonat Med.* 1998;3:346-352.

53. Finer NN, Merritt TA, Bernstein G, Job L, Mazela J, Segal R. An open label, pilot study of Aerosurf(R) combined with nCPAP to prevent RDS in preterm neonates. *J Aerosol Med Pulm Drug Deliv.* 2010;23:303-309.

54. Berggren E, Liljedahl M, Winbladh B, et al. Pilot study of nebulized surfactant therapy for neonatal respiratory distress syndrome. *Acta Paediatr.* 2000;89:460-464.

55. Minocchieri S, Berry CA, Pillow JJ. Nebulised surfactant to reduce severity of respiratory distress: a blinded, parallel, randomised controlled trial. *Arch Dis Child Fetal Neonatal Ed.* 2019;104:F313-F319.

56. Cummings JJ, Gerday E, Minton S, et al. Aerosolized calfactant for newborns with respiratory distress: a randomized trial. *Pediatrics.* 2020;146:e20193967.

57. Gaertner VD, Thomann J, Bassler D, Ruegger CM. Surfactant nebulization to prevent intubation in preterm infants: a systematic review and meta-analysis. *Pediatrics.* 2021;148:e2021052504.

58. Kattwinkel J, Robinson M, Bloom BT, Delmore P, Ferguson JE. Technique for intrapartum administration of surfactant without requirement for an endotracheal tube. *J Perinatol.* 2004;24:360-365.

59. Lamberska T, Settelmayerova E, Smisek J, Luksova M, Maloskova G, Plavka R. Oropharyngeal surfactant can improve initial stabilisation and reduce rescue intubation in infants born below 25 weeks of gestation. *Acta Paediatr.* 2018;107:73-78.

60. Murphy MC, Galligan M, Molloy B, Hussain R, Doran P, O'Donnell C. Study protocol for the POPART study-Prophylactic Oropharyngeal surfactant for Preterm infants: a randomised trial. *BMJ Open.* 2020;10:e035994.

61. Murphy MC, Miletin J, Guthe HJ, et al. A randomised trial of prophylactic oropharyngeal surfactant for preterm infants. *PAS abstract.* 2021;2907-HP-QA.198.

62. Rojas-Reyes MX, Morley CJ, Soll R. Prophylactic versus selective use of surfactant in preventing morbidity and mortality in preterm infants. *Cochrane Database Syst Rev.* 2012;3:CD000510.

63. Schmolzer GM, Agarwal M, Kamlin CO, Davis PG. Supraglottic airway devices during neonatal resuscitation: an historical perspective, systematic review and meta-analysis of available clinical trials. *Resuscitation.* 2013;84:722-730.

64. Wyckoff MH, Aziz K, Escobedo MB, et al. Part 13: Neonatal Resuscitation: 2015 American Heart Association Guidelines Update for Cardiopulmonary Resuscitation and Emergency Cardiovascular Care. *Circulation.* 2015;132:S543-S560.

65. Fraser J, Hill C, McDonald D, Jones C, Petros A. The use of the laryngeal mask airway for inter-hospital transport of infants with type 3 laryngotracheo-oesophageal clefts. *Intensive Care Med.* 1999;25:714-716.

66. Trevisanuto D, Grazzina N, Ferrarese P, Micaglio M, Verghese C, Zanardo V. Laryngeal mask airway used as a delivery conduit for the administration of surfactant to preterm infants with respiratory distress syndrome. *Biol Neonate.* 2005;87:217-220.

67. Attridge JT, Stewart C, Stukenborg GJ, Kattwinkel J. Administration of rescue surfactant by laryngeal mask airway: lessons from a pilot trial. *Am J Perinatol.* 2013;30:201-206.

68. Sadeghnia A, Tanhaei M, Mohammadizadeh M, Nemati M. A comparison of surfactant administration through i-gel and ET-tube in the treatment of respiratory distress syndrome in newborns weighing more than 2000 grams. *Adv Biomed Res.* 2014;3:160.

69. Pinheiro JM, Santana-Rivas Q, Pezzano C. Randomized trial of laryngeal mask airway versus endotracheal intubation for surfactant delivery. *J Perinatol.* 2016;36:196-201.

70. Barbosa RF, Simões e Silva AC, Silva YP. A randomized controlled trial of laryngeal mask airway for surfactant administration in neonates. *Jornal de Pediatria.* 2017;93:in press.

71. Gharehbaghi M, Moghaddam YJ, Radfar R. Comparing the efficacy of surfactant administration by laryngeal mask airway and endotracheal intubation in neonatal respiratory distress syndrome. *Crescent J Med Biol Sci.* 2018;5:222-227.

72. Roberts KD, Brown R, Lampland AL, et al. Laryngeal mask airway for surfactant administration in neonates: a randomized, controlled trial. *J Pediatr.* 2018;193:40-46.

73. Dargaville PA. Administering surfactant without intubation - what does the laryngeal mask offer us? *J Pediatr (Rio J).* 2017; 93:313-316.

74. Dargaville PA, Aiyappan A, De Paoli AG, et al. Minimally-invasive surfactant therapy in preterm infants on continuous positive airway pressure. *Arch Dis Child Fetal Neonatal Ed.* 2013;98:F122-F126.

75. Calevo MG, Veronese N, Cavallin F, Paola C, Micaglio M, Trevisanuto D. Supraglottic airway devices for surfactant treatment: systematic review and meta-analysis. *J Perinatol.* 2019;39: 173-183.

76. Kribs A, Pillekamp F, Hunseler C, Vierzig A, Roth B. Early administration of surfactant in spontaneous breathing with nCPAP: feasibility and outcome in extremely premature infants (postmenstrual age </=27 weeks). *Paediatr Anaesth.* 2007;17: 364-369.

77. Kanmaz HG, Erdeve O, Canpolat FE, Mutlu B, Dilmen U. Surfactant administration via thin catheter during spontaneous breathing: randomized controlled trial. *Pediatrics.* 2013;131: e502-e509.

78. Dargaville PA, Aiyappan A, Cornelius A, Williams C, De Paoli AG. Preliminary evaluation of a new technique of minimally invasive surfactant therapy. *Arch Dis Child Fetal Neonatal Ed.* 2011;96:F243-F248.

79. Aguar M, Cernada M, Brugada M, Gimeno A, Gutierrez A, Vento M. Minimally invasive surfactant therapy with a gastric tube is as effective as the intubation, surfactant, and extubation technique in preterm babies. *Acta Paediatr.* 2014;103:e229-e233.

80. Maiwald CA, Neuberger P, Vochem M, Poets C. QuickSF: A new technique in surfactant administration. *Neonatology.* 2017; 111:211-213.

81. Klotz D, Porcaro U, Fleck T, Fuchs H. European perspective on less invasive surfactant administration-a survey. *Eur J Pediatr.* 2017;176:147-154.

82. Heiring C, Jonsson B, Andersson S, Bjorklund LJ. Survey shows large differences between the Nordic countries in the use of less invasive surfactant administration. *Acta Paediatr.* 2017;106: 382-386.

83. Vento M, Bohlin K, Herting E, Roehr CC, Dargaville PA. Surfactant administration via thin catheter: a practical guide. *Neonatology.* 2019;116:211-226.

84. Embleton ND, Deshpande SA, Scott D, Wright C, Milligan DW. Foot length, an accurate predictor of nasotracheal tube length in neonates. *Arch Dis Child Fetal Neonatal Ed.* 2001;85: F60-F64.

85. Dargaville PA, Kamlin CO, De Paoli AG, et al. The OPTIMIST-A trial: evaluation of minimally-invasive surfactant therapy in preterm infants 25-28 weeks gestation. *BMC Pediatr.* 2014;14:213.

86. Maiwald CA, Neuberger P, Franz AR, et al. Catheter insertion depths in less-invasive surfactant administration. *Arch Dis Child Fetal Neonatal Ed.* 2022;107:222-224.

87. Kribs A, Roll C, Gopel W, et al. Nonintubated surfactant application vs conventional therapy in extremely preterm infants: a randomized clinical trial. *JAMA Pediatr.* 2015;169: 723-730.

88. Hartel C, Herting E, Humberg A, et al. Association of administration of surfactant using less invasive methods with outcomes in extremely preterm infants less than 27 weeks of gestation. *JAMA Netw Open.* 2022;5:e2225810.

89. Herting E, Hartel C, Gopel W. Less invasive surfactant administration: best practices and unanswered questions. *Curr Opin Pediatr.* 2020;32:228-234.

90. Göpel W, Kribs A, Ziegler A, et al. Avoidance of mechanical ventilation by surfactant treatment of spontaneously breathing preterm infants (AMV): an open-label, randomised, controlled trial. *Lancet.* 2011;378:1627-1634.

91. Dargaville PA, Kamlin COF, Orsini F, et al. Effect of minimally invasive surfactant therapy vs sham treatment on death or bronchopulmonary dysplasia in preterm infants with respiratory distress syndrome: The OPTIMIST-A randomized clinical trial. *JAMA.* 2021;326:2478-2487.

92. Mohammadizadeh M, Ardestani AG, Sadeghnia AR. Early administration of surfactant via a thin intratracheal catheter in preterm infants with respiratory distress syndrome: feasibility and outcome. *J Res Pharm Pract.* 2015;4:31-36.

93. Yang G, Hei M, Xue Z, et al. Effects of less invasive surfactant administration (LISA) via a gastric tube on the treatment of respiratory distress syndrome in premature infants aged 32 to 36 weeks. *Medicine (Baltimore).* 2020;99:e19216.

94. Jobe AH. Techniques for administering surfactant. In: Robertson B, Taeusch HW, eds. *Surfactant therapy for lung disease.* New York: Marcel Dekker; 1995;309-324.

95. Niemarkt HJ, Kuypers E, Jellema R, et al. Effects of less-invasive surfactant administration on oxygenation, pulmonary surfactant distribution, and lung compliance in spontaneously breathing preterm lambs. *Pediatr Res.* 2014;76:166-170.

96. Bohlin K, Bouhafs RK, Jarstrand C, et al. Spontaneous breathing or mechanical ventilation alters lung compliance and tissue association of exogenous surfactant in preterm newborn rabbits. *Pediatr Res.* 2005;57:624-630.

97. Ueda T, Ikegami M, Rider ED, et al. Distribution of surfactant and ventilation in surfactant-treated preterm lambs. *J Appl Physiol.* 1994;76:45-55.

98. Hentschel R, Brune T, Franke N, et al. Sequential changes in compliance and resistance after bolus administration or slow infusion of surfactant in preterm infants. *Intensive Care Med.* 2002;28:622-628.

99. Miedema M, de Jongh FH, Frerichs I, et al. Changes in lung volume and ventilation during surfactant treatment in ventilated preterm infants. *Am J Respir Crit Care Med.* 2011;184: 100-105.

100. van der Burg PS, de Jongh FH, Miedema M, et al. Effect of minimally invasive surfactant therapy on lung volume and ventilation in preterm infants. *J Pediatr.* 2016;170:67-72.

101. Goncalves-Ferri WA, Rossi FS, Costa ELV, et al. Lung recruitment and pendelluft resolution after less invasive surfactant administration in a preterm infant. *Am J Respir Crit Care Med.* 2020;202:766-769.

102. Dekker J, Lopriore E, Rijken M, et al. Sedation during minimal invasive surfactant therapy in preterm infants. *Neonatology.* 2016;109:308-313.

103. Dekker J, Lopriore E, van Zanten HA, et al. Sedation during minimal invasive surfactant therapy: a randomised

controlled trial. *Arch Dis Child Fetal Neonatal Ed.* 2019;104: F378-F383.

104. Göpel W, Kribs A, Hartel C, et al. Less invasive surfactant administration is associated with improved pulmonary outcomes in spontaneously breathing preterm infants. *Acta Paediatr.* 2015;104:241-246.

105. Klebermass-Schrehof K, Wald M, Schwindt J, et al. Less invasive surfactant administration in extremely preterm infants: impact on mortality and morbidity. *Neonatology.* 2013;103: 252-258.

106. Peterson J, den Boer MC, Roehr CC. To sedate or not to sedate for less invasive surfactant administration: an ethical approach. *Neonatology.* 2021;118:639-646.

107. Bourgoin L, Caeymaex L, Decobert F, et al. Administering atropine and ketamine before less invasive surfactant administration resulted in low pain scores in a prospective study of premature neonates. *Acta Paediatr.* 2018;107:1184-1190.

108. Bensouda B, St-Hilaire M, Mandel R, et al. Implementation of less-invasive surfactant administration in a Canadian neonatal intensive care unit. *Arch Pediatr.* 2022;29:444-447.

109. Reynolds P, Bustani P, Darby C, et al. Less-invasive surfactant administration for neonatal respiratory distress ayndrome: a consensus guideline. *Neonatology.* 2021;118:586-592.

110. Fiori HH, Fiori RM. Why not use a surfactant test for respiratory distress syndrome? *Neonatology.* 2015;107:312.

111. Herting E, Kribs A, Hartel C, et al. Two-year outcome data suggest that less invasive surfactant administration (LISA) is safe. Results from the follow-up of the randomized controlled AMV (avoid mechanical ventilation) study. *Eur J Pediatr.* 2020;179: 1309-1313.

112. Mehler K, Broer A, Roll C, et al. Developmental outcome of extremely preterm infants is improved after less invasive surfactant application: developmental outcome after LISA. *Acta Paediatr.* 2021;110:818-825.

Respiratory Control and Oxygen Instability in Premature Infants

Juliann M. Di Fiore, Richard J. Martin, Nelson Claure, and Eduardo H. Bancalari

Chapter Outline

Introduction

Biological Challenges in Characterizing Neonatal Respiratory Control

Central Respiratory Control

Central and Peripheral Chemosensitivity

Contribution From Inflammatory Mechanisms

Clinical Challenges in Defining Neonatal Apnea

Mechanisms of Oxygenation Instability

Association Between Intermittent Hypoxemia, Bradycardia, and Outcomes

Mechanistic Insights Into Morbidity

Controversies in Therapy

    Accepted Treatments

    Controversial Approaches

Key Points

- Understanding the physiology of neonatal respiratory control has served as an effective guide to common therapeutic approaches.
- Both the acute and longer-term consequences of intermittent hypoxemia and apnea of prematurity are subjects of intense interest.
- Intermittent hypoxemia may contribute to an inflammatory stress response.
- Although caffeine is the mainstay of apnea therapy, there remains considerable controversy regarding optimal treatment regimens.
- Innovative newer approaches to stabilize respiratory control and improve lung function may hold promise as future interventions.

Introduction

There are a multitude of reasons why immaturity in respiratory control is of interest to scientists and clinicians alike. From a biological perspective, it represents a unique link between the developing respiratory and central nervous systems. The resultant apnea precipitates repetitive hypoxemia episodes, and hence, preterm infants serve as a novel biological model for studying the consequences of such episodic hypoxemia. From a clinical perspective, the combination of immature respiratory control, an immature lung, and the resultant therapeutic ventilatory support predisposes these infants to chronic respiratory morbidity. Finally, there is a need to optimize and provide safe pharmacotherapy that enhances respiratory neural output in this high-risk population of neonates. These are some of the current high-profile issues and controversies that this review will address.

Biological Challenges in Characterizing Neonatal Respiratory Control

The ability to challenge respiratory neural output with hypoxic or hypercapnic exposures is quite limited in human infants. Therefore, one must rely on older studies to better understand the maturation of peripheral and central components of chemoreception. We are also very dependent on neonatal animal models, particularly data derived from rodents, although, unfortunately, such models rarely exhibit long spontaneous apnea or periodic breathing as seen in preterm infants.

Central Respiratory Control

The neural circuitry that generates respiratory rhythm and governs inspiratory and expiratory motor patterns is distributed throughout the pons and medulla. The medulla contains a specialized region known as the pre-Bötzinger complex, which contains neurons that exhibit intrinsic pacemaker activity capable of producing rhythmic respiratory motor output without sensory feedback. Although a fundamental feature of this network is that it enables breathing to occur automatically, this systematic central rhythmicity may fail in preterm infants.[1] Meanwhile, central and peripheral sensory inputs from multiple sources allow adjustments to the patterns of inspiratory and expiratory activity in response to changing metabolic conditions. For example, inhibitory sensory inputs from the upper airway may be particularly prominent in early postnatal life to serve a protective function, although this may trigger potentially clinically significant apnea.

A poorly understood concept is the relationship between periodic breathing, i.e., repetitive cycles of respiratory output and pauses of approximately 5 to 10 seconds' duration, and apneic episodes typically of 10 to 20 seconds' duration that do not exhibit a cyclic pattern. Available data suggest that periodic breathing occurs predominantly in quiet sleep while apnea is more common in active sleep. This would suggest a different central or peripheral biological basis for those breathing patterns as discussed later.

Excitatory and inhibitory neurotransmitters and neuromodulators mediate the rhythmogenic synaptic communications between neurons of the medulla. Glutamate, acting on AMPA and NMDA receptors, is the major neurotransmitter mediating excitatory synaptic input to brainstem respiratory neurons. Gamma-aminobutyric acid (GABA) and glycine are the two primary inhibitory neurotransmitters in the network, mediating the waves of inhibitory postsynaptic potentials during the silent phase of respiratory neurons. Interestingly, during late embryonic and early postnatal development, GABA and glycine can mediate *excitatory* neurotransmission secondary to changes in the chloride gradient across the membrane. It is unclear how this phenomenon relates to the inhibition of respiratory output and resultant apnea seen in preterm infants.[2] Neonatal rodent data suggest that caffeine, which is a nonselective adenosine receptor inhibitor, may block excitatory A_{2A} receptors at GABAergic neurons and so inhibit GABA output and contribute to the ability of caffeine to enhance respiratory drive.[3] Serotonin may be of particular importance in the modulation of respiratory function. Serotonergic neurons and their projections may represent the neuroanatomic substrate for the integration of cardiorespiratory responses. Defects in the medullary serotonergic system likely contribute importantly to the pathogenesis of sudden infant death syndrome (SIDS).[4] For future advances in the pharmacotherapy of neonatal apnea, greater understanding of the maturation of these neurotransmitters/neuromodulators is imperative.

Central and Peripheral Chemosensitivity

Responsiveness to CO_2 is the major chemical driver of respiratory neural output. This is apparent in fetal life where breathing movements increase under hypercapnic conditions in animal models. As in later life, CO_2/H^+ responsiveness is predominantly based in the brainstem, although peripheral chemoreceptors contribute to the ventilatory response and respond more rapidly. The reduced ventilatory response to carbon dioxide in small preterm infants, especially those with apnea, is primarily the result of decreased central chemosensitivity; however, mechanical factors such as poor respiratory function and an unstable, compliant chest wall may contribute.[5] It is difficult to distinguish the neural from mechanical factors that contribute to respiratory failure in this population.[6]

It has been known for many years that preterm infants respond to a fall in inspired oxygen concentration with a transient increase in ventilation over approximately 1 minute, followed by a return to baseline or even depression of ventilation. The characteristic response to low oxygen in infants appears to result from initial peripheral chemoreceptor stimulation, followed by overriding depression of the respiratory center as a result of hypoxemia. Such hypoxic respiratory depression may be useful in the hypoxic intrauterine environment where respiratory activity is only intermittent and not contributing to gas exchange. The nonsustained response to low inspired oxygen concentration may, however, be a disadvantage postnatally. Decreased peripheral chemoreceptor responsiveness to oxygen or central hypoxic depression of respiratory neural output may impair recovery from apnea. In contrast, excessive peripheral chemosensitivity has also been shown to compromise ventilatory stability and predispose to periodic breathing and even apnea in preterm infants.[7,8] Periodic breathing is thought to result from a combination of dominant peripheral chemosensitivity combined with a CO_2 level close to the apneic threshold, resulting in the characteristic cycles of breaths and pauses. These findings are consistent with the observed postnatal delay in onset of periodic breathing as peripheral chemoreceptors may be silenced in the initial postnatal period.[2,9-11]

Contribution From Inflammatory Mechanisms

It is well recognized that apnea may be the first indication of neonatal sepsis. There is also considerable current biological interest in the role of inflammation on respiratory neural output at both central and peripheral levels. Although inflammatory cytokines probably do not readily cross the blood-brain barrier, systemic infection does upregulate inflammatory cytokines at the blood-brain barrier, resulting in activation of prostaglandin signaling and resultant inhibition of respiratory neural output.[12] Chorioamnionitis is a major precipitant of preterm birth. It is possible that antenatal or postnatal exposure of the lung to a proinflammatory stimulus may activate brain circuits that destabilize respiratory neural output. In neonatal rodents, there is a response of proinflammatory cytokine gene expression in the brainstem after intrapulmonary lipopolysaccharide exposure, which is partially vagally mediated.[13] This is accompanied by significant ventilatory depression to hypoxic exposure. An interesting related line of investigation is the role of intermittent hypoxia and resultant oxidant stress on inflammatory pathways that regulate respiratory neural output. Much work needs to be done to explore these potential interrelationships between impaired respiratory neural output and inflammation,

intermittent hypoxemia (IH), and any resultant oxidant stress as discussed later.

Clinical Challenges in Defining Neonatal Apnea

During early postnatal life, apneic events are ubiquitous; they can vary widely in duration and are often accompanied by bradycardia and/or intermittent hypoxemia.[14] Accordingly, American Academy of Pediatrics (AAP) guidelines have historically defined clinical apnea of prematurity as a respiratory pause of >20 seconds or shorter if accompanied by hypoxemia (O_2 sat <80–85%) and/or bradycardia (<80 bpm).[15] It should be noted that even short respiratory pauses, approximating 10 seconds or less, may be associated with hypoxemia and/or bradycardia. Apnea is categorized as (1) central—with loss of central respiratory drive resulting in complete cessation of flow and absence of respiratory effort; (2) obstructive—with absence of flow in the presence of respiratory efforts; and (3) mixed—consisting of both central and obstructive components. Mixed apnea accounts for ~40% to 50% of all events in preterm infants[14,16] and is often initiated by a loss of central drive, followed by a delay in resolution due to upper airway closure.[17] However, airway narrowing and/or collapse, as measured by cardiac signal transmission on the flow waveform, can also occur during central apnea.[18] Unfortunately, standard impedance monitoring, which reflects chest wall motion, may fail to differentiate obstructed versus unobstructed inspiratory efforts.

The true incidence of apnea during early postnatal life has been grossly underestimated due to the historical practice of using nursing documentation, shown to underreport the true frequency of clinical events by >50%.[19] More accurate pneumogram recordings have revealed a high incidence of cardiorespiratory events even in convalescing infants. For example, in very low-birth-weight (VLBW) neonates, 91% of pneumograms performed within 72 hours of anticipated discharge revealed apnea accompanied by a fall in heart rate or oxygen saturation.[20] This has been supported in an expanded cohort of 1211 infants <35 weeks' gestation showing that preterm infants continue to experience short apnea with bradycardia and/or hypoxemia in the week prior to discharge.[21] It is, therefore, not surprising that hospitalization is frequently prolonged due to concern about persistent cardiorespiratory events. NICU EMR databases are beginning to incorporate automated detection of apnea/bradycardia/hypoxemia in contrast to manual entries by the nursing staff. Since hospital discharge is often driven by the presence (or absence) of events, it is unclear how the anticipated increased frequency of documentation with automated bedside monitoring may affect the duration of hospitalization.

Mechanisms of Oxygenation Instability

In extremely preterm infants, intermittent hypoxemia (IH) events are pervasive and transient during early postnatal life with a relatively low incidence during the first week of life, followed by a rapid increase during the second and third weeks and a plateau or decrease thereafter.[22] Intermittent hypoxemia events are almost always preceded by body movement[23] or a respiratory pause.[14] The initiation, duration, and severity of IH can be influenced by many factors including baseline oxygen saturation,[24] oxygen diffusion in the lung pulmonary oxygen stores, total blood oxygen carrying capacity, the slope of the hemoglobin oxygen dissociation curve, cardiac shunts, and oxygen consumption.[25]

Intermittent hypoxemia events in neonates have been traditionally attributed to hypoventilation due to central or obstructive apnea, but these mechanisms mainly apply to spontaneously breathing infants. The occurrence of spontaneous IH in mechanically ventilated infants is often perplexing because they occur in spite of continued cycling of the ventilator and patency of the airway. These episodes of hypoxemia are characterized by a rapid decline in oxygen saturation (SpO_2) that become more frequent with advancing postnatal age.[22,26,27]

One of the most common mechanisms leading to spontaneous IH events in mechanically ventilated preterm infants consists of forced exhalations secondary to contractions of the abdominal musculature that impinge on the respiratory system and impair respiratory mechanics. The resultant decrease in lung volume and hypoventilation cause hypoxemia that becomes more severe and persistent with successive abdominal contractions.[23,28,29]

Electromyographic measurements show that these forced exhalations are caused by contractions of the abdominal muscles that produce a marked increase in abdominal and intrathoracic pressure, some of them in excess of 25 cm H_2O.[29] As shown in Fig. 8.1, repeated contractions of the abdominal muscles can prolong the hypoxemia episodes and increase their severity. It is important to note that in mechanically ventilated infants, the endotracheal tube bypasses the glottis and eliminates the protective upper airway's function to preserve lung volume during the rise in intrathoracic pressure.

The factors that elicit these forced exhalations leading to loss in lung volume and hypoventilation with hypoxemia have not been clearly defined. However, behavioral disturbances appear to trigger IH. Increased body activity, agitation, squirming, and tachycardia are frequently present moments prior to the onset of the episodes.[23] Increased frequency of IH has been observed during awake or indeterminate sleep states than in quiet or active sleep.[30] This is important because indeterminate sleep is the most common sleep state in preterm infants. These observations correlate with the observed increased frequency of IH during the day compared to nighttime in mechanically ventilated extreme premature infants.[31] The higher daytime IH frequency is likely related to increased patient activity accompanied by disrupted sleep as well as by more negative stimulation associated with routine care in the NICU. Prone position has also been associated with fewer and shorter IH episodes compared to supine.[32,33]

The combination of increased activity leading to ventilation changes and poor lung function due to the underlying lung disease may aggravate the frequency and severity of IH. In addition, the low functional residual capacity and decreased lung compliance characteristic of mechanically ventilated infants combined with bypassing of the glottis by the endotracheal tube may increase the likelihood of reaching closing volume in some areas of the lung with even small decreases in lung volume.

The decline in SpO_2 during these episodes of hypoxemia is more abrupt than what is expected from a decline in ventilation alone and often persist after ventilation has been reestablished.[23] This observation suggests that the initial loss in lung volume and

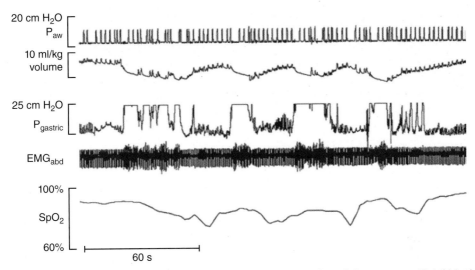

Fig. 8.1 Mechanism triggering an episode of hypoxemia in a ventilated infant. Recordings of airway pressure *(P$_{AW}$)*, tidal volume *(V$_T$)*, gastric pressure *(P$_{gastric}$)*, abdominal muscle electromyography *(EMG$_{abd}$)*, and arterial oxygen saturation *(SpO$_2$)* show multiple decreases in end-expiratory lung volume and minute ventilation associated with contractions of the abdominal muscles causing increases in P$_{gastric}$. Each decline in end-expiratory lung volume and tidal volume, despite continuous cycling of the ventilator, is followed by a decline in Spo$_2$. (From Esquer C, Claure N, D'Ugard C, et al. Role of abdominal muscles activity on duration and severity of hypoxemia episodes in mechanically ventilated preterm infants. *Neonatology.* 2007;92:182-186.)

hypoventilation may produce ventilation-perfusion inequalities and some degree of intrapulmonary shunting causing a rapid decline in SpO$_2$. The onset of hypoxemia can also provoke an increase in pulmonary vascular resistance and induce right-to-left shunting through extrapulmonary channels. These circulatory changes can explain why episodes of IH are frequently observed in infants with chronic lung disease and increased pulmonary vascular reactivity. In many of these infants, normoxemia is restored only after the fraction of inspired oxygen (FiO$_2$) is increased, which may restore oxygenation not only by increasing the alveolar-capillary oxygen gradient but also by attenuating the hypoxia-induced pulmonary vasoconstriction.

Association Between Intermittent Hypoxemia, Bradycardia, and Outcomes

Multiple studies in preterm infants have shown an association between apnea of prematurity and morbidity. However, more recent data in neonatal models suggest that the accompanying hypoxemia and/or bradycardia may be the contributing factor(s) in initiating a pathological cascade (Fig. 8.2). Unfortunately,

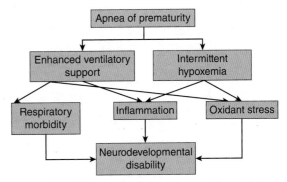

Fig. 8.2 Potential association between apnea of prematurity and longer-term disability in preterm infants.

in infant trials, it is very difficult to implicate causality as opposed to association when relating apnea and IH to outcome. In contrast, animal models have been able to show direct connections between distinct patterns of postnatal IH exposure and long-term sequelae.

Sleep disordered breathing (SDB) is a relatively common condition in children and young adults.[34,35] Former preterm infants are especially at risk, although the mechanisms are currently unknown.[35,36] Early postnatal exposure to chronic intermittent hypoxia in rodents results in a blunted acute ventilatory response to hypoxia during adulthood, suggesting that early IH patterns can have long-lasting effects on respiratory stability.[37] This may be one explanation why former preterm infants have a nearly fourfold increase in the obstructive apnea hypopnea index at 8 to 11 years of age when compared to former healthy term infants.[35] A subsequent trial in former preterm infants assessed the effect of early postnatal caffeine on sleep architecture and breathing patterns at 5 to 12 years of age. Although there were no differences between caffeine groups, ~10% of the infants had obstructive sleep apnea (OSA), again suggesting former preterm birth is a risk factor for SDB in later childhood.[38]

Respiratory morbidities associated with preterm birth are a result of a combination of factors beginning with an immature respiratory control center superimposed on an underdeveloped lung. After birth the preterm infant is further exposed to environmental stressors such as supplemental oxygen and positive pressure support to counter respiratory and oxygen instability. As a result, both FiO_2 and IH have been implicated in poor respiratory outcomes including BPD[39,40] and asthma.[41] More extensive analyses are currently being performed in the prematurity-related ventilatory control study (Pre-Vent)—a multicenter trial of >500 infants <29 weeks' gestation that will incorporate bedside monitoring variables along with biomarkers to elucidate individual cardiopulmonary phenotypes and mechanisms of ventilatory control contributing to adverse outcomes in preterm infants.[42]

IH may be one of many factors that contribute to growth trajectory in preterm infants. Data in neonatal rats have shown that IH induces both brain[43] and body[44] growth restrictions which were followed by catch-up growth after a few weeks of recovery. Limited infant data support the relationship between decreased weight gain and hypoxia,[45,46] but animal models suggest that any potential effects of IH on growth restriction may be short term and reversible. In contrast, the effect of IH on cardiovascular control may be long-lasting and dependent on the pattern of IH exposure. For example, rat pups exposed to a clustered pattern of IH exhibited lower blood pressure which was sustained after 2 months of exposure. In contrast, an equally dispersed paradigm of IH had no effect on blood pressure.[44] Young adult women born

preterm display increased risk of hypertension compared to former healthy term infants,[47] but there are currently no infant studies looking at the interaction between preterm birth, IH, and blood pressure. What role early postnatal IH exposure plays in cardiovascular development has yet to be determined.

There is strong evidence in both animal models and infants suggesting an association between cardiorespiratory events and impaired executive function. In VLBW infants, delayed resolution and increased event severity during early postnatal life are risk factors for severe disabilities at 13 months of age.[48] Apnea during hospitalization has also been shown as a predictor of neurodevelopmental impairment at 2 to 3 years of age[49,50] and diminished adaptive behavior at early school age (Vineland Adaptive Behavior Composite).[51] Many of the infant studies relied on chart documentation of apnea, limiting the reliability of study findings, and do not address the question of whether it is the apnea or the accompanying hypoxemia that initiates the pathological sequelae.

In neonatal rodents, exposure to intermittent hypoxia evokes long-lasting behavioral and neurochemical alterations resulting in impaired working memory,[52] decreased brain weight,[52] increased expression of caspase-3,[52] locomotor hyperactivity, and alterations in dopamine signaling in adulthood,[53] reinforcing long-term effects of IH exposure on brain development. In addition, neonatal exposure to fluctuations in oxygen levels causes retinal neovascularization with the severity of vascular tortuosity and retinal hemorrhage being dependent on the time between subsequent IH cycles.[54] Long-term recordings have now allowed for more reliable and detailed analyses of oxygen saturation patterns and morbidity in infants. For instance, continuous pulse oximetry monitoring over the first 2 months of life revealed an association between severe retinopathy of prematurity and a higher frequency of IH, of longer duration, and distinct timing between IH events.[55] A secondary analysis of infants enrolled in the Canadian Oxygen Trial revealed an association between increased time spent <80% during IH events and a greater probability of death or disability, cognitive or language delay, severe retinopathy of prematurity, and motor impairment at 18 months of age[56] that was limited to IH events of ≥1 minute in duration. Thus, the risk of IH and morbidity may be dependent on the distinct pattern of IH events.

In summary, the potential consequences of apnea of prematurity are most likely associated with the accompanying fall in oxygenation. Pathological cascades may be initiated by specific high-risk patterns of IH and have both short and long-lasting effects, including SDB, growth restriction, retinopathy of prematurity, neurodevelopmental impairment, and alterations in cardiovascular regulation. Identification of high-risk patterns may provide insight into future intervention protocols in the NICU setting.

Mechanistic Insights Into Morbidity

Little information is known regarding the mechanism underlying morbidities associated with IH, although alterations in oxidative stress, inflammatory mediators, and trophic factors may be attributed to initiating a pathophysiological cascade. Low levels of oxygenation alter transcriptional responses which are mediated by hypoxia-inducible factors (HIFs). In animal models, intermittent hypoxia has been shown to initiate accumulation of HIF-1α[57,58] and reactive oxygen species generation[59] during the onset of reoxygenation. At the same time, IH exposure initiates degradation of HIF-2α and downregulation of superoxide dismutase.[58] The net result is overall prooxidant signaling leading to pathophysiology. These effects are supported by data in healthy volunteers demonstrating that chronic IH increases oxidative stress by increasing production of reactive oxygen species without a compensatory increase in antioxidant activity.[60] Future therapeutic interventions could include inhibition of oxidative stress associated with episodes of IH.

The increase in IH events during early postnatal life in extremely preterm infants may also play a role in enhancing inflammatory cytokine levels. In animal models, IH initiates an inflammatory response during early postnatal life[61] with increments in TNF-α, IL-8, and IL-6 from onset of IH exposure. Correspondingly, in extremely low-birth-weight (ELBW) infants, recurrent or persistent elevations of serum inflammatory proteins within the first month of life have been associated with increased frequency of IH events[62] and attention-deficit behavior at 2 years of age.[63]

Therefore, it is reasonable to suggest that IH during early postnatal life may play a role in the inflammatory response associated with later neurodevelopmental dysfunction. This may be one possible explanation why caffeine, a known antiinflammatory, improves rate of survival of VLBW infants without neurodevelopmental impairment at 18 to 21 months.[64]

Controversies in Therapy

There are various pharmacological and nonpharmacological therapies for apnea of prematurity. Therapies are initiated depending on variations in NICU clinical practice, nursing documentation of events, clinical status, and infant respiratory requirements. Some therapies are shown to be beneficial in larger trials while other treatments are controversial requiring further investigation.

ACCEPTED TREATMENTS

Caffeine

Caffeine is the most common therapy used to treat apnea and intermittent hypoxemia. Caffeine and other methylxanthines have been prescribed in preterm infants for the last 40 years[65,66] and have been shown to reduce apnea and need for mechanical ventilation.[67] In a recent study, Rhein et al. demonstrated that caffeine therapy, administered to infants of 25 to 32 weeks' gestation, decreased the number of intermittent hypoxemic events and time with hypoxemia at 35 and 36 weeks' postmenstrual age (PMA).[68]

The largest trial of caffeine (Caffeine for Apnea of Prematurity Trial) randomly assigned 2006 infants with birth weight between 500 and 1250 g to caffeine or placebo in the first 10 days of life. Although apnea of prematurity was not measured in this clinical trial, caffeine administration was associated with a reduction in the duration of positive pressure support, oxygen supplementation, and incidence of bronchopulmonary dysplasia.[69] Caffeine also significantly improved survival without neurodevelopmental disability at 18 to 21 months.[64,70]

There are various pharmacological effects of caffeine in apnea of prematurity. Most importantly, it stimulates the respiratory center in the brainstem and increases sensitivity to carbon dioxide.[71] Mechanisms of action include blockade of adenosine A_1 and A_{2A} receptor subtypes resulting in excitation of respiratory neural output.[72,73] Caffeine has also been shown to enhance peripheral chemoreceptor activation.[74] A loading dose of caffeine showed a rapid (within 5 minutes) and prolonged (2 hours) increase in diaphragmatic activity which was associated with an increase in tidal volume.[75] Caffeine may also have antiinflammatory properties in the lung. For example, rat pups exposed prenatally to lipopolysaccharide had improved lung function and cytokine profiles after caffeine treatment.[76] Lastly, caffeine is a radical scavenger preventing oxidative damage in brain tissue of rabbits[77] and IH induced oxidative stress in the brainstem of newborn rats.[78] Taken as a whole, caffeine has a range of mechanistic pathways to both stabilize respiration and reduce the risk of hypoxia/hyperoxia-induced sequelae.

Optimal strategies of caffeine therapy have yet to be determined (see Table 8.1). For example, common practice entails a caffeine citrate loading dose of 20 mg/kg followed by 5 to 10 mg/kg/day[64,69,70,79] with potential side effects including tachycardia, dysrhythmia, feeding intolerance, GERD, jitteriness, irritability, or rarely observed seizures.[71] However, a higher loading dose of 80 mg/kg in preterm infants has been associated with an increased incidence of cerebellar hemorrhage and hypertonicity and should therefore be avoided.[80]

There have been no randomized control trials addressing the optimal time to start or stop caffeine in spontaneously breathing infants. The ideal time to start caffeine has been examined by a few retrospective cohort studies. Early caffeine administration during the first 2 to 3 days of life was associated with reduction of bronchopulmonary dysplasia,[68,81,82] PDA

TABLE 8.1   Caffeine Therapy Controversies

Prophylactic versus therapeutic: Optimal onset of therapy?
Optimal maintenance dosing: Upper limit?
Role for additional loading dose?
Optimal duration of therapy: When to stop?
Mechanism of action: Optimizing respiratory control, antiinflammatory or antioxidant?

---

requiring treatment,[81-83] and duration of positive pressure ventilation.[82] In contrast, a recent observational study showed that caffeine started on day 1 compared to days 2 to 6 did not influence mortality, BPD, or the rate of continuous positive airway pressure (CPAP) failure leading to invasive mechanical ventilation.[84] A recent randomized controlled trial evaluated the effect of early caffeine to that of placebo in mechanically ventilated preterm infants. This trial, based on the assumption that a consistent respiratory drive is essential to facilitate weaning from mechanical ventilation, did not show a significant effect on the time to achieve the first successful extubation.[85] The findings from these two studies suggest that the underlying lung disease may be a stronger determinant of the need for invasive respiratory support than poor respiratory drive during the first days or weeks after birth.

A recent cohort study in over 81,000 infants <35 weeks' gestational age showed substantial variability among sites in the timing of caffeine discontinuation.[86] However, AAP guidelines suggest discontinuing caffeine when cardiorespiratory events are insignificant for 5 to 7 days or 33 to 34 weeks' PMA, whichever comes first.[72] However, it is important to realize that preterm infants born at very young gestational ages may continue to have apnea and intermittent hypoxemia events well beyond 33 to 34 weeks' PMA.[72]

Noninvasive Respiratory Support

Nasal CPAP is safe and effective and has a prominent role in treatment for apnea of prematurity. CPAP is a noninvasive form of applying a constant distending airway pressure during inhalation and exhalation. It supports infants who are spontaneously breathing but who have airway instability, pulmonary edema, or atelectasis.[83] CPAP enhances functional residual capacity, reduces work of breathing, and decreases mixed and obstructive apnea.[87-89]

There is considerable controversy regarding the best mode of CPAP delivery. This is further complicated by the various low- and high-flow nasal cannulas that are widely used for CPAP delivery despite limited comparative studies. Refinement of techniques to both deliver CPAP and provide effective synchronized noninvasive ventilation (NIV) may be the answer.

NIV is more effective than CPAP in reducing apnea frequency, particularly in premature infants who present with frequent apnea episodes.[90,91] NIV does not offer advantages over CPAP in premature infants with infrequent apnea.[92]

Oxygen Administration

As discussed earlier, centrally mediated hypoxic depression is prominent in early postnatal life. It follows that avoidance of hypoxemia should benefit apnea; additionally, hypoxia increases the pauses associated with periodic breathing. Earlier studies found that increases in FiO_2 decreased apnea of prematurity and periodic breathing.[93,94] More recent data demonstrated that targeting a lower baseline oxygen saturation (85–89%) compared to higher oxygen saturation (91–95%) was associated with an increased rate of intermittent hypoxemic events in preterm infants.[24] Since major complications of oxygen toxicity include retinopathy of prematurity and lung damage with resultant bronchopulmonary dysplasia, it is important to balance the level of supplemental oxygen with potential risks associated with oxygen.

Studies have evaluated the use of systems that automatically adjust FiO_2 in preterm infants with oxygenation instability.[95-101] Automatic FiO_2 control is more effective than the clinical staff or a fully dedicated nurse in maintaining SpO_2 within the target range. Although it did not reduce the number of all IH episodes, it reduced the number of the more severe and prolonged episodes (those with SpO_2 below 80% for more than 1 minute). The reason is that these systems are designed to immediately respond to IH episodes and attenuate their severity and duration by rapidly increasing the FiO_2 but do not prevent their occurrence. In some of these studies, the frequency of brief episodes of hyperoxemia was higher during automatic compared to manual FiO_2 adjustments by the clinical staff. This is likely due to the maintenance of high basal SpO_2 levels during routine care in an attempt to prevent IH. The impact of this new automated strategy on neonatal outcomes is being evaluated in a large randomized controlled trial.[102]

Positioning

Studies have demonstrated that prone positioning may stabilize the chest wall, improve oxygenation, and decrease apnea.[103] Therefore keeping infants prone for periods of time in the NICU is a reasonable approach. Excessive neck flexion needs to be avoided to prevent upper airway obstruction. It is possible that there may be a modest benefit from a head elevated at a 15 degrees tilt position.[104] Despite the possible benefits, the prone position should be avoided close to discharge when infants should be preferentially maintained supine and the parents educated that supine is the recommended sleep position at home where continuous monitoring is no longer available.

CONTROVERSIAL APPROACHES

Kangaroo Care

Multiple studies encompassing various age groups of premature infants have compared the effects of kangaroo care on decreasing apnea of prematurity and intermittent desaturation episodes. In one study, skin-to-skin care increased bradycardia and desaturation episodes.[105] However, a recent meta-analysis showed a decrease in apnea with kangaroo care.[106] Therefore, use of skin-to-skin has benefits in newborn care including bonding between mother and infant, improved breastfeeding, and may show benefit for the treatment of apnea of prematurity.

Olfactory Stimulation

Olfactory sensitivity can be elicited in preterm infants as young as 28 weeks' gestation.[107] Preferential reactions to odors include facial expressions, mouth or limb movement, and changes in breathing frequency making it a potential therapeutic for apnea of prematurity. A small study of 14 infants unresponsive to pharmacologic intervention showed a 44% decline in apnea with the presentation of vanillin on the periphery of the infant's pillow.[108] Advantages of olfactory stimulation are ease of implementation that can accompany current treatments and no known adverse effects. A current randomized trial is underway to investigate three distinct odorants (mint, grapefruit, and vanilla) to reduce the occurrence of apnea in preterm infants.[109] If successful, application of preferential odors could provide a low cost and easily accessible adjunct therapy for apnea of prematurity.

Blood Transfusions

There have been conflicting views regarding blood transfusions to reduce the incidence of apnea of prematurity. Zagol et al. found an association between blood transfusions and a decreased number of apnea/bradycardia/desaturation events in addition to a reduction of apneas at higher hematocrits,[110] while more recent findings in infants with a hematocrit of 20% to 42% packed red blood cell (pRBC) transfusion decreased the frequency of intermittent hypoxemia with no diminution observed with platelet and plasma transfusions.[111] In a separate randomized controlled trial, the frequency of apneas was twice as high in a restrictive-transfusion versus liberal-transfusion group.[112] In contrast, other studies have shown no significant difference in frequency of apnea,[113,114] bradycardia,[113] or hypoxemia.[113] Abu Jawdeh et al. showed that improvement in intermittent hypoxemic events occur only after the first week of life which may explain some of the discrepancy between studies.[115] Although the results among studies are conflicting, they do suggest that severe anemia may contribute to worsening of apnea of prematurity and an increase in hematocrit may protect against the hypoxemia that accompanies apnea. Additionally, it should be noted that blood transfusions have been associated with potentially more complications including increased respiratory support after transfusions, necrotizing enterocolitis, and BPD.[114]

Mechanosensory Stimulation

Kinesthetic stimulation using oscillating mattresses for prevention of apnea has been proposed as a treatment for apnea of prematurity. In a meta-analysis which included 154 infants, there was no clear evidence of effect of this therapy on apnea or bradycardia.[116] By contrast, in a more recent small-scale study of 10 preterm infants, stochastic (random) stimulation reduced desaturation episodes.[117] There may be a future for such novel modes of kinesthetic or related stimulation to improve respiratory drive.

Doxapram

Doxapram stimulates peripheral and central chemoreceptors, which results in augmentation of breathing. Significant reductions in apnea have been shown with increasing dose of doxapram. However, higher doses have been accompanied by elevations in blood pressure,[118] and prolonged use in the neonatal period has been associated with an adverse Mental Developmental Index in infants <1250 g birth weight.[119] In the Caffeine for Apnea of Prematurity Trial, infants in the placebo group were more likely to develop cerebral palsy than the caffeine group; however, in the placebo group, infants were three times more likely to receive doxapram.[64] With limited data to support the efficacy and safety of doxapram[120] and the possibility of long-term adverse effects, this therapy has limited appeal.

Discharge Practice

There is virtually no evidence for practice regarding discharge decisions for infants who have apnea of prematurity. It is known that infants born at a younger gestational age have delayed resolution of apnea and bradycardia events. In a retrospective cohort study that included 1400 infants ≤34 weeks' gestation, a 5- to 7-day apnea/bradycardia-free interval had a success rate between 94% and 96% of predicting no events after discharge. Success rates were dependent on the gestational age and PMA of the infant.[121] In most NICU settings, an apnea event-free period before discharge of 5 to 7 days is commonly used.[72] Often this is based on nursing observation and monitor alarm thresholds for recording of apnea and bradycardia events. Preterm infants have clinically undetected apnea events that may not be apparent unless continuous electronic recording is investigated. However, there is no evidence that they predict acute life-threatening events.[20] At this time, routine home monitoring for resolved apnea of prematurity is not recommended,[72] although this is an option for selected infants who are sent home on oxygen or have certain congenital disorders requiring frequent monitoring.

Acknowledgment

The authors would like to acknowledge Dr. Vidhi Shah for her assistance in the original version of this chapter.

REFERENCES

1. Stryker C, Dylag A, Martin RJ. Apnea and control of breathing. In: Jobe A, Whitsett J, Abman S, eds. *Fetal and Neonatal Lung Development: Clinical Correlates and Technologies for the Future.* Cambridge: Cambridge University Press; 2016:223-237.
2. Gauda EB, Martin RJ. Control of breathing. In: *Avery's Diseases of the Newborn.* 10th ed. Philadelphia: Elsevier Inc.; 2018:600-617.e4.

3. Mayer CA, Haxhiu MA, Martin RJ, et al. Adenosine A2A receptors mediate GABAergic inhibition of respiration in immature rats. *J Appl Physiol*. 2006;100:91-97.

4. Kinney HC, Broadbelt KG, Haynes RL, et al. The serotonergic anatomy of the developing human medulla oblongata: implications for pediatric disorders of homeostasis. *J Chem Neuroanat*. 2011;41:182-199.

5. Gerhardt T, Bancalari E. Apnea of prematurity: I. Lung function and regulation of breathing. *J Pediatrics*. 1984;74:58-62.

6. Martin RJ. Chapter 157: Pathophysiology of apnea of prematurity. In: Polin RA, Abman SH, Rowitch DH, Benitz WE, Fox WW, eds. *Fetal & Neonatal Physiology*. 5th ed. Philadelphia: Elsevier; 2016.

7. Cardot V, Chardon K, Tourneux P, et al. Ventilatory response to a hyperoxic test is related to the frequency of short apneic episodes in late preterm neonates. *Pediatr Res*. 2007;62:591-596.

8. Nock ML, Difiore JM, Arko MK, et al. Relationship of the ventilatory response to hypoxia with neonatal apnea in preterm infants. *J Pediatr*. 2004;144:291-295.

9. Patel M, Mohr M, Lake D, et al. Clinical associations with immature breathing in preterm infants: part 2-periodic breathing. *Pediatr Res*. 2016;80:28-34.

10. Khan A, Qurashi M, Kwiatkowski K, et al. Measurement of the CO_2 apneic threshold in newborn infants: possible relevance for periodic breathing and apnea. *J Appl Physiol*. 2005;98:1171-1176.

11. Al-Matary A, Kutbi I, Qurashi M, et al. Increased peripheral chemoreceptor activity may be critical in destabilizing breathing in neonates. *Semin Perinatol*. 2004;28:264-272.

12. Hofstetter AO, Saha S, Siljehav V, et al. The induced prostaglandin E2 pathway is a key regulator of the respiratory response to infection and hypoxia in neonates. *Proc Natl Acad Sci U S A*. 2007;104:9894-9899.

13. Balan KV, Kc P, Hoxha Z, et al. Vagal afferents modulate cytokine-mediated respiratory control at the neonatal medulla oblongata. *Respir Physiol Neurobiol*. 2011;178:458-464.

14. Di Fiore JM, Arko MK, Miller MJ, et al. Cardiorespiratory events in preterm infants referred for apnea monitoring studies. *Pediatr*. 2001;108:1304-1308.

15. Finer NN, Higgins R, Kattwinkel J, et al. Summary proceedings from the apnea-of-prematurity group. *Pediatr*. 2006;117:S47-S51.

16. Barrington KJ, Finer NN. Periodic breathing and apnea in preterm infants. *Pediatr Res*. 1990;27:118-121.

17. Gauda EB, Miller MJ, Carlo WA, et al. Genioglossus response to airway occlusion in apneic versus nonapneic infants. *Pediatr Res*. 1987;22:683-687.

18. Lemke RP, Idiong N, Al-Saedi S, et al. Evidence of a critical period of airway instability during central apneas in preterm infants. *Am J Resp Crit Care Med*. 1998;157:470-474.

19. Brockmann PE, Wiechers C, Pantalitschka T, et al. Underrecognition of alarms in a neonatal intensive care unit. *Arch Dis Childh Fetal Neonatal Ed*. 2013;98:F524-F527.

20. Barrington KJ, Finer N, Li D. Predischarge respiratory recordings in very low birth weight newborn infants. *J Pediatr*. 1996;129:934-940.

21. Fairchild K, Mohr M, Paget-Brown A, et al. Clinical associations of immature breathing in preterm infants: part 1-central apnea. *Pediatric Res*. 2016;80:21-27.

22. Di Fiore JM, Bloom JN, Orge F, et al. A higher incidence of intermittent hypoxemic episodes is associated with severe retinopathy of prematurity. *J Pediatr*. 2010;157:69-73.

23. Dimaguila MA, Di Fiore JM, Martin RJ, et al. Characteristics of hypoxemic episodes in very low birth weight infants on ventilatory support. *J Pediatr*. 1997;130:577-583.

24. Di Fiore JM, Walsh M, Wrage L, et al. Low oxygen saturation target range is associated with increased incidence of intermittent hypoxemia. *Pediatr*. 2012;161:1047-1052.

25. Sands SA, Edwards BA, Kelly VJ, et al. Mechanism underlying accelerated arterial oxygen desaturation during recurrent apnea. *Am J Resp Crit Care Med*. 2010;182:961-969.

26. Garg M, Kurzner SI, Bautista DB, et al. Clinically unsuspected hypoxia during sleep and feeding in infants with bronchopulmonary dysplasia. *Pediatrics*. 1988;81:635-642.

27. Durand M, McEvoy C, MacDonald K. Spontaneous desaturations in intubated very low birth weight infants with acute and chronic lung disease. *Pediatric Pulmonology*. 1992;13:136-142.

28. Bolivar JM, Gerhardt T, Gonzalez A, et al. Mechanisms for episodes of hypoxemia in preterm infants undergoing mechanical ventilation. *J Pediatr*. 1995;127:767-773.

29. Esquer C, Claure N, D'Ugard C, et al. Role of abdominal muscles activity on duration and severity of hypoxemia episodes in mechanically ventilated preterm infants. *Neonatology*. 2007;92:182-186.

30. Lehtonen L, Johnson MW, Bakdash T, et al. Relation of sleep state to hypoxemic episodes in ventilated extremely-low-birth-weight infants. *J Pediatr*. 2002;141:363-368.

31. Jain D, D'Ugard C, Bello J, et al. Hypoxemia episodes during day and night and their impact on oxygen saturation targeting in mechanically ventilated preterm infants. *Neonatology*. 2018;113:69-74.

32. McEvoy C, Mendoza ME, Bowling S, et al. Prone positioning decreases episodes of hypoxemia in extremely low birth weight infants (1000 grams or less) with chronic lung disease. *J Pediatr*. 1997;130:305-309.

33. Chang YJ, Anderson GC, Dowling D, et al. Decreased activity and oxygen desaturation in prone ventilated preterm infants during the first postnatal week. *Heart Lung*. 2002;31:34-42.

34. Paavonen EJ, Strang-Karlsson S, Raikkonen K, et al. Very low birth weight increases risk for sleep-disordered breathing in young adulthood: the Helsinki Study of Very Low Birth Weight Adults. *Pediatrics*. 2007;120:778-784.

35. Rosen CL, Larkin EK, Kirchner HL, et al. Prevalence and risk factors for sleep-disordered breathing in 8- to 11-year-old children: association with race and prematurity. *J Pediatr*. 2003;142:383-389.

36. Jaleel Z, Schaeffer T, Trinh C, et al. Prematurity: a prognostic factor for increased severity of pediatric obstructive sleep apnea. *Laryngoscope*. 2021;131:1909-1914.

37. Reeves SR, Gozal D. Respiratory and metabolic responses to early postnatal chronic intermittent hypoxia and sustained hypoxia in the developing rat. *Pediatr Res*. 2006;60:680-686.

38. Marcus CL, Meltzer LJ, Roberts RS, et al. Long-term effects of caffeine therapy for apnea of prematurity on sleep at school age. *Am J Respir Crit Care Med*. 2014;190:791-799.

39. Raffay TM, Dylag AM, Sattar A, et al. Neonatal intermittent hypoxemia events are associated with diagnosis of bronchopulmonary dysplasia at 36 weeks postmenstrual age. *Pediatr Res*. 2019;85(3):318-323.

40. Fairchild KD, Nagraj VP, Sullivan BA, et al. Oxygen desaturations in the early neonatal period predict development of bronchopulmonary dysplasia. *Pediatr Res*. 2019;85(7):987-993.

41. Di Fiore JM, Dylag AM, Honomichl RD, et al. Early inspired oxygen and intermittent hypoxemic events in extremely premature infants are associated with asthma medication use at 2 years of age. *J Perinatol*. 2019;39:203-211.

42. Dennery PA, Di Fiore JM, Ambalavanan N, et al. Pre-Vent: the prematurity-related ventilatory control study. *Pediatric research*. 2019;85:769-776.

43. Kanaan A, Farahani R, Douglas RM, et al. Effect of chronic continuous or intermittent hypoxia and reoxygenation on cerebral capillary density and myelination. *Am J Physiol Regul Integr Comp Physiol*. 2006;290:R1105-R1114.

44. Pozo ME, Cave A, Koroglu OA, et al. Effect of postnatal intermittent hypoxia on growth and cardiovascular regulation of rat pups. *Neonatology*. 2012;102:107-113.

45. Warburton A, Monga R, Sampath V, et al. Continuous pulse oximetry and respiratory rate trends predict short-term respiratory and growth outcomes in premature infants. *Pediatr Res*. 2019;85:494-501.

46. Moyer-Mileur LJ, Nielson DW, Pfeffer KD, et al. Eliminating sleep-associated hypoxemia improves growth in infants with bronchopulmonary dysplasia. *Pediatrics*. 1996;98:779-783.

47. Skudder-Hill L, Ahlsson F, Lundgren M, et al. Preterm birth is associated with increased blood pressure in young adult women. *J Am Heart Assoc*. 2019;8:e012274.

48. Pillekamp F, Hermann C, Keller T, et al. Factors influencing apnea and bradycardia of prematurity - implications for neurodevelopment. *Neonatology*. 2007;91:155-161.

49. Janvier A, Khairy M, Kokkotis A, Cormier C, Messmer D, Barrington KJ. Apnea is associated with neurodevelopmental impairment in very low birth weight infants. *J Perinatol*. 2004;24:763-768.

50. Cheung PY, Barrington KJ, Finer NN, et al. Early childhood neurodevelopment in very low birth weight infants with predischarge apnea. *Pediatr Pulmonol*. 1999;27:14-20.

51. Taylor HG, Klein N, Schatschneider C, et al. Predictors of early school age outcomes in very low birth weight children. *J Dev Behav Pediatr*. 1998;19:235-243.

52. Ratner V, Kishkurno SV, Slinko SK, et al. The contribution of intermittent hypoxemia to late neurological handicap in mice with hyperoxia-induced lung injury. *Neonatology*. 2007;92:50-58.

53. Decker MJ, Jones KA, Solomon IG, et al. Reduced extracellular dopamine and increased responsiveness to novelty: neurochemical and behavioral sequelae of intermittent hypoxia. *Sleep*. 2005;28:169-176.

54. Coleman RJ, Beharry KD, Brock RS, et al. Effects of brief, clustered versus dispersed hypoxic episodes on systemic and ocular growth factors in a rat model of oxygen-induced retinopathy. *Pediatr Res*. 2008;64:50-55.

55. Di Fiore JM, Kaffashi F, Loparo K, et al. The relationship between patterns of intermittent hypoxia and retinopathy of prematurity in preterm infants. *Pediatr Res*. 2012;72:606-612.

56. Poets CF, Roberts RS, Schmidt B, et al. Association between intermittent hypoxemia or bradycardia and late death or disability in extremely preterm infants. *JAMA*. 2015;314:595-603.

57. Yuan G, Nanduri J, Khan S, et al. Induction of HIF-1alpha expression by intermittent hypoxia: involvement of NADPH oxidase, Ca_2+ signaling, prolyl hydroxylases, and mTOR. *J Cell Physiol*. 2008;217:674-685.

58. Nanduri J, Wang N, Yuan G, et al. Intermittent hypoxia degrades HIF-2alpha via calpains resulting in oxidative stress: implications for recurrent apnea-induced morbidities. *Proc Natl Acad Sci U S A*. 2009;106:1199-1204.

59. Fabian RH, Perez-Polo JR, Kent TA. Extracellular superoxide concentration increases following cerebral hypoxia but does not affect cerebral blood flow. *Int J Dev Neurosci*. 2004;22:225-230.

60. Pialoux V, Hanly PJ, Foster GE, et al. Effects of exposure to intermittent hypoxia on oxidative stress and acute hypoxic ventilatory response in humans. *Am J Respir Crit Care Med*. 2009;180:1002-1009.

61. Li S, Qian XH, Zhou W, et al. Time-dependent inflammatory factor production and NFkappaB activation in a rodent model of intermittent hypoxia. *Swiss Med Wkly*. 2011; 141:w13309.

62. Abu Jawdeh EG, Huang H, Westgate PM, et al. Intermittent hypoxemia in preterm infants: a potential proinflammatory process. *Am J Perinatol*. 2021;38:1313-1319.

63. O'Shea TM, Joseph RM, Kuban KC, et al. Elevated blood levels of inflammation-related proteins are associated with an attention problem at age 24 mo in extremely preterm infants. *Pediatr Res*. 2014;75:781-787.

64. Schmidt B, Roberts RS, Davis P, et al. Long-term effects of caffeine therapy for apnea of prematurity. *N Engl J Med*. 2007; 357:1893-1902.

65. Kuzemko JA, Paala J. Apnoeic attacks in the newborn treated with aminophylline. *Arch Dis Child*. 1973;48:404-406.

66. Aranda JV, Gorman W, Bergsteinsson H, et al. Efficacy of caffeine in treatment of apnea in the low-birth-weight infant. *J Pediatr*. 1977;90:467-472.

67. Henderson-Smart DJ, Steer P. Methylxanthine treatment for apnea in preterm infants. *Cochrane Database Syst Rev*. 2001: CD000140.

68. Rhein LM, Dobson NR, Darnall RA, et al. Effects of caffeine on intermittent hypoxia in infants born prematurely: a randomized clinical trial. *JAMA Pediatr*. 2014;168:250-257.

69. Schmidt B, Roberts RS, Davis P, et al. Caffeine therapy for apnea of prematurity. *N Engl J Med*. 2006;354:2112-2121.

70. Schmidt B, Anderson PJ, Doyle LW, et al. Survival without disability to age 5 years after neonatal caffeine therapy for apnea of prematurity. *JAMA*. 2012;307:275-282.

71. Abdel-Hady H, Nasef N, Shabaan AE, et al. Caffeine therapy in preterm infants. *World J Clin Pediatr*. 2015;4:81-93.

72. Eichenwald EC. Apnea of prematurity. *Pediatrics*. 2016;137.

73. Wilson CG, Martin RJ, Jaber M, et al. Adenosine A2A receptors interact with GABAergic pathways to modulate respiration in neonatal piglets. *Respir Physiol Neurobiol*. 2004;141:201-211.

74. Chardon K, Bach V, Telliez F, et al. Effect of caffeine on peripheral chemoreceptor activity in premature neonates: interaction with sleep stages. *J Appl Physiol (1985)*. 2004;96:2161-2166.

75. Kraaijenga JV, Hutten GJ, de Jongh FH, et al. The effect of caffeine on diaphragmatic activity and tidal volume in preterm infants. *J Pediatr*. 2015;167:70-75.

76. Koroglu OA, MacFarlane PM, Balan KV, et al. Anti-inflammatory effect of caffeine is associated with improved lung function after lipopolysaccharide-induced amnionitis. *Neonatology*. 2014; 106:235-240.

77. Prasanthi JR, Dasari B, Marwarha G, et al. Caffeine protects against oxidative stress and Alzheimer's disease-like pathology in rabbit hippocampus induced by cholesterol-enriched diet. *Free Radic Biol Med*. 2010;49:1212-1220.

78. Laouafa S, Iturri P, Arias-Reyes C, et al. Erythropoietin and caffeine exert similar protective impact against neonatal intermittent hypoxia: apnea of prematurity and sex dimorphism. *Exp Neurol*. 2019;320:112985.

79. Rosen C, Taran C, Hanna M, et al. Caffeine citrate for apnea of prematurity-One dose does not fit all a prospective study. *J Perinatol*. 2021;41:2292-2297.

80. McPherson C, Neil JJ, Tjoeng TH, et al. A pilot randomized trial of high-dose caffeine therapy in preterm infants. *Pediatr Res*. 2015;78:198-204.

81. Lodha A, Seshia M, McMillan DD, et al. Association of early caffeine administration and neonatal outcomes in very preterm neonates. *JAMA Pediatr*. 2015;169:33-38.

82. Dobson NR, Patel RM, Smith PB, et al. Trends in caffeine use and association between clinical outcomes and timing of therapy in very low birth weight infants. *J Pediatr*. 2014;164:992-998.e3.

83. Patel RM, Leong T, Carlton DP, Vyas-Read S. Early caffeine therapy and clinical outcomes in extremely preterm infants. *J Perinatol.* 2013;33:134-140.

84. Patel RM, Zimmerman K, Carlton DP, et al. Early caffeine prophylaxis and risk of failure of initial continuous positive airway pressure in very low birth weight infants. *J Pediatr.* 2017; 190:108-111.e1.

85. Amaro CM, Bello JA, Jain D, et al. Early caffeine and weaning from mechanical ventilation in preterm infants: a randomized, placebo-controlled trial. *J Pediatr.* 2018;196:52-57.

86. Ji D, Smith PB, Clark RH, et al. Wide variation in caffeine discontinuation timing in premature infants. *J Perinatol.* 2020;40: 288-293.

87. Pantalitschka T, Sievers J, Urschitz MS, et al. Randomized crossover trial of four nasal respiratory support systems on apnoea of prematurity in very low birth weight infants. *Arch Dis Child Fetal Neonat Ed.* 2009;94:F245-F248.

88. Millar D, Kirpalani H. Benefits of non invasive ventilation. *Indian Pediatr.* 2004;41:1008-1017.

89. Zhao J, Gonzalez F, Mu D. Apnea of prematurity: from cause to treatment. *Eur J Pediatr.* 2011;170:1097-1105.

90. Bisceglia M, Belcastro A, Poerio V, et al. A comparison of nasal intermittent versus continuous positive pressure delivery for the treatment of moderate respiratory syndrome in preterm infants. *Minerva Pediatr.* 2007;59:91-95.

91. Lin CH, Wang ST, Lin YJ, Yeh TF. Efficacy of nasal intermittent positive pressure ventilation in treating apnea of prematurity. *Pediatr Pulmonol.* 1998;26:349-353.

92. Ryan CA, Finer NN, Peters KL. Nasal intermittent positive-pressure ventilation offers no advantages over nasal continuous positive airway pressure in apnea of prematurity. *Am J Dis Child.* 1989;143:1196-1198.

93. Weintraub Z, Alvaro R, Kwiatkowski K, et al. Effects of inhaled oxygen (up to 40%) on periodic breathing and apnea in preterm infants. *J Appl Physiol.* 1992;72:116-120.

94. Simakajornboon N, Beckerman RC, Mack C, et al. Effect of supplemental oxygen on sleep architecture and cardiorespiratory events in preterm infants. *Pediatrics.* 2002;110:884-888.

95. Claure N, Gerhardt T, Everett R, et al. Closed-loop controlled inspired oxygen concentration for mechanically ventilated very low birth weight infants with frequent episodes of hypoxemia. *Pediatrics.* 2001;107:1120-1124.

96. Urschitz MS, Horn W, Seyfang A, et al. Automatic control of the inspired oxygen fraction in preterm infants: a randomized crossover trial. *Am J Respir Crit Care Med.* 2004;170: 1095-1100.

97. Claure N, D'Ugard C, Bancalari E. Automated adjustment of inspired oxygen in preterm infants with frequent fluctuations in oxygenation: a pilot clinical trial. *J Pediatr.* 2009;155:640-645.e1-e2.

98. Claure N, Bancalari E, D'Ugard C, et al. Multicenter crossover study of automated control of inspired oxygen in ventilated preterm infants. *Pediatrics.* 2011;127:e76-e83.

99. Waitz M, Schmid MB, Fuchs H, et al. Effects of automated adjustment of the inspired oxygen on fluctuations of arterial and regional cerebral tissue oxygenation in preterm infants with frequent desaturations. *J Pediatr.* 2015;166:240-244.e1.

100. Zapata J, Gómez JJ, Araque Campo R, et al. A randomised controlled trial of an automated oxygen delivery algorithm for preterm neonates receiving supplemental oxygen without mechanical ventilation. *Acta Paediatr.* 2014;103:928-933.

101. van Kaam AH, Hummler HD, Wilinska M, et al. Automated versus manual oxygen control with different saturation targets and modes of respiratory support in preterm infants. *J Pediatr.* 2015;167:545-550.e1-e2.

102. Poets CF, Franz AR. Automated FiO_2 control: nice to have, or an essential addition to neonatal intensive care. *Arch Dis Child Fetal Neonatal Ed.* 2017;102:F5-F6.

103. Miller-Barmak A, Riskin A, Hochwald O, et al. Oxygenation instability assessed by oxygen saturation histograms during supine vs prone position in very low birthweight infants receiving noninvasive respiratory support. *J Pediatr.* 2020;226: 123-128.

104. Di Fiore JM, Poets CF, Gauda E, et al. Cardiorespiratory events in preterm infants: etiology and monitoring technologies. *J Perinatol.* 2016;36:165-171.

105. Bohnhorst B, Gill D, Dördelmann M, et al. Bradycardia and desaturation during skin-to-skin care: no relationship to hyperthermia. *J Pediatr.* 2004;145:499-502.

106. Montealegre-Pomar A, Bohorquez A, Charpak N. Systematic review and meta-analysis suggest that Kangaroo position protects against apnoea of prematurity. *Acta Paediatrica.* 2020;109:1310-1316.

107. Sarnat HB. Olfactory reflexes in the newborn infant. *J Pediatr.* 1978;92:624-626.

108. Marlier L GC, Messer J. Olfactory stimulation prevents apnea in premature newborns. *J Pediatr.* 2005;115:83-88.

109. Duchamp-Viret P, Nguyen HK, Maucort-Boulch D, et al. Protocol of controlled odorant stimulation for reducing apnoeic episodes in premature newborns: a randomised open-label Latin-square study with independent evaluation of the main endpoint (PREMODEUR). *Bmj Open.* 2021;11:e047141.

110. Zagol K, Lake DE, Vergales B, et al. Anemia, apnea of prematurity, and blood transfusions. *J Pediatr.* 2012;161:417-421.e1.

111. Kovatis KZ, Di Fiore JM, Martin RJ, et al. Effect of blood transfusions on intermittent hypoxic episodes in a prospective study of very low birth weight infants. *J Pediatr.* 2020;222: 65-70.

112. Bell EF SR, Widness JA, Mahoney LT, et al. Randomized trial of liberal versus restrictive guidelines for red blood cell transfusion in preterm infants. *Pediatrics.* 2005;115:1685-1691.

113. Poets CF, Pauls U, Bohnhorst B. Effect of blood transfusion on apnea, bradycardia and hypoxemia in preterm infants. *Eur J Pediatr.* 1997;156:311-316.

114. Valieva OA, Strandjord TP, Mayock DE, et al. Effects of transfusions in extremely low birth weight infants: a retrospective study. *J Pediatr.* 2009;155:331-337.e1.

115. Abu Jawdeh EG, Martin RJ, Dick TE, et al. The effect of red blood cell transfusion on intermittent hypoxemia in ELBW infants. *J Perinatol.* 2014;34:921-925.

116. Osborn DA, Henderson-Smart DJ. Kinesthetic stimulation versus theophylline for apnea in preterm infants. *Cochrane Database Syst Rev.* 2000;1998:CD000502.

117. Bloch-Salisbury E, Indic P, Bednarek F, et al. Stabilizing immature breathing patterns of preterm infants using stochastic mechanosensory stimulation. *J Appl Physiol (1985).* 2009;107:1017-1027.

118. Barrington KJ, Finer NN, Torok-Both G, et al. Dose-response relationship of doxapram in the therapy for refractory apnea of prematurity. *J Pediatr.* 1987;80:22-27.

119. Sreenan C EP, Demianczuk N, Robertson CMT. Isolated mental developmental delay in very low birth weight infants: association with prolonged doxapram therapy for apnea. *J Pediatr.* 2001;139:832-837.

120. Vliegenthart RJ, Ten Hove CH, Onland W, et al. Doxapram treatment for apnea of prematurity: a systematic review. *Neonatology.* 2017;111:162-171.

121. Lorch SA, Srinivasan L, Escobar GJ. Epidemiology of apnea and bradycardia resolution in premature infants. *J Pediatr.* 2011;128:e366-e373.

Chapter 9

Pulmonary-Cardiovascular Interaction

Shahab Noori, Elizabeth R. Fisher, and Martin Kluckow

Chapter Outline

Introduction
Cardiorespiratory Interactions at Birth
The Physiology of Cardiovascular and Respiratory Interaction
  Preload
  Contractility
  Afterload
Effect of the Respiratory System on the Cardiovascular System
  Mechanical Ventilation
  Effects of PEEP, CPAP and MAP
  Effect of Tidal Volume and Sustained Lung Inflation
  Effect of Acidosis and Permissive Hypercapnia
Effect of the Cardiovascular System on the Respiratory System
  Pulmonary Hypertension

Patent Ductus Arteriosus
Asphyxia
Congenital Diaphragmatic Hernia
Congenital Heart Disease
Neonatal Sepsis
Interaction During Early Transition and Potential Clinical Implications
  Surfactant
  Carbon Dioxide, CBF and Brain Injury
Interaction After Transition and Potential Clinical Implications
Conclusions

Key Points

- The respiratory and cardiac systems are integrally related both anatomically and functionally, and as a result there are significant interactions, particularly in the newborn period.

- Inappropriately high airway pressure during mechanical ventilation leads to adverse hemodynamic effects including a reduction in left and right ventricular output, a decrease in venous return, and an increase in pulmonary vascular resistance (PVR). Inappropriately low airway pressure can also have detrimental effects by decreasing lung volume and consequently increasing PVR.

- PEEP and MAP in the range commonly used in clinical practice in settings of lung diseases with low compliance and in the absence of low lung volume or hyperexpansion have mild effects on hemodynamics.

- In addition to the direct effects of ventilator settings on the cardiovascular system, the chosen treatment strategy and aims, such as a particular blood gas goal, can have a significant effect on the cardiovascular system. While the impact of acidosis on cardiovascular system is not well studied, there is accumulating evidence that excessive hypercapnia especially in the first few postnatal days attenuates cerebral blood flow autoregulation and likely contributes to reperfusion injury in preterm infants.

Introduction

The cardiorespiratory system consists of two organ systems—the heart and cardiovascular system and the lungs and pulmonary vasculature—which are designed to work together to deliver an adequate supply of oxygen to the tissues to meet the demands of oxygen consumption. There are complex anatomical and physiological relationships between these two organ systems. An understanding as to how they interact both normally and in the presence of pathology or interventions, such as the provision of positive pressure, is essential for any clinician working with sick children and infants. Changes in intrathoracic pressure affect both organ systems, and within the cardiovascular system, there are differential effects on the left- and right-sided structures. A delicate balance needs to be maintained between the distending airway pressure needed to optimize lung volume and thus oxygenation, but avoiding excessive pressure that would compromise global cardiac function that is necessary for adequate systemic blood flow, which is essential for normal oxygen delivery. Both optimal oxygenation and normal cardiac output are required to deliver adequate oxygen to the tissues. Reduced tissue oxygenation often has a multifactorial causation; however, many of the issues will be related to what is happening at the level of the cardiorespiratory interaction.

The initial cardiorespiratory interaction is during birth at the time of the circulatory transition and umbilical cord clamping. A normal relationship between the spontaneously breathing infant with normal lungs and cardiovascular system should ensue—in which case there will be balance between the closely associated lungs and heart. If there is pathology, particularly respiratory distress, then the interventions required to support the respiratory system such as positive pressure ventilation may adversely impact the function of the heart. Similarly, abnormalities of cardiac function such as ventricular failure can result in lung congestion and the need for respiratory support. Finally, changes in the pulmonary vasculature, particularly in the neonatal transition where failure of the normal fall in pulmonary vascular resistance (PVR), can impair cardiac function. The predominant influence on the cardiorespiratory interaction is mean airway pressure (MAP) which most directly affects the intrathoracic pressure. The effect of inspiration/expiration in addition to MAP is minimal. Adjunctive respiratory therapies such as inhaled nitric oxide may also rapidly change the balance between cardiac and respiratory systems.

Cardiorespiratory Interactions at Birth

In utero, the fetus has fluid-filled lungs with a very low pulmonary blood flow—about 10% of postnatal flow[1] and minimal tidal volume changes such that any pressure exerted on the heart physically and via venous return is steady and unchanging. The interposition of the placenta and the unique fetal shunts—the ductus venosus, foramen ovale (FO), and patent ductus arteriosus (PDA)—into the fetoplacental circulation results in a fetal circulation quite different to that of the postnatal infant just minutes after birth. Instead of being two parallel circulations, there is admixture of blood at several levels. Oxygenated blood returning from the placenta via the umbilical vein passes through the ductus venosus and into the inferior vena cava (IVC). Blood then streams into the right atrium where due to the anatomy of the right atrium and FO, the oxygenated blood is directed preferentially across the FO into the left atrium (LA), thus improving the oxygenation level of blood passing from LA into left ventricle and subsequently toward the systemic circulation. The presence of the PDA and fetal conditions (hypoxemia, vasoconstricting factors) that cause increased PVR result in preferential blood flow from the right ventricle via the right to left shunting PDA into the systemic circulation.[2] The significantly reduced blood flow to the pulmonary circulation means that the normal main source of preload to the LA (when there is no placental flow), the pulmonary venous return, is significantly limited in utero.[3] Blood passing from the right ventricle via the PDA and from the left ventricle into the aorta travels down the descending aorta and deoxygenated blood is then sent to the placenta via iliac and eventually umbilical arteries to complete the fetoplacental circulation. The main flow to the LA is provided by the placental return and some flow from lower body via the IVC—this is an important consideration when the timing of umbilical cord clamping in the newborn transition is considered. Interruption of the placental blood flow return prior to establishment of the pulmonary blood flow through the lungs puts the transitioning newborn at risk of a loss of preload to the systemic ventricle with a subsequent fall in systemic cardiac output.[4]

The events of the perinatal cardiopulmonary transition constitute the first, and possibly most crucial, cardiorespiratory interaction and there is potential for significant complications ranging from premature interruption of the placental blood flow resulting in an acute drop in cardiac output[4] to failure to properly transition leading to the syndrome of persistent pulmonary hypertension in the newborn (PPHN, Table 9.1). For premature infants, the complex transition to neonatal physiology is disrupted by varying degrees of cardiac dysfunction, poorly compliant and underdeveloped lungs, and failure of expected closure of fetal channels (particularly the ductus arteriosus). The combination of these insults can result in atelectasis, persistent elevation in PVR, poor cardiac output, and systemic hypotension. It is therefore of particular importance that ventilation and cord management strategies are optimized to limit hemodynamic instability. Keeping

the cardiorespiratory events of the transition in sequence has become an important aspect of management at birth. The key initial event is inflation of the lungs (usually spontaneously by crying, or otherwise augmented with positive pressure devices), resulting in a rapid increase in pulmonary blood flow and reversal of the ductal shunt to become left to right.[5] Additionally, the lung liquid must be rapidly absorbed; animal imaging data suggest that this occurs via transepithelial gradients developed during inspiration.[6,7] With the increased pulmonary blood flow, adequate left atrial filling is established and the umbilical cord can now be cut without acutely reducing the left atrial return. In this sequence, oxygenation is provided by the lungs prior to the placental "lung" being removed by cord clamping.

Failure to allow the natural sequence of events to unfold may result in significant hemodynamic instability, at least in animal models.[8] Umbilical venous blood accounts for 30% to 50% of venous return to the heart.[9,10] Clamping the umbilical cord prior to lung aeration can therefore result in reduced preload, as poor left atrial filling from low pulmonary blood flow is unable to make up for the loss of umbilical venous flow. In combination with raised left ventricular (LV) afterload from a rapid increase in systemic arterial pressure as the low resistance placenta is removed, these acute physiologic changes can result in reduced cardiac output and haemodynamic instability.

These hemodynamic changes are much less marked if the pulmonary blood flow is established by lung aeration prior to cord clamping (termed physiologically based cord clamping).[11] Delaying cord clamping increases the likelihood that the newborn infant will establish breathing/lung inflation before the umbilical cord is clamped.[12,13] In addition, the benefits of a delay in cord clamp time have generally been ascribed to the receipt of a placental transfusion.[13] The volume of placental transfusion may be as high as 20 to 30 mL/kg of birth weight[14] in term infants and up to 15 mL/kg in preterm infants.[15] This is dependent on a number of factors, including gravity, time, flow/patency of the umbilical vessels, and spontaneous breathing efforts. Delayed cord clamping is associated with lower rates of early hypotension, inotropic support, blood transfusion, and surfactant use in premature infants compared to early cord clamping.[16,17]

TABLE 9.1 Clinical Relevance of Cardiorespiratory Interaction at Birth

Event	Intervention	Impact
Inspiration	Stimulation or PPV	Fluid absorption ↑ Pulmonary blood flow Reversal of PDA shunt
Lung aeration prior to cord clamping	Stimulation, CPAP/PPV[a]	Placental transfusion
Establishing FRC	CPAP/PPV	Improved oxygenation, ↓ risk of PPHN
Avoidance of hyperoxia	Judicious use of oxygen	Improved response to iNO

CPAP, Continuous positive airway pressure; *FRC*, functional residual capacity; *iNO*, inhaled nitric oxide; *PDA*, patent ductus arteriosus; *PPHN*, persistent pulmonary hypertension in the newborn; *PPV*, positive pressure ventilation.
[a]Excessively high CPAP and PPV can also negatively impact venous return and cardiovascular function (see text).

Respiratory efforts result in significant fluctuations in umbilical cord blood flow[18] and can potentially enhance the placental transfusion received by preferentially directing umbilical venous return to the right atrium on inspiration.[19] The provision of positive pressure and initial resuscitative measures while the infant is still attached to the umbilical cord has been hypothesized to provide additional benefit to the transitional circulation, and as a means to facilitate placental transfusion for compromised infants where delayed cord clamping would otherwise be abandoned for neonatal resuscitation. In the BabyDUCC trial,[20] nonvigorous infants born over 32 weeks' gestation requiring transitional assistance were randomized to either resuscitation during placental transfusion or early cord clamping. The primary outcome of heart rate at 60 to 120 seconds was similar between the two groups, as were oxygen saturations in the delivery room. Observational data show that the vast majority of preterm infants spontaneously breathe by time of arrival to resuscitaire, regardless of whether cord clamping is early or delayed.[21] Two recent randomized controlled trials (RCTs) have compared delayed cord clamping with and without assisted ventilation in premature infants.[12,22] Apgar scores, oxygen saturations, delivery room interventions, and hemodynamics in the first 24 hours including rates of inotropic support and blood transfusion appear similar whether respiratory support was initiated prior to cord clamping or not. While the hemodynamic benefits of establishing lung aeration with an intact cord have not yet been proven, multiple additional studies addressing this clinical question are currently underway.[23-25]

Umbilical cord milking is another alternative for provision of a placental transfusion to the newborn. As transfusion occurs over a shorter time period, there is less opportunity for the effect of the respiratory system on the volume of transfusion and subsequent cardiac flow on effects.[26] Despite this, there still seem to be cardiovascular benefits such as higher mean blood pressure and less inotrope use compared to immediate cord clamping.[27]

Umbilical cord milking may even encourage greater early oxygenation and lower MAP requirement compared to delayed cord clamping.[28] However, multiple recent studies have identified an association with higher incidence of severe intraventricular hemorrhage compared to delayed cord clamping, primarily in the extremely low birth weight (ELBW) group.[16,29,30] This is likely caused by a rapid surge in cerebral blood flow (CBF), consistent with the effects seen in premature lambs of a large rise in mean carotid artery pressure and blood flow, without any increase in pulmonary blood flow.[31] An RCT[32] reported a greater need for respiratory and hemodynamic support in preterm infants exposed to umbilical cord milking compared to delayed cord clamping—including ventilation, surfactant, inotropic agents, and blood transfusion—though there was discrepancy in gestational ages between the two groups.

For the aforementioned reasons, delayed cord clamping generally remains the preferred cord management approach in premature infants. The 2019 Cochrane Review[33] was largely inconclusive about many of the physiological effects and advantages of the different cord management strategies. Cord clamping to optimize the pulmonary and hemodynamic transition at birth remains an active area of research.

After inflation of the lungs and the commencement of spontaneous negative pressure breathing, there are further cardiorespiratory interactions with venous blood return to the heart being enhanced by the negative pressure generated during normal inspiration. This can be seen on blood flow traces showing a respiratory pattern, more so in adults.[34] If an infant requires positive pressure support, either by continuous positive airway pressure (CPAP) or mechanical ventilation, some degree of impact on the cardiovascular system is inevitable. Mechanical ventilation raises intrathoracic pressure and reduces venous return and preload to the right heart, thus also impairing right ventricular performance, especially if the distending pressure is excessive, relative to the compliance of the lungs. Mechanical ventilation also significantly affects PVR and right ventricular afterload. The left ventricle in contrast receives venous return from within the thorax so is less affected by changes in intrathoracic pressure. Cardiac output from the left ventricle is dependent on blood flow from the right ventricle, so changes in RV output will affect LV output too. Increased pressure in the right ventricle can cause a conformational change in the heart with displacement of the interventricular septum which decreases LV preload and compliance. Although LV contractility is not affected by positive pressure ventilation, the LV output can be significantly affected by changes in the LV myocardial wall tension (difference between LV systolic pressure and mean intrathoracic pressure).[35,36] There is also a potentially positive effect of mechanical ventilation and raised intrathoracic pressure on the LV with lower LV afterload due to a decreased transmyocardial pressure gradient in the setting of higher intrathoracic pressure (Fig. 9.1).[37]

After birth, the neonate is exposed to higher oxygen tension compared to fetal life. Routine use of an oxygen supplement can deleteriously affect the cardiovascular transition. Indeed, animal models have shown a reduction in response to inhaled nitric oxide in sheep with PPHN exposed to high fractional inspiratory oxygen.[38] Each of the elements of cardiovascular function can be affected by the respiratory system—the preload via changes in intrathoracic pressure and pulmonary blood flow, the contractility by

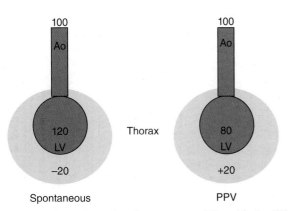

Fig. 9.1 Effects of intrathoracic pressure on left ventricular *(LV)* afterload. This is a schematic drawing of an example of the difference in intrathoracic and left ventricular pressure in spontaneously breathing versus PPV in an adult. On the left side of this example, the left ventricle of a spontaneously breathing patient needs to generate a transmural pressure of 120 mm Hg in response to a systemic systolic pressure of 100 mm Hg and a mean intrathoracic pressure of −20 mm Hg. When this patient is mechanically ventilated with a mean intrathoracic pressure of +20 mm Hg, the left ventricle has to generate a pressure of only 80 mm Hg to result in the same systemic systolic pressure of 100 mm Hg. Thus, an augmentation of mean intrathoracic pressure will reduce left ventricular afterload and potentially improve overall left ventricular function. *Ao,* Aorta; *PPV,* positive pressure ventilation. (From Cheifetz IM. Cardiorespiratory interactions: the relationship between mechanical ventilation and hemodynamics. *Respir Care.* 2014; 59(12):1937-1945.)

direct impingement on ventricles within a confined space, and the afterload by changes in the PVR (both overinflation and underinflation increase PVR)[39] that also translates to inadequate filling of the LA in the setting of reduced pulmonary blood flow.[40,41]

The Physiology of Cardiovascular and Respiratory Interaction

During normal phasic spontaneous breathing with negative intrathoracic pressure, the passive systemic venous return is easily able to fill the right atrium that is at low pressure with the additional augmenting effect of inspiration. The end-diastolic volumes of both ventricles change in different directions—enhanced venous return into the RV from outside the thorax increases RV filling, which makes the LV stiffer and harder to fill.[42] When positive pressure is applied, the opposite happens with impaired RV filling and easier LV filling. The end result of these changes is fluctuations in the systemic arterial pressure. In a ventilated adult, ventilator-induced changes in preload can result in a variable stroke volume and subsequently variation in the pulse pressure. The rise in arterial pressure during a positive pressure breath is counterintuitive as the expectation would be reduction in venous return and subsequently the pulse pressure should decrease. Factors that may account for this include an increase in pulmonary venous return from squeezing of capillaries, decreased LV afterload, mechanical assist of LV contraction by compression, and adrenergic stimulation with increased inotropy.[43] The degree of pulse pressure variation can be used to predict responsiveness to a volume bolus during supportive hemodynamic management.[44] Interestingly, the effect of mechanical ventilation on the right ventricle is opposite—impaired venous return and cardiac output, which in turn reduces the venous return to the LA that will result in a fall in LV output as well. Pulse pressure variation is also seen in neonates in association with cardiopulmonary interactions but is probably not as variable and thus not likely to be as predictive of fluid responsiveness.[45] This may be due to the greater compliance of the newborn chest wall, compared to the adult, which may decrease the transmission of positive pressure to the pleural space and mediastinum.

TABLE 9.2   Impact of Lung Disease and Ventilator Support on Components of Cardiac Output

Component	Respiratory alteration	Resultant effect
Preload	High mean airway pressure	↓ RV preload
	High pulmonary vascular resistance	↓ LV preload
Contractility	High pulmonary vascular resistance	↓ RV contractility
	Acidosis secondary to permissive hypercapnia	↓ Contractility*
Afterload	High pulmonary vascular resistance	↑ RV afterload
	Positive intrathoracic pressure	↓ LV afterload

LV, Left ventricular; *RV*, right ventricular.

PRELOAD

Preload is an important driver of adequate cardiac contractility, and subsequently cardiac output and the newborn heart are particularly sensitive to changes in preload. Worsening respiratory disease can impact on both right and left sides of the heart (Table 9.2). Higher MAP impairs systemic venous return to the right atrium, necessitating higher central venous pressure (CVP) to counteract the increased intrathoracic pressure, particularly in the setting of positive pressure ventilation. If the reduced systemic venous return is not balanced by increased CVP, the preload to the right ventricle is reduced and thus right ventricular output (RVO) will fall. A reduction in RVO results in reduced pulmonary blood flow which, apart from the effect on oxygenation, will also impact upon the preload and filling to the LA and subsequently the systemic cardiac output. The reduction in pulmonary blood flow can be exacerbated by the state of recruitment of the lungs. Underrecruited lungs will result in collapse in the supporting tissues around blood vessels in the lung, thus increasing PVR. If the lungs are overinflated, the increased pressure from the air-filled structures in the lung will cause compression of pulmonary vasculature and also result in impaired pulmonary blood flow and reduced return to the LA (Fig. 9.2). If there is increased

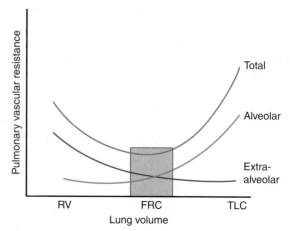

Fig. 9.2 Schematic representation of the relationship between lung volume and pulmonary vascular resistance. As lung volume increases from residual volume *(RV)* to total lung capacity *(TLC)*, the alveolar vessels become increasingly compressed by the distending alveoli, and so their resistance increases, whereas the resistance of the extra-alveolar vessels (which become less tortuous as lung volume increases) falls. The combined effect of increasing lung volume on the pulmonary vasculature produces the typical "U-shaped" curve as shown, with its nadir, or optimum, at around normal functional residual capacity *(FRC)*. (From Shekerdemian L, Bohn D. Cardiovascular effects of mechanical ventilation. *Arch Dis Child.* 1999;80(5):475-480.)

pulmonary vasoconstriction such as in PPHN, this will also impair blood flow through the lungs. An index of severity of raised PVR can be obtained by assessing the pulmonary venous return, in which case the pulmonary venous velocity is reduced.[46] Direct impingement of the heart, either by excessive MAP with overdistended lungs or by dilation of either ventricle, can cause septal bowing and reduction of ventricular cavity, typically of the LV by the RV with PPHN.[47]

With the positive airway pressures, the negative influence on cardiac output is mediated primarily through reduced systemic venous return, while at higher MAPs, direct effects on PVR and myocardial function become important.[40] In the sickest infants, all of these factors are likely to be important. MAP is often very high, hypoxia and acidosis are common, and pulmonary artery pressure is high as suggested by the commonly observed low ductal blood flow velocity. Both ventricles also show the ability to substantially increase output when the preload is increased by a ductal or atrial shunt, confirming a degree of myocardial reserve. The effect of positive pressure ventilation in reducing systemic venous return and cardiac output may be as important in preterm infants as it has been recognized to be in adults. There are few studies on the effect of ventilation on cardiac output in the preterm infant. Hausdorf and Hellwege[48] demonstrated a 25% to 30% reduction in ventricular stroke and cardiac output, with no effect on blood pressure, by increasing positive end-expiratory pressure (PEEP) from 0 to 8 cm of water (cm H_2O) in a group of preterm infants. The clinical importance of this is that an aggressive effort to improve arterial oxygenation may reduce perfusion and thus compromise tissue oxygen delivery. Trang[49] suggested that this occurs at PEEP levels above 6 cm H_2O in preterm infants. However, the absolute level of PEEP or MAP is not as important as the appropriateness of those pressures for the compliance of the lungs; the more compliant the lungs are, the greater the transmission of distending airway pressure to the mediastinum and thus the greater the impairment of cardiac output.

Interventions to counteract the deleterious effects of respiratory diseases and ventilator support on the preload primarily involve judicious use of ventilation settings to avoid excessive MAP and addressing the underlying pathophysiology of the lung disease, for example, reducing PVR. However, there is some evidence from adults[41] and one study in the preterm newborn[50] to suggest that volume expansion can correct some of the preload deficit which results from positive pressure ventilation and improve cardiac output in the short term.

CONTRACTILITY

Mechanical ventilation does not appear to directly affect myocardial contractility. However, through a decrease in LV afterload, it may enhance LV contractility. On the other hand, as discussed earlier, inappropriately high or low lung volume can increase PVR and therefore through an increase in RV afterload can impair right ventricular contractility. In addition, ventilator strategies aimed at permissive hypercapnia with resulting acidosis can decrease myocardial contractility at least in adult (see "Effect of Acidosis and Permissive Hypercapnia"). In the term infant, poor cardiac output is most often the result of an asphyxial insult or sepsis. Poor cardiac output in the preterm infant has been seen primarily as a consequence of

an immature myocardium,[51] especially in the first few postnatal days of the very premature infant.[52] LV ejection fraction, admittedly a broad measure of myocardial function in the preterm infant,[53] was not significantly associated with either ventricular output. The predominantly left to right pattern of ductal shunting will reduce RV output and atrial shunting will reduce left ventricular output (LVO) by shunting blood from the systemic back to the pulmonary circulations. This effect is apparent even in the first postnatal days.

AFTERLOAD

Afterload also potentially has a large effect on cardiac output in the transitioning newborn infant. The afterload that the right ventricle is exposed to is determined primarily by what is happening in the lungs—both in terms of aeration and in terms of the pulmonary vascular pressure. Optimization of lung recruitment and addressing raised PVR are both important strategies to improve right ventricular function. Judicious management of the shunting through the PDA may also be important with strategies to allow the PDA to remain open and promote a right to left shunt sometimes reducing afterload on the RV and allowing improved forward flow out of the ventricle. Although, as discussed earlier, positive pressure ventilation can enhance LV contractility by reducing the LV afterload (wall stress), systemic vascular resistance plays a more important role in changes in LV afterload than mechanical ventilation.

The newborn myocardium and cardiac function are more vulnerable to both preload and afterload changes than older infants and adults and this is even more so in preterm infants. They have a simpler structure with fewer mitochondria and differences in the myofibrils themselves result in less reserve and ability to compensate for changes in blood volume and peripheral resistance.[52,54]

Effect of the Respiratory System on the Cardiovascular System

MECHANICAL VENTILATION

In a normal spontaneously breathing infant during inspiration, the negative intrathoracic pressure increases the transmural pressure in the right atrium

(RA) and right ventricle (RV), thereby increasing the venous return. During expiration, the opposite effects occur; however, due to the presence of valves in the venous system, these effects are relatively small. On the other hand, when a patient is on positive pressure respiratory support, during inspiration the pleural pressure increases and therefore venous return to the RA is impeded while the improvement in venous return occurs during the expiratory phase.

The effect of phases of respiration during mechanical ventilation on the left and right ventricular filling is different. During expiration, both phases of ventricular filling (early passive and atrial) increase on the right side and decrease on the left side.[55] The increase in LV filling during inspiration may be related to the increase intra-/interalveolar pressure improving drainage to the LA and improved LV distensibility due to lower RV volume.

EFFECTS OF PEEP, CPAP, AND MAP

The effects of PEEP, CPAP, and MAP on venous return, PVR, and cardiac function for the most part depend on the lung compliance and lung volume. Both extremes of lung volume can increase PVR (Fig. 9.2).[56] This increase in RV afterload can impair RV function and through ventricular interdependence also adversely affect LV function.

In an experiment on premature lambs with normal lungs ventilated with tidal volume of 5 mL/kg and receiving PEEP of 4 cm H_2O, PEEP was changed randomly to 0, 8, and 12 cm H_2O.[57] Increasing PEEP from 4 to 8 and from 4 to 12 decreased pulmonary blood flow (PBF) by 20.5% and 41%, respectively, and caused corresponding changes in PVR; reducing PEEP from 4 to 0 did not affect PBF. Interestingly, despite decreasing PBF, increasing PEEP from 4 to 8 and then 12 cm H_2O improved oxygenation, presumably due to improvement in lung recruitment and ventilation-perfusion (VQ) matching. Higher PVR and lower PBF with an increase in PEEP have also been shown in a swine model with normal pulmonary function testing.[58] Again, it needs to be emphasized that these animals had normal lung compliance and therefore any PEEP > 4 cm H_2O would be excessive. Indeed, with low lung compliance, a significantly higher CPAP may have little hemodynamic effects.[59] A recent study compared hemodynamic impacts of low (5 cm H_2O), high

(12 cm H_2O), and dynamic CPAP (12 decreasing to 8 cm H_2O) in preterm lamb at birth.[59] Mean pulmonary blood flow was higher in the high and dynamic CPAP groups presumably due to better lung recruitment compared to the low CPAP group. In addition, high CPAP did not adversely affect CBF or cerebral venous drainage as assessed by measuring left carotid blood flow and right jugular venous pressure, respectively.

Although the effects of increase in PEEP/MAP in human neonates are similar to those of animal models, they are less prominent. When the PEEP increased from 0 to 4 and 8 cm H_2O in preterm infants after the acute phase of respiratory distress syndrome, both left and right cardiac output decreased.[48] In a larger study, preterm and term infants on mechanical ventilation with a baseline PEEP of 5 were exposed to a brief period of higher PEEP of 8.[60] They found a statistically nonsignificant 5% decrease in RVO and no effect on systemic circulation as evidenced by unchanged superior vena cava (SVC) flow as a group. However, the effect on SVC flow was variable with a third of the subjects showing a significant (about 25%) increase and another third demonstrating a significant decrease in SVC flow. These divergent effects are probably explained by differences in the underlying lung pathology, those with more compliant lungs having a decrease in flow with higher PEEP while those with more atelectatic lungs showing improved flow with higher PEEP. In this study, no change in ductal diameter or in percentage of right-to-left shunt was noted. Another study assessed the effect of change in PEEP from a baseline of 5 cm H_2O to 2 and 8 on ductal shunting and systemic flow in ventilated extremely preterm infants with a PDA.[61] Reduction of PEEP to 2 had no significant effect. There was no change in SVC flow or cerebral regional oxygen saturation, but there was a mild reduction in LVO with resultant decrease in LVO/SVC ratio when PEEP was increased to 8. This is suggestive of a mild reduction in left-to-right ductal shunting. However, the low LVO could also reflect a reduction in venous return. Interestingly, a study found no difference in LVO, RVO, or SVC flow with CPAP 4, 6, and 8 cm H_2O in stable preterm infants with minimal lung disease.[62] Similarly, a recent study of preterm infants during the first three postnatal days showed no effect on cerebral tissue oxygen saturations, transcutaneous CO_2, and arterial oxygen saturation with changes in CPAP from 4 to 6, then to 8, and finally back to 4 cm H_2O.[63] The lack of any hemodynamic effect observed in these two studies may be attributed at least in part to ineffective pressure transmission via a noninvasive nasal interface. Indeed, this may also explain the lack of difference in hemodynamics between nasal intermittent positive pressure ventilation (NIPPV) and CPAP. Preterm infants requiring respiratory support at median age of 20 days had similar LVO, RVO, SVC flow, and anterior CBF velocity when placed on NIPPV and nasal CPAP each for 30 minutes.[64] Another recent study showed no difference in LVO, RVO, and work of breathing between high CPAP ($\geq$9 cm H_2O) and NIPPV in preterm infants after the third postnatal week.[65] Finally, studies of preterm infants weaning off CPAP have shown variable results with some reporting no effect whereas others demonstrated lower RVO and SVC flow while on CPAP.[66,67]

An investigation of the impact of lung recruitment with high-frequency oscillation on pulmonary, systemic, and ductal blood flow in preterm infants with RDS demonstrates interesting findings.[68] Before giving surfactant, the MAP was increased stepwise until the FiO_2 was <0.25 or no further improvement in oxygenation was noted; this was called opening pressure. Then the MAP was decreased until deterioration in oxygenation was noted; this was called the closing pressure. Then lungs were recruited again and MAP was kept at 2 cm H_2O above the closing pressure which was called the optimal pressure. Despite very high MAP at the optimal pressure (20 cm H_2O), the hemodynamic effects were small. The RVO decreased by 17% but no change in SVC flow, ductal diameter, or flow pattern was noted.

Based on the available literature, the impact of PEEP or CPAP of up to 8 cm H_2O on ductal diameter and flow, systemic, and pulmonary blood flow in preterm infants appears to be negligible or minimal. This is in contrast to animal studies that have demonstrated a significant reduction in venous return and pulmonary blood flow and an increase in PVR. Although this may be the result of interspecies differences, the main reason for the discrepancy is likely to be the difference in lung compliance. Animal studies in general evaluated the impact of PEEP in models with normal lung compliance, whereas in human studies subjects had lung disease with presumably variable decrease in compliance. Indeed, as noted earlier, even a very high MAP appears to have little effect on the hemodynamics in subjects with poor lung compliance.[68] Therefore, the positive airway pressure more readily affects intrapleural pressure and overdistends the alveoli if it is inappropriately high for the degree of reduced compliance. As such, inappropriately high PEEP and MAP can result in increased PVR and reduction in pulmonary blood flow leading to hypoxemia and decreased systemic blood flow.

EFFECT OF TIDAL VOLUME AND SUSTAINED LUNG INFLATION

Little is known about the effect of different tidal volumes on hemodynamics. In a pediatric swine model with normal lung function, increasing tidal volume (up to 25 mL/kg) resulted in progressive and exponential increase in PVR and reduction in RVO and these effects were more pronounced with higher PEEP.[58] These deleterious effects appear to be the result of decreased preload (impaired venous return) and lung overdistention with physical compression of the microvasculature. Clearly, a grossly excessive tidal volume of this degree will have deleterious effects. In addition, as discussed earlier, normal lung compliance in these animal models limits the applicability of the findings to human subjects with lung disease.

A pilot RCT evaluated the impact of sustained lung inflation (30 cm H_2O for 15 seconds for up to 3 times) versus a control group (standard of care) on cerebral hemodynamics in moderately preterm infants during delivery room resuscitation.[69] The two groups had similar cerebral tissue oxygenation. However, unlike the control group, the sustained lung inflation group did not have a decrease in cerebral blood volume. The authors attributed this to decreased cerebral venous drainage which in a vulnerable population may increase the risk of intraventricular hemorrhage.[70] Clearly, more studies are needed to delineate the impact of sustained lung inflation on cardiac function and cerebral hemodynamics.

EFFECT OF ACIDOSIS AND PERMISSIVE HYPERCAPNIA

Although little data are available on its safety and efficacy, permissive hypercapnia is a common lung-protective strategy used in the care of neonates with lung disease.[71,72] Acceptance of higher carbon dioxide than normal allows for use of lower ventilator settings and smaller tidal volumes and as a result decreased volutrauma and lung injury.[73] As the renal compensatory metabolic alkalosis takes several days to take hold and may be further delayed in extremely premature infants due to renal tubular immaturity, permissive hypercapnia leads to acidosis especially in the first few postnatal days. Little is known about the impact of acidosis on cardiovascular function and cerebral hemodynamics in neonates.

The ionic channels in the myocyte are pH sensitive with some promoting and others reducing the influx of calcium, with the net effect of an increase in intracellular calcium with an acidic pH.[74] However, due to inhibition of myofibrillar responsiveness in acidic pH, myocardial contractility decreases despite an increase in intracellular calcium. In adult humans, acidosis and permissive hypercapnia affect the heart and vascular system leading to a decrease in myocardial contractility and a drop in systemic vascular resistance (SVR). Despite the decrease in contractility, cardiac output increases, most likely secondary to low afterload. Most of the effects of hypercapnia on the cardiovascular system appear to be mediated via altering pH as the aforementioned effects tend to attenuate or completely disappear with administration of a base or with passage of time as compensatory metabolic alkalosis sets in.[75,76] Interestingly, animal studies suggest that the myocardial and vascular responses to acidosis are developmentally regulated and different in newborn versus adult subjects. Newborn animals exhibit a more tolerant myocardium but greater vasodilation in response to acidosis.[77-79] Little is known about the effects of acidosis in human neonates. A recent prospective cross-sectional study evaluated the effect of pH and carbon dioxide (CO_2) on cardiovascular function in hemodynamically stable preterm infants.[80] The pH ranged from 7.02 to 7.46 and CO_2 from 28 to 76 mm Hg and base excess from -13 to $+6$ mEq/L. The authors found no relationship between various indices of myocardial contractility and pH in the first 2 weeks after birth. There was no relationship between either LVO or SVR with pH (or CO_2) during the transitional period (first 3 days). However, a weak but significant negative correlation between LVO and pH and positive correlation between SVR and pH was noted after the transitional period (postnatal day 4 to 14). Carbon dioxide had a positive and negative correlation with LVO and SVR, respectively, during the posttransitional period. The observed association remained significant even after adjusting for the effect of base deficit. This lack of reduction in contractility in contrast to the findings in adults may be due to higher intracellular buffer in neonates compared to that of the mature myocardium.[81] As for the effect of pH and CO_2 on cardiac output and SVR, there appears to be a postnatal maturational process in the cardiovascular response with the pattern becoming similar to that seen in adults only after the first 3 postnatal days.[80] Attempts at normalizing pH in the case of metabolic acidosis by giving sodium bicarbonate yield minimal hemodynamic effects. When sodium bicarbonate was given to ventilated preterm infants with metabolic acidosis, despite an increase in pH from mean 7.24 to 7.30, the increase in cardiac output was transient and likely was reflective of volume administration.[82] A study of infusion of sodium bicarbonate in piglets with mild metabolic acidosis showed progressive vasoconstriction of pial arterioles.[83] However, correction of metabolic acidosis with sodium bicarbonate had no effect on cerebral, renal, and splanchnic regional tissue oxygenation in very low birth weight neonates.[84]

Effect of the Cardiovascular System on the Respiratory System

The impact of impaired cardiovascular system function on the respiratory system is primarily through alteration in normal pulmonary blood flow. In the case of myocardial dysfunction, for example, in the setting of perinatal asphyxia, the RVO can be low due to poor contractility. In addition, the concomitant pulmonary hypertension which is common in this setting could lead to a severely compromised pulmonary blood flow and hypoxemic respiratory failure.

Excessive pulmonary flow in the setting of intracardiac shunt or PDA will result in pulmonary edema and decrease lung compliance necessitating an escalation in ventilator support.

Impaired LV diastolic function increases left atrial pressure and can result in pulmonary venous congestion and pulmonary edema. Unfortunately, due to difficulty in noninvasively assessing diastolic function, this problem is often unrecognized.

The close relationship between the cardiovascular and respiratory systems both functionally and anatomically means that these systems interact and influence each other significantly. In the neonates, there are several specific conditions that result in important interactions that can be clinically relevant.

PULMONARY HYPERTENSION

The syndrome of PPHN presenting clinically as an infant with hypoxic respiratory failure out of proportion to the degree of lung abnormality is associated with significant interaction between the lungs and cardiovascular system. It is important to understand that PPHN is a clinical syndrome, not a single entity of raised pulmonary pressures. Early-onset pulmonary hypertension can arise from a variety of clinical conditions, the end result of which is dependent on the relative effect of each of the components. The effect of each component on the respiratory system is also variable. The underlying components of PPHN include lung pathology and VQ mismatch (meconium aspiration, pneumonia), the effect of asphyxia on myocardial function, whether the ductus arteriosus is patent, the relative pressures across the PDA resulting in left to right, right to left, or bidirectional shunt, the PVR, and the systemic vascular resistance. Each of these components has some influence on the respiratory system—some more directly than others. The effect of airspace abnormality causing VQ mismatch is clear and can result in reduced gas exchange with poor oxygenation and carbon dioxide retention, both of which in turn may result in increased PVR. Increased PVR can change the direction of shunting across the PDA depending on what the systemic vascular resistance and blood pressure is, reduce the pulmonary blood flow, and cause right ventricular hypertrophy and dysfunction from increased afterload. Pulmonary blood flow is reduced due to poor RV function and increased afterload from both PVR and lung air space changes, which directly impinge on the patency of pulmonary blood vessels. The iatrogenic effect of mechanical ventilation or increased distending pressure also contributes to this impingement on the pulmonary blood vessels. The effect of reduced pulmonary

blood flow due to multiple underlying causes cascades on to the systemic side of the heart with reduced filling of the LA and subsequently decreased LVO. The reduced LVO may be exacerbated by asphyxial myocardial injury—with up to 70% of asphyxiated infants demonstrating evidence of abnormal cardiac function when cardiac output is measured.[85,86] The reduction in systemic blood flow may then in turn result in reduced systemic blood pressure, which results in more right to left shunting through the PDA. Finally, the ventricular interdependence of the right and left ventricles, which share a septum and fibers and are constrained by the pericardium, can result in further reductions in the LVO due to decreased cavity size and preload from septal bowing away from the right ventricle in the setting of high pulmonary vascular pressures (Fig. 9.3).[87]

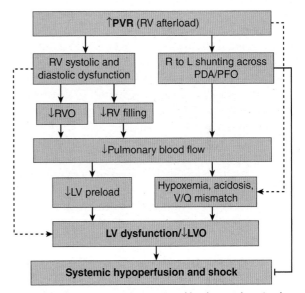

Fig. 9.3 Circulatory changes in neonates with pulmonary hypertension (PPHN) showing the multiple underlying pathophysiologies and the interactions between them, which can lead to a vicious cycle of hypoxemia, V/Q mismatch, and cardiac dysfunction. *LV,* Left ventricular; *LVO,* left ventricular output; *PDA,* patent ductus arteriosus; *PFO,* patent foramen ovale; *PVR,* pulmonary vascular resistance; *R to L,* right to left; *RV,* right ventricular; *RVO,* right ventricular output; *V/Q,* ventilation/perfusion. (Reproduced with permission from McNamara P, Weisz D, Giesinger RE, Jain A. Hemodynamics. In: MacDonald MG, Seshia MK, eds. Avery's Neonatology: Pathophysiology & Management of the Newborn. 7th ed. Philadelphia: Wolters Kluwer; 2016:457-486.)

Acute sequelae of pulmonary hypertension include worsening VQ mismatch, escalation of respiratory support, and detrimental effects on right ventricular function from pressure loading and LVO from reduced preload. This creates an environment of hypoxemia and acidosis, which, due to their pulmonary vasoconstrictive properties, can lead to a cycle of worsening PVR and inflammation. Chronic exposure to hypoxia, hyperoxia, oxidative stress, and inflammation stimulates remodeling of the pulmonary vasculature, resulting in pulmonary vessel narrowing and reduced compliance. As these vascular changes progressively increase the PVR, the pulmonary vascular bed becomes increasingly stiff, right ventricular afterload increases, and function deteriorates. Right ventricular hypertrophy occurs as a compensatory mechanism in order to increase contractility to maintain pulmonary blood flow and coupling to the pulmonary circulation. With time, the high afterload state results in right ventricular dilatation and dysfunction. As PBF and right ventricular performance decline, LVO becomes increasingly compromised. In the presence of an intracardiac shunt, pulmonary-to-systemic flow can help to offload afterload to the right ventricle, but at the expense of exacerbating hypoxemia.

Late-onset pulmonary hypertension can occur due to increased PVR in a subset of infants with bronchopulmonary dysplasia (BPD), from pulmonary overcirculation in persistent unrestrictive systemic-to-pulmonary shunts, or from pulmonary venous congestion due to pulmonary vein stenosis or left heart obstructive lesions. This is a separate entity to early PPHN, which is a disturbance in hemodynamic transition after birth. The pathophysiology underlying pulmonary hypertension in BPD is multifactorial and incompletely delineated but relates to impaired alveolarization, disrupted vascular growth, and abnormal remodeling from smooth muscle proliferation and endothelial dysfunction.[88,89] The presence of pulmonary hypertension substantially worsens chronic respiratory morbidity[90] and overall mortality, with over fourfold increased risk of death in a recent meta-analysis.[91] The interaction between parenchymal and vascular components of neonatal chronic lung disease is discussed further in the "Interaction After Transition and Potential Clinical Implications" section of this chapter. Chronic pulmonary hypertension can result in subclinical pulmonary vascular disease that continues into childhood and early adulthood, with elevated pulmonary arterial pressure and right ventricular dysfunction reported in ex-premature adults.[92]

PATENT DUCTUS ARTERIOSUS

The effect of a PDA on the lung occurs at multiple levels and at differing time points. The initial effect occurs with increasing left to right shunt through a PDA that has failed to constrict fully, usually in the setting of a premature infant. Failure of full constriction in the first few hours in the setting of an infant who has rapidly improving lung compliance results in an increasing left to right shunt through the PDA. The resultant increased pulmonary blood flow has several effects. The first is the physical effect of stiffer lungs, more difficult for the infant to inflate or requiring higher positive pressure if on respiratory support. Premature infants may develop carbon dioxide retention or have increasing apnea and need for respiratory support. Second, the increased blood flow through lung blood vessels and capillaries results in pulmonary venous congestion and fluid leakage into the interstitial tissues. This predisposes infants to additional lung damage and the need for increased respiratory support. Finally, acute increases in pulmonary blood flow can lead to more significant complications including pulmonary hemorrhage (hemorrhagic pulmonary edema)[93] that can cause acute pulmonary injury and clinical deterioration, with a need for high ventilator pressures and eventually long-term pulmonary damage.

The association between PDA and BPD is clear but a causal relationship has not been established. Reduction in the incidence of BPD has not been demonstrated in clinical trials of early treatment to close the PDA. These trials however are problematic in that there were large variations in patient clinical features and a high incidence of open label treatment confounding the results.[94]

A less frequent but important pulmonary complication of PDA, where there is significant lung-heart interaction, is secondary pulmonary hypertension. Prolonged exposure of the pulmonary vasculature to systemic pressures in widely patent PDAs can cause vascular remodeling and ultimately elevated pulmonary arterial pressure.[95] Pulmonary artery vascular changes occur over months to years. Rarely, pulmonary arterial hypertension can become suprasystemic, resulting in Eisenmenger syndrome and reversal of ductal shunting to right to left.

Identification of patients at greatest benefit of ductal closure as well as the optimal treatment regimen and timing of treatment remains contentious and is beyond the scope of this chapter. However, we will consider the impacts of different treatment approaches from the perspective of their cardiorespiratory interactions and effects.

The pulmonary benefits of eliminating systemic to pulmonary ductal shunting include ending excess pulmonary blood flow and subsequent pulmonary edema, improvement in lung compliance, and potential ability to wean ventilatory support and possibly aid recovery in chronic lung disease.[96,97] The respiratory benefits of ductal closure from nonsteroidal anti-inflammatory drugs or paracetamol must be weighed against their safety concerns, including short-term fluid retention and pulmonary edema, variable efficacy, and the risk of unnecessary treatment with possible spontaneous ductal closure. Though surgical ligation enables definitive PDA closure and may improve lung compliance and respiratory support requirement,[98] its long-term benefits in preventing BPD are conflicting. In addition, surgical ligation can cause cardiorespiratory decompensation intraoperatively from open thoracotomy and single lung ventilation and postoperatively in post-ligation cardiac syndrome. Hsu et al. demonstrated that less than 50% of infants undergoing ductal ligation had improvement in respiratory state at 1 week postoperatively, with improvement more likely in high-frequency ventilated neonates.[99] Surgical ligation is increasingly being superseded by percutaneous device closure. This less invasive technique avoids thoracotomy and disruption in gas exchange due to retraction of the left lung. Device closure appears to have a lower incidence of post-ligation cardiac syndrome and faster pulmonary recovery.[100,101] While ductal closure seems physiologically valuable, whether to treat requires consideration of the likelihood of spontaneous closure and the efficacy, safety profiles, and unclear long-term benefits of pharmacological and surgical treatments.

Alternatively, electing to not treat the PDA implies tolerance of systemic to pulmonary shunting, with respiratory sequelae as outlined already. A retrospective study by Schena et al. found that each week with a grade E3 or E4 hemodynamically significant PDA according to McNamara and Sehgal's PDA staging criteria[102] increased the risk of BPD by 70%.[103] While several studies have identified poorer respiratory outcomes and greater risk of BPD with a change in practice toward conservative PDA treatment,[104,105] this association is not consistent. The PDA-TOLERATE trial reported similar rates of BPD with early routine pharmacologic management compared to conservative treatment,[106] though it is worth noting that almost 50% of the conservatively managed neonates received rescue ductal treatment with a cyclooxygenase inhibitor. A secondary analysis of this study found that persistent exposure to a moderate or large PDA was associated with BPD in infants mechanically ventilated for 10 days or longer.[107]

Conservative PDA management focuses on achieving a higher MAP, permissive hypercapnia, fluid restriction, and use of diuretic agents and possibly transfusing toward a higher hematocrit level to limit ductal shunting. Targeting a higher positive end-expiratory pressure of 8 cm compared to 5 cm H_2O was suggested to modestly reduce left-to-right ductal shunting in a small study of mechanically ventilated infants.[61] The mechanism behind this is inducing an elevation in PVR to narrow the transductal pressure gradient between the aorta and pulmonary artery. Similarly, permissive hypercapnia is utilized for its pulmonary vasoconstrictive properties in order to increase the PVR. The purpose of fluid restriction and diuretic use is to limit pulmonary overcirculation and left atrial dilatation through acting directly on pulmonary blood flow volume. The 2014 Cochrane meta-analysis of studies from more than two decades found a reduction in the risk of PDA.[108] However, fluid restriction could negatively impact systemic blood flow when the daily volume administration is below 140 mL/kg. In an observational study of extremely preterm neonates undergoing conservative ductal management with fluid restriction, the mean postnatal day of PDA closure was 53 in infants born at 23 to 24 weeks' gestation, 41 in infants born 25 to 26 weeks' gestation, and 36 in infants born at 27 to 28 weeks' gestation,[109] with 95% of PDAs closing by discharge from hospital. There have been historic concerns that furosemide may in fact promote ductal patency by stimulating renal prostaglandin E_2 production; this is less clear in more recent literature.[110] Pursuing a higher hematocrit has been suggested to increase viscosity and increase the PVR. Most of these practices are extrapolated from animal models or other clinical scenarios and have no or limited evidence for ductal management.[111,112] In addition, there may be inherent harm from these strategies—including barotrauma from aggressive ventilation and poor lung growth and compromised systemic perfusion from diuretics and fluid restriction—as well as harm from exposure to long-term ductal shunting.

ASPHYXIA

The asphyxiated neonate is often in a state of cardiac dysfunction and pulmonary hypertension. The appearance of an asphyxiated infant—pale, tachycardic, with impaired perfusion—suggests cardiovascular compromise and indeed transient myocardial ischemia is commonly associated with asphyxia.[113,114] Myocardial impairment results in respiratory impairment from reduced cardiac output with venous congestion and subsequent respiratory distress.

Hypoxia and acidosis stimulate systemic and pulmonary vasoconstriction in attempt to redirect blood to essential organs, particularly the brain. The elevation in PVR gives rise to acute pulmonary hypertension. As discussed earlier in "Pulmonary Hypertension," this increases afterload to the right ventricle and reduces preload to the left ventricle. In conjunction with ventricular dysfunction from myocardial ischemia, low cardiac output and systemic hypotension can ensue.

Passage of meconium in utero is a common occurrence in fetal distress. Asphyxiated infants at birth may have the added complication of meconium aspiration, which directly causes lung injury through chemical pneumonitis and surfactant inactivation and compounds the risk of PPHN. In addition, both therapeutic hypothermia and seizures may be considered additional insults to the pulmonary vasculature that may worsen pulmonary hypertension. The bradycardia common to therapeutic hypothermia may also reduce cardiac output, though systemic blood pressure is supported by increased systemic vascular tone.

CONGENITAL DIAPHRAGMATIC HERNIA

The pathophysiology of congenital diaphragmatic hernia (CDH) is dominated by the interplay of pulmonary hypoplasia, pulmonary hypertension, and LV dysfunction. Several factors accentuate this interaction, including displacement of the heart due to herniated organs and the need for positive pressure ventilation. Profound

hypoxia can occur from a combination of lung hypoplasia and in utero pulmonary vascular changes which result in raised pulmonary pressures. PPHN, which is expected and can be critical, is exacerbated by postnatal hypoxia and acidosis which stimulate pulmonary vasoconstriction and further reduce pulmonary blood flow.

Pulmonary hypoplasia reduces the surface area available for gas exchange and lung compliance. The disparity in lung volume and functioning parenchyma between the affected and unaffected lungs adds additional complication to the neonate's respiratory state. Aggressive mechanical ventilation is frequently required in response to respiratory failure, despite conventional practice of encouraging permissive hypercapnia. Barotrauma and volutrauma predispose to iatrogenic lung injury to the unaffected "normal" lung that is exposed to high pressure and is often significantly hyperinflated. Ventilation strategies accordingly aim to balance adequate support with protecting and preserving the unaffected lung.

Pulmonary vascular disease is caused by disrupted pulmonary vasculature with pathologic vascular remodeling in utero. The respiratory epithelium is responsible for signaling cascades that regulate endothelial cell growth and development. With abnormal respiratory epithelium in pulmonary hypoplasia, reduction in signaling pathways results in endothelial dysfunction and vascular remodeling.[115] Smooth muscle proliferation results in thickened pulmonary vessels with increased tone and reactivity. Pulmonary vascular changes increase PVR and contribute substantially to pulmonary hypertension postnatally.

Biventricular systolic and diastolic dysfunction can occur in CDH.[116] RV dysfunction is predominantly caused by pressure loading from pulmonary hypertension, whereas the pathophysiology of LV dysfunction is often multifactorial. There is usually a variable degree of LV hypoplasia in infants with CDH.[117] This compounds the deleterious effects of pulmonary hypertension on the left ventricle to worsen cardiac output, but it also can directly exacerbate PPHN by increasing afterload to the lungs and causing pulmonary venous congestion. LV dysfunction complicates decisions around pulmonary vasodilator therapy due to the risk of pulmonary edema.[118] Ventricular dysfunction may be a poor prognostic marker in CDH and has been associated with requirement for extracorporeal membrane oxygenation therapy.[119] Systemic hypotension is commonly seen in this patient population due to decreased venous return, hypoxia, acidosis, and LV dysfunction secondary to abnormal ventricular septal motion. This in turn can exacerbate hypoxemia and reduce pulmonary blood flow further from right-to-left ductal shunting, though in the setting of significant LV dysfunction and poor systemic cardiac output, shunting at the PDA level may have the advantage of supporting systemic blood flow.

CONGENITAL HEART DISEASE

Another potential area where the cardiovascular system interacts with the respiratory system is in infants with congenital heart disease. The physiological effects of positive pressure ventilation on the systemic and pulmonary circulations should be carefully considered. Ductal-dependent cyanotic heart disease presents acutely at the time of ductal closure or earlier if there are signs of desaturation. Disordered blood flow and hypoxia often result in raised pulmonary pressures. Flow to the pulmonary and systemic circulations depends on the cardiac defect and physiology. In the setting of an unbalanced circulation, there is inadequate outflow from one side of the heart with excessive blood flow through the other circulation. Infants who have congenital heart disease that is associated with increased pulmonary blood flow, including severe left heart abnormalities such as hypoplastic left heart syndrome and univentricular physiology, may have pulmonary overcirculation with increased risk of pulmonary edema. This is associated with a reduction in systemic output due to preferential flow into the pulmonary circulation. Clinically, these infants manifest signs of poor systemic perfusion—including weak or absent peripheral pulses, mottling, delayed capillary refill, tachycardia, hypotension, lactic acidosis, and oliguria—as well as evidence of pulmonary overcirculation: respiratory distress, hepatomegaly, and interstitial fluid on chest x-ray. Simplistically, medical management aims to equalize flow through the two circulations with prostaglandin E_1 infusion to augment systemic flow through the PDA, while at the same time employing measures such as use of high PEEP, mechanical ventilation, and diuretic therapy to limit excessive pulmonary blood flow. Maintaining PVR is important to ensure right-to-left ductal shunting. In neonates with inadequate right ventricular outflow due to obstructive right-sided lesions, such as critical Ebstein anomaly or pulmonary stenosis, the focus is on ensuring adequate pulmonary flow to support tissue oxygenation. Titration of prostaglandin dosing is often required in ductal-dependent pulmonary circulations, particularly with postnatal drop in PVR. An important principle of medical management is to create equipoise between the pulmonary and systemic circulations such that there is both acceptable oxygenation by the lungs and systemic output to the tissues.

NEONATAL SEPSIS

The hemodynamic sequelae of sepsis directly impact respiratory function. The pathophysiology of hemodynamic disturbance in sepsis is heterogeneous; it may be dominated by peripheral vasodilatation and "warm" shock, peripheral vasoconstriction, cardiac dysfunction, and low cardiac output, or a combination of these processes. Increasingly this is thought to occur as a continuum with initial distributive "warm" shock progressing to "cold" shock. Systemic vasodilatation results in hypotension from peripheral pooling of blood and poor venous return, unless there is a compensatory increase in cardiac output. This appears to be a common initial hemodynamic response in septic neonates, with multiple observational studies demonstrating high cardiac output states in response to vasoregulatory failure.[120-122] Hypovolemia and low preload will have flow on effects on the volume of pulmonary blood flow, limiting gas exchange in the lungs, as well as on LV systolic performance.[123] As myocardial contractility and maintenance of stroke volume are dependent on adequate coronary perfusion during diastole, tachycardia or low diastolic blood pressure can further exacerbate ventricular dysfunction. As cardiac output falls, vasomotor tone may change from a low to high state, with compensatory systemic vasoconstriction occurring to sustain blood pressure. This may reduce LV systolic function even further from exposure to high afterload. Cardiac dysfunction and inadequate systemic flow or pressure ultimately impairs organ perfusion and oxygen delivery, leading to anaerobic cellular metabolism. This begets acidosis and hypoxia which are potent stimulators for pulmonary vasoconstriction. Pulmonary hypertension caused by a surge in PVR is a well-recognized complication of neonatal sepsis, may cause profound VQ mismatch, and itself can then perpetuate right ventricular failure.[120] A small study found that almost 50% of infants with late onset sepsis had echocardiographic features of pulmonary hypertension (defined as pulmonary artery systolic pressure over 35 mm Hg), compared to no neonates in the age-matched controls.[124]

Apneas are a common manifestation of neonatal sepsis and often necessitate mechanical ventilation. Particularly for premature infants, many of whom have underlying lung disease, reintubation exposes already damaged lungs to volutrauma, barotrauma, atelectrauma, and biotrauma. For many of these infants, lung recovery will be set back and the period of mechanical ventilation may be prolonged before extubation is possible.

In addition, fluid management in sepsis carries additional risk for further respiratory compromise. Fluid resuscitation with crystalloids is frequently first-line treatment for hypotension prior to commencing vasoactive agents. This may well have a place to correct relative intravascular depletion in the clinical picture of peripheral vasodilatation. However, hemodynamic disturbances in sepsis are varied, and in many infants may not involve low systemic vascular resistance. Overzealous intravenous fluid administration can cause fluid overload and pulmonary edema, as well as reduced contractility due to increased end-diastolic ventricular pressure which limits coronary artery perfusion. The 2017 American College of Critical Care Medicine Clinical Practice Parameters for Hemodynamic Support of Pediatric and Neonatal Septic Shock recommends fluid boluses of 10 mL/kg isotonic crystalloid or colloid boluses, up to 40 mL/kg, until improvement in perfusion or presence of hepatomegaly[125] for neonates. However, there is increasing evidence in neonatal, pediatric, and adult sepsis that aggressive fluid resuscitation is harmful.[126,127] Multiple pediatric studies have identified longer duration of mechanical ventilation and higher oxygenation index in the setting of positive fluid balance.[128-130] A large trial of children in Africa with severe infection found 45% higher mortality rate at 48 hours in the groups that received 20 to 40 mL/kg

bolus of either normal saline or albumin compared to control,[131] though generalizability to tertiary neonatal units in developed countries is limited. In separate publications from the AWAKEN study, greater peak fluid balance in both premature and term neonates in the first week of life increased the odds of requiring mechanical ventilation on day 7, while a negative fluid balance at day 7 was protective.[132,133] Clearly, there is a balance to be found for fluid management to restore circulatory volume without causing harm from subsequent fluid overload and pulmonary edema. This balance may be difficult to achieve because in neonates, sepsis is often associated with massive increae in capillary permeability leading to edema and intravascular volume depletion necessitating volume expansion despite positive fluid balance.

Interaction During Early Transition and Potential Clinical Implications

The role of left-to-right PDA shunting in the pathogenesis of BPD and pulmonary hemorrhage was briefly discussed earlier. In this section, we will review the cardiovascular and cerebral hemodynamic effects of surfactant administration and CO_2 alteration in preterm infants.

SURFACTANT

Surfactant administration for respiratory distress syndrome can be associated with significant changes in hemodynamics. Although surfactant may have vasodilatory properties, most of the hemodynamic changes are likely to be due to mechanical effects of the instillation process and rapid improvement in lung compliance and functional residual capacity. As a result, studies have shown variable effects of surfactant on indices of CBF with some showing reduction and others reporting no change or an increase.[134-138] Some of the changes have been attributed to redistribution of blood flow and increase in CO_2.[134,135,137] A recent animal study showed that delivery of surfactant via intubation versus less invasive surfactant administration (LISA) has a more significant effect on cerebral hemodynamics.[139]

The reported effects of surfactant on systemic and pulmonary blood flow are also variable. Animal studies have shown an increase in pulmonary blood flow. Human data on the subject are scarce. In preterm neonates in the delivery room, surfactant administration resulted in an increase in RVO but no change in SVC flow.[140] It is intriguing that despite an increase in ductal diameter in the presence of a completely left to right shunt, an increase in fractional shortening, and an increase in LA to aortic root ratio, the LVO decreased in this study. In more mature preterm infants, rescue surfactant several hours after birth resulted in an increase in SVC flow and RVO but only in those who were considered surfactant-responders defined as having an FiO_2 of 0.21 by 3 hours following surfactant administration.[141] Interestingly, no change in PDA or patent foramen ovale (PFO) flow was noted in this study.

The effect of surfactant on the PDA is of particular interest as the improvement in lung compliance and reduction in PVR can significantly increase left-to-right ductal shunting and theoretically predispose to pulmonary hemorrhage. While animal studies have shown a significant increase in left-to-right ductal shunting after surfactant administration,[142] this has not been demonstrated in humans.[137,140,141] Although there are differences between experimental models and clinical settings, the lack of effect in humans could also be due to difficulty in assessing ductal flow using Doppler techniques.

CARBON DIOXIDE, CEREBRAL BLOOD FLOW, AND BRAIN INJURY

As mentioned earlier, CO_2 values above the normal level are commonly seen in preterm infants. Accepting higher CO_2 allows for use of lower ventilator settings and weaning from respiratory support although this has not been shown to impact development of BPD.[143,144] Furthermore, there are little data on the safety of CO_2 ranges used for permissive hypercapnia.[72]

Changes in CO_2 significantly alter cerebral hemodynamics with hypocapnia reducing and hypercapnia increasing CBF. These changes in CBF could have a significant impact on outcome. Indeed, there is a strong association between high CO_2 and occurrence of periventricular/intraventricular hemorrhage (P/IVH).[145,146] Higher CO_2 has been shown to be an independent predictor of severe P/IVH or death[147] and maximum CO_2 in the first 3 days is a dose-dependent predictor of severe P/IVH.[148] It is postulated that high CO_2 potentiates the reperfusion phase of the ischemia-reperfusion injury that precedes occurrence of P/IVH.[149] Interestingly, the effect of CO_2 on CBF is blunted in the first day. However, by the second postnatal day, the cerebral vasculature becomes very reactive to high CO_2.[150,151] A study showed a breakpoint between middle cerebral artery mean flow velocity, a surrogate for CBF, and CO_2 at about 52 mm Hg with no relationship below and a strong linear relationship above this threshold.[151] A recent study found a 5% increase in cerebral tissue oxygen saturation when CO_2 was higher than 55 mm Hg.[152] Furthermore, high CO_2 not only increases CBF but also, through attenuation of CBF autoregulation, makes the brain more vulnerable to blood pressure swings.[151,153] Both these mechanisms could enhance reperfusion injury.[154] Therefore, permissive hypercapnia above the low 50s in the first few days may put vulnerable extremely premature infants at a higher risk for developing P/IVH. Interestingly, neurodevelopmental follow-up results of an RCT of mild versus high permissive hypercapnia in intubated ELBW infants were not different between the groups.[155] Low CO_2 on the other hand decreases CBF and has been associated with periventricular leukomalacia.[156,157] Unlike permissive hypercapnia, hypocapnia clearly does not confer any benefits in preterm infants and therefore should be avoided. There may be a different effect of hypcapnia on cerebral circulation when the low PCO_2 is the result of normal physiologic compensation for metabolic acidosis and the pH is not alkalotic but this issue has not been adequately studied.

Interaction After Transition and Potential Clinical Implications

Although inappropriate ventilator support and excessive MAP can have similar deleterious effects on cardiovascular function as described earlier, the clinical implications are often less apparent after the transitional period as the preterm infant becomes less vulnerable. In recent years, pulmonary hypertension and RV failure in the setting of BPD have increasingly been recognized. Pathophysiology of the pulmonary hypertension associated with BPD is unclear. It is likely related to lung injury, inflammation, and arrest of pulmonary development associated with BPD, although evidence of pulmonary hypertension has also been reported in preterm infants with seemingly mild or no BPD.[158] The reported prevalence of pulmonary hypertension is variable and depends on the studied population and how pulmonary hypertension was defined on echocardiography. Estimating pressure gradient using tricuspid regurgitation (TR) jet is the most reliable measure of estimating pulmonary pressure using echocardiography. Unfortunately, a TR jet may not be present in up to 25% of cases despite the presence of pulmonary hypertension.[118] Furthermore, estimating pulmonary pressure by assessment of the PDA shunt is often not feasible in patients with BPD, as the ductus is rarely patent. In such cases, qualitative and less reliable markers of pulmonary hypertension such as interventricular septal flattening, RV dilatation, and hypertrophy can be used. It is important to note that even when the TR jet is present, echocardiography may not accurately estimate the severity of pulmonary hypertension.[159] Using the TR jet, the prevalence of pulmonary hypertension after the first month of life was reported to be about 12% among ELBW infants in a prospective observational study.[160] When qualitative indices of pulmonary hypertension were used, the prevalence was about 18%.[160] In retrospective studies, using both quantitative and qualitative echocardiographic indices of pulmonary hypertension, the prevalence 4 weeks after birth was about 8% in all ELBW infants[161] and about 15% in ELBW infants with BPD.[162] A recent prospective study of preterm infants with a birth weight of 500 to 1250 g using both quantitative and qualitative echocardiographic indices of pulmonary hypertension reported a 42% incidence in pulmonary hypertension at 7 days after birth.[158] Interestingly, early pulmonary hypertension was a risk factor for increased severity of BPD and pulmonary hypertension at 36 weeks' postmenstrual age.[158] This suggests that pulmonary vascular disease, independent of BPD, contributes to the development of pulmonary hypertension. Other risk factors for developing pulmonary hypertension in patients with BPD include extreme prematurity, low birth weight, small for gestational age, oligohydramnios, prolonged ventilator support, and PDA ligation.[158,160-164] It is important to screen high-risk preterm infants with BPD, as pulmonary hypertension increases the risk of mortality and poor neurodevelopmental outcome in this population.[158,160,162,165]

Conclusions

Understanding the interaction between the respiratory and cardiovascular systems is important in the management of neonates in the intensive care unit. The impact of respiration on circulatory function and vice versa is most prominently evident at birth and during the early transition. During this period, unsuccessful transition of one system can significantly alter the normal sequence of events in the other system with potential for significant complications. Following the transitional period (first few postnatal days), although the impact of appropriate ventilator settings for the disease condition on the cardiovascular system is small, excessive and inappropriately low ventilator support can severely impair the cardiovascular function and compromise both systemic and pulmonary blood flow. There is an optimal balance between the use of positive pressure ventilation to improve alveolar ventilation and the effects that higher MAP will have on systemic and particularly pulmonary blood flow. As both alveolar oxygenation and systemic blood flow are required for oxygen delivery, this balance must be carefully considered (Fig. 9.4). Finally, we must appreciate that very little is known regarding the effects of different modes of ventilation and common ventilator strategies, such as permissive hypercapnia, on hemodynamics.

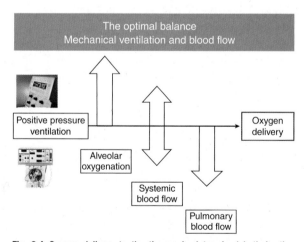

Fig. 9.4 Oxygen delivery to the tissues is determined both by the alveolar ventilation and oxygenation (mainly respiratory contribution) and by the blood flow to those tissues. There is an optimal balance between the use of positive pressure ventilation to improve alveolar ventilation and the effects that higher MAP will have on systemic and particularly pulmonary blood flow. Understanding this balance and particularly the effect of positive pressure on both the respiratory and cardiovascular systems is crucial to good neonatal care. *MAP*, Mean airway pressure. (DeWaal K. 2015, Personal communication)

REFERENCES

1. Rasanen J, Wood DC, Weiner S, et al. Role of the pulmonary circulation in the distribution of human fetal cardiac output during the second half of pregnancy. *Circulation.* 1996;94(5): 1068-1073.
2. Gao Y, Raj JU. Regulation of the pulmonary circulation in the fetus and newborn. *Physiol Rev.* 2010;90(4):1291-1335.
3. Rudolph AM. Fetal and neonatal pulmonary circulation. *Annu Rev Physiol.* 1979;41:383-395.
4. Bhatt S, Polglase GR, Wallace EM, et al. Ventilation before umbilical cord clamping improves the physiological transition at birth. *Front Pediatr.* 2014;2:113.
5. Crossley KJ, Allison BJ, Polglase GR, et al. Dynamic changes in the direction of blood flow through the ductus arteriosus at birth. *J Physiol.* 2009;587(Pt 19):4695-4704.
6. te Pas AB, Davis PG, Hooper SB, et al. From liquid to air: breathing after birth. *J Pediatr.* 2008;152(5):607-611.
7. Hooper SB, Kitchen MJ, Wallace MJ, et al. Imaging lung aeration and lung liquid clearance at birth. *FASEB J.* 2007;21: 3329-3337.
8. Bhatt S, Alison BJ, Wallace EM, et al. Delaying cord clamping until ventilation onset improves cardiovascular function at birth in preterm lambs. *J Physiol.* 2013;591(Pt 8):2113-2126.
9. Linderkamp O. Placental transfusion: determinants and effects. *Clin Perinatol.* 1982;9(3):559-592.
10. Wu TW, Azhibekov T, Seri I. Transitional hemodynamics in preterm neonates: clinical relevance. *Pediatr Neonatol.* 2016; 57(1):7-18.
11. Hooper SB, Binder-Heschl C, Polglase GR, et al. The timing of umbilical cord clamping at birth: physiological considerations. *Matern Health Neonatol Perinatol.* 2016;2:4.
12. Katheria A, Poeltler D, Durham J, et al. Neonatal resuscitation with an intact cord: a randomized clinical trial. *J Pediatr.* 2016; 178:75-80.e73.
13. Katheria AC, Lakshminrusimha S, Rabe H, et al. Placental transfusion: a review. *J Perinatol.* 2017;37:105-111.
14. Farrar D, Airey R, Law GR, et al. Measuring placental transfusion for term births: weighing babies with cord intact. *BJOG.* 2011;118(1):70-75.
15. Aladangady N, McHugh S, Aitchison TC, et al. Infants' blood volume in a controlled trial of placental transfusion at preterm delivery. *Pediatrics.* 2006;117(1):93-98.
16. El-Naggar W, Afifi J, Dorling J, et al. A comparison of strategies for managing the umbilical cord at birth in preterm infants. *J Pediatr.* 2020;225:58-64.e54.
17. Kumbhat N, Eggleston B, Davis AS, et al. Placental transfusion and short-term outcomes among extremely preterm infants. *Arch Dis Child Fetal Neonatal Ed.* 2021;106(1):62-68.
18. Boere I, Roest AA, Wallace E, et al. Umbilical blood flow patterns directly after birth before delayed cord clamping. *Arch Dis Child Fetal Neonatal Ed.* 2015;100(2):F121-F125.
19. Brouwer E, Knol R, Kroushev A, et al. Effect of breathing on venous return during delayed cord clamping: an observational study. *Arch Dis Child Fetal Neonatal Ed.* 2022;107(1):65-69.
20. Badurdeen S, Davis PG, Hooper SB, et al. Physiologically based cord clamping for infants >/=32+0 weeks gestation: a randomised clinical trial and reference percentiles for heart rate and oxygen saturation for infants >/=35+0 weeks gestation. *PLoS Med.* 2022;19(6):e1004029.
21. Murphy MC, McCarthy LK, O'Donnell CPF. Crying and breathing by new-born preterm infants after early or delayed cord clamping. *Arch Dis Child Fetal Neonatal Ed.* 2020;105(3):331-333.
22. Nevill E, Mildenhall LFJ, Meyer MP. Effect of breathing support in very preterm infants not breathing during deferred cord clamping: a randomized controlled trial (The ABC study). *J Pediatr.* 2023;253:94-100.e1.
23. *VentFirst: A Multicenter RCT of Assisted Ventilation During Delayed Cord Clamping for Extremely Preterm Infants.* 2016. Available at: https://clinicaltrials.gov/ct2/show/NCT02742454. Accessed December 6, 2022.
24. *Aeration, Breathing, Clamping Study 3 (ABC3).* 2019. Availale at: https://clinicaltrials.gov/ct2/show/NCT03808051. Accessed December 6, 2022.
25. *Delayed Cord Clamping With Oxygen In Extremely Low Gestation Infants.* 2020. https://clinicaltrials.gov/ct2/show/NCT04413097. Accessed December 6, 2022.
26. Katheria AC, Truong G, Cousins L, et al. Umbilical cord milking versus delayed cord clamping in preterm infants. *Pediatrics.* 2015;136(1):61-69.
27. Katheria A, Blank D, Rich W, et al. Umbilical cord milking improves transition in premature infants at birth. *PloS one.* 2014;9(4):e94085.
28. Katheria AC, Szychowski JM, Essers J, et al. Early cardiac and cerebral hemodynamics with umbilical cord milking compared with delayed cord clamping in infants born preterm. *J Pediatr.* 2020;223:51-56.e1.
29. Kumbhat N, Eggleston B, Davis AS, et al. Umbilical cord milking vs delayed cord clamping and associations with in-hospital outcomes among extremely premature infants. *J Pediatr.* 2021; 232:87-94.e4.
30. Katheria A, Reister F, Essers J, et al. Association of umbilical cord milking vs delayed umbilical cord clamping with death or severe intraventricular hemorrhage among preterm infants. *JAMA.* 2019;322(19):1877-1886.
31. Blank DA, Polglase GR, Kluckow M, et al. Haemodynamic effects of umbilical cord milking in premature sheep during the neonatal transition. *Arch Dis Child Fetal Neonatal Ed.* 2018;103:F539-F546.
32. Atia H, Badawie A, Elsaid O, et al. The hematological impact of umbilical cord milking versus delayed cord clamping in premature neonates: a randomized controlled trial. *BMC pregnancy and childbirth.* 2022;22(1):714.
33. Rabe H, Diaz-Rossello JL, Duley L, et al. Effect of timing of umbilical cord clamping and other strategies to influence placental transfusion at preterm birth on maternal and infant outcomes. *Cochrane Database Syst Rev.* 2019;9(9):CD003248.
34. Feihl F, Broccard AF. Interactions between respiration and systemic hemodynamics. Part II: practical implications in critical care. *Intensive Care Med.* 2009;35(2):198-205.
35. Pinsky MR, Summer WR, Wise RA, et al. Augmentation of cardiac function by elevation of intrathoracic pressure. *J Appl Physiol Respir Environ Exerc Physiol.* 1983;54(4):950-955.
36. Pinsky MR, Summer WR. Cardiac augmentation by phasic high intrathoracic pressure support in man. *Chest.* 1983;84(4): 370-375.
37. Cheifetz IM. Cardiorespiratory interactions: the relationship between mechanical ventilation and hemodynamics. *Respir Care.* 2014;59(12):1937-1945.
38. Lakshminrusimha S, Swartz DD, Gugino SF, et al. Oxygen concentration and pulmonary hemodynamics in newborn lambs with pulmonary hypertension. *Pediatr Res.* 2009;66(5):539-544.
39. Benumof JL. Mechanism of decreased blood flow to atelectatic lung. *J Appl Physiol Respir Environ Exerc Physiol.* 1979;46(6): 1047-1048.

40. Biondi JW, Schulman DS, Soufer R, et al. The effect of incremental positive end-expiratory pressure on right ventricular hemodynamics and ejection fraction. *Anesthesia & Analgesia.* 1988;67:144-151.

41. Dhainaut JF, Devaux JY, Monsallier JF, et al. Mechanisms of decreased left ventricular preload during continuous positive pressure ventilation in ARDS. *Chest.* 1986;90:74-80.

42. Kim BH, Ishida Y, Tsuneoka Y, et al. Effects of spontaneous respiration on right and left ventricular function: evaluation by respiratory and ECG gated radionuclide ventriculography. *J Nucl Med.* 1987;28(2):173-177.

43. Jardin F, Farcot JC, Gueret P, et al. Cyclic changes in arterial pulse during respiratory support. *Circulation.* 1983;68(2):266-274.

44. Marik PE, Cavallazzi R, Vasu T, et al. Dynamic changes in arterial waveform derived variables and fluid responsiveness in mechanically ventilated patients: a systematic review of the literature. *Crit Care Med.* 2009;37(9):2642-2647.

45. Heskamp L, Lansdorp B, Hopman J, et al. Ventilator-induced pulse pressure variation in neonates. *Physiol Rep.* 2016;4(4):e12716.

46. Jain A, McNamara PJ. Persistent pulmonary hypertension of the newborn: Advances in diagnosis and treatment. *Semin Fetal Neonatal Med.* 2015;20(4):262-271.

47. Jain A, Mohamed A, El-Khuffash A, et al. A comprehensive echocardiographic protocol for assessing neonatal right ventricular dimensions and function in the transitional period: normative data and z scores. *J Am Soc Echocardiogr.* 2014;27(12):1293-1304.

48. Hausdorf G, Hellwege HH. Influence of positive end-expiratory pressure on cardiac performance in premature infants: a Doppler-echocardiographic study. *Crit Care Med.* 1987;15:661-664.

49. Trang TT, Tibballs J, Mercier JC, et al. Optimization of oxygen transport in mechanically ventilated newborns using oximetry and pulsed Doppler-derived cardiac output. *Critical Care Medicine.* 1988;16:1094-1097.

50. Maayan C, Eyal F, Mandelberg A, et al. Effect of mechanical ventilation and volume loading on left ventricular performance in premature infants with respiratory distress syndrome. *Crit Care Med.* 1986;14(10):858-860.

51. Gill AB, Weindling AM. Echocardiographic assessment of cardiac function in shocked very low birthweight infants. *Arch Dis Child.* 1993;68:17-21.

52. Takahashi Y, Harada K, Kishkurno S, et al. Postnatal left ventricular contractility in very low birth weight infants. *Pediatr Cardiol.* 1997;18(2):112-117.

53. Lee LA, Kimball TR, Daniels SR, et al. Left ventricular mechanics in the preterm infant and their effect on the measurement of cardiac performance. *J Pediatr.* 1992;120(1):114-119.

54. Teitel DF. Physiologic development of the cardiovascular system in the fetus. In: Polin RA, Fox WW, eds. *Fetal and Neonatal Physiology.* Vol 2nd. Philadelphia: W. B Saunders Company; 1998:827-836.

55. Maroto E, Fouron JC, Teyssier G, et al. Effect of intermittent positive pressure ventilation on diastolic ventricular filling patterns in premature infants. *J Am Coll Cardiol.* 1990;16(1):171-174.

56. Shekerdemian L, Bohn D. Cardiovascular effects of mechanical ventilation. *Arch Dis Child.* 1999;80(5):475-480.

57. Polglase GR, Morley CJ, Crossley KJ, et al. Positive end-expiratory pressure differentially alters pulmonary hemodynamics and oxygenation in ventilated, very premature lambs. *J Appl Physiol.* 2005;99(4):1453-1461.

58. Cheifetz IM, Craig DM, Quick G, et al. Increasing tidal volumes and pulmonary overdistention adversely affect pulmonary vascular mechanics and cardiac output in a pediatric swine model. *Crit Care Med.* 1998;26(4):710-716.

59. Martherus T, Crossley KJ, Rodgers KA, et al. High-CPAP does not impede cardiovascular changes at birth in preterm sheep. *Front Pediatr.* 2020;8:584138.

60. de Waal KA, Evans N, Osborn DA, et al. Cardiorespiratory effects of changes in end expiratory pressure in ventilated newborns. *Arch Dis Child Fetal Neonatal Ed.* 2007;92(6):F444-F448.

61. Fajardo MF, Claure N, Swaminathan S, et al. Effect of positive end-expiratory pressure on ductal shunting and systemic blood flow in preterm infants with patent ductus arteriosus. *Neonatology.* 2014;105(1):9-13.

62. Beker F, Rogerson SR, Hooper SB, et al. The effects of nasal continuous positive airway pressure on cardiac function in premature infants with minimal lung disease: a crossover randomized trial. *J Pediatr.* 2014;164(4):726-729.

63. Zhou H, Hou X, Cheng R, et al. Effects of nasal continuous positive airway pressure on cerebral hemodynamics in preterm infants. *Front Pediatr.* 2020;8:487.

64. Chang HY, Cheng KS, Lung HL, et al. Hemodynamic effects of nasal intermittent positive pressure ventilation in preterm infants. *Medicine (Baltimore).* 2016;95(6):e2780.

65. Mukerji A, Abdul Wahab MG, Razak A, et al. High CPAP vs. NIPPV in preterm neonates - A physiological cross-over study. *J Perinatol.* 2021;41(7):1690-1696.

66. Moritz B, Fritz M, Mann C, et al. Nasal continuous positive airway pressure (n-CPAP) does not change cardiac output in preterm infants. *Am J Perinatol.* 2008;25(2):105-109.

67. Abdel-Hady H, Matter M, Hammad A, et al. Hemodynamic changes during weaning from nasal continuous positive airway pressure. *Pediatrics.* 2008;122(5):e1086-e1090.

68. de Waal K, Evans N, van der Lee J, et al. Effect of lung recruitment on pulmonary, systemic, and ductal blood flow in preterm infants. *J Pediatr.* 2009;154(5):651-655.

69. Schwaberger B, Pichler G, Avian A, et al. Do sustained lung inflations during neonatal resuscitation affect cerebral blood volume in preterm infants? a randomized controlled pilot study. *PLoS one.* 2015;10(9):e0138964.

70. Schmolzer GM, Kumar M, Aziz K, et al. Sustained inflation versus positive pressure ventilation at birth: a systematic review and meta-analysis. *Arch Dis Child Fetal Neonatal Ed.* 2015;100(4):F361-F368.

71. van Kaam AH, De Jaegere AP, Rimensberger PC, et al. Incidence of hypo- and hyper-capnia in a cross-sectional European cohort of ventilated newborn infants. *Arch Dis Child Fetal Neonatal Ed.* 2013;98(4):F323-F326.

72. Wong SK, Chim M, Allen J, et al. Carbon dioxide levels in neonates: what are safe parameters? *Pediatr Res.* 2022;91(5):1049-1056.

73. Miller JD, Carlo WA. Safety and effectiveness of permissive hypercapnia in the preterm infant. *Curr Opin Pediatr.* 2007;19(2):142-144.

74. Orchard CH, Kentish JC. Effects of changes of pH on the contractile function of cardiac muscle. *Am J Physiol.* 1990;258 (6 Pt 1):C967-C981.

75. Weber T, Tschernich H, Sitzwohl C, et al. Tromethamine buffer modifies the depressant effect of permissive hypercapnia on

myocardial contractility in patients with acute respiratory distress syndrome. *Am J Respir Crit Care Med.* 2000;162 (4 Pt 1):1361-1365.

76. Carvalho CR, Barbas CS, Medeiros DM, et al. Temporal hemodynamic effects of permissive hypercapnia associated with ideal PEEP in ARDS. *Am J Respir Crit Care Med.* 1997;156(5):1458-1466.

77. Nakanishi T, Gu H, Momma K. Developmental changes in the effect of acidosis on contraction, intracellular pH, and calcium in the rabbit mesenteric small artery. *Pediatr Res.* 1997;42(6):750-757.

78. Nakanishi T, Gu H, Momma K. Effect of acidosis on contraction, intracellular pH, and calcium in the newborn and adult rabbit aorta. *Heart Vessels.* 1997;12(5):207-215.

79. Nakanishi T, Seguchi M, Tsuchiya T, et al. Effect of acidosis on intracellular pH and calcium concentration in the newborn and adult rabbit myocardium. *Circ Res.* 1990;67(1):111-123.

80. Noori S, Wu TW, Seri I. pH effects on cardiac function and systemic vascular resistance in preterm infants. *J Pediatr.* 2013;162(5):958-963.e1.

81. Nakanishi T, Okuda H, Nakazawa M, et al. Effect of acidosis on contractile function in the newborn rabbit heart. *Pediatr Res.* 1985;19(5):482-488.

82. Fanconi S, Burger R, Ghelfi D, et al. Hemodynamic effects of sodium bicarbonate in critically ill neonates [see comments]. *Intensive Care Med.* 1993;19(2):65-69.

83. Chilakala SK, Parfenova H, Pourcyrous M. The effects of sodium bicarbonate infusion on cerebrovascular function in newborn pigs. *Pediatr Res.* 2022;92(3):729-736.

84. Mintzer JP, Parvez B, Alpan G, et al. Effects of sodium bicarbonate correction of metabolic acidosis on regional tissue oxygenation in very low birth weight neonates. *J Perinatol.* 2015;35(8):601-606.

85. Sehgal A, Wong F, Menahem S. Speckle tracking derived strain in infants with severe perinatal asphyxia: a comparative case control study. *Cardiovasc Ultrasound.* 2013;11:34.

86. Giesinger RE, Bailey LJ, Deshpande P, et al. Hypoxic-ischemic encephalopathy and therapeutic hypothermia: the hemodynamic perspective. *J Pediatr.* 2017;180:22-30.e2.

87. McNamara P, Weisz D, Giesinger RE, Jain A. Hemodynamics. In: MacDonald MG, Seshia MK, eds. *Avery's Neonatology: Pathophysiology & Management of the Newborn.* 7th ed. Philadelphia: Wolters Kluwer; 2016:457-486.

88. Goss K. Long-term pulmonary vascular consequences of perinatal insults. *J Physiol.* 2019;597(4):1175-1184.

89. Malloy KW, Austin ED. Pulmonary hypertension in the child with bronchopulmonary dysplasia. *Pediatr Pulmonol.* 2021; 56(11):3546-3556.

90. Lagatta JM, Hysinger EB, Zaniletti I, et al. The impact of pulmonary hypertension in preterm infants with severe bronchopulmonary dysplasia through 1 year. *J Pediatr.* 2018;203:218-224.e3.

91. Arjaans S, Zwart EAH, Ploegstra MJ, et al. Identification of gaps in the current knowledge on pulmonary hypertension in extremely preterm infants: a systematic review and meta-analysis. *Paediatr Perinat Epidemiol.* 2018;32(3):258-267.

92. Goss KN, Beshish AG, Barton GP, et al. Early pulmonary vascular disease in young adults born preterm. *Am J Respir Crit Care Med.* 2018;198(12):1549-1558.

93. Kluckow M, Evans N. Ductal shunting, high pulmonary blood flow, and pulmonary hemorrhage. *J Pediatr.* 2000;137(1):68-72.

94. Zonnenberg I, de WK. The definition of a haemodynamic significant duct in randomized controlled trials: a systematic literature review. [Review]. *Acta Paediatrica.* 2012;101(3):247-251.

95. Philip R, Nathaniel Johnson J, Naik R, et al. Effect of patent ductus arteriosus on pulmonary vascular disease. *Congenit Heart Dis.* 2019;14(1):37-41.

96. Mirza H, Garcia J, McKinley G, et al. Duration of significant patent ductus arteriosus and bronchopulmonary dysplasia in extremely preterm infants. *J Perinatol.* 2019;39(12):1648-1655.

97. Hamrick SEG, Sallmon H, Rose AT, et al. Patent ductus arteriosus of the preterm infant. *Pediatrics.* 2020;146(5):e20201209.

98. Szymankiewicz M, Hodgman JE, Siassi B, et al. Mechanics of breathing after surgical ligation of patent ductus arteriosus in newborns with respiratory distress syndrome. *Biol Neonate.* 2004;85(1):32-36.

99. Hsu KH, Wong P, Ram Kumar S, et al. Predictors of respiratory improvement 1 week after ligation of patent ductus arteriosus in preterm infants. *J Pediatr.* 2019;205:49-54.e2.

100. Wheeler CR, Vogel ER, Cusano MA, et al. Definitive closure of the patent ductus arteriosus in preterm infants and subsequent short-term respiratory outcomes. *Respir Care.* 2022;67(5):594-606.

101. Rodriguez Ogando A, Planelles Asensio I, de la Blanca ARS, et al. Surgical ligation versus percutaneous closure of patent ductus arteriosus in very low-weight preterm infants: which are the real benefits of the percutaneous approach? *Pediatr Cardiol.* 2018;39(2):398-410.

102. McNamara PJ, Sehgal A. Towards rational management of the patent ductus arteriosus: the need for disease staging. *Arch Dis Child Fetal Neonatal Ed.* 2007;92(6):F424-F427.

103. Schena F, Francescato G, Cappelleri A, et al. Association between hemodynamically significant patent ductus arteriosus and bronchopulmonary dysplasia. *J Pediatr.* 2015;166(6):1488-1492.

104. Relangi D, Somashekar S, Jain D, et al. Changes in patent ductus arteriosus treatment strategy and respiratory outcomes in premature infants. *J Pediatr.* 2021;235:58-62.

105. Liebowitz M, Clyman RI. Prophylactic indomethacin compared with delayed conservative management of the patent ductus arteriosus in extremely preterm infants: effects on neonatal outcomes. *J Pediatr.* 2017;187:119-126.e1.

106. Clyman RI, Liebowitz M, Kaempf J, et al. PDA-TOLERATE Trial: an exploratory randomized controlled trial of treatment of moderate-to-large patent ductus arteriosus at 1 week of age. *J Pediatr.* 2019;205:41-48.e6.

107. Clyman RI, Kaempf J, Liebowitz M, et al. Prolonged tracheal intubation and the association between patent ductus arteriosus and bronchopulmonary dysplasia: a secondary analysis of the PDA-TOLERATE trial. *J Pediatr.* 2021;229:283-288.e2.

108. Bell EF, Acarregui MJ. Restricted versus liberal water intake for preventing morbidity and mortality in preterm infants. *Cochrane Database Syst Rev.* 2014(12):CD000503.

109. Sung SI, Chang YS, Kim J, Choi JH, Ahn SY, Park WS. Natural evolution of ductus arteriosus with noninterventional conservative management in extremely preterm infants born at 23-28 weeks of gestation. *PLoS one.* 2019;14(2):e0212256.

110. Thompson EJ, Greenberg RG, Kumar K, et al. Association between furosemide exposure and patent ductus arteriosus in hospitalized infants of very low birth weight. *J Pediatr.* 2018;199:231-236.

111. De Buyst J, Rakza T, Pennaforte T, Johansson AB, Storme L. Hemodynamic effects of fluid restriction in preterm infants with significant patent ductus arteriosus. *J Pediatr.* 2012;161(3):404-408.

112. Smith A, McNamara PJ, El-Khuffash AF. Non-pharmacological management of a hemodynamically significant patent ductus arteriosus. *Semin Fetal Neonatal Med.* 2018;23(4):245-249.

113. Shah P, Riphagen S, Beyene J, Perlman M. Multiorgan dysfunction in infants with post-asphyxial hypoxic-ischaemic encephalopathy. *Arch Dis Child Fetal Neonatal Ed.* 2004;89(2):F152-F155.

114. Tapia-Rombo CA, Carpio-Hernandez JC, Salazar-Acuna AH, et al. Detection of transitory myocardial ischemia secondary to perinatal asphyxia. *Arch Med Res.* 2000;31(4):377-383.

115. Montalva L, Antounians L, Zani A. Pulmonary hypertension secondary to congenital diaphragmatic hernia: factors and pathways involved in pulmonary vascular remodeling. *Pediatr Res.* 2019;85(6):754-768.

116. Altit G, Bhombal S, Van Meurs K, Tacy TA. Diminished cardiac performance and left ventricular dimensions in neonates with congenital diaphragmatic hernia. *Pediatr Cardiol.* 2018;39(5):993-1000.

117. Kinsella JP, Steinhorn RH, Mullen MP, et al. The Left ventricle in congenital diaphragmatic hernia: implications for the management of pulmonary hypertension. *J Pediatr.* 2018;197:17-22.

118. Abman SH, Hansmann G, Archer SL, et al. Pediatric pulmonary hypertension: guidelines from the American Heart Association and American Thoracic Society. *Circulation.* 2015;132(21):2037-2099.

119. Altit G, Bhombal S, Van Meurs K, Tacy TA. Ventricular performance is associated with need for extracorporeal membrane oxygenation in newborns with congenital diaphragmatic hernia. *J Pediatr.* 2017;191:28-34.e1.

120. Johnston N, de Waal K. Clinical and haemodynamic characteristics of preterm infants with early onset sepsis. *J Paediatr Child Health.* 2022;58(12):2267-2272.

121. Saini SS, Kumar P, Kumar RM. Hemodynamic changes in preterm neonates with septic shock: a prospective observational study*. *Pediatr Crit Care Med.* 2014;15(5):443-450.

122. de Waal KA, Evans N. Hemodynamics in preterm infants with late-onset sepsis. *J Pediatr.* 2010;156(6):918-922.

123. Kharrat A, Jain A. Hemodynamic dysfunction in neonatal sepsis. *Pediatr Res.* 2022;91(2):413-424.

124. Deshpande S, Suryawanshi P, Holkar S, et al. Pulmonary hypertension in late onset neonatal sepsis using functional echocardiography: a prospective study. *J Ultrasound.* 2022;25(2):233-239.

125. Davis AL, Carcillo JA, Aneja RK, et al. The American College of Critical Care Medicine Clinical Practice Parameters for Hemodynamic Support of Pediatric and Neonatal Septic Shock: Executive Summary. *Pediatr Crit Care Med.* 2017;18(9):884-890.

126. Silversides JA, Major E, Ferguson AJ, et al. Conservative fluid management or deresuscitation for patients with sepsis or acute respiratory distress syndrome following the resuscitation phase of critical illness: a systematic review and meta-analysis. *Intensive Care Med.* 2017;43(2):155-170.

127. Wang MP, Jiang L, Zhu B, et al. Association of fluid balance trajectories with clinical outcomes in patients with septic shock: a prospective multicenter cohort study. *Mil Med Res.* 2021;8(1):40.

128. Flori HR, Church G, Liu KD, Gildengorin G, Matthay MA. Positive fluid balance is associated with higher mortality and prolonged mechanical ventilation in pediatric patients with acute lung injury. *Crit Care Res Pract.* 2011;2011:854142.

129. Valentine SL, Sapru A, Higgerson RA, et al. Fluid balance in critically ill children with acute lung injury. *Crit Care Med.* 2012;40(10):2883-2889.

130. Sinitsky L, Walls D, Nadel S, Inwald DP. Fluid overload at 48 hours is associated with respiratory morbidity but not mortality in a general PICU: retrospective cohort study. *Pediatr Crit Care Med.* 2015;16(3):205-209.

131. Maitland K, Kiguli S, Opoka RO, et al. Mortality after fluid bolus in African children with severe infection. *N Engl J Med.* 2011;364(26):2483-2495.

132. Selewski DT, Akcan-Arikan A, Bonachea EM, et al. The impact of fluid balance on outcomes in critically ill near-term/term neonates: a report from the AWAKEN study group. *Pediatr Res.* 2019;85(1):79-85.

133. Selewski DT, Gist KM, Nathan AT, et al. The impact of fluid balance on outcomes in premature neonates: a report from the AWAKEN study group. *Pediatr Res.* 2020;87(3):550-557.

134. Schipper JA, Mohammad GI, van Straaten HL, Koppe JG. The impact of surfactant replacement therapy on cerebral and systemic circulation and lung function. *Eur J Pediatr.* 1997;156(3):224-227.

135. Nuntnarumit P, Bada HS, Yang W, Korones SB. Cerebral blood flow velocity changes after bovine natural surfactant instillation. *J Perinatol.* 2000;20(4):240-243.

136. Kaiser JR, Gauss CH, Williams DK. Surfactant administration acutely affects cerebral and systemic hemodynamics and gas exchange in very-low-birth-weight infants. *J Pediatr.* 2004;144(6):809-814.

137. Saliba E, Nashashibi M, Vaillant MC, Nasr C, Laugier J. Instillation rate effects of exosurf on cerebral and cardiovascular haemodynamics in preterm neonates. *Arch Dis Child Fetal Neonatal Ed.* 1994;71(3):F174-F178.

138. Roll C, Knief J, Horsch S, Hanssler L. Effect of surfactant administration on cerebral haemodynamics and oxygenation in premature infants—a near infrared spectroscopy study. *Neuropediatrics.* 2000;31(1):16-23.

139. Rey-Santano C, Mielgo VE, Gomez-Solaetxe MA, Salomone F, Gastiasoro E, Loureiro B. Cerebral oxygenation associated with INSURE versus LISA procedures in surfactant-deficient newborn piglet RDS model. *Pediatr Pulmonol.* 2019;54(5):644-654.

140. Sehgal A, Mak W, Dunn M, et al. Haemodynamic changes after delivery room surfactant administration to very low birth weight infants. *Arch Dis Child Fetal Neonatal Ed.* 2010;95(5):F345-F351.

141. Katheria AC, Leone TA. Changes in hemodynamics after rescue surfactant administration. *J Perinatol.* 2013;33(7):525-528.

142. Clyman RI, Jobe A, Heymann M, et al. Increased shunt through the patent ductus arteriosus after surfactant replacement therapy. *J Pediatr.* 1982;100(1):101-107.

143. Carlo WA, Stark AR, Wright LL, et al. Minimal ventilation to prevent bronchopulmonary dysplasia in extremely-low-birth-weight infants. *J Pediatr.* 2002;141(3):370-374.

144. Thome UH, Genzel-Boroviczeny O, Bohnhorst B, et al. Permissive hypercapnia in extremely low birthweight infants (PHELBI): a randomised controlled multicentre trial. *Lancet Respir Med.* 2015;3(7):534-543.

145. Fabres J, Carlo WA, Phillips V, Howard G, Ambalavanan N. Both extremes of arterial carbon dioxide pressure and the magnitude of fluctuations in arterial carbon dioxide pressure are

associated with severe intraventricular hemorrhage in preterm infants. *Pediatrics*. 2007;119(2):299-305.

146. McKee LA, Fabres J, Howard G, Peralta-Carcelen M, Carlo WA, Ambalavanan N. PaCO2 and neurodevelopment in extremely low birth weight infants. *J Pediatr*. 2009;155(2):217-221.e1.

147. Ambalavanan N, Carlo WA, Wrage LA, et al. PaCO2 in surfactant, positive pressure, and oxygenation randomised trial (SUPPORT). *Arch Dis Child Fetal Neonatal Ed*. 2015;100(2):F145-F149.

148. Kaiser JR, Gauss CH, Pont MM, Williams DK. Hypercapnia during the first 3 days of life is associated with severe intraventricular hemorrhage in very low birth weight infants. *J Perinatol*. 2006;26(5):279-285.

149. Noori S, McCoy M, Anderson MP, Ramji F, Seri I. Changes in cardiac function and cerebral blood flow in relation to peri/intraventricular hemorrhage in extremely preterm infants. *J Pediatr*. 2014;164(2):264-270.e1-e3.

150. Pryds O, Greisen G, Lou H, Friis HB. Heterogeneity of cerebral vasoreactivity in preterm infants supported by mechanical ventilation. *J Pediatr*. 1989;115(4):638-645.

151. Noori S, Anderson M, Soleymani S, Seri I. Effect of carbon dioxide on cerebral blood flow velocity in preterm infants during postnatal transition. *Acta Paediatr*. 2014;103(8):e334-e339.

152. Hoffman SB, Lakhani A, Viscardi RM. The association between carbon dioxide, cerebral blood flow, and autoregulation in the premature infant. *J Perinatol*. 2021;41(2):324-329.

153. Kaiser JR, Gauss CH, Williams DK. The effects of hypercapnia on cerebral autoregulation in ventilated very low birth weight infants. *Pediatr Res*. 2005;58(5):931-935.

154. Noori S, Seri I. Hemodynamic antecedents of peri/intraventricular hemorrhage in very preterm neonates. *Semin Fetal Neonatal Med*. 2015;20(4):232-237.

155. Thome UH, Genzel-Boroviczeny O, Bohnhorst B, et al. Neurodevelopmental outcomes of extremely low birthweight infants randomised to different PCO2 targets: the PHELBI follow-up study. *Arch Dis Child Fetal Neonatal Ed*. 2017;102(5):F376-F382.

156. Wiswell TE, Graziani LJ, Kornhauser MS, et al. Effects of hypocarbia on the development of cystic periventricular leukomalacia in premature infants treated with high-frequency jet ventilation. *Pediatrics*. 1996;98(5):918-924.

157. Shankaran S, Langer JC, Kazzi SN, et al. Cumulative index of exposure to hypocarbia and hyperoxia as risk factors for periventricular leukomalacia in low birth weight infants. *Pediatrics*. 2006;118(4):1654-1659.

158. Mourani PM, Sontag MK, Younoszai A, et al. Early pulmonary vascular disease in preterm infants at risk for bronchopulmonary dysplasia. *Am J Respir Crit Care Med*. 2015;191(1):87-95.

159. Mourani PM, Sontag MK, Younoszai A, et al. Clinical utility of echocardiography for the diagnosis and management of pulmonary vascular disease in young children with chronic lung disease. *Pediatrics*. 2008;121(2):317-325.

160. Bhat R, Salas AA, Foster C, et al. Prospective analysis of pulmonary hypertension in extremely low birth weight infants. *Pediatrics*. 2012;129(3):e682-e689.

161. Collaco JM, Dadlani GH, Nies MK, et al. Risk factors and clinical outcomes in preterm infants with pulmonary hypertension. *PloS One*. 2016;11(10):e0163904.

162. Slaughter JL, Pakrashi T, Jones DE, et al. Echocardiographic detection of pulmonary hypertension in extremely low birth weight infants with bronchopulmonary dysplasia requiring prolonged positive pressure ventilation. *J Perinatol*. 2011;31(10):635-640.

163. Kim DH, Kim HS, Choi CW, et al. Risk factors for pulmonary artery hypertension in preterm infants with moderate or severe bronchopulmonary dysplasia. *Neonatology*. 2012;101(1):40-46.

164. Check J, Gotteiner N, Liu X, et al. Fetal growth restriction and pulmonary hypertension in premature infants with bronchopulmonary dysplasia. *J Perinatol*. 2013;33(7):553-557.

165. Nakanishi H, Uchiyama A, Kusuda S. Impact of pulmonary hypertension on neurodevelopmental outcome in preterm infants with bronchopulmonary dysplasia: a cohort study. *J Perinatol*. 2016;36(10):890-896.

Ventilator Strategies to Reduce Lung Injury and Duration of Mechanical Ventilation

Martin Keszler and Nelson Claure

Chapter Outline

Introduction
Ventilator-Associated Lung Injury
How Can We Reduce Vali?
Delivery Room Stabilization
Noninvasive Respiratory Support
Strategies of Mechanical Ventilation
Basic Modes of Synchronized Ventilation
Synchronized Intermittent Mandatory Ventilation
Assist Control

Pressure Support Ventilation
Choice of Assisted Ventilation Modes
Volume-Targeted Ventilation
Importance of the Open Lung Strategy
High-frequency Ventilation
    Proportional Assist Ventilation
    Neurally Adjusted Ventilatory Assist
Evidence-Based Approach to Mechanical Ventilation

Key Points

- The immature lungs of extremely preterm infants are susceptible to damage from a variety of factors that are potentially modifiable by the use of lung-protective strategies of respiratory support.
- Avoidance of mechanical ventilation (MV), optimal delivery room stabilization, and early use of noninvasive respiratory support are important elements in minimizing lung injury.
- When MV is needed, it should be employed with care and attention to individual patient's specific pathophysiology and with a goal of extubation at the earliest opportunity.
- Recruitment and maintenance of optimal lung volume is a key element in any lung-protective ventilation strategy, including both conventional and high-frequency ventilation.
- Volume-targeted ventilation maintains more stable tidal volume and minute ventilation, shortens the duration of MV, and is associated with a decrease in both lung and brain injury.

Introduction

Despite appropriate emphasis on noninvasive respiratory support when feasible, mechanical ventilation (MV) remains a mainstay of therapy in many extremely preterm infants.[1-3] Although frequently life-saving, invasive MV has many untoward effects on the brain and the lungs, especially in the most immature infants.[1] The endotracheal tube (ETT) acts as a foreign body, quickly becoming colonized with nosocomial organisms and acting as a portal of entry for pathogens, potentially leading to ventilator-associated pneumonia and late-onset sepsis.[4] For these reasons, avoidance of MV in favor of noninvasive respiratory support is considered one of the most important steps in preventing neonatal morbidity. When MV is required, the goal is to wean the patient from invasive ventilation as soon as feasible in order to minimize ventilator-associated lung injury (VALI). While VALI is a key element in the pathogenesis of bronchopulmonary dysplasia (BPD), many other factors play an important role in its pathogenesis, including the intrauterine environment (inflammation and infection), postnatal infection, oxidative stress, impaired intrauterine and postnatal nutrition, and excessive fluid administration. The long-accepted causative role of patent ductus arteriosus (PDA) has more recently been brought into question.[5] While there is clearly an association between PDA and BPD, there is no clear evidence that medical or surgical closure of the ductus reduces the incidence of BPD, other complication of prematurity, or that it shortens the duration of MV.

Ventilator-Associated Lung Injury

Many terms have been used to describe the mechanism of injury in VALI. *Barotrauma* refers to damage caused by inflation pressure. The conviction that pressure is the major determinant of lung injury has caused clinicians to focus on limiting inflation pressure, often to the point of precluding adequate support. However, available evidence indicates that high inflation pressure by itself, without correspondingly high tidal volume (V_T), does not result in lung injury. Rather, injury related to high inflation pressure is mediated through tissue stretch resulting from excessive V_T or from regional overdistention when ventilating lungs with extensive atelectasis results in maldistribution of the tidal volume.[6] Dreyfuss and colleagues demonstrated more than 30 years ago that severe acute lung injury occurred in small animals ventilated with large V_T, regardless of whether that volume was generated by positive or negative pressure.[7] In contrast, animals exposed to the same high inflation pressure but with an elastic bandage over the chest and abdomen to limit chest wall excursion and thus V_T had much less evidence of lung injury. Similarly, Hernandez et al. demonstrated that animals exposed to pressure as high as 45 cm H_2O did not show evidence of acute lung injury when their chest and abdomen were enclosed in a plaster cast.[8] *Volutrauma* refers to injury caused by overdistention and excessive stretch of tissues, which leads to disruption of alveolar and small airway

epithelium resulting in acute edema, outpouring of protein-rich exudate that inactivates surfactant, and release of proteases, cytokines, and chemokines. This in turn leads to activation of macrophages and invasion of activated neutrophils. Collectively, this latter process is referred to as *biotrauma*. Another important concept is that of *atelectrauma* or lung damage caused by tidal ventilation in the presence of atelectasis.[9] Atelectrauma causes lung injury via several mechanisms. The portion of the lungs that remains atelectatic experiences increased surfactant turnover and has high critical opening pressure. There are shear forces at the boundary between the aerated and atelectatic parts of the lung, leading to structural tissue damage. Ventilation of injured lungs using inadequate end-expiratory pressure results in repeated alveolar collapse and expansion and rapidly injures the immature lungs. Perhaps most importantly, when a portion of the lungs is atelectatic, any gas entering the lungs will preferentially distend the aerated portion of the lung, which is more compliant than the atelectatic lung with its high critical opening pressure. This fact is evident from Laplace's law (pressure = $2 \times$ surface tension/radius) and corroborated by experimental evidence, showing that the most injured portion of the lung was the aerated nondependent lung.[6] This maldistribution of V_T leads to overdistention of that portion of the lungs and regional volutrauma. Thus, VALI is initiated by some form of biophysical injury, which in turn triggers a release of proinflammatory mediators from activated leukocytes leading to biotrauma and initiates the complex cascade of lung injury and eventual repair. A schematic representation of the cycle of VALI is illustrated in Fig. 10.1.

How Can We Reduce Vali?

As is evident from the prior discussion, the process of lung damage from MV is multifactorial and cannot be linked to any single variable. Consequently, any approach to reducing lung injury and minimizing the length of MV must be comprehensive and begin with the initial stabilization of the infant in the delivery room. Because some degree of impairment of normal pulmonary development (i.e., arrest of alveolarization) is probably inevitable when an extremely preterm fetus is suddenly thrust into what by fetal standards is a very hyperoxic environment and must initiate air breathing with lungs that are incompletely developed, it is unlikely

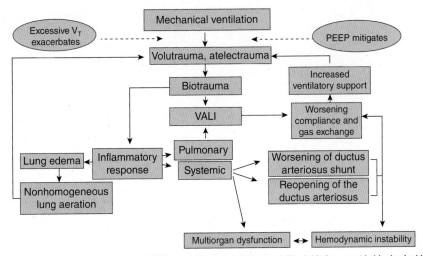

Fig. 10.1 The cycle of ventilator-associated lung injury *(VALI)* is complex and multifactorial. The initiating event is biophysical injury from excessive tissue stretch, which in turn leads to biotrauma and initiates the cascade of lung injury and repair. Both systemic and pulmonary inflammatory responses become operative and lead to secondary adverse effects that in turn worsen pulmonary status, leading to a need for escalating ventilatory settings, which in turn cause more injury. *PEEP,* Positive end-expiratory pressure.

that improved respiratory support can completely prevent impairment of lung structure and function. However, optimal respiratory and general supportive care can minimize the superimposition of VALI on this developmental arrest and together with optimal nutrition can facilitate lung growth and repair.

Delivery Room Stabilization

The time immediately after birth when air breathing is initiated in structurally immature surfactant deficient lungs is known to be a critical time during which the process of lung injury and subsequent repair may be triggered in a matter of minutes. Moments after birth, the newborn infant must rapidly clear lung fluid from the airways and terminal air spaces, aerate their lungs, and sustain a functional residual capacity (FRC), thus facilitating a dramatic increase in pulmonary blood flow. Vigorous full-term infants achieve this critical transition quickly and effectively,[10] but this is a much greater challenge for the very preterm infants who may be unable to generate sufficient critical opening pressure to achieve adequate lung inflation because of their limited muscle strength, excessively compliant chest wall, limited surfactant pool, and incomplete lung development. The excessively compliant chest wall of the preterm infant fails to sustain the lung

aeration that may have been achieved spontaneously or with positive pressure ventilation. For the same reasons, these infants may be unable to generate sufficient negative intrathoracic pressure to effectively move lung fluid from the air spaces to the interstitium, lymphatics, and veins. Subsequent tidal breathing, both spontaneous and that generated by positive pressure ventilation, occurs in lungs that are still partially fluid-filled and incompletely expanded. This situation leads to maldistribution of tidal volume to a fraction of the preterm lung, a phenomenon that can generate excessive tissue stretch even when a tidal volume generally thought to be safe is used.

The use of positive end-expiratory pressure (PEEP) and/or continuous positive airway pressure (CPAP) during the initial stabilization of preterm infants compensates for the excessively compliant chest wall and surfactant deficiency by stabilizing alveoli during the expiratory phase and has been shown to facilitate establishment of FRC.[11] Both NRP and ILCOR guidelines give a qualified endorsement to the use of PEEP/CPAP, but cite lack of high-quality randomized controlled trials (RCTs) to make a stronger recommendation.[12] However, the physiologic rationale and experimental evidence from preclinical studies is so persuasive that this practice has become the de facto standard of care in much of the developed world and thus an RCT would be very difficult to undertake. Although there are no data on the optimal end-expiratory pressure level to maintain FRC without inducing lung injury, there is a strong rationale for continuous application of the end-expiratory pressure and avoidance of any disconnection that results in loss of FRC. Provision of the usual level of end-expiratory pressure alone may not sufficiently address the inadequate muscle strength of the preterm infant or help clear lung fluid rapidly enough to avoid regional volutrauma and atelectrauma. Owing to the much greater viscosity of liquid compared to air, resistance to moving liquid through small airways is much greater than that for air, making the time constants required to move fluid through the airways much longer. These considerations support the concept that a prolonged (AKA "sustained") inflation applied soon after birth should be more effective in clearing lung fluid in the first minutes of life than the typical short inflations used during positive pressure ventilation. It has been proposed that rapid and effective lung recruitment that results in even distribution of V_T immediately after birth should reduce VALI. Early evidence supported the theoretical advantages of sustained inflation in preterm infants,[11,13] but the potential for harm from overdistention was also evident.[14] Subsequent studies did not offer evidence that sustained inflation reduces VALI.[15-17] The largest RCT to date failed to substantiate any benefit of sustained inflation in the most vulnerable infants < 27 weeks' gestation and was terminated early because of an increase in early neonatal mortality in the intervention arm.[18] A subsequent meta-analysis concluded that there is no evidence to support the routine use of sustained inflation in the care of extremely low-birth-weight (ELBW) infants.[19] A novel approach to the effort to facilitate uniform lung expansion soon after birth in preterm infants is being tested in a large multicenter trial, which compares the use of standard static PEEP to a titrated PEEP strategy that seeks to tailor the level of distending pressure to each infant's need based on initial response (Australian New Zealand Clinical Trials Registry ACTRN12618001686291).

Noninvasive Respiratory Support

Avoiding MV reduces iatrogenic lung injury, though the magnitude of this benefit is much more modest than early cohort comparisons of CPAP versus MV suggested.[20] A meta-analysis of four large trials that enrolled nearly 2800 preterm infants[21-24] showed that BPD rates alone were not significantly different between infants randomized to MV and those assigned to nasal CPAP (32.4% vs. 34.0%).[25] However, the more important combined outcome of death or BPD (death and BPD are competing outcomes) showed a nearly 10% reduction (RR, 0.91; 95% CI, 0.84–0.99) with a number needed to treat of 25. There was also a significant decrease in the duration of MV and a trend toward shorter duration of supplemental oxygen with early CPAP in two of the trials.[21,22]

Nasal intermittent positive-pressure ventilation (NIPPV), if delivered effectively, may be able to augment an immature infant's inadequate respiratory effort without the complications associated with endotracheal intubation.[26] This approach has the benefit of avoiding the use of an ETT, thus reducing the incidence of VALI and ventilator-associated pneumonia, and avoiding the contribution of postnatal inflammatory response to the development of BPD.[27] A meta-analysis of several small single-center studies concluded that NIPPV was superior to CPAP in preventing extubation failure, especially when NIPPV was synchronized with the infant's respiratory effort,[28] but a subsequent large multinational randomized trial in ELBW infants failed to show any benefits with no reduction in BPD, mortality, or the combined outcome.[29] Current evidence suggests that unsynchronized NIPPV rarely generates a measurable tidal volume,[30] likely because the vocal cords are closed except when the infant is actively breathing in. The cyclic inflation, however, does result in a higher mean airway pressure and it is likely that this higher distending pressure accounts for some of the observed benefits of NIPPV (primarily in reducing postextubation failure) in the most recent Cochrane Review.[31] Buzzella et al. demonstrated that the use of higher, as opposed to lower CPAP level following extubation significantly reduced CPAP failure, providing the explanation for the apparent superiority of NIPPV over CPAP.[32] Studies are underway to test the hypothesis that CPAP and NIPPV are equivalent when used at the same mean airway pressure. Nasal high-frequency oscillatory ventilation (HFOV) has also been explored by several groups, but as of this writing, the suggestion of efficacy is only based on case reports and small series.[33-35] Noninvasive neurally adjusted ventilatory assist (NIV-NAVA) uses the electrical activity of the diaphragm (EAdi) to trigger ventilator inflations and is thus not affected by leakage of a noninvasive interface; it may thus be the best tool to deliver noninvasive ventilation in small preterm infants.[36] However, definitive studies are still lacking.

Strategies of Mechanical Ventilation

The goal of MV is to maintain acceptable gas exchange with a minimum of adverse effects and to wean from invasive support as expeditiously as possible. There are many devices and modes of ventilation to choose from with limited high-quality evidence to guide the clinician's choice. Because of the wide range of clinical conditions, weights, and gestational ages of neonatal patients, there are no simple rules regarding indications for intubation and initiation of MV. "Standard" indications for intubation and arbitrary initial ventilator settings that are often recommended in texts on this subject have limited utility. Instead, choice of modalities of support and ventilation strategies should be guided by the specific underlying pathophysiologic considerations. Ventilators are nothing but tools in our hands that we need to employ thoughtfully in order to optimize outcomes.

Basic Modes of Synchronized Ventilation

Despite relative paucity of high-quality evidence, the question is no longer whether to use synchronized versus unsynchronized ventilation, but rather which modality of synchronization is best. Synchronization of ventilator inflations with the infant's spontaneous breaths allows the clinician to avoid or minimize sedation/muscle relaxation and to maximally utilize the patient's own spontaneous respiratory effort. Encouraging spontaneous breathing during MV has clear advantages, but it makes managing MV more challenging for the clinician. Optimal use of assisted ventilation requires a clear understanding of the complex interaction between the awake, spontaneously breathing infant, and the various modalities of synchronized ventilation. Appreciation of the additive nature of the patient's inspiratory effort and the positive pressure

generated by the ventilator is key to understanding these interactions. The transpulmonary pressure, the sum of the negative inspiratory effort of the infant, and the positive inflation pressure from the ventilator determines the magnitude of the tidal volume. Because in a preterm infant, the spontaneous effort is often sporadic and highly variable, the resulting transpulmonary pressure and V_T typically fluctuate.

In the following paragraphs, we will briefly review the common modes of synchronized ventilation, the important advantages of volume-targeted ventilation (VTV), and the importance of optimizing lung inflation.

Synchronized Intermittent Mandatory Ventilation

Synchronized intermittent mandatory ventilation (SIMV) is a basic synchronized mode that provides a user-selected number of inflations in synchrony with the infant's breathing. If no spontaneous effort is detected during a trigger window, a mandatory inflation is delivered. Spontaneous breaths in excess of the set ventilator rate receive no support. SIMV allows the operator to control the ventilator rate as well as inflation pressure and PEEP. Weaning is accomplished by gradual lowering of both rate and inflation pressure. In small preterm infants, SIMV results in uneven tidal volumes and high work of breathing because of the high airway resistance of the narrow ETT, limited muscle strength, and mechanical disadvantage of the infant's excessively compliant chest wall. SIMV alone thus is not the optimal mode in this population, but the key shortcomings can be mitigated by the addition of pressure support to the spontaneous breaths of the infant (see below).

Assist Control

In neonatal applications, assist control (AC) is a time-cycled, pressure-controlled mode that supports every spontaneous breath, thus resulting in a smaller and more uniform V_T and lower work of breathing than SIMV. The goal is to have the infant and the ventilator work together with every breath, resulting in lower ventilator pressure and less hemodynamic impairment. A backup ventilator rate provides a minimum rate in case of apnea and should be set just below the infant's spontaneous rate, usually at 40 inflations per minute in a preterm infant. A backup rate that is too low will result in excessive fluctuations in minute ventilation and oxygen saturations during periods of apnea. Because the infant controls the ventilator rate, gradual withdrawal of support is accomplished by lowering the peak inflation pressure (PIP), reducing the support given to each breath, and thus encouraging the infant to gradually take over the work of breathing. Depending on the device used, some vigilance may be necessary to avoid autotriggering. Because ventilators do not commonly have a user-set upper limit to the cycling frequency, there is a risk of hyperventilation due to autotriggering. This is seldom a problem when specialty neonatal ventilators with effective leak adaptation are used, but even with those devices, water condensation in the expiratory limb can cause autotriggering.

Pressure Support Ventilation

Pressure support ventilation (PSV) functions differently in adult and neonatal ventilators, a situation that may cause confusion. In specialty neonatal ventilators, PSV is a pressure-controlled mode that supports every spontaneous breath just like AC but is flow-cycled. Flow cycling means that inflation is terminated when inspiratory flow declines to a preset threshold (usually 5%–20% of peak flow) eliminating inspiratory hold (prolonged inflation time) and thus providing more complete synchrony. Avoiding prolonged inflation time is thought to result in less fluctuation in intrathoracic and intracranial pressure that is a consequence of infants exhaling during inspiratory hold. Additionally, PSV automatically adjusts inspiratory time (T_I) in response to the changing lung mechanics of the patient and is able to deliver a longer inspiratory time when the infant sighs. Changing from time-cycled AC to PSV typically results in a shorter T_I and therefore lower mean airway pressure (P_{AW}); adjustment to PEEP may thus be needed to maintain P_{AW} and avoid atelectasis. A substantial leak around the ETT may affect flow cycling. To prevent excessive inspiratory time during PSV, the inspiratory time limit must be set appropriately. Similar to AC, the risk of autotriggering is also present during PSV, especially when universal ventilators not specifically designed for neonates with uncuffed ETTs are used.

As with AC, a backup rate will maintain a minimum inflation rate. In most devices, PSV can also be used to support spontaneous breathing between low-rate SIMV, in order to overcome the problems associated with inadequate spontaneous respiratory effort, and high ETT resistance (SIMV+PS), or in a fully spontaneous mode (CPAP+PS). When used with SIMV or with CPAP, PSV does not provide a backup mandatory rate, so a reliable spontaneous respiratory effort is required. There is no sound evidence base for choosing the level of pressure support, which is typically ordered as X cm H_2O above PEEP. The recommendation that PIP should be two-thirds of the SIMV PIP advocated by some is not evidence-based. Because the purpose of PS is to allow the infant's spontaneous effort to generate an adequate tidal volume, there is no one level of PS that is appropriate for all patients. PS level should be adjusted to achieve a tidal volume of at least 4 mL/kg in order to avoid excessive dead space rebreathing. Weaning from PSV when it is used as a primary mode is accomplished in the same way as for AC. When used in conjunction with SIMV, both the SIMV inflation rate and PIP should be lowered, leaving the infant increasingly breathing spontaneously with only a modest level of PS, at which point extubation should be attempted.

Choice of Assisted Ventilation Modes

To date, only three small randomized trials compared AC versus SIMV. These trials did not show clear advantages of one mode over the other in regards to weaning and duration of MV, though a recent meta-analysis by Greenough et al. found a strong trend favoring AC with a shorter duration of weaning (mean difference −42.4 hours, 95% CI −94.35 to 9.60).[37-39] In the absence of large randomized trials to provide the necessary evidence base, the choice between AC and SIMV, the two most widely used modalities of synchronized ventilation remains a matter of training, personal preference, or habit. Physiologic considerations and short-term studies indicate that modes that support every spontaneous breath are preferable in small preterm infants breathing through narrow ETTs. Documented benefits of AC over SIMV include smaller and less variable V_T, less tachypnea, more rapid weaning from MV, and smaller fluctuations in blood pressure.[37,40,41] A recent study showed that even when combined with PS, SIMV resulted in higher work of breathing than AC.[42] Despite indications that SIMV does not provide optimal support in extremely low gestational age newborns, many clinicians continue to use it both in the acute phase of illness and during weaning from MV,[43] based on the common assumption that both rate and pressure must be weaned prior to extubation. Preference for the lower inflation rate of SIMV appears to be based on the superficially plausible assumption that a smaller number of inflations are inherently less damaging. This concept ignores the fact that the slower ventilator rate is accomplished at the expense of a larger V_T,[40] a variable that is clearly more injurious than ventilator rate (e.g., consider high-frequency ventilation [HFV]), and is contradicted by available evidence from both preclinical and clinical studies.[44,45] Many clinicians also mistakenly believe that assisting every breath precludes respiratory muscle training. This concern fails to recognize that the infant contributes an increasing amount of inspiratory effort to the transpulmonary pressure during weaning. As the ventilator inflation pressure is decreased, the infant progressively takes over a greater proportion of the work resulting in effective training of the respiratory muscles. As weaning progresses, the inflation pressure is decreased to the point when it only overcomes the added resistance of the ETT and circuit, at which point the infant can be extubated. As previously stated, the shortcomings of SIMV can be mitigated by the addition of PS and most clinicians now use SIMV in this way. However, this is a more complicated modality of support with the only apparent advantage being the greater comfort level of many clinicians with SIMV.

Volume-Targeted Ventilation

Pressure-controlled ventilation became the standard approach to MV in newborn infants because early attempts at volume-controlled ventilation using equipment available at the time in infants with uncuffed ETT were disappointing. Pressure-controlled ventilation remains the dominant mode of ventilation in the NICU because of its simplicity, ability to ventilate despite a large ETT leak, and improved intrapulmonary gas distribution due to a decelerating gas flow pattern.[46,47] The

fear of pressure as the major culprit in lung injury is deeply ingrained and many clinicians continue to believe that directly controlling PIP is important, despite unequivocal evidence that volume, not pressure is the key element in VALI.[48,49] The danger of using pressure control is that V_T is not directly controlled and changes when compliance of the respiratory system is altered. Consequently, minute ventilation may change substantially without any adjustment of ventilator settings with lung volume recruitment or surfactant administration, resulting in hyperventilation and volutrauma. Tidal volume may become insufficient with decreased lung compliance, increased airway resistance, or absence of patient's spontaneous respiratory effort and lead to hypercapnia, tachypnea, increased work of breathing and oxygen consumption, agitation, fatigue, atelectasis/atelectrauma, and acidosis. Rapid, shallow breathing leads to inefficient gas exchange due to increased dead space:V_T ratio. It is therefore evident that relatively tight control of V_T is highly desirable and for this reason, volume-controlled ventilation remains the standard of care in adult and pediatric ventilation.

There are many ways to regulate V_T delivery during MV. Modern ventilators now make it possible to use volume-controlled ventilation in newborn infants by allowing for measurement of exhaled V_T at the airway opening, so that manual adjustment of set V_T at the ventilator end of the patient circuit can be made to achieve a desired exhaled V_T.[50] More convenient are volume-targeted modes that are modifications of pressure-controlled ventilation that automatically adjust inflation pressure and/or time to achieve a target V_T.[51] With V_T as the primary control variable, inflation pressure is automatically reduced as lung compliance and patient inspiratory effort improve, resulting in real-time weaning of pressure. While manual volume targeting can also be achieved with pressure-controlled ventilation by close monitoring of exhaled V_T and manual changes of PIP, VTV results in more timely adjustments with no active effort on the part of the user. The key to effective use of VTV is appreciation of the importance of selecting an appropriate V_T target. Several observational studies defined the typical V_T requirement in various circumstances and patient categories.[52-55] It is important to understand that these values are population means, which represent a good starting point, but that clinical assessment

TABLE 10.1   **Summary Table Listing the Major Outcomes Assessed in the Meta-Analysis of 16 Parallel and Four Crossover Randomized Clinical Trials of Volume-Targeted Versus Pressure-Controlled Ventilation**

	Relative Risk or Mean Difference	95% CI	NNTB (95% CI)
Death or BPD at 36 weeks	0.75	0.53–1.07	NA
BPD at 36 weeks' PMA	0.73	0.59–0.89[a]	8 (5–20)
Grade 3–4 IVH	0.53	0.37–0.77[a]	11 (7–25)
PVL ± severe IVH	0.47	0.27–0.80[a]	11 (7–33)
Pneumothorax	0.52	0.31–0.87[a]	20 (11–100)
Hypocapnia	0.49	0.33–0.72[a]	3 (2–5)
Days of MV	−1.35	−1.83 to −0.86[a]	

[a]Statistically significant differences.

BPD, Bronchopulmonary dysplasia; *CI*, confidence interval; *IVH*, intraventricular hemorrhage; *MV*, mechanical ventilation; *NNTB*, number needed to benefit; *PMA*, postmenstrual age; *PVL*, periventricular leukomalacia.

Adapted from Klingenberg C, Wheeler KI, McCallion N, et al. Volume-targeted versus pressure-limited ventilation in neonates. *Cochrane Database Syst Rev.* 2017;10:CD003666.

of the patient's response to these initial settings must guide subsequent adjustments based on patient's respiratory effort (tachypnea, retractions, or apnea) and of displayed ventilator waveforms.[56] Volume guarantee (VG) is the most extensively studied form of VTV and the basic control algorithm is increasingly being adopted by ventilator manufacturers. Benefits documented in two recent meta-analyses that encompassed several different modalities of VTV include significant decrease in the rate of BPD, pneumothorax, severe intraventricular hemorrhage (IVH), and periventricular leukomalacia, as well as less hypocapnia and shorter duration of MV (Table 10.1).[57,58] Despite these well-documented benefits, adoption of VTV in the United States remains slow and uneven.[59]

Importance of the Open Lung Strategy

Ensuring that gas entering the lungs is evenly distributed into an "open lung," thus avoiding atelectrauma as a key element of any lung-protective ventilation strategy.[60] Adequate PEEP is widely recognized as a means of mitigating lung injury.[60,61] Unfortunately, the impassioned plea of Burkhard Lachman 30 years ago to "OPEN THE LUNG AND KEEP IT OPEN!"[62] has been ignored by many practitioners during conventional MV despite a sound physiologic basis and strong experimental evidence in its favor. In practical terms, the open lung is achieved by applying adequate PEEP.[63] Sufficient inflation pressure to reach the

critical opening pressure of the atelectatic alveoli is also needed; often this is achieved by spontaneous sighs of the infant. One of the most important obstacles to optimizing the way conventional MV is practiced is the persistence of "PEEP-o-phobia," the fear of using adequate levels of end-expiratory pressure. This may be in part due to the fact that the open lung strategy has not been extensively evaluated in the clinical setting.[61] It is important to understand that there is no single optimal PEEP level. The level of end-expiratory pressure must be tailored to the degree of lung injury (i.e., lung compliance). For infants with healthy lungs and thus normal lung compliance, PEEP of 3 cm H_2O may be appropriate; PEEP of 6 cm H_2O may well lead to overexpansion of normal lungs with circulatory impairment and elevated cerebral venous pressure. On the other hand, atelectatic, poorly compliant lungs may transiently require PEEP levels as high as 8 to 10 cm H_2O or more to achieve adequate alveolar recruitment and optimize ventilation/perfusion ratio. Once the lungs are adequately inflated, they become more compliant and the PEEP needs to be reduced to avoid overdistention. As Laplace's law teaches us, less distending pressure is needed to keep well inflated alveoli open than was needed to overcome the critical opening pressure of atelectatic alveoli/terminal air sacs. Because we seldom ventilate infants with healthy lungs, PEEP of < 5 cm H_2O should generally not be used. Interventions that result in interruption of PEEP (e.g., routine suctioning or unnecessary disconnection of the patient circuit) should be kept to a minimum to avoid loss of lung volume recruitment. Maintenance of sufficient lung volume may be particularly important during the critical period post-extubation in infants with significant lung disease.[32]

High-Frequency Ventilation

In contrast to conventional ventilation, the importance of optimizing lung volume has been recognized since its early days of high-frequency ventilation (HFV), where the optimal lung volume strategy has become standard practice and is widely understood to be critical to its success.[64,65] HFV includes several modes of ventilation, including HFOV, high-frequency jet ventilation (HFJV), and high-frequency percussive ventilation (HFPV), which have been used in neonatology since the 1980s. The benefit of HFV is believed to be a function of reduced transmission of pressure and volume swings to the periphery of the lungs. A number of early animal studies demonstrated the short-term benefits of HFOV with an optimal lung volume strategy.[66] Yoder et al. compared the effect of more prolonged HFOV and low V_T positive pressure ventilation using the immature baboon model for BPD, demonstrating that, compared to conventional ventilation, prolonged use of HFOV significantly improved early lung function with sustained improvement in pulmonary mechanics up to 28 days of life and less pulmonary inflammation in the recovery phase of their respiratory distress syndrome (RDS).[67] Clinical results with HFV have been less consistent with several RCTs of various modes of HFV showing improved outcomes, including reduction in BPD and/or duration of MV,[68-72] while other trials showed no improvement.[73-78] Interpretation of RCTs of HFV is made more challenging by the fact that most were done many years ago in patient populations that differ markedly from infants we treat today and compared HFV with less sophisticated (more injurious) strategies of conventional ventilation than those in use today.[61] Importantly, HFV trials that showed benefit were exclusively those that used the optimal lung volume strategy. In those "successful" HFV studies, there were two important differences between study and control groups: high frequency versus low frequency and open lung approach versus low distending

pressure. The latter may be the more important difference; HFOV used without the open lung strategy was relatively ineffective in reducing lung injury.[79] At the same time, several preclinical studies demonstrated that conventional ventilation, when used with the open lung strategy, can achieve similar degrees of lung protection as HFOV, suggesting that optimizing lung volume, rather than frequency, is the key factor.[80-82] However, clinical application of the open lung strategy with conventional ventilation may be more difficult, at least psychologically and the approach has not been adequately evaluated in clinical trials.[83]

With the inclusion of more recent clinical trials that reflect advances in conventional ventilation strategies, the lung-protective effect of HFOV is less clear than earlier studies suggested. Individual patient data meta-analysis from several RCTs failed to demonstrate superiority of HFOV over conventional ventilation and did not suggest that any particular subgroup of preterm infants might uniquely benefit from HFOV.[84] A more recent 2015 Cochrane Review clinical trials of elective HFOV versus conventional ventilation in preterm infants with acute pulmonary dysfunction demonstrated no effect on mortality. However, in contrast to earlier reviews, the risk ratio for BPD was shifted just enough to reach significance due to inclusion of a 2014 study by Sun et al. that suggested an improbably large reduction in the combined outcome of death or BPD.[85] The authors of the Cochrane Review concluded that the overall conclusion was weakened by the inconsistency of benefit across studies.[86] Nonetheless, there may be more subtle benefits of lung-protective HFOV strategies as suggested by the long-term pulmonary follow-up from the United Kingdom Oscillation Study (UKOS), which demonstrated less severe, long-term pulmonary function abnormalities in the HFOV group despite no difference in the primary outcome of BPD at 36 weeks.[87] Important new developments in HFOV include the availability of VTV that can effectively maintain stable minute ventilation despite changes in lung compliance, much like conventional VG, and thus reduce the risk of lung and brain injury.[88]

PROPORTIONAL ASSIST VENTILATION

The respiratory effort of the ventilated preterm infant must overcome increased resistive and/or elastic loads due to the underlying lung disease to generate an adequate V_T. Proportional assist ventilation (PAV) is a modality whereby the ventilator pressure is automatically adjusted in proportion to the volume, flow, or both, generated by the patient. This enhances the infant's ability to generate adequate volume and flow and reduces the elastic or restrictive loads that impede breathing. In PAV, the user determines the degree of mechanical unloading by setting the elastic (volume proportional) and resistive (flow proportional) gains in airway pressure.

The volume and flow proportional gains must be tailored to each infant and require accurate estimation of the respiratory compliance and/or airway resistance. An excessively high elastic (volume) gain that exceeds the elastic recoil of the lungs can lead to a runaway increase in pressure, whereas a resistive (flow) gain that compensates beyond the airway resistance can lead to pressure oscillations.

Operator adjustments of the volume or flow proportional gains during PAV that are needed to maintain adequate ventilation parallel to some extent the adjustments in PIP during PSV or AC ventilation to maintain an adequate V_T. During PAV the airway pressure is automatically adjusted by the ventilator, but the clinician is responsible for setting appropriate limits for peak pressure, delivered volume, inspiratory time, and the backup mandatory inflations in case of apnea.

PAV resulted in reduced breathing effort and improved ventilation and gas exchange with lower peak pressures in comparison with IMV, AC ventilation, and SIMV in preterm infants during the weaning phase of RDS and in the evolving phases of chronic lung disease.[89-91]

It should be noted that the PAV approach assumes mature respiratory control because it is a positive feedback mechanism that unloads the elastic and resistive forces to allow the subject with insufficient strength to generate the desired V_T. The inconsistent and highly variable respiratory drive of the preterm infant may not be optimally suited for this form of assistance. Additionally, because the system, by necessity, responds to inspiratory flow and volume, a large leak around the uncuffed ETT would be interpreted as a large inspiration and given correspondingly high level of inflation pressure, potentially leading to dangerously large V_T. Although PAV has been available for many years, it does not appear to have gained widespread acceptance, possibly because of its complexity and being limited to a single manufacturer platform.

NEURALLY ADJUSTED VENTILATORY ASSIST

Neurally adjusted ventilatory assist (NAVA) is a modality that automatically adjusts ventilator pressure in proportion to the patient's respiratory effort as measured by the EAdi that is detected by an array of microelectrodes mounted on a special feeding tube. The proportionality factor known as the *NAVA number* determines the increase in pressure per microvolt of EAdi. Because the ventilator pressure faithfully mirrors the infant's inspiratory effort, NAVA optimizes synchrony, allowing the patient full control of the respiratory cycle, including onset of inflation, PIP, and onset of exhalation. Like PAV, this is a positive feedback system, with the same concern about amplifying the variability of the immature infant's respiratory effort, but unlike PAV, it is not affected by leak around the ETT, which is an important advantage in patients with uncuffed ETTs.

The ventilator displays the maximal and minimal EAdi, allowing the clinician to monitor the infant's work of breathing and adequacy of the end-expiratory pressure, respectively. High or rising peak EAdi suggests a need for increasing the NAVA level. Minimal EAdi represents the tonic activity of the diaphragm; a relatively high minimal EAdi indicates the need to increase PEEP, which must be done manually. Patients with significant lung disease and intact respiratory control typically generate strong inspiratory effort, but are unable to achieve adequate V_T. With stepwise increases in the NAVA level, the EAdi initially remains stable while the inflation pressure and resulting V_T increase. When the degree of unloading becomes sufficient to achieve adequate minute ventilation, the infant's respiratory effort, as measured by the EAdi, decreases, indicating lower work of breathing. This so-called "break point" indicates optimal unloading of the patient's respiratory system.[92] In subjects with mature respiratory control, further increases in the NAVA number do not increase the V_T or minute ventilation as the patient reduces their respiratory effort. Premature infants may not always respond in this way—recent observations noted that as the NAVA level increased, a higher proportion of excessive V_T was delivered, with 20%

to 25% of V_T greater than 10 mL/kg (measured at the airway opening) at NAVA level of 2.5 cm $H_2O/\mu V$.[93] This likely occurs because preterm infants often respond to external stimuli by briefly generating large inspiratory effort when disturbed, which will be potentiated by the positive feedback of NAVA. Backup pressure or flow-triggered, pressure-controlled ventilation is needed in case of apnea or inadequate EAdi signal.

In short-term studies, NAVA has been shown to be as effective in maintaining gas exchange in premature infants as modalities of conventional pressure-controlled ventilation, sometimes with lower PIP or work of breathing.[94-98] This later effect has been attributed to the better synchrony between the infant's inspiration and the ventilator, but such comparisons are also influenced by the settings selected on the respective modalities. The only randomized trial conducted to date did not demonstrate any reduction in duration of MV, chronic lung disease pneumothorax, or IVH.[99]

The ability to continuously monitor the patient's respiratory effort is an attractive feature of NAVA and allows both physiologic monitoring and appropriate adjustments of respiratory support. The EAdi signal has minimal trigger delay and is unaffected by movement, airflow artifacts, or air leak around uncuffed ETT, making NAVA very attractive for noninvasive ventilation with a high degree of synchrony.[100] Noninvasive NAVA is likely to be safer in immature infants, because excessive V_T is unlikely to be achieved with an open system.

The reported findings on the use of NAVA are promising, but further research is needed to assess its safety and efficacy in premature infants. The level of support depends largely on the NAVA gain setting, but little is known about the effects of different NAVA gain settings or the methods to determine the most appropriate gain. Appropriate limits for PIP should be set to avoid excessive V_T resulting from the positive feedback when the infant becomes agitated and apnea ventilation is necessary when respiratory effort is lacking. Adequately powered prospective trials with important clinical outcomes, such as BPD or IVH, are urgently needed.

Evidence-Based Approach to Mechanical Ventilation

Based on the concepts outlined earlier, certain general guidelines for lung-protective approach to MV can be formulated. The overarching goal is to minimize adverse effects on the infant's lungs, hemodynamics, and brain while supporting adequate gas exchange. Because prolonged duration of ventilation is associated with increased likelihood of chronic lung disease, late-onset sepsis, and neurodevelopmental impairment, successful extubation at the earliest possible time is an important goal. Ventilation settings must be individualized to address each patient's specific condition, but must include the dual objectives of optimizing lung volume/preventing atelectasis and avoiding excessively large V_T. The open lung strategy improves lung compliance, minimizes oxygen requirement, avoids surfactant inactivation, and achieves even V_T distribution. Prevention of excessive V_T delivery minimizes volutrauma and hypocapnia, the two most important and potentially preventable elements of lung and brain injury. Modern neonatal ventilators give clinicians access to effective volume-targeted modes, but not all NICUs in the United States have invested in ventilators specifically designed for newborn infants, relying instead on so-called universal ventilators, which may not provide optimal volume-targeted modes for the smallest infants. Effective use of VTV requires the practitioner to abandon their deeply ingrained "barophobia" and embrace instead the importance of consistent tidal volume delivery. Equally important is familiarity with the appropriate V_T targets, which are a function of patient size, postnatal age, and nature of their lung disease.[51,101]

When relatively high pressures are needed to achieve adequate support, HFV may be a better option. The encouraging results of long-term pulmonary outcome from the UKOS study coupled with the recent availability (at least outside of the United States) of HFOV devices capable of measuring and regulating V_T (HFOV+VG)[102,103] will likely lead to resurgence of enthusiasm for early use of HFOV as a lung-protective prevention strategy.

Proportional assist modalities, such as PAV and NAVA, have not been adequately evaluated in preterm infants and therefore should be used with caution.[104] NAVA may be more suitable in the support of older infants with established BPD who have more mature respiratory control, but more data are needed before recommending this approach.

Mild permissive hypercapnia and lowest FiO_2 consistent with adequate oxygenation are generally considered appropriate, but $PCO_2 > 60$ mm Hg should be avoided in the first 72 hours of life due to increased risk of IVH.[105-107] There is no evidence to support the routine use of sedation and therefore infants should be allowed to breathe spontaneously. Routine suctioning should be avoided, as it leads to derecruitment, transient hypoxemia, and perturbation of cerebral hemodynamics.[108] However, when secretions are detected by auscultation or by perturbation of the flow waveform, rapid gentle suctioning without instillation of normal saline should be performed using a closed suction apparatus.

In the absence of clear evidence from RCTs, the choice of SIMV or AC remains a matter of personal preference and practice style. There is little difference between the two in the acute phase of respiratory failure when the set rate is relatively high with both modes, but becomes more pronounced during weaning, especially in the smallest infants due to high ETT resistance. Prolonged ventilation with low rate SIMV should be avoided in these infants, as it imposes an undesirably high work of breathing. SIMV also results in larger V_T compared to AC, because small preterm infants typically do not generate adequate spontaneous V_T and thus have a high dead space:V_T ratio. To a significant degree, this problem may be overcome by adding pressure support (PS) to the spontaneous breaths during SIMV.[109] While this approach is effective, it adds complexity and does not appear to have any advantage over AC or PSV used alone, as long as atelectasis is avoided by using adequate level of PEEP. Additionally, it is important to recognize that volume targeting will only be applied to the SIMV inflations when using SIMV with PS and VG.

Some degree of arrest of normal lung development is probably inevitable in the most immature infants even with optimized respiratory and therefore "new BPD" is unavoidable at the lowest gestational ages. Suboptimal respiratory support is likely to exacerbate that process and add an element of added lung injury, leading to the superimposition of "old BPD." The wide variation in the risk-adjusted incidence of BPD among the academic medical centers of the Eunice Kennedy Shriver National Institutes of Health Neonatal Research Network suggests that MV and other clinical practices constitute potentially modifiable risk factors.[110] The concepts outlined in this chapter are

based on the best available evidence and physiologic rationale and may provide an opportunity to minimize adverse respiratory outcomes in extremely immature infants requiring respiratory support.

Conflict of Interest Statement

Dr. Keszler has received honoraria for lectures and research grant support from Draeger Medical. Dr. Keszler also chairs the Data Safety Monitoring Board of a clinical trial supported by Chiesi USA.

REFERENCES

1. Walsh MC, Morris BH, Wrage LA, et al. Extremely low birth-weight neonates with protracted ventilation: mortality and 18-month neurodevelopmental outcomes. *J Pediatr*. 2005;146(6):798-804.
2. Network SSGotEKSNNR, Finer NN, Carlo WA, et al. Early CPAP versus surfactant in extremely preterm infants. *N Engl J Med*. 2010;362(21):1970-1979.
3. Morley CJ, Davis PG, Doyle LW, et al. Nasal CPAP or intubation at birth for very preterm infants. *N Engl J Med*. 2008;358(7):700-708.
4. Garland JS. Strategies to prevent ventilator-associated pneumonia in neonates. *Clin Perinatol*. 2010;37(3):629-643.
5. Benitz WE. Treatment of persistent patent ductus arteriosus in preterm infants: time to accept the null hypothesis? *J Perinatol*. 2010;30(4):241-252.
6. Tsuchida S, Engelberts D, Peltekova V, et al. Atelectasis causes alveolar injury in nonatelectatic lung regions. *Am J Respir Crit Care Med*. 2006;174(3):279-289.
7. Dreyfuss D, Soler P, Basset G, et al. High inflation pressure pulmonary edema. Respective effects of high airway pressure, high tidal volume, and positive end-expiratory pressure. *Am Rev Respir Dis*. 1988;137(5):1159-1164.
8. Hernandez LA, Peevy KJ, Moise AA, et al. Chest wall restriction limits high airway pressure-induced lung injury in young rabbits. *J Appl Physiol*. 1989;66(5):2364-2368.
9. Mols G, Priebe HJ, Guttmann J. Alveolar recruitment in acute lung injury. *Br J Anaesth*. 2006;96(2):156-166.
10. Mortola JP, Fisher JT, Smith JB, et al. Onset of respiration in infants delivered by cesarean section. *J Appl Physiol Respir Environ Exerc Physiol*. 1982;52(3):716-724.
11. te Pas AB, Siew M, Wallace MJ, et al. Establishing functional residual capacity at birth: the effect of sustained inflation and positive end-expiratory pressure in a preterm rabbit model. *Pediatr Res*. 2009;65(5):537-541.
12. Aziz K, Lee CHC, Escobedo MB, et al. Part 5: Neonatal Resuscitation 2020 American Heart Association Guidelines for Cardiopulmonary Resuscitation and Emergency Cardiovascular Care. *Pediatrics*. 2021;147(suppl 1):e2020038505E.
13. Schmolzer GM, O'Reilly M, Labossiere J, et al. Cardiopulmonary resuscitation with chest compressions during sustained inflations: a new technique of neonatal resuscitation that improves recovery and survival in a neonatal porcine model. *Circulation*. 2013;128(23):2495-2503.

14. Bjorklund LJ, Ingimarsson J, Curstedt T, et al. Manual ventilation with a few large breaths at birth compromises the therapeutic effect of subsequent surfactant replacement in immature lambs. *Pediatr Res.* 1997;42(3):348-355.

15. Hillman NH, Kemp MW, Miura Y, et al. Sustained inflation at birth did not alter lung injury from mechanical ventilation in surfactant-treated fetal lambs. *PLoS One.* 2014;9(11):e113473.

16. Hillman NH, Kemp MW, Noble PB, et al. Sustained inflation at birth did not protect preterm fetal sheep from lung injury. *Am J Physiol Lung Cell Mol Physiol.* 2013;305(6):L446-L453.

17. Wyckoff MH. Improving neonatal cardiopulmonary resuscitation hemodynamics: are sustained inflations during compressions the answer? *Circulation.* 2013;128(23):2468-2469.

18. Kirpalani H, Ratcliffe SJ, Keszler M, et al. Effect of sustained inflations vs intermittent positive pressure ventilation on bronchopulmonary dysplasia or death among extremely preterm infants: the SAIL randomized clinical trial. *JAMA.* 2019;321(12):1165-1175.

19. Foglia EE, Te Pas AB, Kirpalani H, et al. Sustained inflation vs standard resuscitation for preterm infants: a systematic review and meta-analysis. *JAMA Pediatr.* 2020;174(4):e195897.

20. Ammari A, Suri M, Milisavljevic V, et al. Variables associated with the early failure of nasal CPAP in very low birth weight infants. *J Pediatr.* 2005;147(3):341-347.

21. Morley CJ, Davis PG, Doyle LW, et al. Nasal CPAP or intubation at birth for very preterm infants. *N Engl J Med.* 2008;358(7):700-708.

22. NICHD Neonatal Research Network, Support Study Group of the Eunice Kennedy Shriver. Early CPAP versus surfactant in extremely preterm infants. *N Engl J Med.* 2010;362:1970-1979.

23. Sandri F, Plavka R, Ancora G, et al. Prophylactic or early selective surfactant combined with nCPAP in very preterm infants. *Pediatrics.* 2010;125(6):e1402-e1409.

24. Dunn MS, Kaempf J, de Klerk A, et al. Randomized trial comparing 3 approaches to the initial respiratory management of preterm neonates. *Pediatrics.* 2011;128(5):e1069-e1076.

25. Schmolzer GM, Kumar M, Pichler G, Aziz K, O'Reilly M, Cheung PY. Non-invasive versus invasive respiratory support in preterm infants at birth: systematic review and meta-analysis. *BMJ.* 2013;347:f5980.

26. Moretti C, Gizzi C, Papoff P, et al. Comparing the effects of nasal synchronized intermittent positive pressure ventilation (nSIPPV) and nasal continuous positive airway pressure (nCPAP) after extubation in very low birth weight infants. *Early Hum Dev.* 1999;56(2-3):167-177.

27. Davis PG, Morley CJ, Owen LS. Non-invasive respiratory support of preterm neonates with respiratory distress: continuous positive airway pressure and nasal intermittent positive pressure ventilation. *Semin Fetal Neonatal Med.* 2009;14(1):14-20.

28. Meneses J, Bhandari V, Alves JG. Nasal intermittent positive-pressure ventilation vs nasal continuous positive airway pressure for preterm infants with respiratory distress syndrome: a systematic review and meta-analysis. *Arch Pediatr Adolesc Med.* 2012;166(4):372-376.

29. Kirpalani H, Millar D, Lemyre B, et al. A trial comparing noninvasive ventilation strategies in preterm infants. *N Engl J Med.* 2013;369(7):611-620.

30. Owen LS, Morley CJ, Dawson JA, et al. Effects of non-synchronised nasal intermittent positive pressure ventilation on spontaneous breathing in preterm infants. *Arch Dis Child Fetal Neonatal Ed.* 2011;96(6):F422-F428.

31. Lemyre B, Davis PG, De Paoli AG, et al. Nasal intermittent positive pressure ventilation (NIPPV) versus nasal continuous positive airway pressure (NCPAP) for preterm neonates after extubation. *Cochrane Database Syst Rev.* 2017;2:CD003212.

32. Buzzella B, Claure N, D'Ugard C, et al. A randomized controlled trial of two nasal continuous positive airway pressure levels after extubation in preterm infants. *J Pediatr.* 2014;164(1):46-51.

33. van der Hoeven M, Brouwer E, Blanco CE. Nasal high frequency ventilation in neonates with moderate respiratory insufficiency. *Arch Dis Child Fetal Neonatal Ed.* 1998;79(1):F61-F63.

34. Mukerji A, Singh B, Helou SE, et al. Use of noninvasive high-frequency ventilation in the neonatal intensive care unit: a retrospective review. *Am J Perinatol.* 2015;30(2):171-176.

35. De Luca D, Dell'Orto V. Non-invasive high-frequency oscillatory ventilation in neonates: review of physiology, biology and clinical data. *Arch Dis Child Fetal Neonatal Ed.* 2016;101:F565-F570.

36. Gibu C, Cheng P, Ward RJ, Castro B, Heldt GP. Feasibility and physiological effects of non-invasive neurally-adjusted ventilatory assist (NIV-NAVA) in preterm infants. *Pediatr Res.* 2017;82(4):650-657.

37. Chan V, Greenough A. Comparison of weaning by patient triggered ventilation or synchronous intermittent mandatory ventilation in preterm infants. *Acta Paediatr.* 1994;83(3):335-337.

38. Dimitriou G, Greenough A, Griffin F, Chan V. Synchronous intermittent mandatory ventilation modes compared with patient triggered ventilation during weaning. *Arch Dis Child Fetal Neonatal Ed.* 1995;72(3):F188-F190.

39. Greenough A, Rossor TE, Sundaresan A, Murthy V, Milner AD. Synchronized mechanical ventilation for respiratory support in newborn infants. *Cochrane Database Syst Rev.* 2016;9:CD000456.

40. Hummler H, Gerhardt T, Gonzalez A, Claure N, Everett R, Bancalari E. Influence of different methods of synchronized mechanical ventilation on ventilation, gas exchange, patient effort, and blood pressure fluctuations in premature neonates. *Pediatr Pulmonol.* 1996;22(5):305-313.

41. Mrozek JD, Bendel-Stenzel EM, Meyers PA, Bing DR, Connett JE, Mammel MC. Randomized controlled trial of volume-targeted synchronized ventilation and conventional intermittent mandatory ventilation following initial exogenous surfactant therapy. *Pediatr Pulmonol.* 2000;29(1):11-18.

42. Vervenioti A, Fouzas S, Tzifas S, Karatza AA, Dimitriou G. Work of breathing in mechanically ventilated preterm neonates. *Pediatr Crit Care Med.* 2020;21(5):430-436.

43. Sharma A, Greenough A. Survey of neonatal respiratory support strategies. *Acta Paediatr.* 2007;96(8):1115-1117.

44. Albertine KH, Jones GP, Starcher BC, et al. Chronic lung injury in preterm lambs. Disordered respiratory tract development. *Am J Respir Crit Care Med.* 1999;159(3):945-958.

45. Multicentre randomised controlled trial of high against low frequency positive pressure ventilation. Oxford Region Controlled Trial of Artificial Ventilation OCTAVE Study Group. *Arch Dis Child.* 1991;66(7 Spec No):770-775.

46. Dani C, Bresci C, Lista G, et al. Neonatal respiratory support strategies in the intensive care unit: an Italian survey. *Eur J Pediatr.* 2013;172(3):331-336.

47. van Kaam AH, Rimensberger PC, Borensztajn D, De Jaegere AP. Ventilation practices in the neonatal intensive care unit: a cross-sectional study. *J Pediatr.* 2010;157(5):767-771.e1-e3.

48. Dreyfuss D, Saumon G. Ventilator-induced lung injury: lessons from experimental studies. *Am J Respir Crit Care Med.* 1998;157(1):294-323.

49. Dreyfuss D, Saumon G. Role of tidal volume, FRC, and end-inspiratory volume in the development of pulmonary edema following mechanical ventilation. *Am Rev Respir Dis.* 1993; 148(5):1194-1203.

50. Singh J, Sinha SK, Clarke P, Byrne S, Donn SM. Mechanical ventilation of very low birth weight infants: is volume or pressure a better target variable? *J Pediatr.* 2006;149(3):308-313.

51. Keszler M. Update on mechanical ventilatory strategies. *NeoReviews.* 2013;14(5):e237-e251.

52. Keszler M, Nassabeh-Montazami S, Abubakar K. Evolution of tidal volume requirement during the first 3 weeks of life in infants <800 g ventilated with Volume Guarantee. *Arch Dis Child Fetal Neonatal Ed.* 2009;94(4):F279-F282.

53. Sharma S, Clark S, Abubakar K, Keszler M. Tidal volume requirement in mechanically ventilated infants with meconium aspiration syndrome. *Am J Perinatol.* 2015;32(10):916-919.

54. Sharma S, Abubakar KM, Keszler M. Tidal volume in infants with congenital diaphragmatic hernia supported with conventional mechanical ventilation. *Am J Perinatol.* 2015;32(6):577-582.

55. Nassabeh-Montazami S, Abubakar KM, Keszler M. The impact of instrumental dead-space in volume-targeted ventilation of the extremely low birth weight (ELBW) infant. *Pediatr Pulmonol.* 2009;44(2):128-133.

56. Keszler M. Volume-targeted ventilation: one size does not fit all. Evidence-based recommendations for successful use. *Arch Dis Child Fetal Neonatal Ed.* 2019;104:F108-F112.

57. Peng W, Zhu H, Shi H, Liu E. Volume-targeted ventilation is more suitable than pressure-limited ventilation for preterm infants: a systematic review and meta-analysis. *Arch Dis Child Fetal Neonatal Ed.* 2014;99(2):F158-F165.

58. Klingenberg C, Wheeler KI, McCallion N, Morley CJ, Davis PG. Volume-targeted versus pressure-limited ventilation in neonates. *Cochrane Database Syst Rev.* 2017;10:CD003666.

59. Gupta A, Keszler M. Survey of ventilation practices in the Neonatal Intensive Care Units of the United States and Canada: use of volume-targeted ventilation and barriers to its use. *Am J Perinatol.* 2019;36(5):484-489.

60. Rimensberger PC, Cox PN, Frndova H, Bryan AC. The open lung during small tidal volume ventilation: concepts of recruitment and "optimal" positive end-expiratory pressure. *Crit Care Med.* 1999;27(9):1946-1952.

61. van Kaam AH, Rimensberger PC. Lung-protective ventilation strategies in neonatology: what do we know—what do we need to know? *Crit Care Med.* 2007;35(3):925-931.

62. Lachmann B. Open up the lung and keep the lung open. *Intensive Care Med.* 1992;18(6):319-321.

63. Castoldi F, Daniele I, Fontana P, Cavigioli F, Lupo E, Lista G. Lung recruitment maneuver during volume guarantee ventilation of preterm infants with acute respiratory distress syndrome. *Am J Perinatol.* 2011;28(7):521-528.

64. Bryan AC. The oscillations of HFO. *Am J Respir Crit Care Med.* 2001;163(4):816-817.

65. Froese AB. Role of lung volume in lung injury: HFO in the atelectasis-prone lung. *Acta Anaesthesiol Scand Suppl.* 1989;90: 126-130.

66. Keszler M, Durand DJ. Neonatal high-frequency ventilation. Past, present, and future. *Clin Perinatol.* 2001;28(3):579-607.

67. Yoder BA, Siler-Khodr T, Winter VT, Coalson JJ. High-frequency oscillatory ventilation: effects on lung function, mechanics, and airway cytokines in the immature baboon model for neonatal chronic lung disease. *Am J Respir Crit Care Med.* 2000;162(5): 1867-1876.

68. Clark RH, Gerstmann DR, Null DM Jr, deLemos RA. Prospective randomized comparison of high-frequency oscillatory and conventional ventilation in respiratory distress syndrome. *Pediatrics.* 1992;89(1):5-12.

69. Gerstmann DR, Minton SD, Stoddard RA, et al. The Provo multicenter early high-frequency oscillatory ventilation trial: improved pulmonary and clinical outcome in respiratory distress syndrome. *Pediatrics.* 1996;98(6 Pt 1):1044-1057.

70. Keszler M, Modanlou HD, Brudno DS, et al. Multicenter controlled clinical trial of high-frequency jet ventilation in preterm infants with uncomplicated respiratory distress syndrome. *Pediatrics.* 1997;100(4):593-599.

71. Plavka R, Kopecky P, Sebron V, Svihovec P, Zlatohlavkova B, Janus V. A prospective randomized comparison of conventional mechanical ventilation and very early high frequency oscillatory ventilation in extremely premature newborns with respiratory distress syndrome. *Intensive Care Med.* 1999; 25(1):68-75.

72. Courtney SE, Durand DJ, Asselin JM, Hudak ML, Aschner JL, Shoemaker CT. High-frequency oscillatory ventilation versus conventional mechanical ventilation for very-low-birth-weight infants. *N Engl J Med.* 2002;347(9):643-652.

73. Wiswell TE, Graziani LJ, Kornhauser MS, et al. High-frequency jet ventilation in the early management of respiratory distress syndrome is associated with a greater risk for adverse outcomes. *Pediatrics.* 1996;98(6 Pt 1):1035-1043.

74. Rettwitz-Volk W, Veldman A, Roth B, et al. A prospective, randomized, multicenter trial of high-frequency oscillatory ventilation compared with conventional ventilation in preterm infants with respiratory distress syndrome receiving surfactant. *J Pediatr.* 1998;132(2):249-254.

75. Moriette G, Paris-Llado J, Walti H, et al. Prospective randomized multicenter comparison of high-frequency oscillatory ventilation and conventional ventilation in preterm infants of less than 30 weeks with respiratory distress syndrome. *Pediatrics.* 2001;107(2):363-372.

76. Johnson AH, Peacock JL, Greenough A, et al. High-frequency oscillatory ventilation for the prevention of chronic lung disease of prematurity. *N Engl J Med.* 2002;347(9):633-642.

77. Van Reempts P, Borstlap C, Laroche S, Van der Auwera JC. Early use of high frequency ventilation in the premature neonate. *Eur J Pediatr.* 2003;162(4):219-226.

78. Thome U, Kossel H, Lipowsky G, et al. Randomized comparison of high-frequency ventilation with high-rate intermittent positive pressure ventilation in preterm infants with respiratory failure. *J Pediatr.* 1999;135(1):39-46.

79. McCulloch PR, Forkert PG, Froese AB. Lung volume maintenance prevents lung injury during high frequency oscillatory ventilation in surfactant-deficient rabbits. *Am Rev Respir Dis.* 1988;137(5):1185-1192.

80. Gommers D, Hartog A, Schnabel R, De Jaegere A, Lachmann B. High-frequency oscillatory ventilation is not superior to conventional mechanical ventilation in surfactant-treated rabbits with lung injury. *Eur Respir J.* 1999;14(4):738-744.

81. Vazquez de Anda GF, Hartog A, Verbrugge SJ, Gommers D, Lachmann B. The open lung concept: pressure-controlled ventilation is as effective as high-frequency oscillatory ventilation in improving gas exchange and lung mechanics in surfactant-deficient animals. *Intensive Care Med.* 1999;25(9):990-996.

82. van Kaam AH, de Jaegere A, Haitsma JJ, Van Aalderen WM, Kok JH, Lachmann B. Positive pressure ventilation with the open lung concept optimizes gas exchange and reduces

ventilator-induced lung injury in newborn piglets. *Pediatr Res.* 2003;53(2):245-253.

83. Jobe AH. Lung recruitment for ventilation: does it work, and is it safe? *J Pediatr.* 2009;154(5):635-636.

84. Cools F, Askie LM, Offringa M, et al. Elective high-frequency oscillatory versus conventional ventilation in preterm infants: a systematic review and meta-analysis of individual patients' data. *Lancet.* 2010;375(9731):2082-2091.

85. Sun H, Cheng R, Kang W, et al. High-frequency oscillatory ventilation versus synchronized intermittent mandatory ventilation plus pressure support in preterm infants with severe respiratory distress syndrome. *Respir Care.* 2014;59(2):159-169.

86. Cools F, Offringa M, Askie LM. Elective high frequency oscillatory ventilation versus conventional ventilation for acute pulmonary dysfunction in preterm infants. *Cochrane Database Syst Rev.* 2015;(3):CD000104.

87. Zivanovic S, Peacock J, Alcazar-Paris M, et al. Late outcomes of a randomized trial of high-frequency oscillation in neonates. *N Engl J Med.* 2014;370(12):1121-1130.

88. Sanchez-Luna M, Gonzalez-Pacheco N, Belik J, Santos M, Tendillo F. New ventilator strategies: high-frequency oscillatory ventilation combined with volume guarantee. *Am J Perinatol.* 2018;35(6):545-548.

89. Schulze A, Rieger-Fackeldey E, Gerhardt T, Claure N, Everett R, Bancalari E. Randomized crossover comparison of proportional assist ventilation and patient-triggered ventilation in extremely low birth weight infants with evolving chronic lung disease. *Neonatology.* 2007;92(1):1-7.

90. Schulze A, Gerhardt T, Musante G, et al. Proportional assist ventilation in low birth weight infants with acute respiratory disease: a comparison to assist/control and conventional mechanical ventilation. *J Pediatr.* 1999;135(3):339-344.

91. Shetty S, Bhat P, Hickey A, Peacock JL, Milner AD, Greenough A. Proportional assist versus assist control ventilation in premature infants. *Eur J Pediatr.* 2016;175(1):57-61.

92. Firestone KS, Fisher S, Reddy S, White DB, Stein HM. Effect of changing NAVA levels on peak inspiratory pressures and electrical activity of the diaphragm in premature neonates. *J Perinatol.* 2015;35(8):612-616.

93. Nam SK, Lee J, Jun YH. Neural feedback is insufficient in preterm infants during neurally adjusted ventilatory assist. *Pediatr Pulmonol.* 2019;54(8):1277-1283.

94. Stein H, Howard D. Neurally adjusted ventilatory assist in neonates weighing <1500 grams: a retrospective analysis. *J Pediatr.* 2012;160(5):786-789.e1.

95. Stein H, Alosh H, Ethington P, White DB. Prospective crossover comparison between NAVA and pressure control ventilation in premature neonates less than 1500 grams. *J Perinatol.* 2013; 33(6):452-456.

96. Lee J, Kim HS, Sohn JA, et al. Randomized crossover study of neurally adjusted ventilatory assist in preterm infants. *J Pediatr.* 2012;161(5):808-813.

97. Shetty S, Hunt K, Peacock J, Ali K, Greenough A. Crossover study of assist control ventilation and neurally adjusted ventilatory assist. *Eur J Pediatr.* 2017;176(4):509-513.

98. Rosterman JL, Pallotto EK, Truog WE, et al. The impact of neurally adjusted ventilatory assist mode on respiratory severity score and energy expenditure in infants: a randomized crossover trial. *J Perinatol.* 2018;38(1):59-63.

99. Kallio M, Koskela U, Peltoniemi O, et al. Neurally adjusted ventilatory assist (NAVA) in preterm newborn infants with respiratory distress syndrome-a randomized controlled trial. *Eur J Pediatr.* 2016;175(9):1175-1183.

100. Lee BK, Shin SH, Jung YH, Kim EK, Kim HS. Comparison of NIV-NAVA and NCPAP in facilitating extubation for very preterm infants. *BMC Pediatr.* 2019;19(1):298.

101. Keszler M. Volume-targeted ventilation: one size does not fit all. Evidence-based recommendations for successful use. *Arch Dis Child Fetal Neonatal Ed.* 2019;104(1):F108-F112.

102. Enomoto M, Keszler M, Sakuma M, et al. Effect of volume guarantee in preterm infants on high-frequency oscillatory ventilation: a pilot study. *Am J Perinatol.* 2017;34(1):26-30.

103. Iscan B, Duman N, Tuzun F, Kumral A, Ozkan H. Impact of volume guarantee on high-frequency oscillatory ventilation in preterm infants: a randomized crossover clinical trial. *Neonatology.* 2015;108(4):277-282.

104. Rossor TE, Hunt KA, Shetty S, Greenough A. Neurally adjusted ventilatory assist compared to other forms of triggered ventilation for neonatal respiratory support. *Cochrane Database Syst Rev.* 2017;10:CD012251.

105. Fabres J, Carlo WA, Phillips V, et al. Both extremes of arterial carbon dioxide pressure and the magnitude of fluctuations in arterial carbon dioxide pressure are associated with severe intraventricular hemorrhage in preterm infants. *Pediatrics.* 2007; 119(2):299-305.

106. Kaiser JR, Gauss CH, Pont MM, Williams DK. Hypercapnia during the first 3 days of life is associated with severe intraventricular hemorrhage in very low birth weight infants. *J Perinatol.* 2006;26(5):279-285.

107. Thome UH, Genzel-Boroviczeny O, Bohnhorst B, et al. Permissive hypercapnia in extremely low birthweight infants (PHELBI): a randomised controlled multicentre trial. *Lancet Respir Med.* 2015;3(7):534-543.

108. Kaiser JR, Gauss CH, Williams DK. Tracheal suctioning is associated with prolonged disturbances of cerebral hemodynamics in very low birth weight infants. *J Perinatol.* 2008; 28(1):34-41.

109. Osorio W, Claure N, D'Ugard C, et al. Effects of pressure support during an acute reduction of synchronized intermittent mandatory ventilation in preterm infants. *J Perinatol.* 2005; 25(6):412-416.

110. Ambalavanan N, Walsh M, Bobashev G, et al. Intercenter differences in bronchopulmonary dysplasia or death among very low birth weight infants. *Pediatrics.* 2011;127(1):e106-e116.

Chapter 11

Prenatal and Postnatal Steroids and Pulmonary Outcomes

Augusto F. Schmidt and Alan H. Jobe

Chapter Outline

Antenatal Corticosteroids

Historical Overview

Pharmacokinetics of Antenatal Steroids

Mechanism of Action of ANS on Fetal Lungs

Dated Randomized Controlled Trials and Current Patient Populations

Non-RCT information Regarding ANS and Outcomes

Repeated ANS Treatments

ANS After 34 Weeks' Gestational Age

ANS Before Elective C-section

Concerns Regarding Drug and Dose Choices for ANS

Long-Term Outcomes After ANS

Antenatal Steroid Use in Low-Resource Environments

Postnatal Steroids

Historical Review

Pathophysiology of BPD: What are we Treating with PNS?

Meta-Analyses of Early and Late Treatments

Drug, Dose, Route, and Duration of Therapy

Alternatives to Early Systemic PNS

How PNS are Used

Summary and Future Directions

Key Points

- Antenatal steroids (ANS) are one of the oldest and most effective therapies in perinatal medicine.
- The randomized controlled trials (RCTs) are dated and do not necessarily apply for current clinical populations in high-resource environments where treatments reduce mortality.
- In low-resource environments, there is potential for risk and unclear benefit of ANS.
- There are minimal RCT data to support ANS use for deliveries before 28 weeks' gestational age.
- The risk to benefit ratio for gestations after 34 weeks is unclear.
- The dose and drug choice for ANS has not been optimized to decrease potential risks.
- Postnatal steroids (PNS) can effectively decrease bronchopulmonary dysplasia (BPD), but there are risks.
- The trend is to use lower doses, for shorter periods of treatment, and later, without randomized data to support.
- Four new trials of PNS begun shortly after birth are proof of principle that PNS decrease BPD.
- PNS should only be used for infants at high risk of severe BPD.

This chapter reviews knowledge gaps and new information about the two primary uses of corticosteroids in the perinatal period: antenatal (maternal) treatments (antenatal steroids [ANS]) to decrease respiratory distress syndrome (RDS) and infant mortality, and post-delivery corticosteroid treatments (postnatal steroids [PNS]) to prevent or treat bronchopulmonary dysplasia (BPD). Clinical and experimental information for both treatments is not optimal for current clinical practice as a result of the histories for the development and testing of corticosteroids for both antenatal and postnatal indications. Both therapies were used by clinicians in the early period of modern perinatal medicine without formal drug development and licensure. Thus, optimal drug selection, dose, and patient selection remain poorly defined today. Much of the clinical information is quite old, and patient populations and clinical management have changed strikingly. Further, the therapies were evaluated and adopted before modern molecular techniques were available, leaving large gaps in knowledge about the mechanisms of action and the potential risks of treatment. Corticosteroids are potent drugs with pleotropic effects on multiple organ systems that play essential roles in basal physiology, stress responses, and when used in higher doses, therapeutic effects. The major focus of this chapter is on the fetal and newborn lung, but cardiovascular and mortality outcomes cannot be separated from lung responses.

Antenatal Corticosteroids

HISTORICAL OVERVIEW

While evaluating the role of fetal exposures to corticosteroids on labor in sheep, Liggins reported in 1969 that fetal dexamethasone infusions caused preterm delivery of lambs that had unanticipatedly good lung aeration.[1] That result was consistent with other early reports that corticosteroids could mature developing organ systems in other animal models. His observation in sheep was quickly evaluated in a clinical trial reported in 1972 that randomly assigned 282 women to a maternal intramuscular treatment with the drug betamethasone (Celestone) that is used to suppress inflammation.[2] Celestone Soluspan is a mixture of two prodrug forms of the fluorinated corticosteroid betamethasone: betamethasone phosphate and a micronized suspension of betamethasone acetate. When injected intramuscularly, the betamethasone phosphate is rapidly dephosphorylated while the betamethasone acetate is slowly deacylated over many hours and days. Both compounds yield free betamethasone, which crosses the placenta to achieve a prolonged fetal exposure when given as a two-dose treatment of 12 mg at a 24-hour interval. This level of detail is important to understand today's approach for ANS dosing (see the following text).

The Liggins and Howie trial demonstrated decreased RDS and mortality in infants of an average gestational age of 35 weeks at delivery.[2] More than 20 trials were completed by 1993 that, in aggregate, demonstrated comparable effects without clear risks. However, ANS were not widely used in the United States until recommended by a National Institutes of Health Consensus Conference in 1994.[3] The majority of trials tested Celestone against placebo, but dexamethasone phosphate, a similar drug given as four doses of 6 mg every 12 hours, was used in some trials as summarized by the definitive meta-analysis of Roberts et al. in 2006 that was last updated in 2020.[4,5] The primary outcomes of most of the trials were decreased RDS and mortality, although ANS also had benefits for decreased intraventricular hemorrhage (IVH) and necrotizing enterocolitis. ANS became the standard of care for all women at risk of preterm delivery before 34 weeks and ANS were recognized as a major advancement in perinatal medicine. There was minimal information developed for drug selection or dose in animal models or humans, and ANS remain unapproved by the US Food and Drug Administration.

PHARMACOKINETICS OF ANTENATAL STEROIDS

Widespread adoption of ANS for fetal lung maturation took place without careful consideration of pharmacokinetics of the different drugs available. Moreover, regimens have been modified according to local availability and some were adopted with minimal or no information of clinical efficacy. The regimen initially trialed by Liggins is a mixture of two prodrugs: (1) betamethasone phosphate, which is rapidly dephosphorylated; and (2) betamethasone acetate, which is slowly deacylated. In nonpregnant reproductive-age women, this mixture reaches peak concentration at 3 hours and has a half-life of 59 hours, with detectable levels up to 11 days after an initial 6 mg dose, which was just 25% of the clinically used dose.[6] The other commonly used drug is intramuscular dexamethasone, which is usually given as four doses of 6 mg 12 hours apart. In nonpregnant reproductive age women, this dose reaches peak concentration at 3 hours but has a much shorter half-life of 5.2 hours.[6] Large animal models of preterm pregnancy have provided information on the transfer and

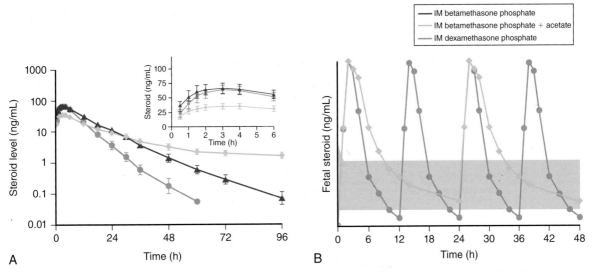

Fig. 11.1 Predicted maternal and schematic representation of fetal plasma concentration of steroids. **A,** Plasma concentration of betamethasone after administration of 6 mg of betamethasone phosphate *(dark blue)*, betamethasone phosphate + acetate *(light blue)*, or dexamethasone phosphate *(orange)* in nonpregnant reproductive-age women (Jobe AH, Milad MA, Peppard T, Jusko WJ. Pharmacokinetics and Pharmacodynamics of Intramuscular and Oral Betamethasone and Dexamethasone in Reproductive Age Women in India. *Clin Transl Sci.* 2020;13(2):391-399. doi:10.1111/cts.12724.) **B,** Predicted fetal concentration profiles after administration of the clinically used regimens with betamethasone acetate + betamethasone-phosphate *(light blue)* and dexamethasone-phosphate *(orange)* and the target concentration range in *shaded green* necessary for fetal lung maturation. (Modified from Schmidt AF, Kemp MW, Milad M, et al. Oral dosing for antenatal corticosteroids in the Rhesus macaque. *PLoS One.* 2019;14(9):e0222817. doi:10.1371/journal.pone.02228177.)

pharmacokinetics of these drugs in the fetus. In order to achieve fetal lung maturation in preterm sheep and rhesus macaques, a low continuous fetal exposure with a concentration of 1 to 3 ng/mL of plasma betamethasone for at least 48 hours is needed for a persistent fetal lung maturation response that lasts 5 to 7 days after initiation of treatment (Fig. 11.1).[7-9]

The current treatment regimens used expose the fetus and the mother to an excess peak concentration of corticosteroids that does not contribute to fetal lung maturation. While a long-acting formulation provides the continuous and prolonged exposure necessary for fetal lung maturation, they may result in prolonged and unnecessary maternal and fetal exposure. Clinicians cannot accurately predict timing of preterm birth in about 50% of the cases, with women often delivering before 24 hours or after 7 days of administration of ANS, when they are no longer effective.[10] In women that deliver soon after administration of Celestone, they will have continued exposure to betamethasone for several days with no benefit and potential side effects of hyperglycemia and hypertension

which may aggravate pregnancies complicated by diabetes and hypertension.

MECHANISM OF ACTION OF ANTENATAL STEROIDS ON FETAL LUNGS

Multiple experimental studies with animals, human fetal lung explants, and isolated lung cells followed the initial Liggins observation in fetal sheep. Exposure to steroids induced the enzymes that contribute to surfactant synthesis and increased surfactant lipid and protein components in tissue and air spaces that became the explanation for the effects of ANS on fetal lungs.[11] However, in large animal models such as sheep and primates, improved lung function as assessed by increased gas volumes and improved lung mechanics occur within 15 to 24 hours, prior to increase in lung surfactant which is only detectable at 3 to 5 days after treatment (Fig. 11.2).[9,12] ANS decrease lung mesenchyme tissue volume, and the barrier function of the air space epithelium improves rapidly after ANS in animal models, which contributed to improved lung function soon after ANS

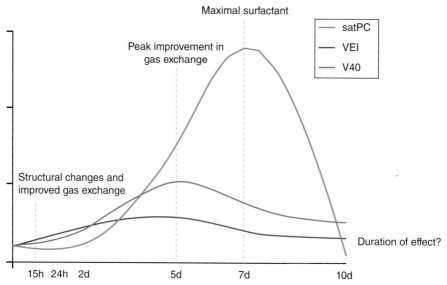

Fig. 11.2 Timeline of changes in static lung compliance *(V40)*, gas exchange (ventilation efficiency index *[VEI]*), and saturated phosphatidylcholine *(satPC)* in the bronchoalveolar lavage fluid based on data from preterm lambs treated with ANS. Lung structural changes can be seen as early as 15 hours after treatment with improvement in gas exchange seen at 24 to 48 hours, and increases in surfactant only seen at 5 days and peaking at 7 days when there is already a decreasing effect on lung compliance and gas exchange. *ANS*, Antenatal steroids; *d*, days; *h*, hours. (Data from Ikegami M, Polk D, Jobe A. Minimum interval from fetal betamethasone treatment to postnatal lung responses in preterm lambs. *Am J Obstet Gynecol.* 1996;174(5):1408-1413.)

treatment.[13] At the cellular level, ANS promote the differentiation of proliferative mesenchymal progenitors into matrix fibroblasts as well as differentiation of alveolar type 1 and type 2 epithelial cells.[14,15] At the molecular level, ANS upregulate and downregulate the expression of thousands of genes within a few hours, with the net effects of improved lung function after preterm delivery.[7] These multiple effects certainly cause improved lung function, but the ANS response is not simply an acceleration of normal lung development. In animal models, fetuses exposed to ANS have a transient decrease in saccular/alveolar septation and microvascular arborization that is similar to the phenotype of delayed lung development associated with BPD with suppression of angiogenesis and lung morphogenesis pathways.[7,16] Alveolarization and microvascular development "catches up" in fetal sheep if they remain undelivered.[17] In a 30-year follow-up, ANS do not seem to alter subsequent lung function after preterm delivery.[18] Empirically very preterm infants exposed to ANS who do not have BPD seem to fare well, although their lung function is not

equivalent to the lung function of term infants.[19] However, term-born infants exposed to ANS have decreased forced vital capacity and forced expiratory volume compared to nonexposed term-born infants.[20] Further work is needed to understand the effects of ANS on the fetal lung and on long-term lung function.

DATED RANDOMIZED CONTROLLED TRIALS AND CURRENT PATIENT POPULATIONS

When ANS were initially used, RDS was a lethal disease for most infants and very preterm infants with or without RDS had very high mortality. The single ANS treatment trials versus placebo reported more than 25 years ago have RDS outcomes for just 102 randomized patients that delivered before 28 weeks' gestational age (Table 11.1). The most recent updates of the Roberts et al.[4] meta-analysis have not provided updated information by gestational age ranges. More recently, the WHO ACTION-I trial in low-resource countries reported 226 infants between 26 and 28 weeks randomized to ANS or placebo with 6% decrease in mortality in the ANS group (relative risk [RR] 0.89,

TABLE 11.1 RCT Data for Antenatal Steroids in Infants Born Before 28 Weeks

Result	Trials	Treated Patients	Controls	Relative Risk (95% CI)
Respiratory distress syndrome	4	48	54	0.79 (0.53–1.18)
Death	2	45	44	0.79 (0.56–1.12)
Intraventricular hemorrhage	1	34	28	0.34 (0.14–0.86)

CI, Confidence interval; RCT, randomized controlled trial.

confidence interval [CI] 0.70–1.14, number needed to treat [NNT] 16), but the rates of RDS were not reported. In contrast, with current practices, RDS in infants more than 28 weeks' gestation is generally easily managed with surfactant and standard techniques for respiratory support. The recommendation at a 1994 Consensus Conference was to administer ANS for women at risk of preterm delivery between 24 and 34 weeks' gestational age, even though there were minimal data to support that recommendation.[3] We lack the randomized controlled trial (RCT) evidence that use of ANS benefits the pulmonary outcomes of the population of infants most targeted to receive ANS today.

NON RANDOMIZED DATA REGARDING ANTENATAL STEROIDS AND OUTCOMES

Other information is available to support ANS use at early gestational ages. Very immature animal models and in vitro explants of human fetal lungs have maturational responses to steroids, indicating that receptors and response pathways are present from early gestational ages.[21] Very large databases from neonatal networks are being extensively mined for outcomes of very low-birth-weight (VLBW) infants who were and were not exposed to ANS.[22-24] These analyses focus on mortality and outcomes such as IVH but not respiratory outcomes soon after birth, presumably because most infants at less than 28 weeks' gestation age receive some respiratory support and are imprecisely coded as having RDS.[25] A weakness of the studies is a lack of information about the severity of the early respiratory distress and any accurate categorization as to whether early deaths are caused by RDS.

Travers et al.[23] reported that ANS decreased mortality for all gestational ages from 24 to 34 weeks. The data are for the period from 2009 to 2013 (n = 61,571 infants) with about 84% of infants exposed to ANS, except at 34 weeks when the percent of exposure was 45% (Fig. 11.3). ANS exposure was associated with a remarkably consistent decreased

Gestational age	Number of infants	% given ANS	NNT
24	2,133	84	6
26	3,046	85	17
28	4,922	86	30
30	7,638	85	139
32	16,273	81	395
34	37,660	45	798

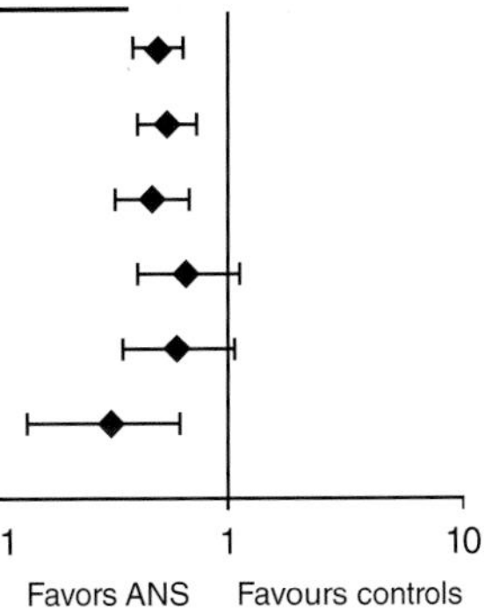

0.1   1   10

Favors ANS   Favours controls

Fig. 11.3 Epidemiology of a large clinical experience for the effect of ANS on infant mortality (2009–2013). Across gestations from 24 to 34 weeks, ANS was associated with a similar decrease in infant death, but the number needed to treat increased greatly as gestational age increased. *ANS,* Antenatal steroids. *NNT,* number needed to treat. (Data from Travers CP, Clark RH, Spitzer AR, et al. Exposure to any antenatal corticosteroids and outcomes in preterm infants by gestational age: prospective cohort study. *BMJ.* 2017;356:j1039.)

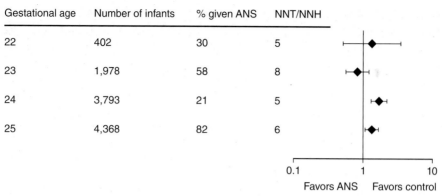

Gestational age	Number of infants	% given ANS	NNT/NNH	
22	402	30	5	
23	1,978	58	8	
24	3,793	21	5	
25	4,368	82	6	

Fig. 11.4 Association of antenatal steroid *(ANS)* use and the bronchopulmonary dysplasia (BPD) outcome. Across very early gestational ages, there was no decrease in BPD, and the overall effect was an increase in BPD. Data for 10,541 infants cared for in the Eunice Kennedy Shriver National Institute of Child Health and Human Development Neonatal Research Network from 1993 to 2009. *NNT/NNH,* number needed to treat or number needed to harm. (Data from Carlo WA, McDonald SA, Fanaroff AA, et al. Association of antenatal corticosteroids with mortality and neurodevelopmental outcomes among infants born at 22 to 25 weeks' gestation. *JAMA.* 2011;306(21):2348-2358.)

mortality even at 34 weeks' gestation. A similar report from Carlo et al.[22] documented decreased mortality and IVH for more than 10,000 infants for the gestational age range from 22 to 25 weeks with 74% of the population exposed to ANS. No respiratory outcomes are reported other than BPD, which is increased with the use of ANS (Fig. 11.4). The association of increased BPD with ANS is common across the RCTs and epidemiology studies. The generally accepted explanation is that ANS improve survival in the most marginal infants who are at increased risk of developing BPD. However, the arrest of septation and microvascular development with ANS may contribute to this adverse lung outcome.[7,16] A more recent cohort of 29,932 infants born at 22 to 25 weeks' gestation, of which 87% received ANS, showed similar positive effects in survival with no association with BPD.[24] The severity of BPD relative to ANS has not been analyzed and is worthy of evaluation.

The optimal interval from ANS treatment to delivery for maximal benefit based on the RCTs is 1 to 7 days.[26] However, the timing of maximal benefit to the lung is unclear and effects on other organs follow different timelines. A new analysis of a large European dataset indicates that maximal benefit for decreasing death may be an exposure interval as short as 18 to 36 hours, with benefit after 3 hours of administration.[27] Such rapid effects would be more consistent with acute steroid effects on cardiovascular function rather than for lung maturation. In preterm

lambs, improved cardiovascular function is observed at 24 hours after ANS and disappears by 2 days (our unpublished observation). However, at 24 hours post steroids, there is increased lung injury and pulmonary interstitial emphysema from mechanical ventilation, and maximal improvement in pulmonary function is seen at 5 days with residual effect up to 10 days.[9,28,29]

A concern with the observational associations between ANS and the clinical outcomes is that the great majority of women are treated with ANS. The women not given ANS differ in ways that cannot be reliably adjusted for in the analyses. The women not exposed to ANS have different causes and severities of problems related to prematurity.[22] Many likely deliver before ANS can be given. The epidemiologic analyses may overestimate the benefits of ANS at early gestational ages. Another concern is treatment creep. The RCT data to support use of ANS at early gestational ages are minimal, and RCTs for the use of ANS at "previable" gestational ages are nonexistent. Again, the epidemiology supports improved outcomes at gestations of 22 and 23 weeks, but that information likely reflects highly selected use of ANS in pregnancies being actively managed to achieve infant survival.[30]

REPEATED ANTENATAL STEROID TREATMENTS

The pregnancies of many women considered likely to deliver 1 to 7 days after ANS may continue for weeks or until term. A recent report noted that more than

50% of women given ANS did not deliver within 7 days.[10] The fact that the majority of women do not deliver in an optimal window for efficacy and many deliver at term is of substantial concern if this "off-target" treatment has adverse effects on the mother or infant. Multiple trials have evaluated predominantly Celestone for repeated ANS given at weekly intervals or at 2-week intervals, or when preterm delivery appeared to be imminent more than 7 days after the initial treatment. The benefits of steroids seem to be optimal at 1 to 7 days after ANS because some of the maturational effects seem to fade after 7 days, and repeated weekly treatments in animal models augment lung benefits.[31] The concerns with repeated treatments are cumulative injury to the fetal lung and neurodevelopment. A meta-analysis of 10 trials that randomized 4733 pregnancies demonstrated modest improvements in respiratory outcomes with no concerns for neurodevelopment.[32] However, several trials reported negative effects of repeated courses of ANS on birth weight and length, and one trial was stopped early for perceived adverse fetal growth effects.[33,34] There are fewer concerns about a single repeated dose of ANS, but the use of multiple weekly treatments likely is excessive. Further, a single dose of Celestone may be adequate for retreatment rather than the two-dose treatment; the results of a trial testing this strategy are pending.[35]

ANTENATAL STEROIDS AFTER 34 WEEKS' GESTATIONAL AGE

Although severe RDS is infrequent after 34 weeks' gestation and the treatment of RDS is generally successful, the odd ratios for RDS and transient tachypnea increase from normalized values of 1 at 38 to 40 weeks to 40 for RDS and 16 for transient tachypnea of the newborn at 34 weeks.[36] These late-gestation infants represent about 6% of the total delivery population and thus consume substantial resources. The definitive trial of ANS for women at risk of preterm delivery at 34/0 to 36/6 weeks' gestation randomly assigned 2831 women to the standard two-dose Celestone treatment or placebo.[37] There was a modest benefit for the composite primary outcome of need for respiratory support, stillbirth, or death, which decreased from 14.4% to 11.6% ($P = 0.023$), with the difference being for respiratory problems. Fewer infants exposed to

ANS than controls had severe respiratory morbidity or received surfactant treatment. However, 24% of ANS-exposed infants had transient hypoglycemia in contrast to 15% of controls. The Society for Maternal-Fetal Medicine statement recommends ANS selectively for late preterm birth,[38] but others have recommended caution because of the lack of follow-up and the relatively modest benefits.[39]

ANTENATAL STEROIDS BEFORE ELECTIVE C-SECTION

Another "late-gestation" use of ANS is before elective cesarean section at early term or term. Stutchfield et al.[40] randomly assigned 998 women to receive two doses of 12-mg betamethasone and found a decrease of about 50% for admittance of infants to a neonatal intensive care unit (NICU) and respiratory problems with the ANS. The benefit was for infants delivered before 39 weeks. A second trial randomly assigned 1280 women to receive three doses of 8-mg dexamethasone before elective cesarean section.[41] Administration of ANS was associated with a decrease in total NICU admissions from 3.9% to 1.6% ($P = 0.014$) and fewer NICU admissions for respiratory morbidity (number needed to treat = 43). From one perspective, the pathologic conditions prevented by ANS for elective cesarean sections are modest, but with cesarean deliveries exceeding 50% of all deliveries in some countries, the potential benefits are considerable. However, the therapy must be safe for use in the majority of women and fetuses, a high bar to confidently achieve.

CONCERNS REGARDING DRUG AND DOSE CHOICES FOR ANTENATAL STEROIDS

Liggins chose the 50/50 mixture of betamethasone phosphate plus betamethasone acetate for maternal intramuscular treatments to match the prolonged exposures with fetal infusions in sheep.[1,2] This dose and treatment interval were not validated by standard pharmacology. The other ANS treatment recommended by the World Health Organization (WHO) is four doses of 6-mg dexamethasone phosphate. There have been fewer clinical evaluations of this less expensive and widely available drug for ANS. Notably, there are no trials for repeated courses of treatment using dexamethasone.[32] Worldwide, different drugs and dosing schedules are used without validation—for example, in the United Kingdom, many centers use two doses of 12 mg of betamethasone phosphate, an untested drug. A similar two-dose regimen using dexamethasone phosphate was recently tested in the ASTEROID trial.[42] Pharmacokinetic studies suggest that drug doses are too high and result in prolonged maternal exposure. In nonpregnant reproductive age women, a single dose of Celestone results in detectable serum levels at 8 days after administration.[6] In preterm sheep and rhesus macaques, 25% lower doses result in similar improvement in lung function to the current clinical dose.[7,8] Further, dexamethasone phosphate or betamethasone phosphate given as two doses is less effective for lung maturation in sheep models.[43] Based on these recent studies, it is likely that the perinatal community is using the wrong drugs at higher doses than necessary to achieve the pulmonary benefits of ANS.[44] Concerns about risks of ANS should be minimized if lower dosing strategies can be developed.

LONG-TERM OUTCOMES AFTER ANTENATAL STEROIDS

The 30-year outcomes of the original Liggins and Howie trial were reassuring,[18,45] but those infants were more mature than current populations. One concern is that the follow-up from the early trials focused on the infants who were delivered before term, with no follow-up of those who received off-target treatments and were delivered close to or at term. Braun et al.[46] observed that newborns delivered after 34 weeks after receiving ANS treatment weighed less than unexposed newborns. There are many other cohort or convenience comparisons of variables (e.g., responses to stress and aortic stiffness) that suggest adverse effects of ANS in later life.[47] There is also increasing evidence of harm in infants exposed to ANS that deliver at term with higher incidence of neurodevelopmental and behavioral problems in those infants compared to term-born infants not exposed to ANS.[48,49] These outcomes are consistent with results from animal models; however, a substantial concern is that the human populations have not been randomly assigned to ANS treatment and followed beyond the newborn period. Because the great majority of women eligible for ANS are treated, a comparison population of unexposed children may not be representative. All observations

are further confounded by prematurity or threatened preterm labor.

ANTENATAL STEROID USE IN LOW-RESOURCE ENVIRONMENTS

Most of the premature infants born worldwide are born in low-resource environments and have a very high mortality rate. The use of ANS is very spotty despite being a priority of the WHO and other groups attempting to improve maternal and infant outcomes. The recently completed Antenatal Corticosteroid Trial illustrated the difficulties and risks of using ANS in low-resource environments.[50] This cluster randomized trial assigned almost 100,000 women in Pakistan, Africa, India, and Guatemala to the WHO-recommended ANS treatment of four doses of betamethasone after identification of risk of preterm delivery. Major problems were a lack of gestational age determination and identification of women at risk. Use of ANS did not improve outcomes for the smallest infants who had a perinatal mortality risk of more than 350 per 1000 births. More problematic was the increased mortality of off-target, ANS-exposed infants who were large and mature, perhaps because of increased infection.[51] This experience is a caution that all exposed infants need to be followed for outcomes, not just those delivered prematurely. A more recent randomized trial of dexamethasone compared to placebo with 3070 infants in low-resource countries showed decreased risk of neonatal death with ANS with no evidence of increased risk.[52] It is important to note, however, that the trial was conducted in secondary and tertiary hospitals with access to modern neonatal respiratory and nutritional interventions. A safe treatment in one environment may be neither safe nor effective in a different environment.

Postnatal Steroids

HISTORICAL REVIEW

There were brief reports of the use of systemic PNS before the first randomized trial by Avery et al. in 1985.[53] Only eight pairs of infants were randomly assigned to a 42-day course of systemic dexamethasone with an initial dose of 0.5 mg/kg vs. standard therapy. The steroid-treated infants improved and came off mechanical ventilation by 72 hours. This high-dose, long-tapering course was validated in a larger trial as superior to an 18-day course of dexamethasone in 1989 by Cummings et al.[54] The team of Doyle, Ehrenkranz, and Halliday has reported meta-analyses of PNS beginning in 2000, with updates continuing to the present.[55,56] These frequently updated reviews were critical to our understanding of a role for PNS in the care of very preterm infants at risk of developing BPD. Because of the frequent use of PNS and concerns about neuroinjury from PNS, the American Academy of Pediatrics and the Canadian Paediatric Association stated the following in 2002: "The routine use of systemic dexamethasone for the prevention or treatment of chronic lung disease in infants with very low birth weight is not recommended."[57] Although epidemiologic studies demonstrated a decrease in steroid use for infants born between 22 and 28 weeks' gestation from a high of 40% in 1996, steroids continue to be used in 10% to 15% of VLBW infants with respiratory failure.[58] A major contribution to the field was the meta-regression analysis in 2005 that was updated in 2014, demonstrating how the baseline risk of BPD in a population modulated the risks of death and cerebral palsy (Fig. 11.5).[59] If

the risks of adverse outcomes may be substantial, why do clinicians continue to use PNS? Shinwell et al.[60] demonstrated that in Israel as the use of PNS decreased, the incidence of BPD increased. The clear answer is that in trials and empirically, PNS facilitate weaning of infants from ventilators and ventilation is associated with poor outcomes.[61,62] However, substantial numbers of infants receive PNS even though they are not receiving significant respiratory support.[63]

PATHOPHYSIOLOGY OF BRONCHOPULMONARY DYSPLASIA: WHAT ARE WE TREATING WITH POSTNATAL STEROIDS?

Although an extensive discussion of BPD is beyond the scope of this chapter, BPD is recognized as the end result of lung injury and repair in VLBW infants.[64] Multiple antenatal variables contribute to postnatal injury mechanisms, such as oxygen exposure, mechanical stretch, and infection, which initiate and maintain chronic lung inflammation over weeks to months.[11] This injury/inflammation must be counteracted by repair mechanisms that support lung development for the infant to survive. PNS are potent synthetic steroids that are given systemically or as

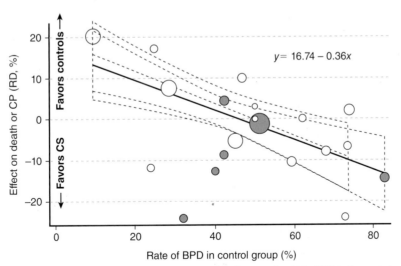

Fig. 11.5 Meta-regression analysis of 20 trials correlating the rate of bronchopulmonary dysplasia *(BPD)* in the control group with the effect of postnatal steroids on death or cerebral palsy *(CP)* expressed as the risk difference *(RD)* between control and steroid-treated infants. Each trial is represented by a *circle* and the size of the circle is proportional to the size of the trial. The higher the rate of BPD in the control group, the greater the likelihood of more benefit to be gained by postnatal steroids. Therefore, at more than 50% BPD in the control population, the benefit of postnatal steroids exceeds the risk. (Figure from Doyle LW, Halliday HL, Ehrenkranz RA, et al. An update on the impact of postnatal systemic corticosteroids on mortality and cerebral palsy in preterm infants: effect modification by risk of bronchopulmonary dysplasia. *J Pediatr.* 2014;165(6):1258-1260.)

aerosols in pharmacologic doses primarily to decrease lung inflammation. However, as mentioned earlier, steroids in developing animal models also interfere with air space septation and microvascular development.[16] Conceptually, PNS have been given from soon after birth to "prevent" BPD, after 7 days of age to "treat" and decrease the incidence of BPD, or more chronically after 36 weeks' gestational age to improve lung function in infants with BPD. The effects of PNS are certainly infant-age-at-treatment–specific and are much more complex than simply suppression of inflammation.

META-ANALYSES OF EARLY AND LATE TREATMENTS

Early treatments, defined by Doyle et al. as treatment at less than 8 days of age, have focused primarily on death and BPD as outcomes.[55] Although the use of PNS did not decrease death in 28 trials, their use did decrease BPD (RR 0.79, 95% CI 0.71–0.88), but the complications of treatment were substantial and included hyperglycemia, hypertension, gastrointestinal perforation, and cerebral palsy. The simultaneous use of indomethacin and dexamethasone was associated with an increased risk of gastrointestinal perforation in several trials.[64] The consensus has been that early PNS are of minimal benefit and their use causes substantial adverse outcomes. However, new trials described in the following sections may change that assessment.

PNS given after 7 days of age did not increase death in 19 trials, and benefits were earlier extubation (RR 0.64, 95% CI 0.56–0.74) and decreased BPD (RR 0.78, 95% CI 0.66–0.88).[56] Although hyperglycemia and hypertension were complications, gastrointestinal perforation and necrotizing enterocolitis were not. The neurodevelopmental outcomes were comparable between PNS-exposed and control infants except for abnormal neurologic examination results in four trials, which may not predict longer-term outcomes. The conclusion of the meta-analysis for late PNS is that the benefits exceed the risks for infants who cannot be weaned from the ventilator before 36 weeks. There is no systematic information about PNS use for infants who require very prolonged ventilation.

DRUG, DOSE, ROUTE, AND DURATION OF THERAPY

Although the trials of PNS are numerous, resulting in meta-analyses that appear to be robust, the trials are quite heterogeneous with varied drug choice, dose, and duration of treatment. Most trials have used dexamethasone phosphate for intervals ranging from 10 to 42 days. Most of the neurodevelopmental outcome data are for infants treated with the high-dose, 42-day treatment beginning at 0.5 mg/kg per day. Many of the adverse outcomes—particularly hyperglycemia and hypertension—likely result from high-dose, prolonged treatments. The adverse neurodevelopmental outcomes may also result from the high dose. A major problem for interpreting trial results is that control infants often were given open-label PNS. Thus, for all outcomes, variable numbers of placebo-treated infants received PNS with poorly documented treatments. As with ANS, formal pharmacologic or pharmacodynamic studies have not been done for PNS.

The recent trend based on small trials has been to decrease the dose and duration of treatment.[65,66] The most influential lower-dose trial is the Dexamethasone: A Randomized Trial (DART) study, which randomly assigned infants to an initial dose of 0.15 mg/kg dexamethasone or placebo.[67] The steroid treatment then was decreased over a 10-day treatment. This international RCT was stopped early because of an inability to enroll patients after the therapy was not recommended by the American Academy of Pediatrics and the Canadian Paediatric Association—a most unfortunate outcome. The trial was planned for 814 patients and ended with just 35 patients in the treatment arm and 35 patients in the control arm. Nevertheless, the dexamethasone-treated infants had striking decreases in oxygen need and fewer PNS-treated infants experienced failed extubation. It is more than ironic that this failed trial has established the default standard of care for PNS use. Hyperglycemia and hypertension were not complications of this low-dose, short-duration PNS protocol. Even lower doses of dexamethasone for PNS may be equally effective but remain to be tested. A recent network meta-analysis of treatments including 62 randomized trials of inhaled, systemic, or intratracheal PNS suggests that short course of less than 8 days of moderate cumulative doses of 2 to 4 mg/kg initiated at 8 to 14 days would be the most appropriate regimen, but the quality of the evidence for this regimen is low.[68]

ALTERNATIVES TO EARLY SYSTEMIC POSTNATAL STEROIDS

Hydrocortisone has been used more frequently in Europe for PNS than dexamethasone. Hydrocortisone is attractive because of its mineralocorticoid potency with relative low glucocorticoid potency. The use of hydrocortisone infusions at 1 mg/kg from day 1 for 7 days followed by 0.5 mg/kg to day 10 was evaluated by Baud et al.[69] in the PREMILOC trial, which included 521 randomly assigned infants of 26.4 weeks average gestational age. The benefits were earlier extubation and more survival without BPD; these benefits were larger for girls and for infants exposed to chorioamnionitis. There was, however, on a subgroup analysis, an increased risk of sepsis in infants born at 24 and 25 weeks' gestation. A recent trial from the National Institute of Child Health and Human Development (NICHD) network for the use of hydrocortisone to facilitate extubation after 14 days of life in infants born before 30 weeks' gestation found that hydrocortisone facilitated extubation compared to placebo but had no effect on survival without moderate or severe BPD or survival without moderate or severe neurodevelopmental impairment.[70]

Aerosolized PNS are frequently used for infants with severe BPD using different steroids and delivery devices with a wide variance in use between neonatal services.[71] In a meta-analysis that evaluated eight trials of inhaled PNS that included 232 infants, the aerosols were begun at more than 7 days of life and did not decrease death or BPD.[72] Of note, there also was no decrease in extubation failure or oxygen use, which are the short-term benefits of systemic PNS for extubation. The aerosolized steroids may have decreased the use of systemic steroids. A second trial evaluated budesonide delivered by metered-dose inhaler.[73] The treatment was two doses/day from day 1 to 14 and one dose per day until 32 weeks or weaned off oxygen and pressure support. This much larger trial randomly assigned 856 patients of 26 weeks' mean gestational age. A nonsignificant 3.3% increase in deaths favored the placebo. The benefit was a significant 10.2% decrease in BPD with the steroid treatment. The authors were cautious about the benefits given the potential risk of increased death.

Surprisingly, although the meta-analysis results and the general consensus are that early use of PNS has a decidedly adverse risk to benefit ratio, innovative trials have recently been published that challenge not using PNS soon after birth to prevent BPD. Two trials used aerosolized steroids. Nakamura et al.[74] randomly assigned 211 infants at a mean gestational age of 26.1 weeks to a fluticasone metered inhaler given twice a day beginning on day 1 after birth and continued to extubation while the other group received placebo. There were no differences in death or the composite outcome of death or oxygen use at discharge overall, but the combined outcome favored PNS for 24 to 26 weeks' gestational age infants and infants exposed to chorioamnionitis.

The most remarkable results were reported by Yeh et al.[75] for a strategy of mixing 0.25 mg/kg of micronized budesonide with surfactant for treatment of infants with RDS versus surfactant alone. They randomly assigned 265 infants of average gestational age of 26.7 weeks for the surfactant treatments at about 2 hours of age. Infants receiving surfactant plus budesonide had no difference in death but a remarkable decrease in BPD from 50% to 29%. Severe BPD also decreased significantly. One strength of this report is that follow-up at 2 to 3 years in a subset of the infants showed no adverse effects of the PNS on neurodevelopment. In animal models, however, intratracheal budesonide does have systemic effects including effects on the brain.[76]

These four trials are proof of principle that early PNS can decrease BPD. In the trials by Nakamura et al. and Bassler et al., the fetal exposure to chorioamnionitis resulted in larger and significant decreases in BPD. This outcome can be interpreted as indicating that early PNS can effectively target the fetal lung inflammation associated with chorioamnionitis. Table 11.2 highlights some of the results from these trials. The aerosol and surfactant plus budesonide treatment strategies target the lungs and thus should have fewer complications. The 10-day hydrocortisone systemic therapy has the advantage of shorter exposures to PNS relative to the aerosols. The surfactant plus budesonide trial was the trial most targeted to the lung, had the shortest exposure, and resulted in the greatest decrease in BPD without increased mortality. The doses for these trials have not been evaluated for optimal effects, admittedly a difficult task in clinical neonatology. These trials challenge the notion that early PNS use is undesirable.

TABLE 11.2   Summary of Recent Early Steroid Trials

Exposures and Outcomes	Fluticasone Inhaler[75]	Budesonide Aerosol[74]	Intravenous Hydrocortisone[70]	Budesonide + Surfactant[76]
Steroid exposure	Targeted to the lungs	Targeted to the lungs	Very low dose, but systemic	Targeted to the lungs
Duration of treatment	Until extubation	Off support or 32 weeks	10 days	With surfactant treatments
Death	Increased by 2.5%	Increased by 3.3%	Decreased by 5%	Decreased by 3%
Bronchopulmonary dysplasia	Decreased by 10.8%	Decreased by 10.2%	Decreased by 4%	Decreased by 21%

While early PNS are also frequently used in neonatology for the management of low blood pressures, presumably due to adrenal insufficiency, Renolleau et al. reported very high cord blood cortisol values in extremely low-birth-weight (ELBW) infants, primarily associated with chorioamnionitis and increased IVH and intestinal perforation.[77] Tolia et al., in an epidemiological study, also reported that higher doses of hydrocortisone were associated with increased death.[78] Therefore, as frequently observed in neonatology, more is not necessarily better.

HOW POSTNATAL STEROIDS ARE USED

Based on our understanding of risks and benefits and the primary mechanism of action of PNS as potent antiinflammatory drugs, we suggest an initial course of PNS only for infants "stuck" on a ventilator and without overt infection. A target time for treatment is 2 to 3 weeks of age with a simple goal: cease ventilation and begin noninvasive respiratory support. We use the DART protocol of 0.15 mg/kg dexamethasone with the dose decreased and stopped by 10 days.[48] However, if the infant has not made progress toward extubation by 3 days, PNS are stopped. Once PNS have been started, then the obligation of the clinical team is to push for an optimized extubation trial. If the PNS fail to improve the infant's condition or the extubation attempt fails, then routine care continues for several more weeks until the infant's condition improves or the team, in desperation, starts another course of PNS. We do not use aerosolized steroids. It is important to note that many preterm infants who are ventilated at 2 to 3 weeks of age will eventually be weaned from the ventilator due to ongoing growth and repair ability of the neonatal lung.

Summary and Future Directions

Corticosteroids are intimately entwined in the care of women at risk of preterm delivery and their preterm infants. Endogenous steroids are essential for fetal and newborn survival. ANS decrease infant death and multiple complications of prematurity, although the standard treatments are likely using the wrong dosing strategies. Caution is warranted for the use of ANS in low-resource environments unless gestation is known and at least basic care is available for the mother and infant. PNS are used because they work, and lower dosing strategies need to be evaluated. An often-overlooked reality is that the majority of very preterm infants are exposed as fetuses to ANS. Other "steroid use opportunities" beyond treatments to prevent or treat BPD with PNS are hydrocortisone to support blood pressure and dexamethasone for airway edema or elective extubation.[79] Thus infants may be exposed to steroids for a number of reasons, and the sickest and most immature infants will have the most reasons. For the future, we need to judiciously use steroids at the lowest doses and for the shortest durations possible. Specific organ targeting such as the addition of budesonide to surfactant is particularly attractive to minimize risk. A perspective on steroids in perinatal medicine is provided by the (modified) apocryphal statement by Galen: "All who receive steroids recover in a short time, except those whom steroids do not help, who all die. It is obvious, therefore, that steroids fail only in incurable cases."

REFERENCES

1. Liggins GC. Premature delivery of foetal lambs infused with glucocorticoids. *J Endocrinol*. 1969;45(4):515-523.
2. Liggins GC, Howie RN. A controlled trial of antepartum glucocorticoid treatment for prevention of the respiratory distress syndrome in premature infants. *Pediatrics*. 1972;50(4):515-525.
3. Effect of corticosteroids for fetal maturation on perinatal outcomes. NIH Consensus Development Panel on the Effect of Corticosteroids for Fetal Maturation on Perinatal Outcomes. *JAMA*. 1995;273(5):413-418.
4. Roberts D, Dalziel S. Antenatal corticosteroids for accelerating fetal lung maturation for women at risk of preterm birth. *Cochrane Database Syst Rev*. 2006(3):CD004454.
5. McGoldrick E, Stewart F, Parker R, et al. Antenatal corticosteroids for accelerating fetal lung maturation for women at risk of preterm birth. *Cochrane Database Syst Rev*. 2020;12:CD004454.
6. Jobe AH, Milad MA, Peppard T, et al. Pharmacokinetics and pharmacodynamics of intramuscular and oral betamethasone and dexamethasone in reproductive age women in India. *Clin Transl Sci*. 2020;13(2):391-399.
7. Schmidt AF, Kannan PS, Bridges JP, et al. Dosing and formulation of antenatal corticosteroids for fetal lung maturation and gene expression in rhesus macaques. *Sci Rep*. 2019; 9(1):9039.
8. Schmidt AF, Kemp MW, Rittenschober-Bohm J, et al. Low-dose betamethasone-acetate for fetal lung maturation in preterm sheep. *Am J Obstet Gynecol*. 2018;218(1):132.e1-132.e9.
9. Kemp MW, Saito M, Schmidt AF, et al. The duration of fetal antenatal steroid exposure determines the durability of preterm ovine lung maturation. *Am J Obstet Gynecol*. 2020;222(2): 183.e1-183.e9.
10. Makhija NK, Tronnes AA, Dunlap BS, et al. Antenatal corticosteroid timing: accuracy after the introduction of a rescue course protocol. *Am J Obstet Gynecol*. 2016;214(1):120.e1-120e6.
11. Jobe AH. Animal models, learning lessons to prevent and treat neonatal chronic lung disease. *Front Med (Lausanne)*. 2015;2:49.
12. Ikegami M, Polk D, Jobe A. Minimum interval from fetal betamethasone treatment to postnatal lung responses in preterm lambs. *Am J Obstet Gynecol*. 1996;174(5):1408-1413.
13. Willet KE, Jobe AH, Ikegami M, et al. Lung morphometry after repetitive antenatal glucocorticoid treatment in preterm sheep. *Am J Respir Crit Care Med*. 2001;163(6):1437-1443.
14. Bridges JP, Sudha P, Lipps D, et al. Glucocorticoid regulates mesenchymal cell differentiation required for perinatal lung morphogenesis and function. *Am J Physiol Lung Cell Mol Physiol*. 2020;319(2):L239-L255.
15. Schmidt AF, Kannan PS, Bridges J, et al. Prenatal inflammation enhances antenatal corticosteroid-induced fetal lung maturation. *JCI Insight*. 2020;5(24):e139452.
16. Massaro D, Massaro GD. Dexamethasone accelerates postnatal alveolar wall thinning and alters wall composition. *Am J Physiol*. 1986;251(2 Pt 2):R218-R224.
17. Jobe AH, Polk DH, Ervin MG, et al. Preterm betamethasone treatment of fetal sheep: outcome after term delivery. *J Soc Gynecol Investig*. 1996;3(5):250-258.
18. Dalziel SR, Rea HH, Walker NK, et al. Long term effects of antenatal betamethasone on lung function: 30 year follow up of a randomised controlled trial. *Thorax*. 2006;61(8):678-683.
19. Fawke J, Lum S, Kirkby J, et al. Lung function and respiratory symptoms at 11 years in children born extremely preterm: the EPICure study. *Am J Respir Crit Care Med*. 2010;182(2):237-245.
20. Bandyopadhyay A, Slaven JE, Evrard C, et al. Antenatal corticosteroids decrease forced vital capacity in infants born fullterm. *Pediatr Pulmonol*. 2020;55(10):2630-2634.
21. Gonzales LW, Ballard PL, Ertsey R, et al. Glucocorticoids and thyroid hormones stimulate biochemical and morphological differentiation of human fetal lung in organ culture. *J Clin Endocrinol Metab*. 1986;62(4):678-691.
22. Carlo WA, McDonald SA, Fanaroff AA, et al. Association of antenatal corticosteroids with mortality and neurodevelopmental outcomes among infants born at 22 to 25 weeks' gestation. *JAMA*. 2011;306(21):2348-2358.
23. Travers CP, Clark RH, Spitzer AR, et al. Exposure to any antenatal corticosteroids and outcomes in preterm infants by gestational age: prospective cohort study. *BMJ*. 2017;356:j1039.
24. Ehret DEY, Edwards EM, Greenberg LT, et al. Association of antenatal steroid exposure with survival among infants receiving postnatal life support at 22 to 25 weeks' gestation. *JAMA Netw Open*. 2018;1(6):e183235.
25. Bancalari EH, Jobe AH. The respiratory course of extremely preterm infants: a dilemma for diagnosis and terminology. *J Pediatr*. 2012;161(4):585-588.
26. Roberts D, Brown J, Medley N, Dalziel SR. Antenatal corticosteroids for accelerating fetal lung maturation for women at risk of preterm birth. *Cochrane Database Syst Rev*. 2017;3:CD004454.
27. Norman M, Piedvache A, Borch K, et al. Association of short antenatal corticosteroid administration-to-birth intervals with survival and morbidity among very preterm infants: results from the EPICE cohort. *JAMA Pediatr*. 2017;171(7):678-686.
28. Willet KE, Jobe AH, Ikegami M, Newnham J, Sly PD. Pulmonary interstitial emphysema 24 hours after antenatal betamethasone treatment in preterm sheep. *Am J Respir Crit Care Med*. 2000;162(3 Pt 1):1087-1094.
29. Schmidt AF, Kemp MW, Rittenschober-Bohm J, et al. Low-dose betamethasone-acetate for fetal lung maturation in preterm sheep. *Am J Obstet Gynecol*. 2017;218:132.e1-132.e9. doi: 10.1016/j.ajog.2017.11.560.
30. Mori R, Kusuda S, Fujimura M, Neonatal Research Network J. Antenatal corticosteroids promote survival of extremely preterm infants born at 22 to 23 weeks of gestation. *J Pediatr*. 2011;159(1):110-114.e1.
31. Ikegami M, Jobe AH, Newnham J, Polk DH, Willet KE, Sly P. Repetitive prenatal glucocorticoids improve lung function and decrease growth in preterm lambs. *Am J Respir Crit Care Med*. 1997;156(1):178-184. doi:10.1164/ajrccm.156.1.9612036.
32. Crowther CA, McKinlay CJ, Middleton P, Harding JE. Repeat doses of prenatal corticosteroids for women at risk of preterm birth for improving neonatal health outcomes. *Cochrane Database Syst Rev*. 2015(7):CD003935. doi:10.1002/14651858. CD003935.pub4.
33. Murphy KE, Hannah ME, Willan AR, et al. Multiple courses of antenatal corticosteroids for preterm birth (MACS): a randomised controlled trial. *Lancet*. 2008;372(9656):2143-2151. doi:10.1016/S0140-6736(08)61929-7.
34. Wapner RJ, Sorokin Y, Thom EA, et al. Single versus weekly courses of antenatal corticosteroids: evaluation of safety and efficacy. *Am J Obstet Gynecol*. 2006;195(3):633-642.
35. Schmitz T, Alberti C, Ursino M, et al. Full versus half dose of antenatal betamethasone to prevent severe neonatal respiratory distress syndrome associated with preterm birth: study protocol for a randomised, multicenter, double blind, placebo-controlled, non-inferiority trial (BETADOSE). *BMC Pregnancy Childbirth*. 2019;19(1):67.

36. Consortium on Safe L, Hibbard JU, Wilkins I, et al. Respiratory morbidity in late preterm births. *JAMA*. 2010;304(4):419-425. doi:10.1001/jama.2010.1015.

37. Gyamfi-Bannerman C, Thom EA, Blackwell SC, et al. Antenatal Betamethasone for women at risk for late preterm delivery. *N Engl J Med*. 2016;374(14):1311-1320. doi:10.1056/NEJMoa1516783.

38. Society for Maternal-Fetal Medicine Publications C. Implementation of the use of antenatal corticosteroids in the late preterm birth period in women at risk for preterm delivery. *Am J Obstet Gynecol*. 2016;215(2):B13-B15. doi:10.1016/j.ajog.2016.03.013.

39. Kamath-Rayne BD, Rozance PJ, Goldenberg RL, Jobe AH. Antenatal corticosteroids beyond 34 weeks gestation: what do we do now? *Am J Obstet Gynecol*. 2016;215(4):423-430. doi:10.1016/j.ajog.2016.06.023.

40. Stutchfield P, Whitaker R, Russell I, Antenatal Steroids for Term Elective Caesarean Section Research T. Antenatal betamethasone and incidence of neonatal respiratory distress after elective caesarean section: pragmatic randomised trial. *BMJ*. 2005; 331(7518):662. doi:10.1136/bmj.38547.416493.06.

41. Nada AM, Shafeek MM, El Maraghy MA, Nageeb AH, Salah El Din AS, Awad MH. Antenatal corticosteroid administration before elective caesarean section at term to prevent neonatal respiratory morbidity: a randomized controlled trial. *Eur J Obstet Gynecol Reprod Biol*. 2016;199:88-91. doi:10.1016/j.ejogrb.2016.01.026.

42. Crowther CA, Ashwood P, Andersen CC, et al. Maternal intramuscular dexamethasone versus betamethasone before preterm birth (ASTEROID): a multicentre, double-blind, randomised controlled trial. *Lancet Child Adolesc Health*. 2019;3(11):769-780. doi:10.1016/S2352-4642(19)30292-5.

43. Schmidt AF, Kemp MW, Kannan PS, et al. Antenatal dexamethasone vs. betamethasone dosing for lung maturation in fetal sheep. *Pediatr Res*. 2017;81(3):496-503. doi:10.1038/pr.2016.249.

44. Kemp MW, Schmidt AF, Jobe AH. Optimizing antenatal corticosteroid therapy. *Semin Fetal Neonatal Med*. 2019;24:176-181. doi:10.1016/j.siny.2019.05.003.

45. Dalziel SR, Walker NK, Parag V, et al. Cardiovascular risk factors after antenatal exposure to betamethasone: 30-year follow-up of a randomised controlled trial. *Lancet*. 2005;365(9474):1856-1862. doi:10.1016/S0140-6736(05)66617-2.

46. Braun T, Sloboda DM, Tutschek B, et al. Fetal and neonatal outcomes after term and preterm delivery following betamethasone administration. *Int J Gynaecol Obstet*. 2015;130(1):64-69. doi:10.1016/j.ijgo.2015.01.013.

47. Kelly BA, Lewandowski AJ, Worton SA, et al. Antenatal glucocorticoid exposure and long-term alterations in aortic function and glucose metabolism. *Pediatrics*. 2012;129(5):e1282-e1290. doi:10.1542/peds.2011-3175.

48. Melamed N, Asztalos E, Murphy K, et al. Neurodevelopmental disorders among term infants exposed to antenatal corticosteroids during pregnancy: a population-based study. *BMJ Open*. 2019;9(9):e031197. doi:10.1136/bmjopen-2019-031197.

49. Raikkonen K, Gissler M, Kajantie E. Associations between maternal antenatal corticosteroid treatment and mental and behavioral disorders in children. *JAMA*. 2020;323(19):1924-1933. doi:10.1001/jama.2020.3937.

50. Althabe F, Aleman A, Berrueta M, et al. A multifaceted strategy to implement brief smoking cessation counseling during antenatal care in argentina and uruguay: a cluster randomized trial. *Nicotine Tob Res*. 2016;18(5):1083-1092. doi:10.1093/ntr/ntv276.

51. Althabe F, Thorsten V, Klein K, et al. The Antenatal Corticosteroids Trial (ACT)'s explanations for neonatal mortality: a secondary analysis. *Reprod Health*. 2016;13(1):62. doi:10.1186/s12978-016-0175-3.

52. Collaborators WAT, Oladapo OT, Vogel JP, et al. Antenatal dexamethasone for early preterm birth in low-resource countries. *N Engl J Med*. 2020;383(26):2514-2525. doi:10.1056/NEJMoa2022398.

53. Avery GB, Fletcher AB, Kaplan M, Brudno DS. Controlled trial of dexamethasone in respirator-dependent infants with bronchopulmonary dysplasia. *Pediatrics*. 1985;75(1):106-111. Available at: https://www.ncbi.nlm.nih.gov/pubmed/3880879.

54. Cummings JJ, D'Eugenio DB, Gross SJ. A controlled trial of dexamethasone in preterm infants at high risk for bronchopulmonary dysplasia. *N Engl J Med*. 1989;320(23):1505-1510. doi:10.1056/NEJM198906083202301.

55. Doyle LW, Ehrenkranz RA, Halliday HL. Early (< 8 days) postnatal corticosteroids for preventing chronic lung disease in preterm infants. *Cochrane Database Syst Rev*. 2014(5): CD001146. doi:10.1002/14651858.CD001146.pub4.

56. Doyle LW, Ehrenkranz RA, Halliday HL. Late (> 7 days) postnatal corticosteroids for chronic lung disease in preterm infants. *Cochrane Database Syst Rev*. 2014(5):CD001145. doi:10.1002/14651858.CD001145.pub3.

57. Committee on F, Newborn. Postnatal corticosteroids to treat or prevent chronic lung disease in preterm infants. *Pediatrics*. 2002;109(2):330-338. doi:10.1542/peds.109.2.330.

58. Stoll BJ, Hansen NI, Bell EF, et al. Trends in care practices, morbidity, and mortality of extremely preterm neonates, 1993-2012. *JAMA*. 2015;314(10):1039-1051. doi:10.1001/jama.2015.10244.

59. Doyle LW, Halliday HL, Ehrenkranz RA, et al. An update on the impact of postnatal systemic corticosteroids on mortality and cerebral palsy in preterm infants: effect modification by risk of bronchopulmonary dysplasia. *J Pediatr*. 2014;165(6):1258-1260.

60. Shinwell ES, Lerner-Geva L, Lusky A, Reichman B. Less postnatal steroids, more bronchopulmonary dysplasia: a population-based study in very low birthweight infants. *Arch Dis Child Fetal Neonatal Ed*. 2007;92(1):F30-F33. doi:10.1136/adc.2006.094474.

61. Barnett ML, Tusor N, Ball G, et al. Exploring the multiple-hit hypothesis of preterm white matter damage using diffusion MRI. *Neuroimage Clin*. 2018;17:596-606. doi:10.1016/j.nicl.2017.11.017.

62. Vliegenthart RJS, Onland W, van Wassenaer-Leemhuis AG, De Jaegere APM, Aarnoudse-Moens CSH, van Kaam AH. Restricted ventilation associated with reduced neurodevelopmental impairment in preterm infants. *Neonatology*. 2017; 112(2):172-179. doi:10.1159/000471841.

63. Virkud YV, Hornik CP, Benjamin DK, et al. Respiratory support for very low birth weight infants receiving dexamethasone. *J Pediatr*. 2017;183:26-30.e3. doi:10.1016/j.jpeds.2016.12.035.

64. Higgins RD, Jobe AH, Koso-Thomas M, et al. Bronchopulmonary dysplasia: executive summary of a workshop. *J Pediatr*. 2018;197:300-308. doi:10.1016/j.jpeds.2018.01.043.

65. Stark AR, Carlo WA, Tyson JE, et al. Adverse effects of early dexamethasone treatment in extremely-low-birth-weight infants. National Institute of Child Health and Human Development Neonatal Research Network. *N Engl J Med*. 2001; 344(2):95-101. doi:10.1056/NEJM200101113440203.

66. Durand M, Mendoza ME, Tantivit P, Kugelman A, McEvoy C. A randomized trial of moderately early low-dose dexamethasone therapy in very low birth weight infants: dynamic pulmonary

mechanics, oxygenation, and ventilation. *Pediatrics*. 2002; 109(2):262-268. doi:10.1542/peds.109.2.262.

67. Doyle LW, Davis PG, Morley CJ, McPhee A, Carlin JB, Investigators DS. Low-dose dexamethasone facilitates extubation among chronically ventilator-dependent infants: a multicenter, international, randomized, controlled trial. *Pediatrics*. 2006;117(1): 75-83. doi:10.1542/peds.2004-2843.

68. Ramaswamy VV, Bandyopadhyay T, Nanda D, et al. Assessment of postnatal corticosteroids for the prevention of bronchopulmonary dysplasia in preterm neonates: a systematic review and network meta-analysis. *JAMA Pediatr*. 2021;175(6):e206826. doi:10.1001/jamapediatrics.2020.6826.

69. Baud O, Maury L, Lebail F, et al. Effect of early low-dose hydrocortisone on survival without bronchopulmonary dysplasia in extremely preterm infants (PREMILOC): a double-blind, placebo-controlled, multicentre, randomised trial. *Lancet*. 2016;387(10030):1827-1836. doi:10.1016/S0140-6736(16)00202-6.

70. Watterberg K, Walsh M, Li L, et al. Hydrocortisone to improve survival without bronchopulmonary dysplasia. *N Engl J Med*. 2022;386(12):1121-1131. doi:10.1056/NEJMoa2114897.

71. Slaughter JL, Stenger MR, Reagan PB, Jadcherla SR. Utilization of inhaled corticosteroids for infants with bronchopulmonary dysplasia. *PLoS One*. 2014;9(9):e106838. doi:10.1371/journal.pone.0106838.

72. Onland W, Offringa M, van Kaam A. Late (>/= 7 days) inhalation corticosteroids to reduce bronchopulmonary dysplasia in preterm infants. *Cochrane Database Syst Rev*. 2017;8:CD002311. doi:10.1002/14651858.CD002311.pub4.

73. Bassler D, Plavka R, Shinwell ES, et al. Early inhaled budesonide for the prevention of bronchopulmonary dysplasia. *N Engl J Med*. 2015;373(16):1497-1506. doi:10.1056/NEJMoa1501917.

74. Nakamura T, Yonemoto N, Nakayama M, et al. Early inhaled steroid use in extremely low birthweight infants: a randomised controlled trial. *Arch Dis Child Fetal Neonatal Ed*. 2016;101(6): F552-F556. doi:10.1136/archdischild-2015-309943.

75. Yeh TF, Chen CM, Wu SY, et al. Intratracheal administration of budesonide/surfactant to prevent bronchopulmonary dysplasia. *Am J Respir Crit Care Med*. 2016;193(1):86-95. doi:10.1164/rccm.201505-0861OC.

76. Hillman NH, Kothe TB, Schmidt AF, et al. Surfactant plus budesonide decreases lung and systemic responses to injurious ventilation in preterm sheep. *Am J Physiol Lung Cell Mol Physiol*. 2020;318(1):L41-L48. doi:10.1152/ajplung.00203.2019.

77. Renolleau C, Toumazi A, Bourmaud A, et al. Association between baseline cortisol serum concentrations and the effect of Prophylactic hydrocortisone in extremely preterm infants. *J Pediatr*. 2021;234:65-70.e3. doi:10.1016/j.jpeds.2020.12.057.

78. Tolia VN, Bahr TM, Bennett MM, et al. The association of hydrocortisone dosage on mortality in infants born extremely premature. *J Pediatr*. 2019;207:143-147.e3. doi:10.1016/j.jpeds.2018.11.023.

79. Finer NN, Powers RJ, Ou CH, et al. Prospective evaluation of postnatal steroid administration: a 1-year experience from the California Perinatal Quality Care Collaborative. *Pediatrics*. 2006;117(3):704-713. doi:10.1542/peds.2005-0796.

Chapter 12

Cell-Based Therapy for Neonatal Lung Diseases

Karen Cecile Young, Bernard Thebaud, and Won Soon Park

Chapter Outline

Introduction
Endogenous Lung Stem Cells
  Alveolar Stem Cells
  Lung Mesenchymal Stem Cells
  Lung Endothelial Progenitors
Cell Therapies for Neonatal Lung Diseases
  The Evidence from Preclinical Studies

Mechanisms of Repair
From Bench to Bedside: The Evidence from Clinical Trials
Barriers and Opportunities for Implementation
Conclusion

Key Points

- The postnatal lung contains populations of stem cells that reconstitute the lung following injury.
- Prematurity and its antecedent factors alter endogenous stem cells leading to dysfunctional lung repair.
- Preterm infants who develop bronchopulmonary dysplasia (BPD) exhibit decreased and/or dysfunctional lung stem cells.
- Mesenchymal stem cells augment lung repair by supporting endogenous lung progenitors, promoting angiogenesis, and reducing inflammation, apoptosis, and fibrosis.
- Cell-free approaches such as stem cell–derived extracellular vesicles preserve lung development in experimental BPD models.
- Early evidence from clinical trials suggest that mesenchymal stem cell therapy is safe in preterm infants at high risk for developing BPD.
- Induced pluripotent stem cell–derived three-dimensional structures are effective platforms for lung disease modeling and drug development.

Introduction

Stem cells are unspecialized cells with two fundamental properties: the ability to divide and make more copies of themselves through a process of self-renewal and the ability to differentiate into various mature specialized progenies depending on their potency (Fig. 12.1). Totipotent stem cells are capable of differentiating into all adult and embryonic tissues, including extraembryonic tissues such as trophectoderm.[1,2] In mammals, only the zygote and the first cleavage blastomeres are totipotent.[2] Pluripotent stem cells are capable of differentiating into derivatives of all three germ layers (ectoderm, mesoderm, and endoderm) and are typically derived from embryos at different embryonic stages of development.[3] They are not able to form extraembryonic tissues such as the placenta. Multipotent stem cells are able to differentiate into multiple cell types of one lineage.[4] The most prominent example remains hematopoietic stem cells, which are capable of differentiating into all cell types of the hematopoietic system.[5]

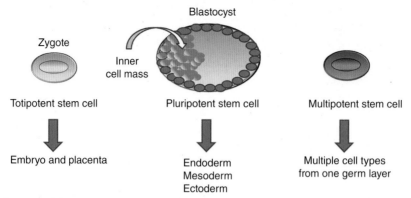

Fig. 12.1 Stem cell potency. Totipotent stem cells (zygote or first cleavage blastomeres) can give rise to all cells in the embryo and placenta. Pluripotent stem cells (e.g., embryonic stem cells) can give rise to the entire embryo and all cell lineages (endoderm, mesoderm, and ectoderm). Multipotent stem cells typically give rise to cells in one cell lineage.

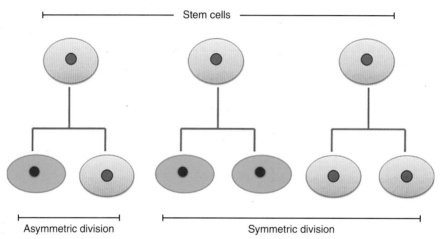

Fig. 12.2 Stem cell division. Stem cells may divide asymmetrically or symmetrically. During symmetric division, the stem cells divide and produce two daughter stem cells or two differentiated daughter progeny. Alternatively, during asymmetric division, the stem cell produces one differentiated daughter progeny and one stem cell.

Stem cells may also be categorized as embryonic or adult stem cells. Embryonic stem cells are derived from blastocysts and are pluripotent.[6] In 2006, Japanese scientists discovered that mouse skin cells could be reprogrammed to function like embryonic stem cells.[7] These cells named "induced pluripotent stem cells" (iPSCs) are being used as a platform to recapitulate some of the crucial differentiation cues that promote cell lineage commitment, to model diseases, engineer new tissues, and test drug efficacy.[8]

On the other hand, adult stem cells are typically multipotent cells. Following asymmetric cell division (Fig. 12.2), adult stem cells produce a population of transit-amplifying progenitor cells.[9] The latter acts as an intermediate between dedicated stem cells and mature differentiated cells. Another population termed facultative stem cells or progenitors are normally quiescent differentiated cells, but following injury, they self-renew and give rise to other differentiated progeny.[10,11] The postnatal lung contains multiple stem and progenitor cell populations located in complex anatomic niches. These cells are activated following injury, but chronic insults deplete this endogenous progenitor cell pool.[12,13] In newborn rodents, hyperoxia exposure alters lung stem and progenitor cell populations morphologically and functionally.[14,15] Conversely, administration of stem cells prevents neonatal lung injury by replenishing the endogenous stem/progenitor cell niche.[16,17] Discoveries such as these have revolutionized the stem cell field. Clinical trials utilizing mesenchymal stem cell (MSC)–based therapies suggest that stem cells are safe and potentially efficacious in neonatal lung diseases.[18,19] Alternative cell-free approaches such as stem cell–derived extracellular vesicles are also promising as they lack tumorigenicity and allow easier biodistribution.[20] Studies evaluating tissue engineering strategies to manufacture functional tissue ex vivo are also underway.[21] This chapter will discuss recent advances in lung stem cell biology, our current understanding of the impact of perinatal exposures on endogenous stem cells, and the application as well as challenges of implementing stem cell–based therapies for neonatal lung diseases.

Endogenous Lung Stem Cells

Attempts to identify a dedicated lung stem cell capable of regenerating all cells within the lung have remained elusive. Instead, lineage tracing studies and single cell transcriptomic methodologies suggest that there are unique anatomic niches of multipotent alveolar, endothelial, and MSC/progenitors that support lung homeostasis and facilitate repair.

ALVEOLAR STEM CELLS

It is now well appreciated that alveolar type 2 epithelial cells (AEC2) are the stem cells for the alveoli.[22-25] Not only are AEC2 capable of self-renewal but they also replenish the alveolar type 1 epithelial cells (AEC1) population under both steady state and injury conditions.[26] In 3D culture, AEC2 form alveolospheres containing cells which express both AEC2 and AEC1 markers.[26] Subsets of AEC2, however, have variable regenerative potential. In whole lung and primary cultures of adult rat AEC2, a hyperoxia-resistant subpopulation of telomerase-positive AEC2 expands in response to injury.[27] In contrast, a

subpopulation of AEC2 with high surface levels of telomerase but low E-cadherin are more proliferative and less likely to undergo hyperoxic damage as compared to AEC2 which express high levels of . E-cadherin.[28] More recent evidence suggests that a rare population of AEC2 that express Axin2[+] are the main alveolar progenitor cells of the distal lung.[29] Axin2[+] AEC2 are in close proximity to fibroblasts expressing Wnt ligands. During severe lung injury, Axin2[+] AEC2 proliferate in response to Wnt ligand and transiently expand the stem cell pool for repair.[30] On the other hand, in the absence of Wnt ligand, AEC2 differentiate into AEC1.

Other rare populations of undifferentiated basally located distal airway stem cells expressing cytokeratin 5, transcription factor 63, and cytokeratin 14 have been also identified as potential alveolar progenitors.[31-33] These cells originate from SOX2[+] airway progenitors,[34] are inactive under steady-state conditions but proliferate and migrate into the alveoli following severe influenza-induced lung injury, differentiating into both airway and alveolar lineages.[31-33] Moreover, in an ovine chorioamnionitis model, acute intrauterine inflammation reduces lung P63[+] alveolar progenitor cell population.[35] The role of P63[+] alveolar progenitor cells in neonatal lung disease, however, remains poorly understood as these cells do not give rise to AEC.

Rare populations of epithelial cells located at the bronchoalveolar duct junction, so-called bronchoalveolar stem cells (BASCS), are another candidate alveolar progenitor population.[36] These cells express both surfactant protein C (SP-C) and secretoglobulin (Scgb1a1), are resistant to naphthalene, and proliferate rapidly after bleomycin-induced lung injury.[37] Although BASCs are unchanged in hyperoxia-induced lung injury,[38] BASCs are able to give rise to AEC2 cells following bleomycin-induced lung injury.[39,40] In specialized culture media, BASCs give rise to cells which express pro–SP-C, aquaporin 5, and Scgb1a1, suggesting that these cells could give rise to cells in the conducting as well as gas exchange portion of the lung. More research is however needed to elucidate the regenerative capacity of these alveolar progenitor cells in BPD, their interactions with cells in the lung vasculature and mesenchymal compartment, and the molecular mechanisms that drive these alveolar progenitors toward quiescence or activation.

LUNG MESENCHYMAL STEM CELLS

Emerging evidence suggests that the fetal lung is enriched with MSCs.[41] Lung MSCs are similar to bone marrow (BM)–derived MSCs in their adherence to plastic, expression of cell surface markers such as CD105, CD90, and CD73, and their capacity to differentiate into osteoblasts, chondroblasts, and adipocytes under appropriate in vitro conditions.[42] However, compared with BM-MSCs, lung MSCs seem to be constitutively more prone to epithelial differentiation[43] and have a distinct pattern of *Hox* gene expression implicated in lung development.[44] Lung MSCs produce proangiogenic and epithelial cell growth factors and appear to be directly involved in regulating the growth and function of endothelial and epithelial cells.[41,45] Lung MSCs are decreased in newborn rodents exposed to hyperoxia[41,46] and supraphysiologic oxygen levels alter the morphology and secretome of lung MSCs.[41] Unlike steady-state conditions, lung MSCs exposed to oxygen secrete less proangiogenic factors and have increased expression of myofibroblast markers.[41] Intriguingly, increased MSCs in the tracheal aspirate of preterm infants predict an increased risk for BPD by more than 25-fold.[47] Moreover, MSCs isolated from the lungs of preterm infants differentiate into myofibroblasts under the influence of the profibrotic factor, transforming growth factor-β.[48] Conceivably, lung microenvironmental cues may influence MSC behavior and function, potentially driving them toward a more dysfunctional fibrotic phenotype.

LUNG ENDOTHELIAL PROGENITORS

Endothelial dysfunction is a key player in the pathogenesis of preterm lung diseases. Thus, the identification of a population of peripheral blood mononuclear cells capable of differentiating into endothelial cells, termed endothelial progenitor cells (EPCs) by Asahara et al., provided an exciting opportunity for lung endothelial cell regeneration.[49] These putative EPCs, which expressed CD34 and VEGFR2, were however later found to be actually myeloid cells with angiogenic properties and they had relatively low capacity to regenerate the lung endothelium.[49,50] Almost a decade later, Alvarez et al. demonstrated that the lung microvascular endothelium is enriched with progenitor cells that exhibit vasculogenic capability.[51] These cells are highly proliferative and quite similar to endothelial colony forming cells (ECFCs), which were identified in umbilical cord blood (UCB).[52,53]

More recently, elegant lineage tracing studies have demonstrated that another population of alveolar capillary stem cells, so-called "gCap" cells, play a role in maintenance and repair of the endothelium.[54] gCap cells express c-kit and increase during development, but neonatal hyperoxia significantly reduces the number of these cells.[55] Interestingly, a unique subset of gCaps which express c-kit and FOXF1 are also reduced in murine alveolar capillary dysplasia.[56] Another population of endothelial cells that express high levels of carbonic anhydrase 4 (Car4) and CD34 were also found to significantly contribute to the proliferative response of the endothelium following lung injury.[57] The exact functional role of Car4[high] endothelial cells in neonatal lung injury is however unclear. Intriguingly, adoptive transfer of c-kit⁺ EPCs increases angiogenesis and prevents alveolar simplification in neonatal mice exposed to hyperoxia.[14] This suggests that these c-kit⁺ EPCs play a pivotal role in neonatal lung endothelial cell homeostasis and repair.[14]

Cell Therapies for Neonatal Lung Diseases

THE EVIDENCE FROM PRECLINICAL STUDIES

The above insights into stem cell biology have unraveled the therapeutic potential of stem cells. Specifically, MSCs have attracted much attention because of their ease of isolation, culture and expansion, allogeneic use, and pleiotropic therapeutic effects.[42] MSCs are of particular interest for a multifactorial disease, such as BPD, in which multiple pathophysiologic mechanisms contribute to impaired alveolar and lung vascular development. Early proof-of-concept studies in neonatal rodents exposed to hyperoxia showed that rodent BM-MSCs administered intravenously (IV) or intratracheally (IT) prevent the arrest in lung vascular and alveolar growth (Fig. 12.3).[46,58] An interesting source of MSCs, especially when treating neonatal diseases, is represented by perinatal tissue. The placenta and umbilical cord (UC) are usually discarded after birth, yet they contain a large number of various cells, including MSCs, with therapeutic potential and can be harvested without harm to the

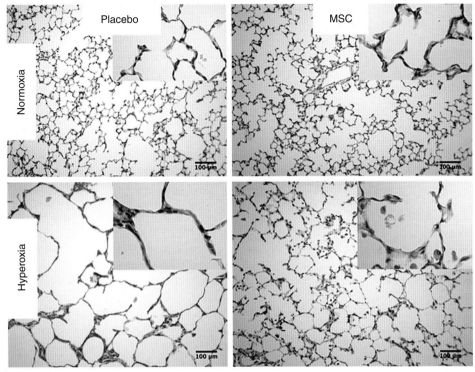

Fig. 12.3 MSCs improve hyperoxia-induced alveolar simplification. Lung sections demonstrating improved alveolar structure following administration of MSCs to neonatal rats with hyperoxia-induced lung injury. *MSC*, Mesenchymal stem cell.

mother or the newborn. After the aforementioned proof-of-concept studies, MSCs derived from the UC (Wharton Jelly) and UCB have been studied extensively in experimental BPD models. Similar to the therapeutic benefit reported for BM-MSCs, UC and UCB-derived MSCs demonstrated comparable effects in hyperoxia-induced neonatal lung injury in rodents.[59-63] These include improved alveolar and lung vascular structures, restoration of alveolar growth, attenuation of lung fibrosis, reduced lung inflammation, and improved exercise capacity. The therapeutic benefit persisted into adulthood with no evidence of tumor formation or adverse effects on lung architecture.[59,63] Since then, numerous investigators have attempted to optimize the use of MSCs by exploring the best timing, dose, and route of administration. A consistent finding however is the low rate of lung engraftment of MSCs. Increasing evidence suggests that MSCs act via a paracrine mechanism to protect the developing lung from injury.[64]

MECHANISMS OF REPAIR

Similar observation of low organ engraftment of transplanted MSC had already been observed in the heart and the central nervous system. The working hypothesis became that MSCs release bioactive molecules that modulate organ repair. Proof-of-concept experiments in vitro showed that cell-free conditioned media derived from MSCs prevent hyperoxia-induced alveolar epithelial cell apoptosis, accelerate alveolar epithelial cell wound healing, and preserve endothelial cord formation on matrigel during hyperoxia.[46]

This paracrine effect was then confirmed in vivo. The efficacy of intraperitoneal administration of MSCs in protecting the neonatal rodent lung suggested a paracrine activity of these cells.[60,65] Direct in vivo evidence was provided by studies in which a single IV injection of cell-free MSC-derived conditioned media improved lung function, alveolar injury, and pulmonary hypertension.[58,66] A single IT injection of BM-MSCs or BM-MSC–free conditioned media offered protected from oxygen-induced alveolar and vascular injury with a persistent benefit up to 3 months.[67] Likewise, cell-free conditioned media derived from human UCB-MSCs injected intraperitoneally prevented and reversed arrested alveolar growth and lung function in hyperoxic-exposed rats with persistent safety and therapeutic benefit up to 6 months.[59]

Thus, rather than replacing injured cells and differentiating into lung cells, MSCs release factors that protect resident lung cells from injury or modulate the function of inflammatory cells. For example, BM-MSC and BM-MSC–derived conditioned media increase the number of BASCs in neonatal mice exposed to hyperoxia.[17] In addition, MSCs can modulate the phenotype of macrophages from a M1 (proinflammatory) to a M2 (healer) phenotype in various disease conditions.[68,69] The interactions between MSC and other immune cells, however, remain unexplored in neonates.

The identification of soluble factors in the conditioned media may allow the discovery of novel repair mechanisms and therapeutic interventions.[70] Likewise, the variety of factors released by MSCs explains their pleiotropic effects and further underscores the rationale for MSC therapy for BPD. MSCs produce factors known to promote lung growth and repair such as keratinocyte growth factors,[71] vascular endothelial growth factor,[72,73] and adiponectin.[74] Novel molecules secreted by MSCs have already been identified, such as stanniocalcin-1[75]—a potent antioxidant—or tumor necrosis factor-alpha–stimulated gene/protein 6 (TSG-6)[76]—a potent antiinflammatory protein, and shown therapeutic benefit in various disease models. These discoveries open interesting therapeutic avenues into manufacturing superior therapeutic cells. For example, preconditioning of BM-MSCs ex vivo in hyperoxia for 24 hours enhanced the release of stanniocalcin-1 in the conditioned media and boosted the therapeutic benefit of preconditioned MSCs on lung architecture in hyperoxic neonatal rodents compared to nonpreconditioned media.[77]

The recognition of the paracrine effect of MSCs has also renewed the excitement into extracellular vesicles, which are crucial for cell-to-cell communication. In particular, MSCs, like many other cells, release membrane-derived nanosize extracellular vesicles, acting as cargos that contain not only the combination of bioactive molecules but also microRNAs (miRNAs).[78] miRNAs are small noncoding RNA molecules involved in transcriptional regulation of gene expression and this may explain the long-term effect of single injections of MSC-derived conditioned media. miRNAs may represent interesting therapeutic targets in the prevention of BPD through activation or silencing of specific genes with beneficial or deleterious effects on lung development.[79] In adult lung injury models, MSC-derived extracellular vesicles attenuate lung macrophage influx, decrease proinflammatory cytokine levels in the bronchoalveolar lavage, and prevent pulmonary vascular remodeling and hypoxic-induced pulmonary hypertension in mice.[80] In hyperoxia models of BPD, MSC-derived extracellular vesicles restore normal lung development,[81-84] alter lung macrophage polarization toward a more antiinflammatory phenotype, and reprogram bone marrow–derived myeloid cells.[85] The therapeutic effects of MSC-derived extracellular vesicles persist long after the acute hyperoxic injury. Intriguingly, antenatal administration of MSC-derived extracellular vesicles in experimental chorioamnionitis[86] and preeclampsia models[87] also promote normal lung development.[88]

FROM BENCH TO BEDSIDE: THE EVIDENCE FROM CLINICAL TRIALS

The aforementioned preclinical evidence supporting the role of MSC transplantation as a potential therapy for BPD without short- and long-term toxicity or tumorigenicity[59,60,62,63,89] provided the foundation for the first clinical trial in preterm newborn infants.[19] This study was an open-label, single-center clinical trial that assessed the safety and feasibility of a single intratracheal transplantation of allogenic human UCB–derived MSCs for BPD. MSCs were transplanted into nine very preterm infants at high risk for developing BPD (mean gestational age 25.3 ± 0.9 weeks, range 24–26 weeks; mean birth weight 793 ± 127 g, range 630–1030 g) at a mean age of 10.4 ± 2.6 days (range 7–14 days) after birth. All of the infants were on ventilator support, the settings of which could not be decreased due to significant respiratory distress within 24 hours prior to enrollment. The first three patients received a low dose of MSCs (1×10^7 cells/kg in 2 mL/kg of saline), while the remaining six patients received a high dose (2×10^7 cells/kg in 4 mL/kg of saline). The

MSCs were administered intratracheally into the left and right lungs in two fractions via a gavage tube, the same method used to administer surfactant. The treatment was well tolerated without any serious adverse effects or dose-limiting toxicity up to 84 days following transplantation. The incidence of serious adverse effects did not significantly differ in the low- and high-dose groups. The levels of IL-6, IL-8, matrix metalloproteinase (MMP)-9, tumor necrosis factor alpha (TNF-α), and transforming growth factor beta 1 (TGF-β1) in the tracheal aspirates collected on day 7 were significantly reduced compared to baseline and day 3 post-transplantation levels. Furthermore, compared to a historical gestational age–, birth weight–, and respiratory severity score–matched control group, BPD severity was significantly lower in transplant recipients. Overall, these findings suggested that IT allogenic human UCB–derived MSC transplantation in very preterm infants at high risk for developing BPD is safe and feasible.

Long-term follow-up studies extending up to 2 years showed no adverse effects.[90] A recently completed phase II double-blind, randomized, multicenter, controlled clinical trial investigating the efficacy and safety of low-dose MSC transplantation compared with a control group for the treatment of BPD in preterm infants 23 to 28 weeks' gestational age showed no difference in the primary outcome of death or moderate/severe BPD between the groups.[18] MSC transplantation however reduced tracheal aspirate inflammatory cytokine levels, and on subgroup analysis, 23 to 24 weeks preterm infants showed a lower incidence of severe BPD with MSC transplantation.[18]

BARRIERS AND OPPORTUNITIES FOR IMPLEMENTATION

Clinical introduction of cell-based therapies could be a paradigm shift in neonatal medicine and in the treatment of BPD and other neonatal lung diseases. However, barriers to clinical implementation, including optimization of the cells delivered to the right patients via the right route, at the right time and dose, need to be overcome for the success of future clinical translation.[19,91–97]

The Ideal Cell

Determining the optimal cells for transplantation is the most critical issue for successful clinical translation.

MSCs have been extensively investigated, and their therapeutic efficacy has consistently been proven in animal models of BPD.[46,60,98–100] Since donor cells do not engraft,[77] allogenic transplantation of MSCs is considered to be safe. Moreover, considering the time-consuming and costly isolation and expansion processes involved in the generation of autologous MSCs, allogenic therapy might have a logistical advantage for its ability to be used off-the-shelf in a clinical setting.

MSCs are also broadly distributed in the body; UCB-derived MSCs exhibit better efficacy in attenuating hyperoxic lung injuries and greater paracrine potency compared to fat-derived MSCs in newborn rats.[99] UCB and UC-derived MSCs are both attractive for therapy as they are easily harvested, more proliferative,[101] and potentially more immunomodulatory[102] as compared to BM-derived MSCs. The yield of MSCs in term UCB is however quite low and isolation of these cells has not always been successful.[101,103] UC-derived MSCs are isolated with significantly more efficiency than BM or UCB-derived MSCs.[104] There is also some evidence that UC-MSCs have greater antiinflammatory effects, potentially due to differences in its expression of surface immunomodulatory molecules and cytokines.[102,105] UC-MSCs do not express CD80, CD40, or CD86, surface molecules involved in T-lymphocyte activation.[106] They also have a higher expression of several antiinflammatory cytokines than BM-derived MSCs.[101,107,108] In one small study, UC-MSCs had better antiinflammatory effects than BM-MSCs in a rodent model of BPD, but the cells tested were obtained from only three donors.[109]

The impact of gender in MSC efficacy has also been explored. Female BM-MSCs secrete more proangiogenic and antiinflammatory factors than BM-MSCs derived from males.[110] In neonatal rats with hyperoxia-induced lung injury, female BM-MSCs are superior to male BM-MSCs in reducing lung inflammation, improving pulmonary hypertension, and attenuating vascular remodeling.[110] These beneficial effects are particularly more pronounced in male recipients, suggesting that female cells[110] maybe a potent BM-MSC population for BPD complicated by severe PH.

Production of a high-quality, standardized, clinical-grade product using good manufacturing practice (GMP) criteria is important in the success of MSCs in a clinical setting.[95] One concern is that the expansion of stem cells in media containing fetal bovine serum (FBS) may increase the risk of zoonotic infections and immunological reactions. Platelet concentrates are an alternative, but obtaining sufficient quantities of autologous platelets from children is challenging. An emerging possibility is Xeno-free synthetic media as there is evidence of increased viable cell yield as compared to FBS-containing expansion media.[111]

Another important issue is the influence of high passage number, freezing, and thawing on stem cell behavior. There is substantial evidence that extended cell passages may induce senescence and genetic instability[112] and thus most clinical trials utilize early passage cells. The effect of cryopreservation on MSC behavior has yielded controversial results. In one animal study, freshly isolated stem cells have a higher therapeutic value than cryopreserved cells as the latter impairs immunosuppressive properties and disrupts the actin cytoskeleton, altering their biodistribution.[113] Other studies however report similar efficacy of fresh and cryopreserved cells.[114] Most preclinical and clinical studies to date utilize cryopreserved cells but some investigators suggest that cryopreserved cells should be recovered in culture prior to administration. Whether this alters stem cell behavior and potency needs further investigation. Based on present evidence, both the Korean and US FDAs approved the use of allogenic human UCB–derived MSCs manufactured with strict GMP compliance for use in phase I/II BPD clinical trials conducted in Korea[19] and the United States.[115]

ECFCs,[116] amniotic fluid stem cells,[117] BM-derived c-kit+ cells[118] have also been evaluated in preclinical models of BPD with varying beneficial effects. A recent systematic review and meta-analysis of 53 preclinical studies assessing 15 different cell-based therapies for BPD concluded that MSCs were the most effective cell therapy although there were few head-to-head comparisons and substantial risk of bias was identified.[119] In a first human phase I study to evaluate the safety and tolerability of allogeneic human amnion epithelial cells in preterm infants at high risk of BPD, the cells were shown to be safe, with no treatment-associated complications at 2-year follow-up.[120]

iPSCs are another autologous source being investigated for neonatal lung regeneration. iPSCs are derived by directly reprogramming mature somatic cells to an embryonic pluripotent state, unidentifiable from embryonic stem cells.[7,121] Yamanaka and colleagues demonstrated that by overexpressing Oct4, Sox2, Klf4, and c-myc, in murine fibroblasts, they were transformed into embryonic stem–like pluripotent stem cells, free of the ethical concerns of embryonic stem cells, but capable of differentiating into derivatives of all three germ layers. iPSCs have been generated from multiple somatic cell sources, and using specific cell differentiation cocktails, iPSCs can be differentiated into any cell of interest. The inherent pluripotency of iPSCs however increases their risk of tumor formation; thus "iPSC-derived" cell-based strategies are being evaluated. For instance, airway delivery of iPSC-derived type 2 alveolar epithelial cells or iPSC-derived lung progenitor cells improve lung function and structure in an experimental model of BPD.[122] The use of gene-editing technology in combination with iPSC technology is also a promising approach to cure monogenic disorders. Gene correction of iPSCs derived from patients carrying a homozygous surfactant mutation restores surfactant processing in type 2 alveolar epithelial cells.[123] iPSC differentiation efficiency however needs improvement as it may take months to get adequate quantities of differentiated cell populations for transplantation. Another important issue is that potentially some pluripotent cells could remain in the iPSC-derived differentiated cell population and lead to malignancy in the recipient. There is also evidence that the process used to reprogram somatic cells to iPSCs alters DNA methylation. Whether this is also evident in iPSC cell derivatives needs to be clarified and screening iPSC-derived cells for any genetic variants will be crucial in moving this therapy forward.

Cell-free approaches will also need further optimization. Willis et al. showed similar lung alveolar protective effects using BM-MSC or UC-MSC–derived extracellular vesicles in a murine BPD model.[29] But extracellular vesicles lack the ability to respond to microenvironmental cues potentially limiting their efficacy. Standardization of extracellular vesicle isolation, purification, manufacturing techniques, potency assays, industrial scale up, circulation kinetics, and biodistribution will be critical.

The Ideal Recipient

Despite its potential benefits, cautious risk benefit evaluations must be made. Identification of preterm infants at highest risk for BPD is a very important step in the application of these potentially beneficial rescue/preventive strategies. Since early gestational age and prolonged respiratory support have be cited as the most important predictors of BPD development among extremely preterm infants,[97] infants of 24 to 26 weeks' gestation needing continuous ventilator support were enrolled in the phase I clinical trial conducted by Chang et al.[19] However, evidence from a multicenter phase II study suggests that preterm infants of 23 to 24 weeks may have the most significant benefit.[18] Additional clinical predictors and/or biomarkers[96] will be necessary to further stratify these infants and determine which infants will ultimately progress to BPD, thus avoiding unnecessary treatment exposure.

Other lung diseases with significant neonatal mortality may also benefit from cell-based therapies. Intraamniotic injection of amniotic fluid–derived stem cells promotes lung growth in experimental CDH models.[124] But interestingly, while amniotic fluid–derived stem cell extracellular vesicles promote fetal lung regeneration in CDH, BM-MSC extracellular vesicles did not have similar beneficial effects. This is potentially secondary to differences in their RNA cargo.[125] The ideal stem cell source may therefore need to be patient- and disease-specific. It should however be noted that even the most rigorously sorted stem cell population might be heterogeneous. Deciphering the biological and functional significance of the variable subpopulations will provide an opportunity for more targeted therapies.

The Ideal Time

While the therapeutic efficacy of MSC transplantation in the prevention and rescue of experimental BPD has already been shown, the optimal timing of their administration is a key issue that remains to be clarified. To date, most published studies have been performed in neonatal rodent hyperoxia-induced lung injury models, which closely mimic the phenotype of severe BPD complicated by pulmonary hypertension. Pierro et al.[100] reported that MSCs or their conditioning media were not only effective for prevention at postnatal day 4 but also their use at postnatal day 14 as a rescue approach both prevented and rescued hyperoxic alveolar growth arrest in newborn rats with

experimental BPD. Chang and colleagues compared the therapeutic efficacy of early versus late MSC administration in newborn rats at postnatal day 3 or postnatal day 10 as well as at both of these time points.[62] This study found significant attenuation of neonatal hyperoxic lung injuries only with early but not with late MSC transplantation, and combined early and late transplantation did not have a synergistic effect. In a study by van Haaften et al.,[46] MSC transplantation at postnatal day 4 for prevention significantly attenuated hyperoxic lung injuries in neonatal rodents, while transplantation at postnatal day 14 for regeneration showed no effect. Based on these preclinical data, the therapeutic time window for MSC transplantation in the treatment of BPD appears to be narrow. It however seems prudent that, in a clinical setting, early identification of the highest risk preterm infants and administration of MSCs within the first few days of life seems preferable over later administration in infants with established BPD.

The Ideal Route

To determine the optimal route of MSC transplantation, several routes, including local IT instillation,[46,60] systemic IV injection,[58,126] and intraperitoneal administration,[60] have been tested. As injured lung tissue produces chemotactic factors, systemically transplanted MSCs migrate[127] and localize to the injured lung.[128] The most convenient and minimally invasive systemic IV approach might be more therapeutically advantageous compared with a local IT approach, especially in very unstable preterm infants with BPD. There is, however, substantial evidence that stem cells are often trapped in the pulmonary capillaries.[129] Despite this limitation, IV delivery of stem cells and their extracellular vesicles has shown efficacy in neonatal lung diseases.[85] In one recent study, monocytes engulfed MSCs trapped in the lung and these circulating monocytes mediated MSC antiinflammatory effects.[130] Yet, most preterm infants at high risk of BPD are intubated and receive ventilator support, and since MSCs can be instilled in the same way as surfactant, IT MSC transplantation during the first days of life might not be so invasive in the extremely preterm infants.[19] Furthermore, despite a fourfold lower dose and more frequent donor cell engraftment, better paracrine potency and attenuation of hyperoxic lung injuries were observed with local IT MSC transplantation than with systemic administration.[60,126] Based on superior therapeutic efficacy observed with local IT compared with systemic IV or intraperitoneal transplantation as demonstrated in this preclinical data, MSCs were delivered IT in the most recent phase I and phase II clinical trials.[18,19]

The Ideal Dose

As previous studies[60,126] have shown that the MSC therapeutic dose could be reduced more than fourfold by choosing a local IT route over systemic IV or intraperitoneal administration, the route of MSC administration might be a major determinant of optimal dosing. Chang et al.[89] compared the therapeutic efficacy of three different doses of human UCB–derived MSCs (5×10^3, 5×10^4, and 5×10^5 cells per animal, reflecting $0.5–50 \times 10^6$ cells per kg body weight) given IT to hyperoxic newborn rat pups at postnatal day 5. The best therapeutic effects were seen in the mid- and high-dose treatment groups. Based on this evidence, a single IT administration of 1×10^7 cells/kg (low-dose, three infants) and 2×10^7 cells (high-dose, six infants) was used in the phase I clinical trial; no dose-limiting toxicity or serious adverse events was observed with either dose.[19] In light of these findings, further preclinical and clinical studies examining the optimal MSC dose of resulting in clinical benefit to human preterm neonates with BPD are anticipated.

Conclusion

In recent years, various translational studies have broadened the knowledge and understanding of stem cell therapy in neonatal lung injury, and clinical trials are harnessing the therapeutic potential of stem cell therapies for neonatal lung diseases, particularly BPD. The exciting progress in both preclinical and clinical research has brought human stem cell therapy for neonatal lung diseases one step closer to clinical translation. It is, however, important to recognize that while stem cells and their derivatives have medicinal properties, they are biologics with complex and dynamic behaviors. A better understanding of the potential protective mechanism of stem cells and the resolution of several issues, such as manufacturing processes, clinical indication, timing, and dose, is required to permit safe clinical translation of stem cell therapy. Potency assays predicting the therapeutic efficacy of stem cells in neonatal lung diseases have been challenging to develop. Ideally, potency testing should evaluate the ability of cell therapy to achieve a specific biological effect, but since stem cell function is driven by microenvironmental cues, potency assays need to be patient- and disease-specific. Combining stem technologies with new gene-editing approaches and tissue engineering techniques has tremendous promise. It will be essential to proceed sequentially rather than in haste with relentless efforts to overcome all obstacles in making stem cell therapy the next treatment breakthrough for neonatal lung diseases.

REFERENCES

1. Kelly SJ. Studies of the developmental potential of 4- and 8-cell stage mouse blastomeres. *J Exp Zool.* 1977;200(3):365-376.
2. Modlinski JA. The fate of inner cell mass and trophectoderm nuclei transplanted to fertilized mouse eggs. *Nature.* 1981;292(5821):342-343.
3. Donovan PJ, Gearhart J. The end of the beginning for pluripotent stem cells. *Nature.* 2001;414(6859):92-97.
4. Rawlins EL, Okubo T, Xue Y. The role of Scgb1a1+ Clara cells in the long-term maintenance and repair of lung airway, but not alveolar, epithelium. *Cell Stem Cell.* 2009;4:525-534.
5. Wu AM, Siminovitch L, Till JE, et al. Evidence for a relationship between mouse hemopoietic stem cells and cells forming colonies in culture. *Proc Natl Acad Sci U S A.* 1968;59(4):1209-1215.
6. Thomson JA, Itskovitz-Eldor J, Shapiro SS, et al. Embryonic stem cell lines derived from human blastocysts. *Science.* 1998;282(5391):1145-1147.
7. Takahashi K, Yamanaka S. Induction of pluripotent stem cells from mouse embryonic and adult fibroblast cultures by defined factors. *Cell.* 2006;126(4):663-676.
8. Shi Y, Inoue H, Wu JC, Yamanaka S. Induced pluripotent stem cell technology: a decade of progress. *Nat Rev Drug Discov.* 2017;16(2):115-130.
9. Potten CS, Loeffler M. Stem cells: attributes, cycles, spirals, pitfalls and uncertainties. Lessons for and from the crypt. *Development.* 1990;110(4):1001-1020.
10. Rawlins EL, Hogan BL. Epithelial stem cells of the lung: privileged few or opportunities for many? *Development.* 2006;133(13):2455-2465.
11. Rawlins EL, Okubo T, Que J, et al. Epithelial stem/progenitor cells in lung postnatal growth, maintenance, and repair. *Cold Spring Harb Symp Quant Biol.* 2008;73:291-295.
12. Whitsett J. A lungful of transcription factors. *Nat Gen.* 1998;20:7.
13. Maeda Y, Dave V, Whitsett JA. Transcriptional control of lung morphogenesis. *Physiol Rev.* 2007;87:219-244.
14. Ren X, Ustiyan V, Guo M, et al. Postnatal alveologenesis depends on FOXF1 signaling in c-KIT+ endothelial progenitor cells. *Am J Respir Crit Care Med.* 2019;200(9):1164-1176.
15. Alphonse RS, Vadivel A, Fung M, et al. Existence, functional impairment, and lung repair potential of endothelial colony-forming

cells in oxygen-induced arrested alveolar growth. *Circulation*. 2014;129(21):2144-2157.

16. Leeman KT, Pessina P, Lee JH, et al. Mesenchymal stem cells increase alveolar differentiation in lung progenitor organoid cultures. *Sci Rep*. 2019;9(1):6479.

17. Tropea KA, Leder E, Aslam M, et al. Bronchioalveolar stem cells increase after mesenchymal stromal cell treatment in a mouse model of bronchopulmonary dysplasia. *Am J Physiol Lung Cell Mol Physiol*. 2012;302(9):L829-L837.

18. Ahn SY, Chang YS, Lee MH, et al. Stem cells for bronchopulmonary dysplasia in preterm infants: a randomized controlled phase II trial. *Stem Cells Transl Med*. 2021;10(8):1129-1137.

19. Chang YS, Ahn SY, Yoo HS, et al. Mesenchymal stem cells for bronchopulmonary dysplasia: phase 1 dose-escalation clinical trial. *J Pediatr*. 2014;164(5):966-972.e6.

20. Willis GR, Kourembanas S, Mitsialis SA. Toward exosome-based therapeutics: isolation, heterogeneity, and fit-for-purpose potency. *Front Cardiovasc Med*. 2017;4:63.

21. Mao AS, Mooney DJ. Regenerative medicine: current therapies and future directions. *Proc Natl Acad Sci U S A*. 2015;112(47): 14452-14459.

22. Adamson IY, Bowden DH. The type 2 cell as progenitor of alveolar epithelial regeneration: a cytodynamic study in mice after exposure to oxygen. *Lab Invest*. 1974;30(1):35-42.

23. Tryka AF, Witschi H, Gosslee DG, et al. Patterns of cell proliferation during recovery from oxygen injury: species differences. *Am Rev Respir Dis*. 1986;133(6):1055-1059.

24. Adamson IY, Bowden DH. The type 2 cell as progenitor of alveolar epithelial regeneration: a cytodynamic study in mice after exposure to oxygen. *Lab Invest*. 1974;30:35.

25. Adamson IY, Bowden DH. Derivation of type 1 epithelium from type 2 cells in the developing rat lung. *Lab Invest*. 1975;32:736.

26. Barkauskas CE, Cronce MJ, Rackley CR, et al. Type 2 alveolar cells are stem cells in adult lung. *J Clin Invest*. 2013;123(7):3025-3036.

27. Driscoll B, Buckley S, Bui KC, et al. Telomerase in alveolar epithelial development and repair. *Am J Physiol Lung Cell Mol Physiol*. 2000;279(6):L1191-L1198.

28. Reddy R, Buckley S, Doerken M, et al. Isolation of a putative progenitor subpopulation of alveolar epithelial type 2 cells. *Am J Physiol Lung Cell Mol Physiol*. 2004;286(4):L658-L667.

29. Zacharias WJ, Frank DB, Zepp JA, et al. Regeneration of the lung alveolus by an evolutionarily conserved epithelial progenitor. *Nature*. 2018;555(7695):251-255.

30. Nabhan AN, Brownfield DG, Harbury PB, et al. Single-cell Wnt signaling niches maintain stemness of alveolar type 2 cells. *Science*. 2018;359(6380):1118-1123.

31. Vaughan AE, Brumwell AN, Xi Y, et al. Lineage-negative progenitors mobilize to regenerate lung epithelium after major injury. *Nature*. 2015;517(7536):621-625.

32. Zuo W, Zhang T, Wu DZA, et al. p63+Krt5+ distal airway stem cells are essential for lung regeneration. *Nature*. 2015; 517(7536):616-620.

33. Kumar Pooja A, Hu Y, Yamamoto Y, et al. Distal airway stem cells yield alveoli in vitro and during lung regeneration following H1N1 influenza infection. *Cell*. 2011;147(3):525-538.

34. Ray S, Chiba N, Yao C, et al. Rare SOX2(+) airway progenitor cells generate KRT5(+) cells that repopulate damaged alveolar parenchyma following influenza virus infection. *Stem Cell Reports*. 2016;7(5):817-825.

35. Widowski H, Ophelders DRMG, van Leeuwen AJCN, et al. Chorioamnionitis induces changes in ovine pulmonary endogenous epithelial stem/progenitor cells in utero. *Pediatr Res*. 2021; 90(3):549-558.

36. Kim CF, Jackson EL, Woolfenden AE. Identification of bronchioalveolar stem cells in normal lung and lung cancer. *Cell*. 2005;121:823-835.

37. Kim CFB, Jackson EL, Woolfenden AE, et al. Identification of bronchioalveolar stem cells in normal lung and lung cancer. *Cell*. 2005;121(6):823-835.

38. Rawlins EL, Okubo T, Xue Y, et al. The role of Scgb1a1(+) Clara cells in the long-term maintenance and repair of lung airway, but not alveolar, epithelium. *Cell Stem Cell*. 2009;4(6):525-534.

39. Rock JR, Barkauskas CE, Cronce MJ, et al. Multiple stromal populations contribute to pulmonary fibrosis without evidence for epithelial to mesenchymal transition. *Proc Natl Acad Sci U S A*. 2011;108(52):E1475-E1483.

40. Zheng D, Limmon GV, Yin L, et al. Regeneration of alveolar type I and II cells from Scgb1a1-expressing cells following severe pulmonary damage induced by bleomycin and influenza. *PLos One*. 2012;7(10):e48451.

41. Möbius MA, Freund D, Vadivel A, et al. Oxygen disrupts human fetal lung mesenchymal cells: implications for bronchopulmonary dysplasia. *Am J Respir Cell Mol Biol*. 2019;60(5):592-600.

42. Dominici M, Le Blanc K, Mueller I, et al. Minimal criteria for defining multipotent mesenchymal stromal cells. The International Society for Cellular Therapy position statement. *Cytotherapy*. 2006;8(4):315-317.

43. Ricciardi M, Malpeli G, Bifari F, et al. Comparison of epithelial differentiation and immune regulatory properties of mesenchymal stromal cells derived from human lung and bone marrow. *PLoS One*. 2012;7(5):e35639.

44. Bozyk PD, Popova AP, Bentley JK, et al. Mesenchymal stromal cells from neonatal tracheal aspirates demonstrate a pattern of lung-specific gene expression. *Stem Cells Dev*. 2011;20(11): 1995-2007.

45. McQualter JL, Yuen K, Williams B, Bertoncello I. Evidence of an epithelial stem/progenitor cell hierarchy in the adult mouse lung. *Proc Natl Acad Sci U S A*. 2010;107(4):1414-1419.

46. van Haaften T, Byrne R, Bonnet S, et al. Airway delivery of mesenchymal stem cells prevents arrested alveolar growth in neonatal lung injury in rats. *Am J Respir Crit Care Med*. 2009; 180(11):1131-1142.

47. Popova AP, Bozyk PD, Bentley JK, et al. Isolation of tracheal aspirate mesenchymal stromal cells predicts bronchopulmonary dysplasia. *Pediatrics*. 2010;126(5):e1127-e1133.

48. Popova AP, Bozyk PD, Goldsmith AM, et al. Autocrine production of TGF-beta1 promotes myofibroblastic differentiation of neonatal lung mesenchymal stem cells. *Am J Physiol Lung Cell Mol Physiol*. 2010;298(6):L735-L743.

49. Asahara T, Murohara T, Sullivan A, et al. Isolation of putative progenitor endothelial cells for angiogenesis. *Science*. 1997; 275(5302):964-966.

50. Rehman J, Li J, Orschell CM, March KL. Peripheral blood "endothelial progenitor cells" are derived from monocyte/macrophages and secrete angiogenic growth factors. *Circulation*. 2003;107(8):1164-1169.

51. Alvarez DF, Huang L, King JA, et al. Lung microvascular endothelium is enriched with progenitor cells that exhibit vasculogenic capacity. *Am J Physiol Lung Cell Mol Physiol*. 2008; 294(3):L419-L430.

52. Ingram DA, Mead LE, Tanaka H, et al. Identification of a novel hierarchy of endothelial progenitor cells using human peripheral and umbilical cord blood. *Blood*. 2004;104(9):2752.

53. Mead LE, Prater D, Yoder MC, Ingram DA. Isolation and characterization of endothelial progenitor cells from human blood. *Curr Protoc Stem Cell Biol.* 2008;Chapter 2:Unit 2C.1.

54. Gillich A, Zhang F, Farmer CG, et al. Capillary cell-type specialization in the alveolus. *Nature.* 2020;586(7831):785-789.

55. Hurskainen M, Mizikova I, Cook DP, et al. Single cell transcriptomic analysis of murine lung development on hyperoxia-induced damage. *Nat Commun.* 2021;12(1):1565.

56. Wang G, Wen B, Ren X, et al. Generation of pulmonary endothelial progenitor cells for cell-based therapy using interspecies mouse–rat chimeras. *Am J Respir Crit Care Med.* 2021;204(3):326-338.

57. Niethamer TK, Stabler CT, Leach JP, et al. Defining the role of pulmonary endothelial cell heterogeneity in the response to acute lung injury. *Elife.* 2020;9:e53072.

58. Aslam M, Baveja R, Liang OD, et al. Bone marrow stromal cells attenuate lung injury in a murine model of neonatal chronic lung disease. *Am J Respir Crit Care Med.* 2009;180(11):1122-1130.

59. Pierro M, Ionescu L, Montemurro T, et al. Short-term, long-term and paracrine effect of human umbilical cord-derived stem cells in lung injury prevention and repair in experimental bronchopulmonary dysplasia. *Thorax.* 2013;68(5):475-484.

60. Chang YS, Oh W, Choi SJ, et al. Human umbilical cord blood-derived mesenchymal stem cells attenuate hyperoxia-induced lung injury in neonatal rats. *Cell Transplant.* 2009;18(8):869-886.

61. Chang YS, Choi SJ, Sung DK, et al. Intratracheal transplantation of human umbilical cord blood derived mesenchymal stem cells dose-dependently attenuates hyperoxia-induced lung injury in neonatal rats. *Cell Transplant.* 2011;20(11):1843-1854.

62. Chang YS, Choi SJ, Ahn SY, et al. Timing of umbilical cord blood derived mesenchymal stem cells transplantation determines therapeutic efficacy in the neonatal hyperoxic lung injury. *PLoS One.* 2013;8(1):e52419.

63. Ahn SY, Chang YS, Kim SY, et al. Long-term (postnatal day 70) outcome and safety of intratracheal transplantation of human umbilical cord blood-derived mesenchymal stem cells in neonatal hyperoxic lung injury. *Yonsei Med J.* 2013;54(2):416-424.

64. Fung ME, Thebaud B. Stem cell-based therapy for neonatal lung disease: it is in the juice. *Pediatr Res.* 2014;75(1-1):2-7.

65. Zhang X, Wang H, Shi Y, et al. Role of bone marrow-derived mesenchymal stem cells in the prevention of hyperoxia-induced lung injury in newborn mice. *Cell Biol Int.* 2012;36(6):589-594.

66. Hansmann G, Fernandez-Gonzalez A, Aslam M, et al. Mesenchymal stem cell-mediated reversal of bronchopulmonary dysplasia and associated pulmonary hypertension. *Pulm Circ.* 2012;2(2):170-181.

67. Sutsko RP, Young KC, Ribeiro A, et al. Long-term reparative effects of mesenchymal stem cell therapy following neonatal hyperoxia-induced lung injury. *Pediatr Res.* 2013;73(1):46-53.

68. Ionescu L, Byrne RN, van Haaften T, et al. Stem cell conditioned medium improves acute lung injury in mice: in vivo evidence for stem cell paracrine action. *Am J Physiol Lung Cell Mol Physiol.* 2012;303(11):L967-L977.

69. Nemeth K, Leelahavanichkul A, Yuen PS, et al. Bone marrow stromal cells attenuate sepsis via prostaglandin E(2)-dependent reprogramming of host macrophages to increase their interleukin-10 production. *Nat Med.* 2009;15(1):42-49.

70. Caplan AI, Correa D. The MSC: an injury drugstore. *Cell Stem Cell.* 2011;9(1):11-15.

71. Lee JW, Fang X, Gupta N, et al. Allogeneic human mesenchymal stem cells for treatment of E. coli endotoxin-induced acute lung injury in the ex vivo perfused human lung. *Proc Natl Acad Sci U S A.* 2009;106(38):16357-16362.

72. Chang YS, Ahn SY, Jeon HB, et al. Critical role of vascular endothelial growth factor secreted by mesenchymal stem cells in hyperoxic lung injury. *Am J Respir Cell Mol Biol.* 2014;51(3):391-399.

73. Thebaud B, Ladha F, Michelakis ED, et al. Vascular endothelial growth factor gene therapy increases survival, promotes lung angiogenesis, and prevents alveolar damage in hyperoxia-induced lung injury: evidence that angiogenesis participates in alveolarization. *Circulation.* 2005;112(16):2477-2486.

74. Ionescu LI, Alphonse RS, Arizmendi N, et al. Airway delivery of soluble factors from plastic-adherent bone marrow cells prevents murine asthma. *Am J Respir Cell Mol Biol.* 2012;46(2):207-216.

75. Block GJ, Ohkouchi S, Fung F, et al. Multipotent stromal cells are activated to reduce apoptosis in part by upregulation and secretion of stanniocalcin-1. *Stem Cells.* 2009;27(3):670-681.

76. Lee RH, Pulin AA, Seo MJ, et al. Intravenous hMSCs improve myocardial infarction in mice because cells embolized in lung are activated to secrete the anti-inflammatory protein TSG-6. *Cell Stem Cell.* 2009;5(1):54-63.

77. Waszak P, Alphonse R, Vadivel A, et al. Preconditioning enhances the paracrine effect of mesenchymal stem cells in preventing oxygen-induced neonatal lung injury in rats. *Stem Cells Dev.* 2012;21:2789-2797.

78. Chaput N, Thery C. Exosomes: immune properties and potential clinical implementations. *Semin Immunopathol.* 2011;33(5):419-440.

79. Olave N, Lal CV, Halloran B, et al. Regulation of alveolar septation by microRNA-489. *Am J Physiol Lung Cell Mol Physiol.* 2016;310(5):L476-L487.

80. Lee C, Mitsialis SA, Aslam M, et al. Exosomes mediate the cytoprotective action of mesenchymal stromal cells on hypoxia-induced pulmonary hypertension. *Circulation.* 2012;126(22):2601-2611.

81. Chaubey S, Thueson S, Ponnalagu D, et al. Early gestational mesenchymal stem cell secretome attenuates experimental bronchopulmonary dysplasia in part via exosome-associated factor TSG-6. *Stem Cell Res Ther.* 2018;9(1):173.

82. Porzionato A, Zaramella P, Dedja A, et al. Intratracheal administration of mesenchymal stem cell-derived extracellular vesicles reduces lung injuries in a chronic rat model of bronchopulmonary dysplasia. *Am J Physiol Lung Cell Mol Physiol.* 2021;320(5):L688-L704.

83. Porzionato A, Zaramella P, Dedja A, et al. Intratracheal administration of clinical-grade mesenchymal stem cell-derived extracellular vesicles reduces lung injury in a rat model of bronchopulmonary dysplasia. *Am J Physiol Lung Cell Mol Physiol.* 2019;316(1):L6-L19.

84. Ahn SY, Park WS, Kim YE, et al. Vascular endothelial growth factor mediates the therapeutic efficacy of mesenchymal stem cell-derived extracellular vesicles against neonatal hyperoxic lung injury. *Exp Mol Med.* 2018;50(4):1-12.

85. Willis GR, Reis M, Gheinani AH, et al. Extracellular vesicles protect the neonatal lung from hyperoxic injury through the epigenetic and transcriptomic reprogramming of myeloid cells. *Am J Respir Crit Care Med.* 2021;204(12):1418-1432.

86. Abele AN, Taglauer ES, Almeda M, et al. Antenatal mesenchymal stromal cell extracellular vesicle treatment preserves lung development in a model of bronchopulmonary dysplasia due to chorioamnionitis. *Am J Physiol Lung Cell Mol Physiol.* 2022;322(2):L179-L190.

87. Taglauer ES, Fernandez-Gonzalez A, Willis GR, et al. Antenatal mesenchymal stromal cell extracellular vesicle therapy prevents preeclamptic lung injury in mice. *Am J Respir Cell Mol Biol.* 2022;66(1):86-95.

88. Willis GR, Fernandez-Gonzalez A, Anastas J, et al. Mesenchymal stromal cell exosomes ameliorate experimental bronchopulmonary dysplasia and restore lung function through macrophage immunomodulation. *Am J Respir Crit Care Med.* 2018;197(1):104-116.

89. Chang YS, Choi SJ, Sung DK, et al. Intratracheal transplantation of human umbilical cord blood-derived mesenchymal stem cells dose-dependently attenuates hyperoxia-induced lung injury in neonatal rats. *Cell Transplant.* 2011;20(11-12):1843-1854.

90. Ahn SY, Chang YS, Kim JH, et al. Two-year follow-up outcomes of premature infants enrolled in the phase I trial of mesenchymal stem cells transplantation for bronchopulmonary dysplasia. *J Pediatr.* 2017;185:49-54.e42.

91. Ahn SY, Chang YS, Park WS. Stem cell therapy for bronchopulmonary dysplasia: bench to bedside translation. *J Korean Med Sci.* 2015;30(5):509-513.

92. Strueby L, Thebaud B. Mesenchymal stromal cell-based therapies for chronic lung disease of prematurity. *Am J Perinatol.* 2016;33(11):1043-1049.

93. Mitsialis SA, Kourembanas S. Stem cell-based therapies for the newborn lung and brain: Possibilities and challenges. *Semin Perinatol.* 2016;40(3):138-151.

94. Mobius MA, Thebaud B. Cell therapy for bronchopulmonary dysplasia: promises and perils. *Paediatr Respir Rev.* 2016;20: 33-41.

95. Mendicino M, Bailey AM, Wonnacott K, et al. MSC-based product characterization for clinical trials: an FDA perspective. *Cell Stem Cell.* 2014;14(2):141-145.

96. D'Angio CT, Ambalavanan N, Carlo WA, et al. Blood cytokine profiles associated with distinct patterns of bronchopulmonary dysplasia among extremely low birth weight infants. *J Pediatr.* 2016;174:45-51.e5.

97. Laughon MM, Langer JC, Bose CL, et al. Prediction of bronchopulmonary dysplasia by postnatal age in extremely premature infants. *Am J Respir Crit Care Med.* 2011;183(12): 1715-1722.

98. Abman SH, Matthay MA. Mesenchymal stem cells for the prevention of bronchopulmonary dysplasia: delivering the secretome. *Am J Respir Crit Care Med.* 2009;180(11):1039-1041.

99. Ahn SY, Chang YS, Sung DK, et al. Cell type-dependent variation in paracrine potency determines therapeutic efficacy against neonatal hyperoxic lung injury. *Cytotherapy.* 2015; 17(8):1025-1035.

100. Pierro M, Ionescu L, Montemurro T, et al. Short-term, long-term and paracrine effect of human umbilical cord-derived stem cells in lung injury prevention and repair in experimental bronchopulmonary dysplasia. *Thorax.* 2013;68(5):475-484.

101. Kern S, Eichler H, Stoeve J, et al. Comparative analysis of mesenchymal stem cells from bone marrow, umbilical cord blood, or adipose tissue. *Stem Cells.* 2006;24(5):1294-1301.

102. Bárcia RN, Santos JM, Filipe M, et al. What makes umbilical cord tissue-derived mesenchymal stromal cells superior immunomodulators when compared to bone marrow derived mesenchymal stromal cells? *Stem Cells Int.* 2015;2015:583984.

103. Javed MJ, Mead LE, Prater D, et al. Endothelial colony forming cells and mesenchymal stem cells are enriched at different gestational ages in human umbilical cord blood. *Pediatr Res.* 2008;64(1):68-73.

104. Secunda R, Vennila R, Mohanashankar AM, et al. Isolation, expansion and characterisation of mesenchymal stem cells from human bone marrow, adipose tissue, umbilical cord blood and matrix: a comparative study. *Cytotechnology.* 2015;67(5):793-807.

105. Vieira Paladino F, de Moraes Rodrigues J, da Silva A, et al. The immunomodulatory potential of Wharton's jelly mesenchymal stem/stromal cells. *Stem Cells Int.* 2019;2019:3548917.

106. Weiss ML, Anderson C, Medicetty S, et al. Immune properties of human umbilical cord Wharton's jelly-derived cells. *Stem cells.* 2008;26(11):2865-2874.

107. Chen MY, Lie PC, Li ZL, Wei X. Endothelial differentiation of Wharton's jelly–derived mesenchymal stem cells in comparison with bone marrow–derived mesenchymal stem cells. *Exp Hematol.* 2009;37(5):629-640.

108. Li X, Bai J, Ji X, et al. Comprehensive characterization of four different populations of human mesenchymal stem cells as regards their immune properties, proliferation and differentiation. *Int J Mol Med.* 2014;34(3):695-704.

109. Benny M, Courchia B, Shrager S, et al. Comparative effects of bone marrow–derived versus umbilical cord tissue mesenchymal stem cells in an experimental model of bronchopulmonary dysplasia. *Stem Cells Transl Med.* 2022;11(2):189-199. doi:10.1093/stcltm/szab011.

110. Sammour I, Somashekar S, Huang J, et al. The effect of gender on Mesenchymal Stem Cell (MSC) efficacy in neonatal hyperoxia-induced lung injury. *PLoS One.* 2016;11(10):e0164269.

111. Lensch M, Muise A, White L, et al. Comparison of synthetic media designed for expansion of adipose-derived mesenchymal stromal cells. *Biomedicines.* 2018;6(2):54.

112. Yang YK, Ogando CR, Wang See C, et al. Changes in phenotype and differentiation potential of human mesenchymal stem cells aging in vitro. *Stem Cell Res Ther.* 2018;9(1):131.

113. Chinnadurai R, Garcia MA, Sakurai Y, et al. Actin cytoskeletal disruption following cryopreservation alters the biodistribution of human mesenchymal stromal cells in vivo. *Stem Cell Reports.* 2014;3(1):60-72.

114. Gramlich OW, Burand AJ, Brown AJ, et al. Cryopreserved mesenchymal stromal cells maintain potency in a retinal ischemia/reperfusion injury model: toward an off-the-shelf therapy. *Sci Rep.* 2016;6:26463.

115. Powell SB, Silvestri JM. Safety of intratracheal administration of human umbilical cord blood derived mesenchymal stromal cells in extremely low birth weight preterm infants. *J Pediatr.* 2019;210:209-213.e2.

116. Alphonse RS, Vadivel A, Fung M, et al. Existence, functional impairment, and lung repair potential of endothelial colony-forming cells in oxygen-induced arrested alveolar growth. *Circulation.* 2014;129(21):2144-2157.

117. Zhu D, Tan J, Maleken AS, et al. Human amnion cells reverse acute and chronic pulmonary damage in experimental neonatal lung injury. *Stem Cell Res Ther.* 2017;8(1):257.

118. Ramachandran S, Suguihara C, Drummond S, et al. Bone marrow-derived c-kit+ cells attenuate neonatal hyperoxia-induced lung injury. *Cell Transplant.* 2015;24(1):85-95.

119. Augustine S, Cheng W, Avey MT, et al. Are all stem cells equal? Systematic review, evidence map, and meta-analyses of preclinical stem cell-based therapies for bronchopulmonary dysplasia. *Stem Cells Transl Med.* 2020;9(2):158-168.

120. Malhotra A, Lim R, Mockler JC, et al. Two-year outcomes of infants enrolled in the first-in-human study of amnion cells for bronchopulmonary dysplasia. *Stem Cells Transl Med.* 2020; 9(3):289-294.

121. Lengner CJ. iPS cell technology in regenerative medicine. *Ann N Y Acad Sci.* 2010;1192:38-44.

122. Shafa M, Ionescu LI, Vadivel A, et al. Human induced pluripotent stem cell-derived lung progenitor and alveolar epithelial cells attenuate hyperoxia-induced lung injury. *Cytotherapy.* 2018;20(1):108-125.

123. Jacob A, Morley M, Hawkins F, et al. Differentiation of human pluripotent stem cells into functional lung alveolar epithelial cells. *Cell Stem Cell.* 2017;21(4):472-488.e10.

124. Takayama S, Sakai K, Fumino S, et al. An intra-amniotic injection of mesenchymal stem cells promotes lung maturity in a rat congenital diaphragmatic hernia model. *Pediatr Surg Int.* 2019; 35(12):1353-1361.

125. Antounians L, Catania VD, Montalva L, et al. Fetal lung underdevelopment is rescued by administration of amniotic fluid stem cell extracellular vesicles in rodents. *Sci Transl Med.* 2021; 13(590):eaax5941.

126. Sung DK, Chang YS, Ahn SY, et al. Optimal route for human umbilical cord blood-derived mesenchymal stem cell transplantation to protect against neonatal hyperoxic lung injury: gene expression profiles and histopathology. *PLoS One.* 2015;10(8):e0135574.

127. Rojas M, Xu J, Woods CR, et al. Bone marrow-derived mesenchymal stem cells in repair of the injured lung. *Am J Respir Cell Mol Biol.* 2005;33(2):145-152.

128. Ortiz LA, Gambelli F, McBride C, et al. Mesenchymal stem cell engraftment in lung is enhanced in response to bleomycin exposure and ameliorates its fibrotic effects. *Proc Natl Acad Sci U S A.* 2003;100(14):8407-8411.

129. Fischer UM, Harting MT, Jimenez F, et al. Pulmonary passage is a major obstacle for intravenous stem cell delivery: the pulmonary first-pass effect. *Stem Cells Dev.* 2009;18(5):683-692.

130. de Witte SFH, Luk F, Sierra Parraga JM, et al. Immunomodulation by therapeutic Mesenchymal Stromal Cells (MSC) is triggered through phagocytosis of MSC by monocytic cells. *Stem Cells.* 2018;36(4):602-615.

Definitions and Diagnostic Criteria of Bronchopulmonary Dysplasia: Clinical and Research Implications

Eduardo H. Bancalari, Nelson Claure, Erik A. Jensen, and Alan H. Jobe

Chapter Outline

Abbreviations

Clinical Presentation of BPD

BPD Diagnosis

Existing Diagnostic Criteria for BPD

   Diagnosis Based on Various Supplemental Oxygen Criteria.

   Severity Graded Diagnostic Criteria

   Impact of the Arterial Oxygenation Targets

Impact of Oxygen Delivery Device

Impact of Timing on BPD Diagnosis

Competing Outcomes

Defining the Populations at Risk for BPD

Prognosis for Long-Term Pulmonary Impairment

Implications for Future Research

Conclusion

Key Points

- Bronchopulmonary dysplasia (BPD) is a common complication of prematurity that results from abnormal lung development and injury that leads to chronic impairment of lung function.

- Use of standardized diagnostic classifications of BPD and its severity is important in clinical trials that evaluate therapeutic strategies and in epidemiologic cohorts to benchmark respiratory outcomes in neonatal centers.

- Current criteria to diagnose BPD do not consistently predict long-term lung health. This is because of the potential for lung repair and recovery on one side and postdischarge events that can affect lung structure and function on the other.

- Objective markers of lung injury that more precisely predict long-term lung health in this population are needed.

Abbreviations

BPD:	Bronchopulmonary dysplasia
BW:	Birth weight
FGR:	Fetal growth restriction
GA:	Gestational age
NC:	Nasal cannula
NCPAP:	Nasal continuous positive airway pressure
NICHD:	National Institute of Child Health and Human Development
NIH:	National Institutes of Health
PMA:	Postmenstrual age
PPV:	Positive pressure ventilation
RDS:	Respiratory distress syndrome
VLBW:	Very low birth weight

Bronchopulmonary dysplasia (BPD) is a heterogeneous disease that results from disruption of lung growth secondary to premature birth and lung damage with aberrant post-injury repair. Harmful perinatal and postnatal exposures that contribute to the development of BPD include prolonged respiratory support, infection, and other proinflammatory factors, fetal growth restriction, and maternal smoking. BPD progresses from variable degrees of early respiratory insufficiency that evolve into more chronic forms of persistent lung disease. The impaired lung function associated with BPD frequently endures through childhood and into adulthood. Therefore, it is important that the diagnostic criteria for BPD accurately define the severity of pulmonary dysfunction in preterm infants and provide prognostic indicators of the degree of respiratory impairment anticipated after the initial hospital discharge. Standardized BPD diagnostic and severity criteria are also important to compare outcomes in infants included in clinical trials, for epidemiological identification of risk factors, and to compare outcomes between centers or within centers for quality improvement activities.

In this chapter, we provide a brief update of the epidemiology of BPD, describe the most frequent diagnostic criteria of BPD, and discuss their possible advantages and limitations in the context of changing clinical presentation and management of respiratory disease in very preterm infants.

Clinical Presentation of Bronchopulmonary Dysplasia

The term "bronchopulmonary dysplasia" was introduced by Northway and collaborators to describe a clinical, radiographic, and pathological entity that occurred predominately in moderate and late preterm infants who survived severe respiratory distress syndrome (RDS) after aggressive mechanical ventilation without positive end-expiratory pressure (PEEP) and exposure to high concentrations of inspired oxygen used in the 1960s and 1970s.[1] These infants developed severe respiratory failure shortly after birth, and most required aggressive mechanical ventilation and supplemental oxygen for long periods. The severity of the respiratory failure and the radiographic images from these infants were clear evidence of their serious lung derangement that resulted in poor short- and long-term outcomes. With the introduction of prenatal corticosteroid therapy, postnatal surfactant, and the many advances in respiratory support and neonatal care, the presentation of BPD changed over the years.[2]

BPD now predominately affects extremely premature infants for whom survival rates continue to increase but chronic respiratory morbidity is common.

The underlying abnormality in the lungs of the premature infant with BPD is a disruption of the normal processes of alveolar and capillary development.[3] The more severe cases are also associated with postnatal airway and vascular remodeling leading to airway obstruction and pulmonary hypertension that can be accompanied by interstitial edema and fibrous tissue proliferation.[4]

Although the classic severe forms of BPD are less common today, some infants still have a clinical course with significant lung damage, a prolonged need for respiratory support resulting in severe respiratory failure, pulmonary hypertension, and marked alterations in the chest radiographs. These infants offer little diagnostic or prognostic dilemma. Unfavorable outcomes are common in these infants, and enduring deficits in respiratory health are expected. Greater difficulty lays with the diagnosis in infants with less severe forms of BPD who have a milder initial respiratory course and require lower levels of respiratory support. The clinical and radiographic evidence in these infants is less conclusive than that in infants with severe BPD, and most have better long-term outcomes. The chest radiographs in less severely affected infants can show diffuse haziness due to loss of gas volume or fluid accumulation, and denser areas of segmental or lobar atelectasis or pneumonic infiltrates are occasionally observed, but there are no areas of severe overinflation typical of the severe forms of BPD. Lethal, severe cases of BPD are characterized by significant morphologic alterations in lung architecture, including emphysema, atelectasis, fibrosis, and marked epithelial squamous metaplasia and smooth muscle hypertrophy in the airways and in the pulmonary vasculature.[5] These alterations are often associated with airway obstruction, pulmonary hypertension, and cor pulmonale, which contribute to prolonged and severe respiratory failure.

Infants developing BPD today are considerably more immature than the earlier cases of severe BPD, and the incidence among infants born after 32 weeks' gestation has become negligible in modern neonatal centers except for some survivors with hypoplastic lungs who need long-term ventilatory support. Today,

BPD predominantly occurs in infants of less than 29 weeks' gestation, but the reported incidence varies considerably between centers and studies. This variability may reflect different populations and management strategies, but it is also due to major inconsistencies in how the disease is defined. The incidence of BPD in infants of less than 29 weeks' gestational age (GA) in the centers of the Eunice Kennedy Shriver National Institute of Child Health and Human Development (NICHD) Neonatal Research Network was 42% during the years 2003 to 2007.[6] According to a recent report from stratified samples of nearly one-fifth of US hospitals, the incidence of BPD among surviving infants of birth weight (BW) below 1500 g declined from 50% to 60% in the 1990s to nearly 40% in the years 2000 to 2006.[7] However, between 1993 and 2012, the incidence of BPD in infants born before 28 weeks in the centers of the NICHD Neonatal Research Network slightly increased.[8] In 2018, 10.3% of infants in the Vermont Oxford Network born less than 30 weeks' gestations died prior to 36 weeks postmenstrual age (PMA) and 40.6% were diagnosed with BPD based on the use of supplemental oxygen or respiratory support at 36 weeks PMA.[9]

The initial presentation of the infants who develop BPD, even among the least mature infants, is more variable than in earlier years. Most infants who developed BPD 40 to 50 years ago had severe RDS, and it is likely that the incidence of BPD would have been even higher absent the relatively high early mortality resulting from severe respiratory failure in those early years of neonatal intensive care. At present, premature infants who develop BPD may present with no or only mild RDS after birth. Based on autopsy and animal models, BPD today is characterized by a reduction in alveolar septation and vascular development,[2,3,5,10-12] suggesting that underlying lung immaturity and abnormal lung development are key contributors to the pathogenesis and the clinical presentation of BPD.

Bronchopulmonary Dysplasia Diagnosis

Clinicians are typically confident with a diagnosis of BPD when encountering severe forms of the disease. Such infants often have persistent, severe respiratory failure and require supplemental oxygen and respiratory support for prolonged periods of time. These support needs are consistent with the severe chronic lung injury observed on chest imaging and convey a poor long-term prognosis. In contrast, many infants who develop BPD today have mild initial respiratory distress,[13-15] and although many may still receive prolonged respiratory support, they typically do not require high levels of assistance and the support is not always continuous. This results in inconsistencies when diagnosing BPD based on the levels of respiratory support.[16]

Because diagnostic criteria for BPD are intended to be used by clinicians not only to diagnose individual infants but also for benchmarking clinical outcomes and as endpoints for clinical and epidemiological studies, such criteria will ideally fulfill several requirements:

1. They should capture both the presence and severity of lung damage. This is particularly important because the lung dysfunction associated with BPD is a continuum from mild to severe disease rather than a categorical presence or absence of disease.
2. They should provide meaningful information to clinicians, serve as a reliable outcome to researchers, and ideally predict long-term lung health.
3. They should be based on objective and verifiable data that can be easily obtained from the medical record. This is necessary for standardization purposes for benchmarking clinical outcomes within and between neonatal centers and in epidemiological or interventional studies.
4. They should not be affected by distinct confounding pathologies that can produce respiratory failure but are independent of BPD or by therapies that may acutely but transiently improve lung function at the time of assessment.

While some of the current diagnostic criteria of BPD fulfill most of these requirements, none fulfill all of them. This is in part because current criteria rely on treatments for the respiratory failure rather than on assessments of lung structure or function. The diagnostic criteria for BPD are primarily based on the need for supplemental oxygen as the marker of respiratory failure with the duration of supplemental oxygen and the fraction of inspired oxygen (FiO_2) needed for adequate arterial oxygen levels used as surrogates of the severity of BPD. There are some important limitations in using oxygen supplementation as the main criterion to diagnose BPD. Although exposure to oxygen therapy is a simple variable to assess, oxygen is also linked to the pathogenesis of BPD and is the main therapy used to maintain adequate oxygenation in respiratory failure from any cause.

The indications for supplemental oxygen can vary from center to center, but after the oxygen saturation targeting trials, there is now more consistency among clinicians on the optimal arterial oxygen saturation range for these infants. However, there are interventions such as steroids, diuretics, and respiratory stimulants that can acutely change oxygen requirement without necessarily changing long-term respiratory outcomes. Different forms of respiratory support can influence gas exchange and oxygenation, thereby reducing the need for oxygen. For this reason, any diagnostic criteria of BPD must also include the use of other forms of respiratory support.

Existing Diagnostic Criteria for Bronchopulmonary Dysplasia

DIAGNOSIS BASED ON VARIOUS SUPPLEMENTAL OXYGEN CRITERIA

Continuous Oxygen Use for the First 28 Days

A workshop sponsored by the NIH in 1979 proposed the BPD diagnosis based on continuous use of supplemental oxygen during the first 28 days plus clinical and radiographic findings compatible with chronic lung disease.[17] These criteria are not suitable for today's preterm infants who develop chronic lung disease, because only a small proportion of them require continuous supplemental oxygen during the first 28 days after birth. Nevertheless, many infants who initially need oxygen for only a few days will subsequently have a deterioration in their respiratory status and receive prolonged supplemental oxygen and develop chronic respiratory failure. These infants present a diagnostic dilemma because they have early mild but persistent respiratory insufficiency that cannot be directly attributed to their initial RDS but still culminates in chronic lung changes.[18]

Supplemental Oxygen at Day 28

To simplify the diagnosis of BPD, some clinicians and investigators have classified BPD as infants who require supplemental oxygen at day 28.[19] This approach avoids the needs for longitudinal data collection but carries the inherent limitations of diagnosing BPD based on data collected at a single time point. Some infants may require supplemental oxygen for a short period of time due to a transient deterioration and not due to chronic lung damage. On the other hand, in less mature infants, the 4-week postnatal age assessment time point may be too early to be a reliable indicator of chronic lung disease.

Oxygen at 36 Weeks Postmenstrual Corrected Age

The use of supplemental oxygen at 36 weeks PMA has become the most frequent criterion to diagnose BPD.[19] This criterion was introduced in 1988 to define abnormal respiratory status at near-term corrected age and to better predict early childhood outcomes among very premature infants who were increasingly surviving the initial hospitalization. In recent years, this definition has at times been modified to also include exposure to supplemental respiratory support at 36 weeks PMA to avoid exclusion of infants receiving respiratory support with 21% FiO_2.[20]

SEVERITY GRADED DIAGNOSTIC CRITERIA

Cumulative Oxygen Supplementation Combined With Oxygen and Respiratory Support at 36 Weeks Postmenstrual Corrected Age

The diagnostic classification of BPD based on the cumulative exposure to supplemental oxygen greater than 28 days and at 36 weeks PMA as recommended by the NIH workshop in 2001[21] addressed the limitations of using oxygen requirement at a single time point or the duration of oxygen dependency as the only indicators of BPD. The recommendations included a cumulative duration of oxygen supplementation for at least 28 days to indicate the chronicity of the lung damage plus the concentration of inspired oxygen at 36 weeks PMA to define the severity of the lung damage at near-term corrected age before discharge. These criteria classify BPD as mild, moderate, or severe based on the FiO_2 and use of positive airway pressure support at 36 weeks PMA (Table 13.1).

The NIH workshop criteria recommended classifying as severe BPD infants who require supplemental oxygen at 30% or higher or receive any form of

TABLE 13.1	NIH Workshop Definition of BPD	
Gestational Age	**<32 Weeks**	**≥32 Weeks**
Time point of assessment	36 weeks PMA or discharge to home, whichever comes first	>28 days but <56 days postnatal age or discharge to home, whichever comes first
Treatment with oxygen >21% for at least 28 days plus:		
Mild BPD	Breathing room air at 36 weeks PMA or discharge, whichever comes first	Breathing room air by 56 days postnatal age or discharge, whichever comes first
Moderate BPD	Need for <30% at 36 weeks PMA or discharge, whichever comes first	Need for <30% at 56 days postnatal age or discharge, whichever comes first
Severe BPD	Need for ≥ 30% oxygen and/or positive pressure (PPV or NCPAP) at 36 weeks PMA or discharge, whichever comes first	Need for ≥ 30% oxygen and/or positive pressure (PPV or NCPAP) at 56 days postnatal age or discharge, whichever comes first

BPD, Bronchopulmonary dysplasia; *NCPAP*, nasal continuous positive airway pressure; *PMA*, postmenstrual age; *PPV*, positive pressure ventilation.
Adapted from Jobe AH, Bancalari E. Bronchopulmonary dysplasia. *Am J Respir Crit Care Med.* 2001;163(7):1723-1729.

positive pressure respiratory support at 36 weeks PMA. Nearly half of the infants who need supplemental oxygen at 36 weeks PMA meet this definition of severe BPD. Most infants meet these criteria based on their need for oxygen and few because of the need for positive pressure respiratory support. However, this is likely to vary significantly between institutions depending on respiratory support practices. Data from the centers of the Prematurity and Respiratory Outcomes Program (PROP) of the National Heart Lung and Blood Institute[22] showed that the proportion of infants who receive invasive mechanical ventilation is about one-fourth of the infants who receive supplemental oxygen at 36 weeks PMA.[9,23] In contrast, the proportion of infants receiving noninvasive respiratory support is closer to that of the infants who remain oxygen dependent at 36 weeks PMA.

In recent years, the use of nasal cannula (NC) has increased considerably in most centers. As evidenced in the data from PROP centers, 47% of infants under 29 weeks of gestation received oxygen via NC at 36 weeks PMA.[22] Because the effective FiO_2 and airway pressure can vary widely and are not objectively measured with NC, this therapy has introduced a new variable to the diagnosis of BPD. This is particularly evident among infants who receive low flows or low oxygen concentrations. The use of a higher concentration of supplemental oxygen as a criterion to diagnose BPD severity reduces the ambiguity resulting from the use of low supplemental oxygen, nasal continuous positive airway pressure (NCPAP), or NCs as indicators of lung disease, but the effective inspired oxygen can still vary depending on the flow and type of canula used.

Adapting Severity Criteria to Changing Respiratory Support Practices

The increased use of noninvasive respiratory support including NC in extremely preterm infants has led to proposed revisions of the diagnostic classifications of BPD. Participants of a 2018 NICHD workshop developed a definition that accounts for NC and other more recent noninvasive forms of respiratory support.[24] This proposed definition (Table 13.2) grades the severity of BPD according to the combination of FiO_2 in the gases delivered by different NC flows, CPAP, noninvasive, and invasive mechanical ventilation. This proposed grading is expected to account to a large extent for the uncertainty of the effective FiO_2 delivered at lower NC flows. This definition also differentiates invasive from noninvasive respiratory support as indicators of disease severity.

Diagnosis of Bronchopulmonary Dysplasia Severity Based on the Mode of Respiratory Support Only

Similarly motivated by the evolving respiratory support practices in very preterm infants and concern over limitations in the prognostic accuracy of existing diagnostic criteria for BPD, investigators from the

TABLE 13.2	Suggested Refinements to the Definition of BPD				
Severity	Mechanical Ventilation	N-CPAP, NIPPV, or Nasal Cannula ≥3 L/min	Nasal Cannula Flow of 1–<3 L/min	Hood O_2	Nasal Cannula Flow of <1 L/min
Grade I		21% O_2	22%–29% O_2	22%–29% O_2	22%–70% O_2
Grade II	21% O_2	22%–29% O_2	≥30% O_2	≥30% O_2	>70% O_2
Grade III	>21% O_2	≥30% O_2			

BPD, Bronchopulmonary dysplasia; NCPAP, nasal continuous positive airway pressure; NIPPV, nasal intermittent positive pressure ventilation.

Adapted from Higgins RD, Jobe AH, Koso-Thomas M, et al. Bronchopulmonary Dysplasia: Executive Summary of a Workshop. J Pediatr. 2018;197:300-308.

NICHD Neonatal Research Network published a data-derived definition of BPD in 2019.[25] This analysis evaluated the prognostic accuracy of 18 different definitions that variably classified BPD presence and severity according to the level and duration of oxygen therapy and the mode of respiratory support administered at 36 weeks PMA. The definition that produced the highest accuracy for predicting death or serious respiratory morbidity and death or moderate-to-severe neurodevelopmental impairment at 18 to 26 months corrected age classified BPD according only to the mode of respiratory support administered at 36 weeks PMA (Table 13.3). Additional consideration for the presence or absence of oxygen exposure for at least 28 days prior to 36 weeks PMA and for the

TABLE 13.3	2019 NICHD Neonatal Research Network Diagnostic Criteria for BPD
BPD Severity	Mode of Respiratory Support at 36 Weeks PMA
No BPD	Room air (no support)
Grade 1	Nasal cannula ≤2 L/min
Grade 2	Nasal cannula >2 L/min, NCPAP, or NIPPV
Grade 3	Invasive mechanical ventilation

BPD severity classified irrespective of prior duration or current level of oxygen therapy.

BPD, Bronchopulmonary dysplasia; NCPAP, nasal continuous positive airway pressure; NIPPV, nasal intermittent positive pressure ventilation; PMA, postmenstrual age.

Adapted from Jensen EA, Dysart K, Gantz MG, et al. The diagnosis of bronchopulmonary dysplasia in very preterm infants. An evidence-based approach. Am J Respir Crit Care Med. 2019;200(6):751-759.

level of oxygen therapy administered at 36 weeks PMA (assessed as FiO_2 <30% vs. ≥30%) did not improve prediction of either composite outcome. Post hoc analyses indicated these evidence-based criteria provided a modest but statistically significant increase in prognostic accuracy as compared to previously published consensus definitions. Recent studies performed in external cohorts also suggest these diagnostic criteria may improve prediction of adverse in-hospital outcomes and resource utilization.[9,26,27]

When interpreting or adopting the different diagnostic classifications of BPD, it is important to consider the contribution and possible interaction between the individual components of these classifications. This is illustrated in Fig. 13.1 that shows the proportion of infants who meet the individual components utilized by different diagnostic criteria. All proportions decrease with GA, which underscores the key role of prematurity in the pathogenesis of BPD. While a large proportion of infants received supplemental oxygen for ≥ 28 days, a prerequisite in the NIH consensus definition, only about half of them received oxygen at 36 weeks PMA and one-fourth received >30% oxygen. The proportion of infants who received noninvasive respiratory support, which in these data were mainly NC, was very similar to that of supplemental oxygen. Only a small proportion of infants received invasive mechanical ventilation at 36 weeks PMA. Fig. 13.2 shows that most infants receiving noninvasive respiratory support were also on supplemental oxygen but at relatively low concentrations (<30%). In contrast, most infants receiving invasive mechanical ventilation were also on higher oxygen concentrations (≥30%) reflecting the severity of their lung disease.

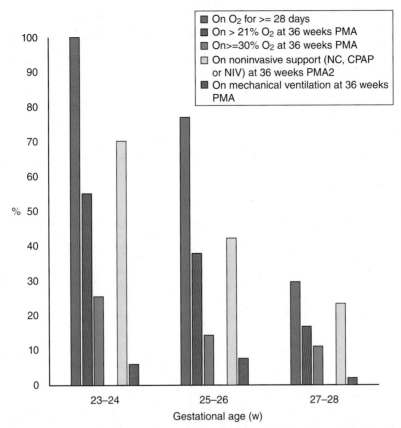

Fig. 13.1 Proportion of infants who meet the individual components of the different BPD diagnostic classifications: supplemental oxygen for at least 28 days, at 36 weeks PMA and on different modes of respiratory support at 36 weeks PMA. The figure shows the proportion of infants who received supplemental oxygen for ≥ 28 days, who received any supplemental oxygen, ≥ 30% oxygen, noninvasive respiratory support (NC at ≥ 1 lpm flow, CPAP, or NIV), or invasive mechanical ventilation at 36 weeks PMA, across different strata of GA. As expected, all proportions are higher at lower GA. Approximately half of the infants who received oxygen supplementation at 36 weeks PMA required >30% oxygen. The proportion of infants who received noninvasive respiratory support, which is mostly NC, is very similar to that receiving supplemental oxygen across GA strata. A relatively small proportion is still receiving invasive mechanical ventilation at 36 weeks PMA. Data were obtained from 383 infants, 23–28 weeks GA, admitted to the neonatal ICU at Holtz Children's Hospital, University of Miami/Jackson Memorial Medical Center during years 2015–2018 who were alive at 36 weeks PMA. *BPD*, Bronchopulmonary dysplasia; *CPAP*, continuous positive airway pressure; *GA*, gestational age; *NC*, nasal cannula; *NIV*, noninvasive ventilation; *PMA*, postmenstrual age.

IMPACT OF THE ARTERIAL OXYGEN TARGETS

The provision of supplemental oxygen to ill newborns has vacillated between periods of liberal and restrictive oxygen use over the past 50 years as clinicians sought to appropriately balance the risks and benefits of this therapy. Intercenter and interprovider variability in target arterial oxygen saturation levels have also been widespread. Such variability in care practice influences oxygen supplementation and the diagnosis of BPD.[28] Centers that target higher oxygen saturation levels will keep infants longer and on higher supplemental oxygen and vice versa.[29] To minimize the influence of different oxygen targets on the incidence of BPD, Walsh et al. in 2003 developed a test to standardize the need for oxygen at 36 weeks PMA as part of the BPD assessment.[30,31] Infants receiving oxygen at a concentration less than 30% are challenged by incrementally decreasing the inspired oxygen to 21%. Infants who maintain arterial oxygen saturation at or above 90% while breathing in room air are not classified as BPD cases.

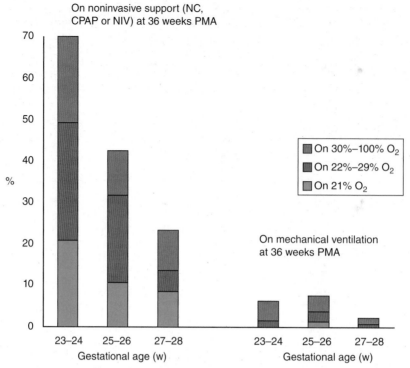

Fig. 13.2 Proportion of infants receiving different supplemental oxygen concentrations according to the mode of respiratory support. The figure shows the proportions of infants who received 21% oxygen, 22%–29% oxygen, or ≥ 30% oxygen while on noninvasive respiratory support (NC at ≥ 1 lpm flow, CPAP, or NIV) or invasive mechanical ventilation at 36 weeks PMA, across different GA strata. Most infants receiving noninvasive support were also on supplemental oxygen and approximately half were on >30% oxygen. In contrast, most infants receiving mechanical ventilation were on >30% oxygen at 36 weeks PMA. Data were obtained from 383 infants, 23–28 weeks GA, admitted to the neonatal ICU at Holtz Children's Hospital, University of Miami/Jackson Memorial Medical Center during years 2015–2018 who were alive at 36 weeks PMA. *CPAP,* Continuous positive airway pressure; *GA,* gestational age; *NC,* nasal cannula; *NIV,* noninvasive ventilation; *PMA,* postmenstrual age.

Applying this test to a cohort of premature infants from the NICHD Neonatal Research Network reduced the BPD incidence from 35% based on the clinical use of oxygen to 25% with the standardized test.[30]

Subsequently, a series of large trials compared outcomes among extremely preterm infants randomized to lower (85%–89%) versus higher (91%–95%) target oxygen saturation ranges. The results of these studies were published between 2012 and 2016 and were incorporated into an individual patient meta-analysis in 2018.[32] The individual trials and pooled analyses suggest there is a trade-off between these two target ranges: an increased incidence of death or necrotizing enterocolitis among infants assigned to the lower SpO_2 target but an increased risk of retinopathy of prematurity and BPD among infants assigned to the higher SpO_2 target. To avoid the increased risk of mortality associated with lower saturation targets, goal ranges are now more uniform between centers and regions, and the impact of the oxygen reduction test on variability in the diagnosis of BPD is less relevant.[32] The oxygen reduction test also does not readily accommodate the high NC flows that are used today without a more complex testing scheme that includes both oxygen and flow reduction. In practice, oxygen and/or flow reduction tests are difficult to do even for clinical trials.[22,33,34]

Despite growing consistency in oxygen saturation targeting, important interactions between oxygen saturation goals and patient and/or center-based characteristics may continue to affect the need for oxygen supplementation. For instance, the altitude above sea level can significantly influence arterial oxygen saturation and need for supplemental oxygen, with bias against centers at higher elevations. In some individual infants, supplemental oxygen may primarily serve to stabilize breathing. A recent study showed that nearly half of the infants who failed an oxygen weaning challenge developed periodic breathing.[35] As such, test failure may result because an acute reduction in FiO_2 induces periodic breathing and apnea with resultant decrease in arterial oxygen saturation. Some premature infants may therefore require higher oxygen saturation targets to stabilize their respiratory control function and not because of frequent desaturations owing to more severe parenchymal lung abnormalities.

IMPACT OF OXYGEN DELIVERY DEVICE

The use of positive airway pressure in infants with respiratory control issues or airway problems but with minimal parenchymal involvement may carry important prognostic implications. This is particularly important in view of the definition of severity of BPD recommended by the 2001 NIH workshop. Based on that definition, infants receiving minimal or no supplemental oxygen but positive pressure support at 36 weeks PMA are classified as having severe BPD. If the control of breathing problem eventually subsides, these infants may have better long-term pulmonary outcomes than infants receiving invasive respiratory support owing to severe parenchymal lung disease. This has become a particularly important issue due to the increased use of NC flow. When used at higher flows than those required for oxygen supplementation alone, flow can generate positive airway pressure that can stabilize lung volume. On the other hand, when the NC flow is insufficient to meet the infant's inspiratory demand, the cannula itself may produce an obstructive effect and increase the need for inspired oxygen. In addition, with NC there is uncertainty of the effective inspired oxygen, and the classification of BPD severity becomes difficult to assess. The use of low flow rates with high oxygen concentrations or high flow rates with 21% oxygen are major confounders in the diagnosis of BPD and may explain the increased incidence of BPD recently reported in some centers.[22,36] Many of the smaller infants receive some form of positive pressure respiratory support for long periods and some of them even beyond 36 weeks

PMA. In these infants this is likely due to a combination of poor respiratory control, week respiratory pump, unstable airways, and evolving chronic lung disease. This is less likely in infants who need high oxygen concentrations while undergoing noninvasive positive pressure respiratory support, which reflects more severe lung disease and predicts worse long-term outcomes.

IMPACT OF TIMING ON BRONCHOPULMONARY DYSPLASIA DIAGNOSIS

The time point when BPD is diagnosed has evolved with changes in the epidemiology and outcomes associated with premature birth.

In recent years, some clinicians and investigators have suggested using 40 weeks corrected age as the time point to establish the diagnosis of BPD instead of 36 weeks.[37] The advantage of using the term "corrected age" is that a later diagnosis will select a group of infants with more severe disease and may improve overall prediction of later outcomes among contemporary infants. Recent data from the Canadian Neonatal Network (CNN),[20] applying the diagnostic criteria of BPD (supplemental oxygen or respiratory support) at 40 weeks PMA, showed that BPD diagnosed at this age better correlated with long-term respiratory outcomes than when the diagnosis was made at an alternative age, between 34 and 44 weeks PMA. Prediction of adverse neurologic outcomes was optimized with classification of BPD status at 37 weeks PMA. Importantly, while diagnosing BPD at later postmenstrual ages may increase total accuracy and specificity, it will decrease sensitivity resulting in more infants who do not carry a diagnosis of BPD but will experience childhood respiratory and neurologic morbidity.[19,20,38] An additional limitation of diagnosing BPD at later time points is that a larger number of infants are transferred or discharged home before classification. In the cohort reported by the CNN, the BPD rate declined from 46% at 36 weeks PMA to 28% at 40 weeks PMA, but more than a third of the decline resulted from attrition in the cohort. This limitation might be addressed by classifying these infants at the time of discharge to home, but infants transferred earlier to alternative care settings may pose additional diagnostic dilemmas.

By defining BPD according to the respiratory support administered at a postmenstrual rather than chronological age, the definition inherently requires longer exposure times for more immature infants. An infant born at 24 weeks of gestation must be on oxygen at 12 weeks after birth to meet criteria while one born at 30 weeks is labeled as having BPD if receiving supplemental oxygen at 6 weeks of age. As mentioned earlier, a limitation of BPD classified only by supplemental respiratory therapy administered at a specific time point is that it may misdiagnose infants who do not have chronic lung disease but are receiving respiratory therapy only briefly for other reasons. Conversely, infants who transiently wean off respiratory support around the time of diagnosis may be incorrectly classified as disease free.

An alternative approach that avoids assessment at a single time point is the use of cumulative oxygen supplementation. This allows classification of infants with mild initial respiratory courses who may have only intermittent oxygen needs during the first weeks but still end up with protracted respiratory support needs and prolonged oxygen supplementation. Infants with more severe lung damage could be classified using a combination of the duration and concentration of inspired oxygen (e.g., the area under the curve or mean oxygen exposure over time). Calculating the cumulative supplemental oxygen to assess the severity of lung disease can be time-consuming, but now this information may be readily abstracted from electronic medical records. Future studies will be required to determine whether such diagnostic approaches improve classification of disease severity and prediction of long-term outcomes relative to current BPD definitions.

Competing Outcomes

Differences in mortality rates before the time of diagnosis can influence the incidence of BPD in surviving infants. A composite outcome such as "BPD or death before 36 weeks PMA" has been used to account for the effect of early mortality.[39] With this approach, one typically assumes that if the infants had survived they would have developed BPD. Although this is a common statistical approach, it is important that the rates of the individual components—death and BPD—are also reported separately because of the obvious difference in importance. In addition, the causes of death

may be independent of respiratory illness and differ between treatment groups in randomized trials. For example, a therapy may shift death etiology from severe, evolving BPD to sepsis by immune suppression without changing the death rate between treatment arms. The same concept applies to other major outcomes such as neurologic development in the preterm infant. For instance, high-dose postnatal steroids improve short-term respiratory outcomes but may increase the risk of cerebral palsy.[40] Changes in death rates and major neurodevelopmental outcomes carry greater importance than the possible effects of an intervention on BPD, but reporting of composite outcomes only may mask important treatment effects.

Deaths prior to 36 weeks PMA will include most infants with respiratory failure from severe progressive lung injury.[22] These infants most likely would have been diagnosed with BPD had they survived, but not always. To improve outcomes among infants susceptible to respiratory deaths prior to 36 weeks, these infants should be considered for the most innovative and high-risk therapies for BPD. Objective means to quantify early respiratory disease severity before the conventional diagnostic criteria for BPD are applied will aid assessment of the risks and benefits of novel therapies studied in critically ill infants.

Defining the Populations at Risk for Bronchopulmonary Dysplasia

An important aspect to consider when interpreting data using a BPD diagnostic classification for benchmarking purposes or in clinical trials is the baseline characteristics of the cohort or population from which the incidence of BPD is being reported. Benchmarking comparisons should also account for differences in early mortality between populations. The reported incidence per total live born infants is likely to be lower than the incidence among premature infants surviving the neonatal period, at 36 weeks PMA, or at discharge.

Because BPD is greatly influenced by the degree of prematurity, stratification by GA or BW is necessary for comparative interpretations between trials or cohorts. Also important is the approach used to define the range of BW or GA used for study inclusion. For instance, a cohort that includes only infants born within a specific BW threshold, e.g., below 1000 g, may inadvertently include a high proportion of growth-restricted infants of more advanced GA that meet the BW cutoff for inclusion. The risk for BPD in these more mature infants may differ from that of appropriate for GA infants who are in the same weight strata but were born at lower GA. A better approach would be to use a given range of GA for eligibility regardless of BW.

When interpreting the findings of clinical trials or epidemiologic cohorts, other entry criteria that could change the basal risk for BPD should also be considered. For example, studies that include only ventilated preterm infants would have higher BPD rates than studies in which all preterm infants are eligible. This is also true for studies that deliberately enroll infants at higher risk of BPD based on their initial respiratory course. The findings from those studies may not be directly applicable to infants of lesser risk or comparable to other studies with different entry criteria. Trials of infants for whom consent for randomization was obtained before birth will differ from those with infants for whom consent is obtained postnatally. The generalizability of study findings must be weighed in the context of these study characteristics.

Prognosis for Long-Term Pulmonary Impairment

As highlighted throughout this chapter, one key purpose of having diagnostic criteria for BPD is to provide a prognosis for long-term respiratory morbidity. BPD at 36 weeks PMA is associated with adverse health outcomes in childhood and later adult years. The costs of BPD are both social and economic and are measured in impaired childhood health and quality of life, family stress and economic hardship, and increased health care costs.[41-43] Premature infants with BPD have a longer initial hospitalization than their peers without BPD. After discharge, half or more of infants diagnosed with BPD will require hospital readmission in the first 2 years of life, most for respiratory reasons.[44,45] Children and adults diagnosed with BPD during infancy are more likely to receive respiratory drug therapies than similar preterm born infants without BPD.[46,47] Impairments in respiratory function and intolerance to physical activities can persist throughout

life in survivors with BPD and predict early onset of chronic obstructive pulmonary disease and adult mortality.[48]

The sensitivity and specificity of different diagnostic criteria of BPD for predicting adverse outcomes at 18 to 22 months' corrected age were evaluated in a cohort of infants born between 1995 and 1999 in the NICHD Neonatal Research Network.[49] Definitions based on the cumulative duration of oxygen for at least 28 days, exposure to oxygen at 36 weeks PMA, and the 2001 NIH workshop criteria were compared. The criteria including oxygen supplementation for at least 28 days were more sensitive in detecting postdischarge respiratory complications than oxygen dependency at 36 weeks PMA, but the specificity was considerably lower. Both criteria using oxygen dependency at 36 weeks PMA were more specific but at a cost of not classifying as BPD some infants that may later need additional respiratory care. This was in agreement with a report showing that discontinuation of supplemental oxygen after day 28 was a more sensitive test (although less specific) than after 36 weeks PMA in predicting poor long-term pulmonary outcomes.[50] Similar results have been observed in other cohorts, where moving the diagnosis of BPD to later chronological or postmenstrual ages increases specificity but reduces sensitivity.

Definitions that classify BPD severity demonstrate greater specificity for predicting adverse long-term respiratory impairments and will avoid some of the limitations of simpler dichotomous classifications of BPD. These findings underscore the importance of analyzing not only the incidence of BPD but also the severity of disease when conducting clinical trials or epidemiologic studies. Despite this benefit, very few studies report the incidence of BPD graded by severity. Increased use of such diagnostic criteria may better characterize longitudinal changes in the epidemiology of BPD and help determine whether therapies impact BPD severity, even when the overall rate of BPD is unaffected.

The intended use of diagnostic criteria of BPD has been to characterize chronic lung disease in infancy and to predict the respiratory course later in life. However, it is important to recognize that very preterm infants without a diagnosis of BPD are still at risk for abnormal lung development and function. Multiple studies have shown that long-term lung function in former premature infants is often abnormal when compared to term infants.[51,52] These alterations can occur in preterm infants irrespective of BPD diagnosis but are more common and severe among survivors with BPD. These alterations are more striking among cases classified as moderate or severe BPD.[53] Therefore, current diagnostic criteria of BPD can help differentiate patients with more severe lung damage from less affected individuals, but the absence of a BPD diagnosis does not assure normal lung function. Most preterm infants can maintain adequate arterial oxygen levels without supplemental oxygen at 36 weeks PMA, but this does not rule out underlying alterations in lung structure and function that could manifest later in life or when exposed to higher demands or injurious factors such as infection or secondhand smoke.

The fact that many premature infants have altered respiratory function later in life, irrespective of their BPD classification, suggests that the lung damage associated with premature birth and the impact of the many factors that can interfere with lung development cannot be defined as a simple dichotomized outcome. Like most biological processes, BPD is more appropriately represented by a continuum spanning spectrum between normal lung development and the profound alterations in lung structure and function seen in the most severe cases.

The correlation between the diagnosis of BPD and lung function later in life can be affected by many events that positively or negatively influence lung development and function after discharge from the hospital.[54] While having a single, early diagnostic criterion of BPD that reliably predicts long-term outcome is desirable, it is not realistic. For this reason, it is important to use short- and long-term endpoints in the assessment of outcomes among very preterm infants. Initial measures should reflect the neonatal respiratory evolution and shorter-term outcomes while later assessments should account for the postnatal respiratory course and longer-term outcomes.

Implications for Future Research

The criteria used to define BPD have evolved over time in response to changes in neonatal care practices and outcomes. Yet deficiencies in the diagnostic criteria remain. Arterial oxygenation or the need for supplemental oxygen to keep saturation levels in the prescribed range provides a practical but relatively crude measure of lung function. Supplemental oxygen alone does not fully reflect the complex alterations in respiratory function that can be at play in premature infants. Oxygen delivery device and device settings may impact prescribed oxygen therapy. Severity-based diagnostic criteria that consider modes of respiratory support administered at 36 weeks PMA improve prediction of adverse childhood outcomes but do not address all limitations in the diagnostic criteria. The mode of administered respiratory support is only a surrogate marker of disease severity, provides limited information about the etiology of respiratory failure, and in some instances may reflect physician treatment preferences rather than actual respiratory function.

Objective diagnostic testing that accurately quantifies abnormalities in lung structure and function may provide a solution to these concerns and must remain a focus of ongoing research. Tests measuring different aspects of lung function including lung volumes, pulmonary mechanics, gas distribution, diffusion capacity, and ventilation/perfusion abnormalities that can be used individually or as a battery could lead to more specific and sensitive ways to predict lung function later in life. Investigators have proposed a noninvasive assessment of pulmonary gas exchange to quantify the degree of pulmonary V/Q mismatch and shunt and grade the disease severity in infants with BPD.[55] Unfortunately, most of these tests at present are too complex for routine clinical use and their interpretation is not simple. Until there are more practical and simpler tests to evaluate lung structure and function, the only tools available are basic indicators of gas exchange to classify BPD and predict long-term lung function.

Recent data suggest that quantitative lung imaging with computed tomography (CT) or magnetic resonance (MR) techniques may improve diagnostic evaluation in BPD.[56-58] Performance of these studies in conjunction with airway evaluation and echocardiography can distinguish phenotypes in severely affected infants.[23] However, the utility and cost-effectiveness of these tests for routine performance in infants with milder disease forms remains uncertain. Future research will ideally identify noninvasive bedside or laboratory diagnostic measures for use in these infants. A particular focus should be evaluation of infants receiving oxygen therapy or respiratory support for conditions other than parenchymal lung disease. Transient conditions such as abnormal control of breathing, acute respiratory illness, and the use of medications such as caffeine, diuretics, or steroids can acutely influence the need for supplemental oxygen and respiratory support, and thereby the classification of BPD. Research into diagnostic tests that can objectively distinguish between etiologies of respiratory insufficiency across the disease spectrum may enable important refinements in BPD diagnostic criteria.

Conclusion

In summary, the use of standard diagnostic classifications of BPD and its severity is important to define the predischarge respiratory condition of infants at near-term corrected age. These standard criteria should be utilized to select endpoints for clinical trials that evaluate therapeutic strategies and to compare clinical outcomes between centers and within centers over time. Most diagnostic criteria of BPD use the need for supplemental oxygen and respiratory support to identify the degree of chronic lung dysfunction. Although the need for supplemental oxygen largely reflects the severity of lung damage present at near-term corrected age, a clear need exists for more precise markers of lung injury and function and better predictors of long-term pulmonary health in premature infants.

REFERENCES

1. Northway Jr WH, Rosan RC, Porter DY. Pulmonary disease following respirator therapy of hyaline-membrane disease: bronchopulmonary dysplasia. *N Engl J Med*. 1967;276(7):357-368.
2. Jobe AJ. The new BPD: an arrest of lung development. *Pediatr Res*. 1999;46(6):641-643.
3. Husain AN, Siddiqui NH, Stocker JT. Pathology of arrested acinar development in postsurfactant bronchopulmonary dysplasia. *Hum Pathol*. 1998;29(7):710-717.
4. McEvoy CT, Jain L, Schmidt B, et al. Bronchopulmonary dysplasia: NHLBI Workshop on the Primary Prevention of Chronic Lung Diseases. *Ann Am Thorac Soc*. 2014;11(suppl 3):S146-S153.
5. Margraf LR, Tomashefski Jr JF, Bruce MC, et al. Morphometric analysis of the lung in bronchopulmonary dysplasia. *Am Rev Respir Dis*. 1991;143(2):391-400.
6. Stoll BJ, Hansen NI, Bell EF, et al. Neonatal outcomes of extremely preterm infants from the NICHD Neonatal Research Network. *Pediatrics*. 2010;126(3):443-456.
7. Stroustrup A, Trasande L. Epidemiological characteristics and resource use in neonates with bronchopulmonary dysplasia: 1993-2006. *Pediatrics*. 2010;126(2):291-297.
8. Stoll BJ, Hansen NI, Bell EF, et al. Trends in care practices, morbidity, and mortality of extremely preterm neonates, 1993-2012. *JAMA*. 2015;314(10):1039-1051.
9. Jensen EA, Edwards EM, Greenberg LT, et al. Severity of bronchopulmonary dysplasia among very preterm infants in the United States. *Pediatrics*. 2021;148(1):e2020030007.
10. Thibeault DW, Mabry SM, Ekekezie II, et al. Collagen scaffolding during development and its deformation with chronic lung disease. *Pediatrics*. 2003;111(4 Pt 1):766-776.
11. Coalson JJ, Winter V, deLemos RA. Decreased alveolarization in baboon survivors with bronchopulmonary dysplasia. *Am J Respir Crit Care Med*. 1995;152(2):640-646.
12. Abman S. *Pulmonary hypertension in chronic lung disease of infancy. Pathogenesis, pathophysiology and treatment*. New York: Dekker; 2000.
13. Parker RA, Lindstrom DP, Cotton RB. Improved survival accounts for most, but not all, of the increase in bronchopulmonary dysplasia. *Pediatrics*. 1992;90(5):663-668.
14. Rojas MA, Gonzalez A, Bancalari E, et al. Changing trends in the epidemiology and pathogenesis of neonatal chronic lung disease. *J Pediatr*. 1995;126(4):605-610.
15. Charafeddine L, D'Angio CT, Phelps DL. Atypical chronic lung disease patterns in neonates. *Pediatrics*. 1999;103(4 Pt 1):759-765.
16. Bancalari E, Claure N, Sosenko IR. Bronchopulmonary dysplasia: changes in pathogenesis, epidemiology and definition. *Semin Neonatol*. 2003;8(1):63-71.
17. Bancalari E, Abdenour GE, Feller R, et al. Bronchopulmonary dysplasia: clinical presentation. *J Pediatr*. 1979;95(5 Pt 2):819-823.
18. Bancalari EH, Jobe AH. The respiratory course of extremely preterm infants: a dilemma for diagnosis and terminology. *J Pediatr*. 2012;161(4):585-588.
19. Shennan AT, Dunn MS, Ohlsson A, et al. Abnormal pulmonary outcomes in premature infants: prediction from oxygen requirement in the neonatal period. *Pediatrics*. 1988;82(4):527-532.
20. Isayama T, Lee SK, Yang J, et al. Revisiting the definition of bronchopulmonary dysplasia: effect of changing panoply of respiratory support for preterm neonates. *JAMA Pediatr*. 2017;171(3):271-279.
21. Jobe AH, Bancalari E. Bronchopulmonary dysplasia. *Am J Respir Crit Care Med*. 2001;163(7):1723-1729.
22. Poindexter BB, Feng R, Schmidt B, et al. Comparisons and limitations of current definitions of bronchopulmonary dysplasia for the prematurity and respiratory outcomes program. *Ann Am Thorac Soc*. 2015;12(12):1822-1830.
23. Wu KY, Jensen EA, White AM, et al. Characterization of disease phenotype in very preterm infants with severe bronchopulmonary dysplasia. *Am J Respir Crit Care Med*. 2020;201(11):1398-1406.
24. Higgins RD, Jobe AH, Koso-Thomas M, et al. Bronchopulmonary dysplasia: executive summary of a workshop. *J Pediatr*. 2018;197:300-308.
25. Jensen EA, Dysart K, Gantz MG, et al. The diagnosis of bronchopulmonary dysplasia in very preterm infants: an evidence-based approach. *Am J Respir Crit Care Med*. 2019;200(6):751-759.
26. Vyas-Read S, Logan JW, Cuna AC, et al. A comparison of newer classifications of bronchopulmonary dysplasia: findings from the Children's Hospitals Neonatal Consortium Severe BPD Group. *J Perinatol*. 2022;42(1):58-64.

27. Kurihara C, Zhang L, Mikhael M. Newer bronchopulmonary dysplasia definitions and prediction of health economics impacts in very preterm infants. *Pediatr Pulmonol.* 2021; 56(2):409-417.

28. Hines D, Modi N, Lee SK, et al. Scoping review shows wide variation in the definitions of bronchopulmonary dysplasia in preterm infants and calls for a consensus. *Acta Paediatr (Oslo, Norway: 1992).* 2017;106(3):366-374.

29. Ellsbury DL, Acarregui MJ, McGuinness GA, et al. Variability in the use of supplemental oxygen for bronchopulmonary dysplasia. *J Pediatr.* 2002;140(2):247-249.

30. Walsh MC, Yao Q, Gettner P, et al. Impact of a physiologic definition on bronchopulmonary dysplasia rates. *Pediatrics.* 2004;114(5):1305-1311.

31. Walsh MC, Wilson-Costello D, Zadell A, et al. Safety, reliability, and validity of a physiologic definition of bronchopulmonary dysplasia. *J Perinatol.* 2003;23(6):451-456.

32. Askie LM, Darlow BA, Finer N, et al. Association between oxygen saturation targeting and death or disability in extremely preterm infants in the neonatal oxygenation prospective meta-analysis collaboration. *JAMA.* 2018;319(21):2190-2201.

33. Foglia EE, Carper B, Gantz M, et al. Association between policy changes for oxygen saturation alarm settings and neonatal morbidity and mortality in infants born very preterm. *J Pediatr.* 2019;209:17-22.e12.

34. Huizing MJ, Villamor-Martínez E, Vento M, et al. Pulse oximeter saturation target limits for preterm infants: a survey among European neonatal intensive care units. *Eur J Pediatr.* 2017; 176(1):51-56.

35. Coste F, Ferkol T, Hamvas A, et al. Ventilatory control and supplemental oxygen in premature infants with apparent chronic lung disease. *Arch Dis Child Fetal Neonatal Ed.* 2015;100(3):F233-F237.

36. Kim F, Bateman DA, Goldstrom N, et al. Revisiting the definition of bronchopulmonary dysplasia in premature infants at a single center quaternary neonatal intensive care unit. *J Perinatol.* 2021;41(4):756-763.

37. Ballard RA, Keller RL, Black DM, et al. Randomized trial of late surfactant treatment in ventilated preterm infants receiving inhaled nitric oxide. *J Pediatr.* 2016;168:23-29.e4.

38. Davis PG, Thorpe K, Roberts R, Schmidt B, Doyle LW, Kirpalani H. Evaluating "old" definitions for the "new" bronchopulmonary dysplasia. *J Pediatr.* 2002;140(5):555-560.

39. Parekh SA, Field DJ, Johnson S, et al. Accounting for deaths in neonatal trials: is there a correct approach? *Arch Dis Child Fetal Neonatal Ed.* 2015;100(3):F193-F197.

40. Doyle LW, Ehrenkranz RA, Halliday HL. Dexamethasone treatment in the first week of life for preventing bronchopulmonary dysplasia in preterm infants: a systematic review. *Neonatology.* 2010;98(3):217-224.

41. Vohr BR, Wright LL, Dusick AM, et al. Neurodevelopmental and functional outcomes of extremely low birth weight infants in the National Institute of Child Health and Human Development Neonatal Research Network, 1993-1994. *Pediatrics.* 2000;105(6):1216-1226.

42. Wood NS, Costeloe K, Gibson AT, et al. The EPICure study: associations and antecedents of neurological and developmental disability at 30 months of age following extremely preterm birth. *Arch Dis Child Fetal Neonatal Ed.* 2005;90(2):F134-F140.

43. Fily A, Pierrat V, Delporte V, et al. Factors associated with neurodevelopmental outcome at 2 years after very preterm birth: the population-based Nord-Pas-de-Calais EPIPAGE cohort. *Pediatrics.* 2006;117(2):357-366.

44. Smith VC, Zupancic JA, McCormick MC, et al. Rehospitalization in the first year of life among infants with bronchopulmonary dysplasia. *J Pediatr.* 2004;144(6):799-803.

45. Greenough A, Alexander J, Burgess S, et al. Health care utilisation of prematurely born, preschool children related to hospitalisation for RSV infection. *Arch Dis Child.* 2004;89(7):673-678.

46. Ryan RM, Keller RL, Poindexter BB, et al. Respiratory medications in infants <29 weeks during the first year postdischarge: the Prematurity and Respiratory Outcomes Program (PROP) Consortium. *J Pediatr.* 2019;208:148-155.e3.

47. Skromme K, Vollsæter M, Øymar K, et al. Respiratory morbidity through the first decade of life in a national cohort of children born extremely preterm. *BMC Pediatr.* 2018;18(1):102.

48. Sillers L, Alexiou S, Jensen EA. Lifelong pulmonary sequelae of bronchopulmonary dysplasia. *Curr Opin Pediatr.* 2020;32(2): 252-260.

49. Ehrenkranz RA, Walsh MC, Vohr BR, et al. Validation of the National Institutes of Health consensus definition of bronchopulmonary dysplasia. *Pediatrics.* 2005;116(6):1353-1360.

50. Davis PG, Thorpe K, Roberts R, et al. Evaluating "old" definitions for the "new" bronchopulmonary dysplasia. *J Pediatr.* 2002;140(5):555-560.

51. Fawke J, Lum S, Kirkby J, et al. Lung function and respiratory symptoms at 11 years in children born extremely preterm: the EPICure study. *Am J Respir Crit Care Med.* 2010;182(2): 237-245.

52. Hjalmarson O, Sandberg K. Abnormal lung function in healthy preterm infants. *Am J Respir Crit Care Med.* 2002;165(1): 83-87.

53. Rite S, Martín de Vicente C, García-Iñiguez JP, et al. The consensus definition of bronchopulmonary dysplasia is an adequate predictor of lung function at preschool age. *Front Pediatr.* 2022;10:830035.

54. Stevens TP, Dylag A, Panthagani I, et al. Effect of cumulative oxygen exposure on respiratory symptoms during infancy among VLBW infants without bronchopulmonary dysplasia. *Pediatr Pulmonol.* 2010;45(4):371-379.

55. Svedenkrans J, Stoecklin B, Jones JG, et al. Physiology and predictors of impaired gas exchange in infants with bronchopulmonary dysplasia. *Am J Respir Crit Care Med.* 2019;200(4): 471-480.

56. Higano NS, Spielberg DR, Fleck RJ, et al. Neonatal pulmonary magnetic resonance imaging of bronchopulmonary dysplasia predicts short-term clinical outcomes. *Am J Respir Crit Care Med.* 2018;198(10):1302-1311.

57. van Mastrigt E, Kakar E, Ciet P, et al. Structural and functional ventilatory impairment in infants with severe bronchopulmonary dysplasia. *Pediatr Pulmonol.* 2017;52(8):1029-1037.

58. van Mastrigt E, Logie K, Ciet P, et al. Lung CT imaging in patients with bronchopulmonary dysplasia: a systematic review. *Pediatr Pulmonol.* 2016;51(9):975-986.

A Physiology-Based Approach to the Respiratory Care of Children With Severe Bronchopulmonary Dysplasia

Leif D. Nelin, Steven H. Abman, and Howard B. Panitch

Chapter Outline

Introduction

Definitions and Scope of Severe BPD

Pathogenesis of Severe BPD

Pathophysiology of Severe BPD

  Respiratory Function

  Lung Mechanics in Severe BPD

  Lung Volumes in Severe BPD

  Forced Flows in Severe BPD

Lung Imaging in Severe BPD

The Cardiovascular System in Severe BPD

Evaluation and Treatment of Severe BPD

  Mechanical Ventilation

  Drug Therapies

  Treatment of Pulmonary Hypertension

  Interdisciplinary Care

Long Term Outcomes

Key Points

- Despite advances in perinatal care, including many innovations in cardiorespiratory management of extremely preterm infants, the incidence of bronchopulmonary dysplasia (BPD) and its severity has not decreased over time and remains a major public health problem.

- Severe BPD (sBPD) is characterized by abnormalities of large and small airways with reduced distal lung surface area with heterogeneous lung units, leading to marked regional variations in airway resistance and tissue compliance throughout the lung. As a result, mechanical ventilation of infants with sBPD requires strikingly different ventilator strategies from those commonly used early in infants with respiratory distress syndrome (RDS) to prevent BPD.

- Disease severity in patients with sBPD can be due to multiple cardiorespiratory problems, including variable contributions from central and peripheral airways disease, altered lung parenchyma, pulmonary hypertension, cardiac dysfunction, altered control of breathing, and chest wall mechanics.

- Optimal care of infants with established BPD requires interdisciplinary teams, consisting of neonatologists, pulmonologists, cardiologists, respiratory therapists, nutritionists, occupational therapists, speech therapists, physical therapists, social workers, pharmacists, psychologists, and others.

- BPD is associated with lifelong changes in pulmonary structure and function, and more studies are needed to determine the long-term cardiorespiratory course across the lifespan.

Introduction

Bronchopulmonary dysplasia (BPD), the chronic lung disease of infancy that follows preterm birth, was first characterized by Northway and colleagues over

50 years ago.[1] In that era, prematurity-associated lung disease contributed to high mortality (60%) in relatively late-gestation preterm infants by today's standards (32–34 weeks gestation). Currently, survival for these moderate to late preterm infants is nearly 100%, with a 94% survival of preterm infants born even at 28 weeks gestation.[2,3] This remarkable success of modern care has increased survival of even the most extremely low gestational age newborns at the limits of viability (currently 22–23 weeks gestation), which likely accounts for the increasing rate of BPD in preterm infants born below 29 weeks gestation.[3] As a result, BPD remains the most common morbidity of preterm birth, occurring in an estimated 10 to 15,000 infants per year in the United States alone.[4] This has important health care implications, as infants with BPD require prolonged NICU hospitalizations; frequent readmissions for respiratory infections, wheezing, and related problems; and often have persistent lung function abnormalities and exercise intolerance as adolescents and young adults.

The overall incidence of BPD has increased over the last 10 to 20 years.[5] However, most infants with chronic lung disease after preterm birth now have a different clinical course and pathology from that described by Northway and that was observed in infants dying with BPD during the presurfactant era.[3,6,7,8] The classic progressive stages of disease, including prominent fibroproliferative changes, which first characterized BPD, are now just one phenotype of the disease that has been termed "old BPD." The phenotype of "old BPD" is no longer the most common manifestation of BPD, the most common disease phenotype now is defined as a disruption of distal lung growth, which has been referred to as "the new BPD."[9] However, it is important to remember that both "old BPD" and "new BPD" are phenotypes still seen today. The "new BPD" phenotype can develop even in preterm newborns who have required minimal or even no ventilator support and relatively low inspired oxygen concentrations during the early postnatal days.[8,9] At autopsy, the lung histology of infants who die with "the new BPD" displays lung injury, but impaired alveolar and vascular growth are the most prominent findings.[9] The "new BPD" is likely the result of disrupted antenatal and postnatal lung growth, which along with abnormalities of central and small airways causes persistent abnormalities of lung architecture

and function. Long-term pulmonary outcomes in BPD are incompletely understood, but recent work suggests persistent high rates of abnormal lung function through late childhood to early adulthood.[10] Indeed, recent studies have demonstrated that BPD is a risk factor for developing chronic obstructive pulmonary disease (COPD) in adults,[11,12] giving rise to the concept that BPD may be a novel COPD endotype.[13]

Although improved care has generally led to milder respiratory courses, infants with BPD can still develop severe lung disease, as reflected by chronic respiratory failure with high mortality and related morbidities (Fig. 14.1). The management of infants with sBPD has received less attention regarding clinical studies and interventions when compared with preventive strategies, yet these infants constitute a critical population who remain at high risk for extensive morbidities and late mortality. Therefore, the goal of this chapter is to characterize the epidemiology, pulmonary, and cardiovascular pathophysiology of sBPD, especially ventilator-dependent infants, and to discuss therapeutic strategies for their management based on best available evidence and/or the underlying physiology.

Definitions and Scope of Severe Bronchopulmonary Dysplasia

BPD has historically been defined by the presence of chronic respiratory signs, a persistent requirement for supplemental oxygen, and an abnormal chest radiograph at 1 month of age or at 36 weeks postmenstrual age (PMA) in patients born at <32 weeks gestation. This definition lacks specificity and fails to account for important clinical distinctions related to the extremes of prematurity and wide variability in how clinicians use prolonged oxygen therapy. The need for supplemental oxygen at 1 month in infants born at 24 or 25 weeks gestation may represent lung or respiratory control immaturity and not reflect the results of "lung injury,"[14] and such infants may or may not develop chronic respiratory disease. A National Institutes of Health (NIH) sponsored conference in 2000 led to a definition of BPD that categorizes the severity of BPD according to the level of respiratory support required at 36 weeks PMA, which has been widely used in the literature.[6] An advantage of this classification is that BPD is defined as a spectrum of disease and may be

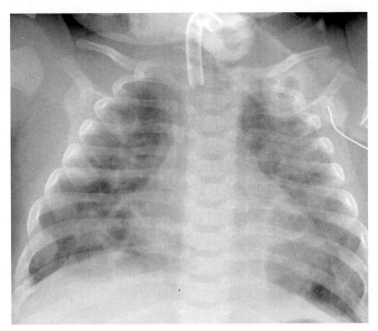

Fig. 14.1 Chest x-ray showing advanced findings of severe, ventilator-dependent BPD. *BPD,* Bronchopulmonary dysplasia.

predictive of long-term pulmonary morbidity. The NIH grading system, however, does not account for newer methods of respiratory support for neonates, like the use of high-flow nasal cannula (HFNC) or more aggressive use of noninvasive ventilation with or without supplemental oxygen. Past studies suggest that this grading of BPD severity is associated with the degree of abnormal lung function during infancy[15]; however, recent studies suggest that antenatal factors are key determinants for late respiratory disease independent of the diagnosis of BPD.[16] With the advent of newer therapies and approaches to respiratory support, the NIH system is also less able to predict mortality and important morbidities accurately.[17]

Another approach to determine the severity of BPD is to assess chest radiographs, but for many infants with chronic supplemental oxygen dependency, the chest x-ray only demonstrates small volumes with hazy lung fields. Various scoring systems have been developed and may predict chronic oxygen dependency and troublesome respiratory symptoms at follow-up.[18,19] Further work is clearly needed to identify early physiologic, structural, and genetic or biochemical markers of BPD that are predictive of critical long-term endpoints, such as the presence of late respiratory disease evidenced by prolonged mechanical ventilation and oxygen therapy, recurrent hospitalizations, wheezing, respiratory medications, and/or exercise intolerance during childhood.

The original NIH classification system defines sBPD as the need for supplemental oxygen with an FiO_2 ≥ 0.30 with or without positive pressure respiratory support at 36 weeks PMA in patients born at <32 weeks gestation.[6] Using the NIH criteria, studies from the Eunice Kennedy Shriver National Institute of Child Health and Human Development Neonatal Research Network and The Children's Hospitals Neonatal Consortium described a 16% incidence of sBPD among infants born < 32 weeks gestation,[15,20] but this proportion can vary based on the definition of sBPD used. Of note, early respiratory deaths after the first week of life but prior to 36 weeks PMA may represent the most severe form of BPD yet are not typically included in databases since they fail to reach the standard endpoint.

In addition, the NIH classification system's designation of sBPD pertained both to those infants who merely required supplemental oxygen ≥ 0.30 FiO_2

and to those infants who continued to require invasive mechanical ventilation. To help distinguish the latter infants from others with sBPD, members of the BPD Collaborative proposed a refinement to the NIH classification, designating those infants born <32 weeks GA who were treated with supplemental oxygen for at least 28 days and who required $FiO_2 \geq 0.30$, or nasal constant positive airway pressure (nCPAP) or HFNC at ≥ 36 weeks as having type 1 sBPD, and those who required invasive mechanical ventilation at ≥ 36 weeks as having type 2 sBPD.[4] Thus, the proportion of infants with the most severe disease requiring high levels of respiratory support have only recently been explored and optimal approaches to their care are incompletely understood. This is an important issue as mortality may increase with the duration of mechanical ventilation.[21]

Recognizing similar shortcomings to the original classification, the NIH convened an expert panel whose workshop publication in 2018 suggested changing the severity of BPD from mild, moderate, and severe, to Grade I, Grade II, Grade III, and Grade III(A).[22] In this classification, infants born <32 weeks GA who have clinical and radiographic evidence of parenchymal lung disease are assessed at 36 weeks PMA for the type of respiratory support required: those with Grade I disease require noninvasive ventilation or HFNC ≥ 3 LPM but no supplemental oxygen, or lower flow oxygen with FiO_2 ranging from 0.22 to 0.79, depending on the flow of gas. Those with Grade II could be treated with invasive mechanical ventilation as long as they do not require supplemental oxygen, use noninvasive ventilation with supplemental oxygen <0.30 FiO_2, or use supplemental oxygen ≥ 0.30 FiO_2 if flow is 1 to <3 LPM or >0.70 FiO_2 if flow is <1 LPM. Infants with Grade III BPD require either invasive mechanical ventilation with supplemental oxygen or noninvasive ventilation with ≥ 0.30 FiO_2, and those with Grade III(A) died between 14 days postnatal age and 36 weeks PMA from respiratory causes.

The need to categorize the severity of BPD is not only important for epidemiological purposes, but having a common definition can also help with the design of clinical trials aimed at those infants most likely to benefit from advanced therapies, help identify mechanisms of injury, or help clinicians predict longer term outcomes. Focusing on this last goal, members of the Canadian Neonatal Network evaluated several definitions of BPD being used for clinical and epidemiological studies focusing on pulmonary and neurodevelopmental outcomes at 18 to 21 months of age.[19] They concluded that need for supplemental oxygen and/or respiratory support at 40 weeks PMA best predicted respiratory morbidity at 18 to 24 months. Once again, however, use of HFNC without supplemental oxygen or standard nasal cannula therapy using very low-flow rates resulted in some infants who could not be classified using this system.

More recently, members of the Eunice Kennedy Shriver National Institute of Child Health and Human Development Neonatal Research Network applied 18 prespecified severity-graded BPD definitions to a population of 2677 very preterm infants.[23] The definition that best predicted late death or serious respiratory morbidity at 18 to 26 months was independent of supplemental oxygen use at 36 weeks PMA. Instead, Grade 1 infants required any kind of nasal cannula therapy at a flow ≤ 2 LPM; Grade 2 infants required >2 LPM nasal cannula (HFNC) or noninvasive ventilation; and Grade 3 infants required invasive ventilation. This definition accurately predicted late death or serious respiratory morbidity in 81% of the infants studied, and late death or serious neurodevelopmental disability in 69%. Further, the incidence of late death or serious respiratory morbidity rose from 10% among those infants classified as not having BPD to 77% among those with Grade 3 BPD. These same criteria were subsequently retrospectively applied to 24,896 infants born between 22 and 29-6/7 weeks in the Vermont Oxford Network.[24] In this group, 10% died before 36 weeks PMA and 49% did not develop BPD while 37% were classified as having either Grade 1 or Grade 2 BPD. Grade 3 BPD developed in 4% of the cohort. Late deaths before NICU discharge occurred in 1% of those infants who survived beyond 36 weeks PMA; among those, 62% carried a diagnosis of Grade 3 BPD, while 35% had either Grade 1 or Grade 2 BPD, and 3% did not have BPD. The frequency of all the evaluated neonatal morbidities increased with severity of BPD, so that they occurred 2 to 3 times more commonly among those with Grade 3 BPD compared with those with Grade 1 or 2 BPD, and more than 4 times as commonly as among those without BPD. Length of stay, supplemental oxygen use at discharge, and need for tracheostomy were all greatest in the infants classified with Grade 3 BPD.

Separately, several of the various grading systems have been compared within populations of extremely preterm infants. Applying the original NIH 2000 definition, the 2018 NIH Workshop refinement of the original definition, and the 2019 Neonatal Research Network (NRN) grading system to 2,380 extremely preterm infants in the Korean National Network, investigators sought to determine which system would best predict respiratory and neurodevelopmental impairments at 18 to 24 months and again at 3 years of age.[25] The original 2000 NIH severity classification did not show any severity-related increased risk for respiratory, neurodevelopmental, or growth impairments. Both the refined NIH Workshop system and the NRN system showed severity-related increases in risk for those impairments at both 18 to 24 months and at 3 years of age, but they noted that the NRN system was easier to apply, given the lack of need to determine supplemental oxygen use at 36 weeks PMA or over the first 28 days of life.

Members of the Children's Hospitals Neonatal Consortium performed another retrospective comparison of the 2018 NIH Workshop and 2019 NRN systems, along with that of the Canadian Neonatal Network among 4161 preterm infants in their network to assess short-term outcomes.[26] All three systems demonstrated a significant severity-based increase in risk of in-hospital mortality or need for tracheostomy, even when gestational age, gender, and center were controlled. Once again, the NRN system was found to be the easiest to apply, and it also had the strongest discrimination of the three for poor short-term outcomes. Investigators from the BPD Collaborative applied their refinement of the original 2001 NIH classification to explore short-term outcomes among 584 infants in their registry.[27] The risk for mortality among those infants with type 2 sBPD was significantly higher than for those with type 1 sBPD (RR 13.8, 95% CI 4.3–44.5, P <0.0001). The infants with type 2 sBPD also had a significantly greater risk for tracheostomy, gastrostomy, impaired growth, and greater use of inhaled bronchodilators and corticosteroids than those with type 1 sBPD. This classification aligned well with the NRN severity

classification, but less well with the 2018 NIH Workshop classification for severe BPD. In addition, 6% of the cohort could not be classified by the 2018 NIH Workshop classification scheme because of unreliable FiO_2 data at 36 weeks PMA.

Using an estimated incidence of sBPD of 16% for infants born at <32 weeks suggests that ~13,000 patients develop sBPD annually in the United States alone.[4] Epidemiologic data are limited, but estimates suggest that roughly 8000 children in the United States receive mechanical ventilation at home.[28] Based on 2011 data from the state of Pennsylvania's Ventilator Assisted Children's Home Program, 36% of ventilator-dependent children were diagnosed with chronic lung disease: 77% of these specifically with the diagnosis of sBPD.[28] From these data it can be extrapolated that ~2000 infants and children with sBPD are dependent on mechanical ventilation at home in the United States.

Severe BPD is directly linked with worse long-term outcomes, such as need for rehospitalization, need for pulmonary medications, poor neurodevelopmental outcomes, need for home ventilation, and others. In one study, the incidence of cerebral palsy was 11% and 27% in those with mild and severe BPD, respectively.[15] A report of patients cared for in the Comprehensive Center for BPD at Nationwide Children's Hospital showed that 12% of patients with moderate BPD had cognitive scores on the Bayley Scales of Infant Development at 18 to 24 months of <70, while 15% of patients with severe BPD had cognitive scores <70.[29]

Pathogenesis of Severe Bronchopulmonary Dysplasia

Preterm infants are especially susceptible to lung injury from mechanical ventilation, oxidative stress, and inflammation due to the extreme structural and biochemical immaturity of the preterm lung. As Northway first observed, BPD has multifactorial etiologies, including hyperoxia, ventilator-induced lung injury, inflammation, and infection.[1] Animal studies suggest that lung injury due to each of these adverse stimuli is at least partly mediated through increased oxidative stress that further augments inflammation, promotes lung injury, and impairs growth factor signaling pathways.[30,31] Antenatal factors, such as maternal smoking, chorioamnionitis, preeclampsia, and intra-uterine growth restriction (IUGR), are clear contributing factors to the risk for BPD and perhaps its severity.[16,32-38] A recent longitudinal study of 587 preterm infants found that maternal smoking increased the risk for BPD twofold and was associated with prolonged mechanical ventilation and respiratory support during the NICU stay.[16] In this study, preexisting maternal hypertension was associated with a twofold increase in odds for BPD. Further studies are needed to determine how different etiologic mechanisms alter the risk for BPD as well as its severity.

Among at-risk infants, the duration and approach to mechanical ventilation, including the use of high inspired oxygen, high peak inspiratory pressures, lower positive end-expiratory pressures (PEEPs), and higher ventilation rate, are also associated with BPD, relationships that could be causal or simply reflect the underlying severity of acute respiratory disease.[39] Mechanical ventilation can induce lung injury through volutrauma, in which phasic stretch or overdistension of the lung can induce lung inflammation, permeability edema, and subsequent structural changes that mimic human BPD, even in the absence of high levels of supplemental oxygen.[40,41] Aggressive mechanical ventilation with hypocarbia has been associated with the development of BPD, as reports have shown an association between low $PaCO_2$ levels and BPD development.[42] High tidal volumes should be avoided both during mechanical ventilation in the early stages of respiratory distress syndrome (RDS) in the NICU and during resuscitation in the delivery room.[43] Although small tidal volumes may reduce the risk for ventilator-induced lung injury in preterm infants, failure to recruit and maintain adequate functional residual capacity (FRC) even with low tidal volumes is injurious in experimental models.[44] Despite some data suggesting that alternate strategies such as nCPAP and other noninvasive ventilation modes may reduce the risk for BPD, there remains striking center-to-center variability and meta-analysis has not shown uniform benefits.[45]

The association of volutrauma with the development of BPD has led to the use of strategies such as permissive hypercapnia to minimize lung injury.[46] Various ventilator devices and strategies have been assessed regarding their ability to reduce BPD.

Meta-analysis of randomized trials has demonstrated that patient-triggered ventilation does not reduce the incidence of BPD but, if started in the recovery phase of RDS, it significantly shortens weaning from mechanical ventilation. The results of randomized trials of highfrequency oscillatory ventilation (HFOV) or high-frequency jet ventilation (HFJV) have been inconsistent.[47,48] Two large studies that incorporated prenatal steroid and surfactant replacement therapy yielded different results. In one, which restricted entry to very low-birth-weight infants with moderate-to-severe hypoxemic respiratory failure following surfactant administration, HFOV was associated with higher survival without BPD and shorter duration of ventilation.[49] No substantial benefit or adverse effects of HFOV were found in the other study, however, which randomized premature infants (<29 weeks) within 1 hour of birth regardless of the degree of lung disease.[50] An explanation for those conflicting results may be that in the current era that includes the use of modified conventional ventilation strategies, pulmonary benefit from HFOV may only be demonstrable in infants with moderate-to-severe disease. Clearly, the strategies applied for either conventional or HFOV are more important than the device itself. HFOV is frequently used as "rescue" therapy in premature newborns with severe respiratory failure despite treatment with exogenous surfactant and conventional ventilation. Whether such an approach reduces the risk to develop BPD or improves long-term outcomes requires additional investigation.

An optimal ventilation mode has not yet emerged to prevent BPD, but it is clear from physiological studies that tidal volumes and inspired oxygen concentrations should be reduced as low as possible to avoid hypocarbia, volutrauma, and oxygen toxicity, while applying strategies to optimize lung recruitment. Two meta-analyses suggest that volume-targeted ventilation reduces the duration of mechanical ventilation and reduces the incidence of BPD.[51,52] An alternative approach to reduce the risk of developing BPD has been to avoid intubation and mechanical ventilation by using early nCPAP. For example, the SUPPORT study found that patients who received early nCPAP without intubation and surfactant therapy had decreased need for intubation or postnatal corticosteroids for BPD, required fewer days of mechanical ventilation, and were more likely to be alive and free from the need for mechanical ventilation by 7 days of age.[53] Many centers now minimize their use of mechanical ventilation, preferring nCPAP with or without administration of exogenous surfactant and report low incidences of BPD in high-risk infants. Since the risk for BPD is associated with the need for mechanical ventilation and centers that use less mechanical ventilation have a lower incidence of BPD, avoiding or minimizing mechanical ventilation during the early course of extreme prematurity may prevent BPD or lessen its severity. As discussed below, however, ventilator strategies during the early stages of respiratory distress are strikingly different from approaches needed to optimize gas exchange and treat chronic respiratory failure in the setting of established BPD.

Pathophysiology of Severe Bronchopulmonary Dysplasia

RESPIRATORY FUNCTION

Multiple abnormalities of lung structure and function contribute to late respiratory disease in BPD. Chronic respiratory signs in children with moderate and severe BPD include tachypnea with shallow breathing, retractions, and paradoxical breathing pattern; coarse rhonchi, rales, and wheezes are typically heard on auscultation. The increased respiratory rate and shallow breathing increase dead space ventilation. Nonuniform damage to the airways and distal lungs results in variable time constants for different areas of the lungs, and inspired gas may be distributed to relatively poorly perfused lung, thereby worsening ventilation-perfusion (V/Q) matching. Dynamic lung compliance is markedly reduced in infants with established BPD, even in those who no longer require oxygen therapy.[54] The reduction in dynamic compliance is due to small airway narrowing, interstitial fibrosis, edema, and atelectasis.

Newer mechanical ventilation strategies have resulted in less central airway damage in infants with the "new BPD," but significant tracheomalacia and abnormalities of conducting airway structure persist in the current era. Increases in airway smooth muscle have been found within the first month of life in BPD infants,[55,56] and epithelial cell height was found to be greater than in controls.[55] The combination of smooth muscle hypertrophy and thickened airway walls, together with fewer alveolar wall attachments supporting small airway patency predispose BPD infants to increased airway resistance, which can be demonstrated even during the first week after birth in preterm neonates at risk for BPD.[57] Although there is not complete agreement among various studies, most have demonstrated that pulmonary or respiratory system resistance is elevated within the first 2 weeks in those ventilator-dependent infants who subsequently develop BPD compared with those who do not develop BPD.[57-61] This abnormality in lung mechanics persists in older infants with BPD and has been found to have an increased total respiratory and expiratory resistance with severe flow limitation, especially at low lung volumes.[60] When resistance is so high that it slows expiratory flows to the point that the lung cannot fully empty before the next breath ensues, dynamic hyperinflation and intrinsic PEEP can occur.[62] Intrinsic PEEP can cause significant trigger asynchrony and dyspnea among ventilator-dependent infants with sBPD.

The presence of tracheobronchomalacia may also result in airflow limitation. It is important for the clinician to recognize this entity because the airflow limitation may be worsened by bronchodilator therapy.[63] Significant tracheomalacia increases respiratory work and energy expenditure related to increased tracheal resistance.[64] The presence of tracheobronchomalacia in BPD infants has been associated with longer courses of mechanical ventilation, longer NICU stays, and more complicated NICU courses.[65] It is not always easy to determine if a collapsible central airway represents excessive compliance of the tracheal wall or is the result of increased transmural (collapsing) pressure across the airway wall caused by severe small airway obstruction: in the latter case, the intraluminal pressure gradient from alveolus to mouth falls more quickly, and simultaneously the infant may generate positive pleural pressure to overcome the obstruction. Both of these situations serve to accentuate the pressure gradient across the airway wall and favor its collapse. While current methods to detect tracheomalacia do not account for transmural pressure assessment, a recent approach attempts to circumvent this by using ultrashort echo time magnetic resonance imaging (MRI) to diagnose tracheomalacia when large changes in central airway cross-sectional area are present in nonsedated infants during quiet tidal breathing.[66]

Recognizing that outcomes of very preterm infants with sBPD depend on more than degree of parenchymal lung disease alone, one center retrospectively assessed 76 infants born <32 weeks GA with sBPD who underwent echocardiography and chest computed tomography with angiography (CTA) between 40 and 50 weeks PMA[67] for a composite outcome of death before NICU discharge or tracheostomy or the need for systemic pulmonary vasodilator therapy at discharge. Moderate-to-severe parenchymal lung disease was based on an Ochiai score ≥8 on the CTA.[68] The presence of pulmonary hypertension (PH) was based on echocardiographic findings. Large airway collapse was based on findings on tracheoscopy or bronchoscopy, or >50% reduction in airway caliber between inspiratory and expiratory images on CTA. Of the cohort, 73 could be classified into at least one of the phenotypes: 57 had moderate-to-severe parenchymal disease, 48 had PH, 44 had large airway disease, and 23 of these infants had all three phenotypes. The presence of PH or large airway disease, but not moderate-to-severe parenchymal lung disease, was associated with an increased risk of the composite outcome (PH, OR 5.4, 95% CI 1.8–16.6; large airway disease OR 5.1, 95% CI 1.7–15.9). Furthermore, an increasing number of disease phenotypes was associated with greater risk for pulmonary vasodilator use at discharge and with tracheostomy, but not with in-hospital mortality.

In the early stages of neonatal respiratory failure, the functional lung volume is often reduced due to atelectasis, but during the later stages of BPD, there is gas trapping with hyperinflation.[58,59,69] This increased resting lung volume caudally depresses the diaphragm and places it at a mechanical disadvantage for generating adequate tidal volumes. One group used infant pulmonary function testing to phenotype infants with sBPD still dependent on invasive or noninvasive mechanical ventilation at the time of testing.[70] The cohort was subsequently divided into three phenotypes: obstructive, restrictive, and mixed, based on pulmonary function values. The majority of the cohort had obstructive disease, defined as a forced expiratory volume in 0.5 seconds (FEV 0.5) <80%

predicted and total lung capacity (TLC) >90% of predicted. They also had significantly greater residual volume (RV) and RV/TLC ratio than either of the other groups, suggesting a component of air trapping. The obstructive group also tended to require tracheostomy and require mechanical ventilation at the time of discharge more frequently compared with the other groups.

Although the new BPD has been characterized as an arrest of distal lung and vascular growth, most of these observations were based on lung histology and evidence that provided direct physiologic data to support this finding was lacking. Tepper and colleagues have demonstrated reduced lung surface area in infants with BPD by utilizing novel methods of assessing diffusion capacity.[71] Thus, established BPD is primarily characterized by reduced surface area and heterogeneous lung units, in which regional variations in airway resistance and tissue compliance lead to highly variable time constants throughout the lung.[72] As a result, mechanical ventilation of infants with sBPD requires strikingly different ventilator strategies from those commonly used early in infants with RDS to prevent BPD. Strategies for severe BPD generally favor longer inspiratory times, larger tidal volumes, higher PEEP, and lower rates to allow more effective gas exchange and respiratory function.

LUNG MECHANICS IN SEVERE BRONCHOPULMONARY DYSPLASIA

Diverse methods have been used to assess lung mechanics in infants with established BPD during tidal breathing. These include measurements of dynamic resistance and compliance of the lung with the use of esophageal pressure catheters; single and multiple breath occlusion for measuring respiratory system resistance and compliance; plethysmography measurement of airway resistance; interrupter and forced oscillation methods for measuring respiratory system resistance; and weighted spirometry. Airway obstruction has also been determined from respiratory inductive plethysmography measurements of phase angle differences in chest wall and abdominal dimensions. These approaches have been reviewed in detail.[73-75] Normalized measures of both static and dynamic lung compliance are reduced in established BPD. This may be due to fibrosis, atelectasis, changes in parenchyma and airway properties, or diminished coupling between lung parenchyma and airways due to edema.[76,77]

Past studies have reported increased airway resistance in infants with established BPD.[58,59,70,78,79] Specific compliance and conductance generally improve over the first 2 to 3 years of life.[80] However, concerns persist regarding limitations of infant pulmonary function testing, especially for routine clinical use given the difficulty in obtaining and using the appropriate equipment, and the need for sedation. Measures of compliance and resistance can be variable as these values are generally determined over a limited tidal volume range and are dependent upon the lung volume at which these measurements are made. Additionally, in BPD patients with airway obstruction, measurements of dynamic compliance are markedly affected by respiratory rate (e.g., "frequency dependence") because of the heterogeneity of time constants of regional lung units. This heterogeneity is reflected in the substantial curvilinearity of the passive expiratory flow-volume curve obtained by the single breath occlusion method in infants with BPD. The respiratory system mechanics in these patients can be well characterized using a "two-compartment" rather than a linear "one-compartment" model.[72,81,82] The abnormalities in compliance and especially resistance in BPD infants significantly alter how the lung fills and empties. For example, the respiratory system time constant of 24 BPD infants mechanically ventilated for 38 ± 4 days increased from 0.14 ± 0.01 seconds at 10 to 20 days of life to 0.33 ± 0.02 seconds at 6 months, 0.48 ± 0.03 seconds at 1 year, and 0.50 ± 0.03 seconds at 2 years.[58]

LUNG VOLUMES IN SEVERE BRONCHOPULMONARY DYSPLASIA

FRC has been measured in infants with BPD by body plethysmography and with nitrogen washout and gas dilution methods.[73] In contrast with plethysmography, washout and gas dilution methods measure only gas that communicates with the conducting airways during tidal breathing. These measurements may underestimate the actual lung volume at FRC because they do not measure volumes of gas trapped behind closed airways and can underestimate volumes in severely obstructed poorly ventilated areas.[83-86] Measurements before 1 year of age using gas dilution and

washout methods have consistently reported reduced FRC in infants with both old and new BPD.[58,78,84,85] In contrast, plethysmography studies have demonstrated normal or elevated FRC values.[87,88] Reductions in gas dilution and nitrogen washout measurements of FRC probably reflect the amount of noncommunicating trapped gas not measured in infants with obstructive disease rather than being indicative of a true restrictive defect. Reduction in the difference between the two methods is probably indicative of improvements in airway function, less gas trapping, and better gas exchange.[69] Thus, functional abnormalities in infants with severe BPD are primarily obstructive rather than restrictive, but precise measurements are especially complicated in severe disease due to the heterogeneity of airway and lung parenchymal abnormalities.

Recently, the use of the raised volume rapid thoracic compression (RVRTC) method for performing spirometry in sedated infants has provided an alternative approach to measure fractional lung volumes, including TLC and RV.[89] Robin et al. have reported the results of fractional lung volume measurements in 28 patients with new BPD.[88] Mean RV and RV/TLC ratio were found to be significantly elevated in infants with BPD compared to normal control infants while mean TLC was in the normal range. In contrast, FRC as measured by plethysmography was found to be only marginally elevated compared to the normal control infants. In addition, TLC continued to increase over the second year of life in infants with BPD, yet the severity of air trapping, as reflected by the RV/TLC ratio, remained unchanged.[89] Thus, infants with the BPD have obstructive airway disease with gas trapping that persists over time and is strikingly abnormal in severe BPD.

As discussed, one of the major goals for providing successful chronic respiratory support is to address the challenge of improving the distribution of gas to optimize lung volumes and gas exchange in the setting of striking heterogeneous lung disease. A potentially useful and exciting advance in enhancing bedside decision-making with adjustments of ventilator support to match evolving changes in physiology is the use of serial point-of-care lung ultrasound (LUS) or electrical impedance tomography (EIT) to address regional areas of hyperinflation.[90,91] Ongoing work with LUS and EIT will explore their potential utility in addition to other clinical and physiologic assessments including clinical status, flow-volume loops, serial chest x-rays, and other markers.

FORCED FLOWS IN SEVERE BRONCHOPULMONARY DYSPLASIA

Measurements of forced flows have been made in infants with BPD using the rapid thoracic compression (RTC) method to produce partial flow-volume curves over the tidal range and the forced deflation and RVRTC techniques to produce forced expiratory flows over the full vital capacity range. The use of these tests in infants with BPD has been reviewed and guidelines for the two RTC methods have been published.[92,93] The RTC technique to produce partial expiratory flow-volume curves was applied to infants with BPD, demonstrating that average maximal flows measured at FRC (Maxar) were reduced by approximately 50% when compared to normal infants.[87] A reduction in V'maxFRC in infants with BPD has been a consistent finding in subsequent studies, and longitudinal measurements over the first 2 years of life demonstrated very modest increases in absolute flows in individual infants with BPD that often do not keep pace with the expected rate of increase with growth.[54] On average, the rate of increase for infants with BPD was substantially below that measured in normal infants over the same interval. Thus, at follow-up, measurements of V'maxFRC in the infants with BPD had fallen even farther below those measured in normal infants.

When airways and lung parenchyma do not grow proportionally, lung growth is considered "dysanaptic."[94] One type of dysanaptic lung growth is characterized by lower than normal expiratory flows despite normal lung volume, reflecting reduced airway size for a given lung volume. This pattern of dysanaptic lung growth has been implicated as one cause of airflow obstruction seen in subjects born extremely prematurely with or without BPD.[95] The ratio of a measurement sensitive to airway size (the forced expiratory flow at 50% of the vital capacity, or FEF_{50}) normalized to the static lung recoil at 50% of the vital capacity ($Pst(L)_{50}$), to a measurement sensitive to lung volume (the vital capacity, VC) is indicative of airway size at a given lung volume.[96] This dysanapsis ratio (DR) is described by the equation $DR = FEF_{50} \div (VC \times Pst(L)_{50})$ and is decreased when airways are

small or elevated if the airways are large for a given lung volume. Investigators examining the presence of bronchodilator responsiveness (BDR) in a group of 93 infants with BPD during their initial NICU stay found that the median DR was significantly smaller among those who demonstrated significant BDR compared with those who did not.[97] Of the group, 62% of the infants had Grade 3 sBPD and 24% had Grade 2 BPD. The DR also correlated significantly with the FEV0.5 ($R^2 = 0.39$, $P < 0.001$) and inversely with the TLC ($R^2 = 0.19$, $P < 0.001$). These data suggest that dysanaptic lung growth, with smaller airways for a given lung volume, could contribute to BDR, lower baseline forced expiratory flows, and degree of lung inflation in infants with BPD. Whether dysanaptic lung growth occurs as a result of early airway injury in infants with BPD or is a marker for infants more likely to develop sBPD remains unknown.

Reduction in forced flow can also reflect severity of the underlying disease. Toddlers with BPD still dependent on supplemental oxygen use after 2 years of age had significantly lower volume-corrected forced flows (V'maxFRC/FRC) than those BPD toddlers who had weaned from supplemental oxygen.[98]

LUNG IMAGING IN SEVERE BRONCHOPULMONARY DYSPLASIA

The chest radiographic characteristics of infants with BPD have changed substantially since the original description by Northway et al.[1] Although the chest x-ray of BPD as classically described is still seen in those infants with severe disease, the usual radiographic changes in today's smaller, less mature infants are much more variable and are often characterized by irregularly distributed areas of fine infiltrates and mild hyperlucency. Chest radiographs often underestimate and correlate poorly with the extent of the pathological changes in infants with established BPD.[99,100] High-resolution computed tomography (HRCT) is a more sensitive technique for detecting structural abnormalities in the lungs of patients with established BPD compared to plain chest radiography (Fig. 14.2).[101,102] Correlations between abnormalities seen on HRCT and measures of lung function and clinical severity suggest that HRCT may be useful in clinical management and as an outcome measure in this population. CT imaging is helpful for identifying unsuspected abnormalities in

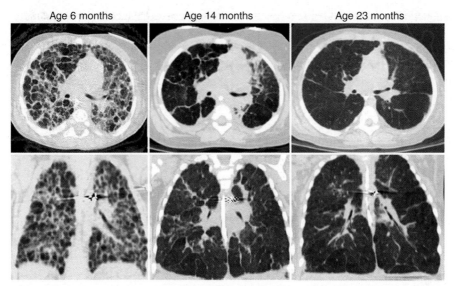

Fig. 14.2 HRCT scans done at 25 cm H_2O during a breath hold in the same patient with severe BPD at three different ages. The top are transverse sections and the bottom are coronal sections taken from the same area. These scans demonstrate that despite ongoing mechanical ventilator support with lung growth and repair, the findings on HRCT improve over time, although the scan at 23 months of age remains abnormal. *BPD*, Bronchopulmonary dysplasia; *HRCT*, high-resolution computed tomography.

the lungs of individual patients with BPD, but its ultimate utility as a tool for clinical management and as an outcome measure for research investigations is not yet clear. Radiation exposure from CT imaging has been substantially greater than that received from standard chest x-rays.[103] However, through the development of novel scanning algorithms, the radiation exposure from CT imaging has been greatly reduced, such that diagnostic HRCT can be done at a radiation dose similar to a chest radiograph.[104,105]

More recently, MRI has undergone dramatic technological improvements, including the use of ultrashort echo times, which has reduced the need for sedation, and these images may provide important lung structure in BPD.[106] Furthermore, MRI strategies to measure lung function are also emerging. For example, Dyke et al.[107] recently demonstrated that MRI could be used to calculate pulmonary ventilation parameters in infants with BPD in the NICU. Gouwens et al.[108] using respiratory-gated, ultrashort echo time MRI measured total lung tidal volume and the tidal volume from noncystic and cystic parts of the lung and found that the cystic areas averaged larger tidal volumes than noncystic areas, and cyst tidal

volume was correlated with cyst size. They also found that peak inspiratory pressure was positively correlated with total lung tidal volume and noncystic tidal volumes.[108] These types of studies demonstrate the potential for MRI scanning in BPD, and as more evidence is generated, the next few years may see lung MRI become an important part of the clinical toolbox for BPD. Other imaging modalities are also being studied for better understanding BPD. For example, single-photon emission computed tomography (SPECT) scanning may be a potential way of directly measuring V/Q matching in infants with BPD in the NICU setting.[109,110]

THE CARDIOVASCULAR SYSTEM IN SEVERE BRONCHOPULMONARY DYSPLASIA

Acute lung injury impairs growth, structure, and function of the developing pulmonary circulation after premature birth.[111,112] Endothelial cells are particularly susceptible to oxidant injury due to hyperoxia or inflammation. The media of small pulmonary arteries may also undergo striking changes, including smooth muscle cell proliferation, precocious maturation of immature pericytes into mature smooth muscle cells, and incorporation of fibroblasts into the vessel wall and surrounding adventitia.[113] Structural changes in the lung vasculature contribute to high pulmonary vascular resistance (PVR) due to narrowing of the vessel diameter and decreased vascular compliance. Decreased angiogenesis may limit vascular surface area, causing further elevations of PVR, especially in response to high cardiac output with exercise or stress. The pulmonary circulation in BPD patients is further characterized by abnormal vasoreactivity, which also increases PVR.[112] Abnormal pulmonary vasoreactivity is evidenced by a marked vasoconstrictor response to acute hypoxia.[112,113] Cardiac catheterization studies have shown that even mild hypoxia causes marked elevations in pulmonary artery pressure, even in infants with modest basal levels of PH. Maintaining oxygen saturation levels above 92% to 94% effectively lowers the pulmonary artery pressure.[112] Strategies to lower pulmonary artery pressure or to minimize lung injury to the pulmonary vasculature may limit the subsequent development of PH in BPD.

Early injury to the lung circulation leads to the rapid development of PH, which contributes significantly to the morbidity and mortality of severe BPD. Even in early reports of BPD, PH and cor pulmonale were recognized as being associated with high mortality.[114,115] Persistent echocardiographic evidence of PH beyond the first few months has been associated with up to 40% mortality in infants with BPD.[116,117] High mortality rates have also been reported in infants with BPD and severe PH, especially in those who require prolonged ventilator support.[112,116] In addition to the adverse effects of PH on the clinical course of infants with BPD, the lung circulation is further characterized by persistence of abnormal or "dysmorphic" growth of the pulmonary circulation, including a relative paucity of small pulmonary arteries with an altered pattern of distribution within the interstitium of the distal lung.[118-120] In infants with severe BPD, decreased vascular growth occurs in conjunction with marked reductions in alveoli, suggesting that the "new BPD" is primarily characterized by growth arrest of the developing lung. This reduction of alveolar-capillary surface area impairs gas exchange, thereby increasing the need for prolonged supplemental oxygen and ventilator therapy, causing marked hypoxemia with acute

respiratory infections and late exercise intolerance, and further increases the risk for developing severe PH. Experimental studies have further shown that early injury to the developing lung can impair angiogenesis,[121-123] which further contributes to decreased alveolarization and simplification of distal lung airspace (the "vascular hypothesis"[119]). Thus, abnormalities of the lung circulation in BPD are not only related to the presence or absence of PH, but more broadly, pulmonary vascular disease after premature birth as manifested by decreased vascular growth and structure also contributes to the pathogenesis and abnormal cardiopulmonary physiology of BPD.

An emerging cause of PH in patients with BPD is pulmonary vein stenosis (PVS).[124-126] Mahgoub et al.[125] described 39 former preterm infants with a median gestational age at birth of 28 weeks and a median birth weight of 1100 g with PVS; 74% of these infants had BPD. In their cohort, freedom from death or restenosis was 73% at 1 year and 55% at 2 years. Another retrospective review of 213 patients with sBPD found that 5% had PVS with a survival to discharge of 50% as compared to 86% survival of sBPD patients with PH without PVS.[124]

In addition to pulmonary vascular disease and right ventricular hypertrophy, other cardiovascular abnormalities associated with BPD include left ventricular hypertrophy (LVH), systemic hypertension, and the development of prominent systemic-to-pulmonary collateral vessels.[127,128] Infants with sBPD can develop LVH in the absence of right ventricular hypertrophy. Systemic hypertension in BPD may be mild, transient, or striking and usually responds to medication. Left ventricular diastolic dysfunction can contribute to lung edema, diuretic dependency, and PH in some infants with BPD.[129] In addition, atrial septal defects commonly complicate the course of infants with BPD and have variable contributions to underlying disease severity. Prominent bronchial or other systemic-to-pulmonary collateral vessels were noted in early morphometric studies of infants with BPD and can be readily identified in many infants during cardiac catheterization. Although these collateral vessels are generally small, large collaterals may contribute to significant shunting of blood flow to the lung, resulting in edema and the need for higher levels of supplemental oxygen. Collateral vessels have been associated with high mortality in some patients with both sBPD and PH. Some infants have improved after embolization of large collateral vessels, as reflected by a reduced need for supplemental oxygen, ventilator support, or diuretics. The contribution of collateral vessels to the pathophysiology of BPD, however, is poorly understood.

Evaluation and Treatment of Severe Bronchopulmonary Dysplasia

A general evaluation and treatment for infants with significant BPD is described below (Table 14.1). An important consideration in the treatment of sBPD is that recovery from this disease will be relatively slow, i.e., months to years rather than days to weeks. Therefore, patience is required when caring for these complicated patients. In other words, management of

---

TABLE 14.1   General Treatment Strategies for Severe Bronchopulmonary Dysplasia

- Family-centered chronic care model
- Focus on neurodevelopment:
  - Optimize pulmonary status/respiratory support.
  - Long-term ventilator settings
  - Consider need for tracheostomy if long-term mechanical ventilation is necessary.
  - Optimize oxygenation, targeting SpO_2 at 92–95%.
  - Use short courses of diuretics to treat episodes of pulmonary edema.
  - Treat airway reactivity with inhaled bronchodilators and/or inhaled steroids.
  - Reserve systemic steroids for acute deteriorations.
- Pulmonary hypertension:
  - Avoid hypoxemia.
  - Use inhaled nitric oxide (NO) for short-term therapy.
  - Treatment will need to be long-term, sildenafil most studied.
  - If response to sildenafil alone is poor, consider adding bosentan and/or prostacyclin.
  - Determine need for cardiac catheterization (see text).
- Nutritional status:
  - Optimize nutrition: fluid restriction with high-caloric density feeds.
- Gastroesophageal reflux (GER):
  - Medical management
  - Consider surgical management if severe or unresponsive to medical management.

---

infants with severe BPD requires a chronic care model, which is strikingly different in philosophy and treatment goals from the approach used in the acute care model that is generally followed in the NICU. This includes strategies for weaning from mechanical ventilation, assessing the need for chronic ventilator support, the role of tracheostomy, and related issues.

Supplemental oxygen remains a mainstay of therapy for infants with BPD, yet the most appropriate target for oxygen saturation levels remains controversial. Growing concern regarding the adverse effects of even moderate levels of oxygen therapy has led many neonatologists to accept oxygen saturations below 90% early after birth of preterm newborns. However, it should also be kept in mind that patients with established sBPD are usually beyond 36 weeks PMA, past the time when retinopathy of prematurity is a major concern. Prolonged monitoring of oxygenation while awake, asleep, and during feeds to ensure the avoidance of hypoxemia is necessary while adjusting oxygen therapy. In those infants with established sBPD, we recommend targeting O_2 saturation above 94% to provide more consistent treatment of underlying PH, to minimize lability and cyanotic episodes, and to enhance growth.

In most NICUs, nCPAPs and/or HFNCs are used to maintain adequate oxygenation and ventilation while avoiding the need for prolonged ventilation or reintubation for ventilator support. Whereas several studies have examined the role of early nCPAP in lieu of endotracheal intubation during the first week after birth, there are no studies regarding benefits of the prolonged use of nCPAP in established BPD with chronic respiratory failure. Although nCPAP may provide adequate support, in some infants with BPD, signs of severe respiratory distress persist despite nCPAP or HFNC therapy, including marked dyspnea, head bobbing, retractions, tachypnea, intermittent cyanosis, and CO_2 retention. These infants may benefit from reintubation and considerations of tracheostomy for chronic ventilator support if subsequent attempts at weaning are not successful. The timing and patient selection for tracheostomy and commitment to more prolonged ventilator support is highly variable between centers.[130,131] Tracheostomy and chronic ventilator support may provide a stable airway to allow for more effective ventilation and less respiratory distress and to enhance cardiopulmonary

TABLE 14.2	Ventilator Strategies in Bronchopulmonary Dysplasia
Acute phase Early in course (prevention)	Strategies to prevent acute lung injury: 1. Low tidal volumes (4–6 mL/kg) 2. Short inspiratory times 3. Increased PEEP as needed for lung recruitment without overdistention (as reflected by high peak airway pressures) 4. Achieve lower FiO$_2$ Goals for gas exchange: 1. Adjust FiO$_2$ to target lower O$_2$ saturations (88%–92%) 2. Permissive hypercapnia

Chronic phase
Late (established
BPD)
	Strategies for effective gas exchange:
	1. Marked regional heterogeneity:
	  • Larger tidal volumes (10–12 mL/kg)
	  • Longer inspiratory time ($\geq$0.6 seconds)
	2. Airways obstruction:
	  • Slower rates allow better emptying, especially with larger tidal volumes.
	  • Complex roles for PEEP with dynamic airway collapse
	3. Interactive effects of vent strategies:
	  • Changes in rate, tidal volume, inspiratory and expiratory times, and pressure support are highly interdependent.
	  • Overdistention can increase agitation and paradoxically worsen ventilation.
	4. Permissive hypercapnia to facilitate weaning

PEEP, Positive end-expiratory pressure.

function as reflected by lower oxygen requirements and less PH. Greater respiratory stability often improves tolerance of respiratory treatments, physical therapies, and handling by staff and family members, thereby improving maternal-infant interactions and neurodevelopmental outcomes. Successful management of chronic ventilator–dependent children requires well-organized, multidisciplinary teams to address the complexity of issues.[4,29]

MECHANICAL VENTILATION

In contrast with a low tidal volume and high PEEP approach to acute RDS for minimizing acute lung injury (acute phase), most clinicians favor a strategy of larger tidal volumes delivered at slower rates with longer inspiratory and expiratory times in sBPD, and this strategy has recently been termed chronic phase ventilation (CPV) (Table 14.2).[82] The CPV strategy is directly related to the striking differences in lung physiology that characterize infants with established BPD from newborns with acute respiratory failure.[82] As described earlier, the striking heterogeneity of lung disease, characterized by marked regional variability in time constants, provides the physiologic rationale for

this strategy in established BPD for improving the distribution of ventilation, minimizing physiologic dead space and gas trapping, and improving gas exchange (Fig. 14.3). This represents a distinct change in strategy from the higher rates and lower tidal volumes commonly utilized early in the course of respiratory distress in the premature infant. No objective studies have, however, been published to substantiate this approach. The overall goal of this ventilator strategy is to provide support while preventing complications and optimizing lung growth and recovery for patients with the most severe form of BPD, i.e., those patients who continue to require invasive mechanical ventilation many weeks into their initial hospitalization.

Ventilation with larger tidal volumes and increased inspiratory times often improves the distribution of ventilation while minimizing dead space ventilation (Fig. 14.3). This strategy can reduce chronic retractions and respiratory distress and may decrease recurrent cyanotic spells in some patients. However, hyperinflation is typically present in severe, ventilator-dependent BPD. As a result, the patient is breathing on a relatively flat portion of the pressure-volume loop,

HETEROGENEITY OF LUNG DISEASE IN ESTABLISHED BPD: ROLE OF VARIABLE TIME CONSTANTS

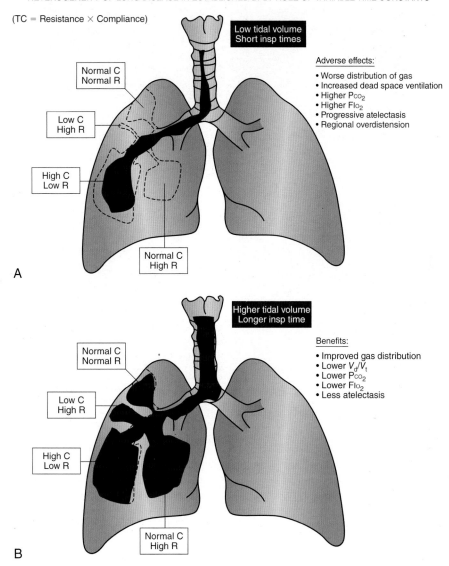

(TC = Resistance × Compliance)

Low tidal volume Short insp times

Normal C
Normal R

Low C
High R

High C
Low R

Normal C
High R

Adverse effects:

- Worse distribution of gas
- Increased dead space ventilation
- Higher P_{CO_2}
- Higher FIo_2
- Progressive atelectasis
- Regional overdistension

A

Higher tidal volume Longer insp time

Normal C
Normal R

Low C
High R

High C
Low R

Normal C
High R

Benefits:

- Improved gas distribution
- Lower V_d/V_t
- Lower P_{CO_2}
- Lower FIo_2
- Less atelectasis

B

Fig. 14.3 Theoretical effects of mechanical ventilator strategies for severe BPD. As illustrated in the top panel (3A), small tidal volume breaths often increase dead space ventilation leading to atelectasis, hypercapnia, and high oxygen requirements in the setting of heterogenous lung disease in severe BPD, while greater tidal volumes and longer inspiratory times (3B) may enhance distribution of gas, leading to lower oxygen requirements, improved ventilation, and less atelectasis. *BPD*, Bronchopulmonary dysplasia.

such that generating large pressures results in only small changes in tidal volumes. Furthermore, lung hyperinflation will increase PVR due to compression of the alveolar vessels. Thus, hyperinflation of the lung worsens not only lung mechanics but also V/Q matching and pulmonary hemodynamics. To effectively

reduce hyperinflation in sBPD, ventilation strategies must also allow for adequate time for exhalation in order to allow all parts of the lung to empty, and this requires relatively low ventilator rates and long expiratory times. Thus, slower rates are needed to accommodate increases in tidal volume and inspiratory time, allowing

Dynamic hyperinflation in severe BPD

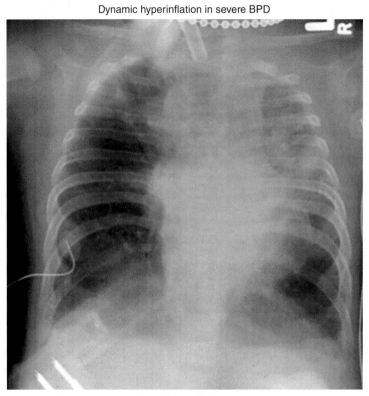

Fig. 14.4 Chest x-ray demonstrating marked gas trapping and dynamic hyperinflation in severe bronchopulmonary dysplasia *(BPD).*

adequate expiratory time and avoiding gas trapping, inadvertent PEEP, and dynamic hyperinflation (Fig. 14.4). Requirements for PEEP are highly variable among ventilator-dependent BPD infants, but generally higher than in the acute phase of RDS. Infants with sBPD often have evidence of tracheomalacia or bronchomalacia, for which increased PEEP will decrease central airway closure (Fig. 14.5).[132-135] However, high PEEP can complicate gas trapping and will not be tolerated without sufficient expiratory times and low ventilator rates. In some BPD infants, the combination of marked alteration in lung mechanics and increase in respiratory drive results in dynamic hyperinflation and intrinsic PEEP even with a large tidal volume-low mandatory rate strategy. When identified, increasing the set PEEP to at least 80% of the intrinsic PEEP may improve the infant's ability to trigger the ventilator, thereby enhancing patient-ventilator synchrony and reducing the infant's respiratory work.

The obvious question in terms of ventilator strategies has now become: When should CPV be started? There are no high-level studies that provide an evidence base for when to transition to CPV in patients with BPD or with "evolving BPD" (i.e., BPD-like physiology prior to definitive diagnosis at 36 weeks PMA). From a physiological basis, at and shortly after birth, most preterm infants with respiratory failure have a relatively homogenous lung disease characterized by low compliance and low resistance resulting in short time constants, and acute phase ventilation is appropriate (Fig. 14.6). Those preterm infants that go on to develop sBPD at 36 weeks PMA now have a heterogenous lung disease characterized by a significant obstructive component and therefore CPV is appropriate (Fig. 14.6). However, there is not a particular time point or PMA when the lung suddenly changes from the relatively homogenous acute lung disease to the predominantly obstructive pattern

BRONCHOGRAM/PEEP STUDY

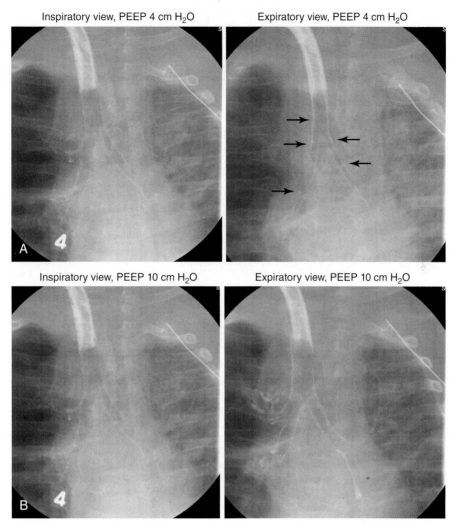

Fig. 14.5 Bronchogram studies for assessing effects of PEEP on central airways caliber. As shown on the top (A), low PEEP support is associated with small airway diameter on inspiration and expiratory airway closure (as marked by *arrows*). Higher PEEP (B) appears to reduce airway closure during expiration. *PEEP*, Positive end-expiratory pressure.

characteristic of chronic sBPD. In other words, it is not one or the other, but rather a continuum over time as BPD progresses (Fig. 14.6). Although preterm infants who go on to develop sBPD may have different courses resulting in lung injury, most of them continue to require some form of respiratory support and supplemental oxygen. If we consider the subgroup of preterm infants who remain on the ventilator, then the adequacy of acute phase ventilation may be assessed using the FiO_2 required to maintain the SpO_2 in range. If this FiO_2 requirement begins to increase on the same settings or in the face of increased tidal volume, then it is likely that the patient is beginning to develop V/Q mismatch due to obstruction. At this point, consideration should be given to beginning to transition to more CPV-like settings. It is also very likely that this transition should be a slow and deliberate process rather than a sudden switch from acute

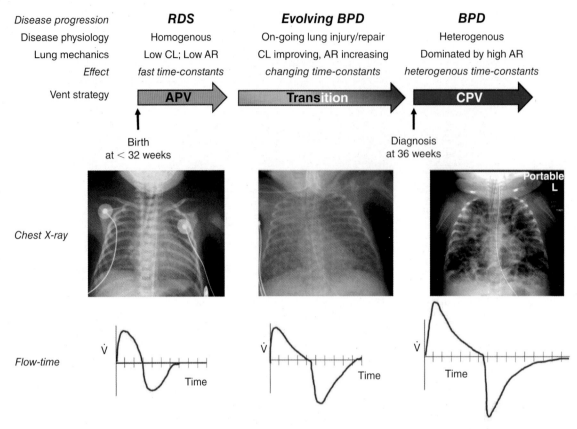

Fig. 14.6 Disease progression in preterm infants going on to develop BPD. At the time of preterm birth at <32 weeks, most preterm infants have respiratory distress syndrome *(RDS)*, while bronchopulmonary dysplasia *(BPD)* is first diagnosed at 36 weeks, and between the acute RDS and the BPD diagnosis is a transition phase (evolving BPD) that is characterized by ongoing lung injury/repair with the development of obstructive lung disease. The lung physiology changes during the transition necessitate a gradual change from acute phase ventilation *(APV)* to chronic phase ventilation *(CPV)*. Shown in the figure are disease physiology, lung mechanics in terms of lung compliance *(CL)*, and airway resistance *(AR)*, as well as effects of the changes on lung mechanics on time constants. Also shown are representative chest x-rays and flow scalars as would be seen on the ventilator screens.

phase settings to CPV. Beginning to slowly increase the tidal volume, slowly decrease the rate, and slowly prolong the inspiratory time will most likely begin to improve V/Q matching, which will be manifest as a decrease in the FiO_2 required to maintain the SpO_2 in range.

As discussed earlier, patients with type 2 sBPD are likely to either have prolonged need for mechanical ventilation or marginal respiratory status on "less in-vasive" forms of support like HFNC or CPAP, thus necessitating a tracheostomy. Indeed, the BPD Collab-orative reported a point prevalence of tracheostomy in sBPD of 12%[130] and the Children's Hospitals Neonatal Consortium (CHNC) reported that 14% of patients

with sBPD underwent tracheostomy placement.[131] There are no data or evidence regarding the optimal timing of tracheostomy in infants with sBPD. Further-more, the majority of NICU providers equate trache-ostomy with a poor outcome.[131] Interestingly, in adult ICU care, early tracheostomy, as defined as ≤10 days, is associated with lower mortality and in-creased likelihood of discharge from the ICU at 28 days compared to late tracheostomy.[136] Similar conclusions have been reached in pediatric ICU care.[137] Furthermore, in a review of the NRN database involving 304 infants who underwent tracheostomy among a group of 8,683 preterm neonates followed to

18 to 22 months corrected age, risk of death or neurodevelopmental impairment was less in those who underwent tracheostomy placement before versus after 120 days.[138] This leads us to wonder if "earlier" tracheostomy would improve survival, neurodevelopmental outcome, and/or time to discharge from the hospital for patients with sBPD in the NICU, as suggested by retrospective studies from one center.[139,140]

Tracheostomy placement is obviously a difficult and complicated decision. Tracheostomy should be viewed as a means for delivering sustained respiratory support to relieve respiratory distress and provide the respiratory stability necessary to optimize neurodevelopmental outcomes in the sub-set of sBPD patients requiring continued mechanical ventilation.[141] In a recent survey of centers participating in the Children's Hospitals Neonatal Consortium, tracheostomy was strongly considered when airway malacia was present, the PCO_2 was consistently ≥ 76 to 85 mm Hg, FiO_2 was consistently ≥ 0.6, PEEP was ≥ 9 to 11 cm H_2O, and/or the PMA was ≥ 44 weeks, demonstrating the wide range of potential indications and the lack of standardization in recommending tracheostomy.[142] Further, complicating the decision to place a tracheostomy is recent data suggesting that there are racial disparities, with non-Hispanic black patients being more likely to receive a tracheostomy compared to non-Hispanic whites and Hispanic infants.[143]

The optimal timing of tracheostomy placement remains to be determined, and various single-center studies have reported a very wide range in the median age at tracheostomy placement.[144] However, we suggest that if a patient born at <28 weeks remains on continuous mechanical ventilatory support through 40 weeks, discussions about tracheostomy should begin with the parents realizing that it will likely take several weeks to reach a definitive decision on tracheostomy. Although, there are likely to be benefits to early tracheostomy in severe BPD, it should be noted that placement of tracheostomy in pediatric patients has been associated with complications in 24% of patients following tracheostomy placement.[145] The overall mortality rate for patients with BPD post-NICU discharge has been reported to be 1-2%[146-148]; however the mortality rate for BPD patients post-tracheostomy ranged from 1% to 26%.[143,144,149,150] Furthermore, recent study[151] found that children with

sBPD who required a tracheostomy had greater cognitive delays at >12 months of age than did children with sBPD without a tracheostomy.

The contribution of gastroesophageal reflux (GER) in sBPD remains controversial. In patients with sBPD consideration should be given to evaluation for GER with radiologic studies (barium swallow studies, upper gastrointestinal series), pH or impedance probes, and/or swallow studies. Since GER with chronic aspiration may contribute to ongoing lung injury, we recommend considering gastrostomy with fundoplication in the patients with the severest form of sBPD. Many would also recommend gastrostomy and fundoplication in the setting of sBPD that is failing to improve if clinical suspicion remains high in the face of negative studies. Jadcherla, et al. reported that GER may cause symptoms in infants with BPD even without the refluxate reaching the pharynx, and that the likelihood of symptoms was related to the clearance time of the acid refluxate.[152] These findings suggest that medical treatment of GER may improve symptoms in patients with BPD.

DRUG THERAPIES

Multiple pharmacologic therapies have been used in the management of BPD, including diuretics, bronchodilators, and steroids. In most cases, despite observations suggesting acute improvement with many of these interventions, there is little or no data regarding long-term safety and efficacy of drugs used in infants with BPD.

Diuretics can improve lung compliance and airway resistance by reducing pulmonary edema. The need for chronic diuretic use may also reflect a contribution of LV diastolic dysfunction to recurrent pulmonary edema.[129] Furosemide has beneficial effects that are independent of its diuretic properties; it induces prostaglandin formation from renal and vascular endothelium that results directly in vasodilation, promoting a shift of fluid from alveoli to the venous compartment.[153] Aerosolized furosemide can acutely improve lung mechanics, but data are lacking regarding its chronic use.[154] The use of alternate-day furosemide may sustain improvements in lung function while minimizing risks for electrolyte imbalance and nephrocalcinosis.[155] A Cochrane review assessing the effects of loop diuretics (furosemide) for preventing or treating BPD in preterm infants concluded that while chronic use of furosemide improves both oxygenation and pulmonary mechanics, there are few data to demonstrate the benefit of chronic administration on need for ventilatory support, duration of hospitalization, or mortality.[156] A second Cochrane review assessing the effects of diuretics acting on the distal renal tubule (thiazides and spironolactone) in the same population concluded that chronic administration of a thiazide and spironolactone improves lung compliance at 4 weeks and reduces the need for furosemide; in intubated patients one study also demonstrated a significant reduction in mortality and extubation failure.[157] The authors concluded that based on their review, there was little evidence to support the use of these diuretics in non-intubated patients. Perhaps because of the lack of consensus regarding the role of diuretics in established BPD, there is great variability in their use. One retrospective observational study of 3252 subjects across 43 NICUs in the United States found that the adjusted mean proportion of days with loop diuretic exposure in infants with Grade 2 or Grade 3 BPD varied from 7.3% to 49.4% ($p < 0.0001$).[158] Furthermore, there was no difference in mortality or PMA at discharge between centers with low versus high use of loop diuretics, although infants from high use centers were more likely to be prescribed loop diuretics at discharge. Noting a lack of studies on the effects of diuretic use following NICU discharge, an expert panel from the European Respiratory Society (ERS) recommended allowing those patients discharged on diuretic therapy to outgrow their doses, given the lack of data supporting the long-term efficacy of diuretics in BPD.[159] Active weaning of diuretics has been shown not to prolong the use of supplemental oxygen among infants with BPD discharged from the NICU with home oxygen therapy when both interventions were done by protocol.[160]

Infants with BPD have airway smooth muscle hypertrophy and often have signs of bronchial hyper-reactivity that acutely improves with bronchodilator therapy but response rates are variable.[161-163] In one single-center study, 59 of 93 (63%) infants with sBPD demonstrated a significant increase in forced expiratory flows following inhaled bronchodilator administration. Data showing long-term benefit of bronchodilators, including β-agonists and anti-cholinergic agents for the prevention or treatment of BPD, however, are lacking.[163] A recent trial among extremely preterm infants showed no benefit of prophylactic use of bronchodilators alone or in combination with inhaled steroids in the prevention of death or development of BPD at 36 weeks PMA.[164] Nevertheless, inhaled bronchodilator use is widespread among hospitalized infants with BPD; one retrospective study of 4986 BPD infants across 44 centers reported that 25% of BPD infants received at least one dose of inhaled bronchodilators between 28 days of life and either NICU discharge or death.[165] Inhaled bronchodilator use increased with severity of disease, so that 48% of those infants with severe BPD received a bronchodilator. Some factors associated with a greater likelihood of inhaled bronchodilator exposure in that study included lower gestational age, lower birth weight, male sex, longer duration of respiratory support, longer duration of diuretic therapy, systemic steroid exposure, and need for tracheostomy. Inhaled bronchodilator use, however, varied widely by center, from 0-59% of infants. In addition to their roles in apnea, aminophylline and caffeine can reduce airway resistance in infants with BPD and may have an additive effect with diuretics. Methylxanthines can improve weaning of infants from mechanical ventilation,[166] but jitteriness, seizures, and gastroesophageal reflux are known side effects.

Corticosteroid therapy, primarily directed at reducing lung inflammation, is one of the most controversial areas of BPD care.[167,168] The use of systemic corticosteroids to prevent BPD early in the course of care of preterm infants was discouraged by the American Academy of Pediatrics (AAP) due to adverse effects on neurodevelopment.[169] A meta-analysis of studies assessing the efficacy of airway administration of corticosteroids, either by inhalation or by direct instillation, however, demonstrated a significant reduction in the incidence of BPD, or BPD or death among preterm infants.[170] Treatment was not associated with worse neurodevelopmental outcomes when compared either to a placebo group or those treated with systemic steroids. Prevention of BPD was greatest among those infants treated with direct airway instillation of budesonide with surfactant as a vehicle. The lack of consistency in dose, timing and duration of therapy across studies requires further investigation to establish recommendations for this therapy. Additionally, no studies to date have addressed long-term safety of this therapy.

In established BPD, corticosteroids are generally used to reduce lung inflammation. The side effects of poor head growth and neurocognitive outcomes with early and prolonged high dose strategies are unacceptable risks for preterm infants at risk for BPD. However, steroid bursts (e.g., prednisone 1–2 mg/kg/day for 3–5 days) may be helpful in the management of sBPD infants with acute deteriorations of lung function. Although commonly used in infants with asthma, inhaled steroids have not consistently shown improvement in lung function in BPD.[171] However, two small studies have shown that inhaled steroids can improve the rate of successful extubation and reduce the need for systemic steroids.[172,173] Two other small randomized controlled trials among infants with moderate-to-severe BPD failed to demonstrate a salutary effect of chronic inhaled corticosteroid use. Among infants treated from 36 weeks PMA through 3 months post-NICU discharge with twice-daily inhaled beclomethasone, there was no significant difference in length of hospital stay, need for supplemental oxygen at discharge, or number of respiratory-related rehospitalizations following discharge.[174] Similarly, routine twice daily administration of fluticasone over 1 year did not reduce the number of symptom-free days or duration of supplemental oxygen use among BPD infants dependent on supplemental oxygen at the time of enrollment.[175]

Despite experience with improvements with inhaled steroid therapy in selected cases or in symptomatic infant who fail to improve sufficiently on bronchodilator therapy, these findings suggest that data are lacking to support the routine use of inhaled corticosteroids in this population. Intriguingly, older children and adolescents with BPD and a history of recurrent wheezing do not demonstrate elevated markers of eosinophilic inflammation[176] or experience bronchospasm in response to mast cell stimulation,[177] making the role of inhaled corticosteroid therapy in these patients less certain. Despite these findings, in a multicenter retrospective review involving 4551 infants with evolving BPD across 44 centers, inhaled corticosteroid use among hospitalized subjects was found in 25% of all BPD infants, and in 43% of those with severe BPD.[178] As with other therapies, inhaled steroid use varied widely across centers, from 0 to 66% of patients. Risk factors for inhaled corticosteroid use involved several markers of disease severity, including lower birth weight and gestational age, longer duration of bronchodilator and diuretic therapies, longer duration of respiratory support and greater need for invasive ventilation or tracheostomy.

TREATMENT OF PULMONARY HYPERTENSION

Recommendations for the evaluation and care of PH-associated BPD have recently been published and are briefly discussed here (Table 14.3).[179,180] The initial clinical strategy for the management of PH in infants with BPD begins with treating the underlying lung disease, including an extensive evaluation for chronic reflux and aspiration, structural airway abnormalities (such as tonsillar and adenoidal hypertrophy, vocal cord paralysis, subglottic stenosis, tracheomalacia, and other lesions), assessments of bronchial reactivity, improving lung edema and airway function, or any other intervening factors. Periods of acute hypoxemia, whether intermittent or prolonged, can often contribute to late PH in BPD. A sleep study may be necessary to determine the presence of noteworthy episodes of hypoxemia and whether hypoxemia has predominantly

---

TABLE 14.3 Pulmonary Hypertension in Severe Bronchopulmonary Dysplasia

- Screening echocardiography:
  - Septal flattening, tricuspid regurgitant jet velocity, cor pulmonale
- If no PH, perform echocardiography every 1–2 months until significant improvement in respiratory status.
- If PH/cor pulmonale present:
  - Optimize respiratory support, avoid hypoxemia.
  - Start inhaled nitric oxide (iNO) at 20 ppm.
- Switch to sildenafil:
  - Start at 0.5 mg/kg q8h and advance as needed to 2 mg/kg q6h if no systemic hypotension.
  - Wean patient off iNO.
- If unable to wean patient off iNO:
  - Continue iNO and sildenafil or consider endothelin receptor antagonist (ETRA) or prostacyclin analog.
- Cardiac catheterization:
  - Evaluate pulmonary hemodynamics, left heart function, presence of pulmonary vein stenosis, aortopulmonary collaterals, and response to acute vasodilator challenge.

obstructive, central, or mixed causes. Additional studies that may be required include flexible bronchoscopy for the diagnosis of anatomical and dynamic airway lesions (such as tracheomalacia) that can contribute to hypoxemia and poor clinical responses to oxygen therapy. Upper gastrointestinal series, pH or impedance probe, and swallow studies may be indicated to evaluate for gastroesophageal reflux and aspiration that can contribute to ongoing lung injury. For patients with BPD and severe PH who fail to maintain near normal ventilation or require high levels of FiO_2 despite conservative treatment, strong consideration should be given to chronic mechanical ventilatory support in an attempt to halt progression of PH.

Despite the growing use of pulmonary vasodilator therapy for the treatment of PH in BPD, data demonstrating efficacy are extremely limited, and the use of these agents should only follow thorough diagnostic evaluations and aggressive management of the underlying lung disease. We strongly encourage cardiac catheterization prior to the initiation of chronic pulmonary vasodilator therapy. Current therapies used for PH therapy in infants with BPD generally include inhaled NO (iNO), sildenafil, endothelin receptor antagonists (ETRAs), and calcium channel blockers (CCB). Note that if PVS is an important contributor to PH in the patient with sBPD, these vasodilators will either have little effect or could worsen the patient's clinical status, underscoring the importance of cardiac catheterization prior to initiation of vasodilator therapy. Calcium channel blockers (such as nifedipine) benefit some patients with PH, and short-term effects of CCB in infants with BPD have been reported.[181] In comparison with an acute study of iNO reactivity in infants with BPD, the acute response to CCB was poor and some infants developed systemic hypotension.[182]

In general, we use sildenafil or bosentan (an ETRA) for chronic therapy of PH in infants with BPD. Sildenafil, a highly selective type 5 phosphodiesterase (PDE-5) inhibitor, augments cyclic GMP content in vascular smooth muscle, and has been shown to benefit adults with PH as monotherapy and in combination with standard treatment regimens.[183] In a study of 25 infants with chronic lung disease and PH (18 with BPD), prolonged sildenafil therapy as part of an aggressive program to treat PH was associated with improvement in PH by echocardiogram in most (88%) patients without significant rates of adverse events.[184] Although the time to improvement was variable, many patients were able to wean off mechanical ventilator support and other PH therapies, especially iNO, during the course of sildenafil treatment without worsening of PH. The recommended starting dose for sildenafil is 0.5 mg/kg/dose every 8 hours. If there is no evidence of systemic hypotension, this dose can be gradually increased over 2 weeks to achieve the desired pulmonary hemodynamic effect or a maximum of 2 mg/kg/dose every 6-8 hours. Other agents, such as ETRAs and prostacyclin analogs, are sometimes used in BPD infants who fail to respond to other approaches, but data on their dosage, safety and efficacy in this population are largely lacking. Serial assessments of chronic PH and cardiac performance generally include echocardiography with measurements of circulating levels of brain natriuretic peptide (BNP) or NT-proBNP at regular intervals. Cardiac catheterization is generally reserved for difficult cases in which PH fails to improve or with adverse effects with PH-targeted therapies (e.g., worsening pulmonary edema) and to further assess left ventricular diastolic dysfunction, PVS, the contribution of shunt lesions such as patent ductus arteriosus, atrial septal defects or ventricular septal defects or with plans for prolonged use of systemic prostanoid therapy.[185]

INTERDISCIPLINARY CARE

Severe BPD is associated with poor nutritional and neurodevelopmental outcomes and increased family stress. Therefore, optimal care of infants with established BPD requires a multidisciplinary team consisting of neonatologists, pulmonologists, respiratory therapists, nutritionists, occupational therapists, speech therapists, physical therapists, social workers, pharmacists, psychologists, etc.[4,29] It is imperative to involve the family in the interdisciplinary care of the patient with established BPD early in the hospitalization to improve the family's comfort with, and understanding of, the disease process. This family-centered care will hasten discharge home, decrease need for rehospitalization, and improve family dynamics. Regular team meetings should occur throughout the NICU course, not simply at the time of discharge.

Nutritional care is critical not only to maintain growth for the patient but also to foster lung healing and repair. We recommend using a growth chart during daily rounds for patients hospitalized with established BPD, to facilitate the assessment of nutritional needs. The goal for weight gain should be an average of 15 to 20 g/kg/day for infants <37 weeks PMA and 20 to 30 g/day for infants ≥37 weeks PMA. Patients with BPD are often fluid restricted. However, they usually require 120 to 150 kcal/kg/day to achieve adequate growth and lung repair, such that high-caloric density feedings are usually required. Whenever possible, the mother's own breast milk should be used in these patients, even if it needs to be heavily fortified.

In patients with established BPD, neurodevelopmental assessments and care are of marked benefit in optimizing care.[4,29] Consultation and application of behavioral interventions are often important factors in many aspects of the care plan. Patients with sBPD require respiratory support that prevents persistent distress and recurrent cyanotic episodes in order to interact well with the parents, caregivers, and environment or to be able to work on motor skills. Intensive neurodevelopmental care for patients with established BPD should include developmental therapies several times a week while hospitalized. These developmental treatments should focus on creating an age-appropriate sensory and social environment. A formal neurodevelopmental assessment should be carried out at approximately 40 weeks PMA so that therapies can then be directed at improving any identified areas of delay. Behavioral aspects of nursing care and routine positive interactions with caregivers can minimize the frequency or severity of recurrent hypoxemia episodes and irritability with agitation. Noxious stimuli should be minimized in these patients (e.g., arterial sampling or heel sticks); and opioids and sedatives should be used with caution.

Long-Term Outcomes

Most children with sBPD who require prolonged mechanical ventilation via tracheostomy eventually can be liberated from ventilatory support and can undergo tracheal decannulation. In a single-center study involving 102 ventilator-dependent subjects with sBPD born at 25 to 27 weeks and weighing 560 to 974 g who were supported at home, survival was 81.4%.[186] Of the 83 subjects alive at the time of the study, 69 (83.1%) were liberated from mechanical ventilation and 60 (72.2%) underwent tracheal decannulation. The median age at liberation from mechanical ventilation was 24 months (IQR, 19–33). In a more recent multicenter study involving 12 centers, 155 infants with a mean gestational age of 25.9 ± 2.5 weeks, birth weight of 757 ± 371 g, and Grade 3 BPD underwent prolonged mechanical ventilation via tracheostomy.[187] In that cohort, 99 (66%) were liberated from mechanical ventilation and 49 (32.6%) had undergone tracheal decannulation. The median age of liberation from mechanical ventilation was 27 months, and the median age of tracheal decannulation was 49 months. One-third of the group was treated outpatient for PH.

The data examining the long-term respiratory outcomes of patients with sBPD have expanded over the last few years and include both structural and functional information. Imaging studies employing chest radiographs, CT imaging, lung MRI, and SPECT have examined radiological changes among BPD survivors throughout childhood and into early adulthood.[188] Common themes across studies include the persistence of radiographic abnormalities like bronchial wall thickening, linear or triangular opacities, and areas of hypoattenuation among subjects with a history of BPD, and greater or more severe changes in those with more severe disease compared with subjects born prematurely without BPD or those born at term. A study of 86 survivors of extreme preterm birth (<1000 g or gestational age ≤28 weeks) at 10 or 18 years of age found significantly higher HRCT scores as well as more opacities and hypoattenuated areas in subjects with a history of moderate or severe BPD than in those with a history of no or mild BPD.[189] Similarly, Wong et al.[190] described abnormal HRCT scans with emphysematous changes in 19 subjects aged 17 to 33 years born at <1500 g between 1980 and 1987 with the diagnosis of moderate-to-severe BPD, and these abnormal CT scans were correlated with abnormalities in pulmonary function. Similar findings were reported among 25 subjects with BPD aged 19 to 33 years born at 23 to 30 weeks GA and 510 to 1490 g.[191] In that study, subjects with BPD were also far more likely to report respiratory symptoms like nocturnal cough or breathlessness with wheezing than term control subjects.

While numerous studies report persistent evidence of airway obstruction and gas trapping among patients with a history of BPD, only a small number of subjects with Grade 3 BPD have been studied during childhood. When comparing 23 subjects who required tracheostomy placement for prolonged mechanical ventilation to 50 subjects with sBPD who did not require tracheostomy, those with tracheostomy were found to have evidence of greater obstructive lung disease, with a lower percent predicted FEV-1 and FEV-1/FVC ratio.[7] Among 19 subjects aged 4.9 to 8.3 years who were born at 26.2 to 28.8 weeks GA and who required mechanical ventilation for 2.1 to 2.8 years, spirometry demonstrated evidence of obstruction with reduced flows and a low FEV-1/FVC ratio.[192,193] Furthermore, serial spirometric studies in those children demonstrated that the airflow obstruction remained static over time, suggesting that such changes would result in lower attained maximum values in early adulthood. These observations have led to the concern that individuals born extremely preterm, and especially those with BPD, contribute to the population of adults who develop fixed airway obstruction, or COPD.[194] Studies suggest that persistent airway obstruction in these subjects can be demonstrated into the fourth decade of life.[195,196]

Thus, there is evidence that sBPD is associated with lifelong changes in pulmonary structure and function.[197,198] However, more studies are needed to accurately determine the long-term course of premature neonates with sBPD and their relative contribution to the growing adult population with COPD.

Acknowledgments

The authors would like to express their gratitude to members of the BPD Collaborative, whose ongoing works and collaborations have been inspirational and play a major role in improving the care and research for neonates, infants, and children with severe BPD.

REFERENCES

1. Northway Jr WH, Rosan RC, Porter DY. Pulmonary disease following respirator therapy of hyaline-membrane disease: bronchopulmonary dysplasia. *N Engl J Med.* 1967;276:357-368.
2. Stoll BJ, Hansen NI, Bell EF, et al. Trends in care practices, morbidity, and mortality of extremely preterm neonates, 1993-2012. *JAMA.* 2015;314:1039-1051.
3. Bell EF, Hintz SR, Hansen NI, et al. Mortality, in-hospital morbidity, care practices, and 2-year outcomes for extremely preterm infants in the US, 2013-2018. *JAMA.* 2022;327(3):248-263.
4. Abman SH, Collaco JM, Shepherd EG, et al. Bronchopulmonary Dysplasia Collaborative. Interdisciplinary care of children with severe bronchopulmonary dysplasia. *J Pediatr.* 2017;181:12-28.e1.
5. Regin Y, Gie A, Eerdekens A, et al. Ventilation and respiratory outcome in extremely preterm infants: trends in the new millennium. *Eur J Pediatr.* 2022;181(5):1899-1907.
6. Jobe AH, Bancalari E. Bronchopulmonary dysplasia. *Am J Respir Crit Care Med.* 2001;163:1723-1729.
7. Rojas MA, Gonzalez A, Bancalari E, et al. Changing trends in the epidemiology and pathogenesis of neonatal chronic lung disease. *J Pediatr.* 1995;126:605-610.
8. Charafeddine L, D'Angio CT, Phelps DL. Atypical chronic lung disease patterns in neonates. *Pediatrics.* 1999;103:759-765.
9. Jobe AH. The new bronchopulmonary dysplasia. *Curr Opin Pediatr.* 2011;23:167-172.
10. Doyle LW, Carse E, Adams AM, et al. Ventilation in extremely preterm infants and respiratory function at 8 years. *N Engl J Med.* 2017;377:329-337.
11. Pulakka A, Risnes K, Metsälä J, et al. Preterm birth and asthma and COPD in adulthood: a nationwide register study from two Nordic countries. *Eur Respir J.* 2023;61(6):2201763.

12. Um-Bergström P, Pourbazargan M, Brundin B, et al. Increased cytotoxic T-cells in the airways of adults with former bronchopulmonary dysplasia. *Eur Respir J.* 2022;60:2102531.
13. Bonadies L, Papi A, Baraldi E. Is bronchopulmonary dysplasia in adult age a novel COPD endotype? *Eur Respir J.* 2022; 60(3):2200984.
14. Mammel D, Kemp J. Prematurity, the diagnosis of bronchopulmonary dysplasia, and maturation of ventilatory control. *Pediatr Pulmonol.* 2021;56(11):3533-3545.
15. Ehrenkranz RA, Walsh MC, Vohr BR, et al. Validation of the National Institutes of Health consensus definition of bronchopulmonary dysplasia. *Pediatrics.* 2005;116:1353-1360.
16. Morrow LA, Wagner BD, Ingram DA, et al. Antenatal determinants of bronchopulmonary dysplasia and late respiratory disease in preterm infants. *Am J Respir Crit Care Med.* 2017; 196:364-374.
17. Poindexter BB, Feng R, Schmidt B, et al. Comparisons and limitations of current definitions of bronchopulmonary dysplasia for the prematurity and respiratory outcomes program. *Ann Am Thorac Soc.* 2015;12(12):1822-1830.
18. Laughon MM, Langer JC, Bose CL, et al. Prediction of bronchopulmonary dysplasia by postnatal age in extremely premature infants. *Am J Respir Crit Care Med.* 2011;183:1715-1722.
19. Isayama T, Lee SK, Yang J, et al. Revisiting the definition of bronchopulmonary dysplasia: effect of changing panoply of respiratory support for preterm neonates. *JAMA Pediatr.* 2017;171:271-279.
20. Padula MA, Grover TR, Brozanski B, et al. Therapeutic interventions and short-term outcomes for infants with severe bronchopulmonary dysplasia born at <32 weeks' gestation. *J Perinatol.* 2013;33:877-881.
21. Walsh MC, Morris BH, Wrage LA, et al. Extremely low birthweight neonates with protracted ventilation: mortality and

18-month neurodevelopmental outcomes. *J Pediatr.* 2005; 146:798-804.

22. Higgins RD, Jobe AH, Koso-Thomas M, et al. Bronchopulmonary dysplasia: executive summary of a workshop. *J Pediatr.* 2018;197:300-308.

23. Jensen EA, Dysart K, Gantz MG, et al. The diagnosis of bronchopulmonary dysplasia in very preterm infants. An evidence-based approach. *Am J Respir Crit Care Med.* 2019;200(6): 751-759.

24. Jensen EA, Edwards EM, Greenberg LT, et al. Severity of bronchopulmonary dysplasia among very preterm infants in the United States. *Pediatrics.* 2021;148(1):e2020030007.

25. Jeon GW, Oh M, Lee J, et al. Comparison of definitions of bronchopulmonary dysplasia to reflect the long-term outcomes of extremely preterm infants. *Sci Rep.* 2022;12(1):18095.

26. Vyas-Read S, Logan JW, Cuna AC, et al. A comparison of newer classifications of bronchopulmonary dysplasia: findings from the Children's Hospitals Neonatal Consortium Severe BPD Group. *J Perinatol.* 2022;42(1):58-64.

27. Guaman MC, Pishevar N, Abman SH, et al. Invasive mechanical ventilation at 36 weeks post-menstrual age, adverse outcomes with a comparison of recent definitions of bronchopulmonary dysplasia. *J Perinatol.* 2021;41(8):1936-1942.

28. Boroughs D, Dougherty JA. Decreasing accidental mortality of ventilator-dependent children at home: a call to action. *Home Healthc Nurse.* 2012;30:103-111; quiz 112-113.

29. Shepherd EG, Knupp AM, Welty SE, et al. An interdisciplinary bronchopulmonary dysplasia program is associated with improved neurodevelopmental outcomes and fewer rehospitalizations. *J Perinatol.* 2012;32:33-38.

30. Delaney C, Wright RH, Tang JR, et al. Lack of EC-SOD worsens alveolar and vascular development in a neonatal mouse model of bleomycin-induced bronchopulmonary dysplasia and pulmonary hypertension. *Pediatr Res.* 2015;78:634-640.

31. Salaets T, Richter J, Brady P, et al. Transcriptome analysis of the preterm rabbit lung after seven days of hyperoxic exposure. *PloS One.* 2015;10:e0136569.

32. Keller RL, Feng R, DeMauro SB, et al. Bronchopulmonary dysplasia and perinatal characteristics predict 1-year respiratory outcomes in newborns born at extremely low gestational age: a prospective cohort study. *J Pediatr.* 2017;187:89-97.e3.

33. Reiss I, Landmann E, Heckmann M, et al. Increased risk of bronchopulmonary dysplasia and increased mortality in very preterm infants being small for gestational age. *Arch Gynecol Obstet.* 2003;269:40-44.

34. Van Marter LJ, Leviton A, Kuban KC, et al. Maternal glucocorticoid therapy and reduced risk of bronchopulmonary dysplasia. *Pediatrics.* 1990;86:331-336.

35. Zeitlin J, El Ayoubi M, Jarreau PH, et al. Impact of fetal growth restriction on mortality and morbidity in a very preterm birth cohort. *J Pediatr.* 2010;157:733-739.e1.

36. Bose C, Van Marter LJ, Laughon M, et al. Fetal growth restriction and chronic lung disease among infants born before the 28th week of gestation. *Pediatrics.* 2009;124:e450-e458.

37. Lee HJ, Kim EK, Kim HS, et al. Chorioamnionitis, respiratory distress syndrome and bronchopulmonary dysplasia in extremely low birth weight infants. *J Perinatol.* 2011;31:166-170.

38. Hansen AR, Barnes CM, Folkman J, et al. Maternal preeclampsia predicts the development of bronchopulmonary dysplasia. *J Pediatr.* 2010;156:532-536.

39. Keszler M. Mechanical ventilation strategies. *Semin Fetal Neonatal Med.* 2017;22:267-274.

40. Deptula N, Royse E, Kemp MW, et al. Brief mechanical ventilation causes differential epithelial repair along the airways of fetal, preterm lambs. *Am J Physiol Lung Cell Mol Physiol.* 2016;311:L412-L420.

41. Hillman NH, Polglase GR, Pillow JJ, et al. Inflammation and lung maturation from stretch injury in preterm fetal sheep. *Am J Physiol Lung Cell Mol Physiol.* 2011;300:L232-L241.

42. Thome UH, Dreyhaupt J, Genzel-Boroviczeny O, et al. Influence of PCO2 control on clinical and neurodevelopmental outcomes of extremely low birth weight infants. *Neonatology.* 2018;113(3):221-230.

43. Keszler M, Sant'Anna G. Mechanical ventilation and bronchopulmonary dysplasia. *Clin Perinatol.* 2015;42:781-796.

44. Tingay DG, Lavizzari A, Zonneveld CE, et al. An individualized approach to sustained inflation duration at birth improves outcomes in newborn preterm lambs. *Am J Physiol Lung Cell Mol Physiol.* 2015;309:L1138-L1149.

45. Isayama T, Iwami H, McDonald S, et al. Association of noninvasive ventilation strategies with mortality and bronchopulmonary dysplasia among preterm infants: a systematic review and meta-analysis. *JAMA.* 2016;316:611-624.

46. Ryu J, Haddad G, Carlo WA. Clinical effectiveness and safety of permissive hypercapnia. *Clin Perinatol.* 2012;39:603-612.

47. Cools F, Offringa M, Askie LM. Elective high frequency oscillatory ventilation versus conventional ventilation for acute pulmonary dysfunction in preterm infants. *Cochrane Database Syst Rev.* 2015:CD000104.

48. Rojas-Reyes MX, Orrego-Rojas PA. Rescue high-frequency jet ventilation versus conventional ventilation for severe pulmonary dysfunction in preterm infants. *Cochrane Database Syst Rev.* 2015:CD000437.

49. Courtney SE, Durand DJ, Asselin JM, et al. High-frequency oscillatory ventilation versus conventional mechanical ventilation for very-low-birth-weight infants. *N Engl J Med.* 2002;347:643-652.

50. Johnson AH, Peacock JL, Greenough A, et al. High-frequency oscillatory ventilation for the prevention of chronic lung disease of prematurity. *N Engl J Med.* 2002;347:633-642.

51. Peng W, Zhu H, Shi H, Liu E. Volume-targeted ventilation is more suitable than pressure-limited ventilation for preterm infants: a systematic review and meta-analysis. *Arch Dis Child Fetal Neonatal Ed.* 2014;99:F158-F165.

52. Klingenberg C, Wheeler KI, McCallion N, et al. Volume-targeted versus pressure-limited ventilation in neonates. *Cochrane Database Syst Rev.* 2017;10(10):CD003666.

53. Finer NN, Carlo WA, Walsh MC, et al. Early CPAP versus surfactant in extremely preterm infants. *N Engl J Med.* 2010;362:1970-1979.

54. Thunqvist P, Gustafsson P, Norman M, et al. Lung function at 6 and 18 months after preterm birth in relation to severity of bronchopulmonary dysplasia. *Pediatr Pulmonol.* 2015;50:978-986.

55. Sward-Comunelli SL, Mabry SM, Truog WE, et al. Airway muscle in preterm infants: changes during development. *J Pediatr.* 1997;130:570-576.

56. Tiddens HA, Hofhuis W, Casotti V, et al. Airway dimensions in bronchopulmonary dysplasia: implications for airflow obstruction. *Pediatr Pulmonol.* 2008;43:1206-1213.

57. Goldman SL, Gerhardt T, Sonni R, et al. Early prediction of chronic lung disease by pulmonary function testing. *J Pediatr.* 1983;102:613-617.

58. Baraldi E, Filippone M, Trevisanuto D, et al. Pulmonary function until two years of life in infants with bronchopulmonary dysplasia. *Am J Respir Crit Care Med.* 1997;155:149-155.

59. Gerhardt T, Hehre D, Feller R, et al. Serial determination of pulmonary function in infants with chronic lung disease. *J Pediatr*. 1987;110:448-456.

60. Lui K, Lloyd J, Ang E, et al. Early changes in respiratory compliance and resistance during the development of bronchopulmonary dysplasia in the era of surfactant therapy. *Pediatr Pulmonol*. 2000;30:282-290.

61. Van Lierde S, Smith J, Devlieger H, et al. Pulmonary mechanics during respiratory distress syndrome in the prediction of outcome and differentiation of mild and severe bronchopulmonary dysplasia. *Pediatr Pulmonol*. 1994;17:218-224.

62. Napolitano N, Jalal K, McDonough JM, et al. Identifying and treating intrinsic PEEP in infants with severe bronchopulmonary dysplasia. *Pediatr Pulmonol*. 2019;54:1045-1051.

63. Panitch HB, Keklikian EN, Motley RA, et al. Effect of altering smooth muscle tone on maximal expiratory flows in patients with tracheomalacia. *Pediatr Pulmonol*. 1990;9:170-176.

64. Gunatilaka CC, Higano NS, Hysinger EB, et al. Increased Work of Breathing due to Tracheomalacia in Neonates. *Ann Am Thorac Soc*. 2020;17:1247-1256.

65. Hysinger EB, Friedman NL, Padula MA, et al. Tracheobronchomalacia is associated with increased morbidity in bronchopulmonary dysplasia. *Ann Am Thorac Soc*. 2017;14(9):1428-1435.

66. Hysinger EB, Bates AJ, Higano NS, et al. Ultrashort echo-time MRI for the assessment of tracheomalacia in neonates. *Chest*. 2020;157:595-602.

67. Wu KY, Jensen EA, White AM, et al. Characterization of disease phenotype in very preterm infants with severe bronchopulmonary dysplasia. *Am J Respir Crit Care Med*. 2020;201:1398-1406.

68. Ochiai M, Hikino S, Yabuuchi H, et al. A new scoring system for computed tomography of the chest for assessing the clinical status of bronchopulmonary dysplasia. *J Pediatr*. 2008;152:90-95, 95.e1-e3.

69. Wauer RR, Maurer T, Nowotny T, et al. Assessment of functional residual capacity using nitrogen washout and plethysmographic techniques in infants with and without bronchopulmonary dysplasia. *Intensive Care Med*. 1998;24:469-475.

70. Shepherd EG, Clouse BJ, Hasenstab KA, et al. Infant pulmonary function testing and phenotypes in severe bronchopulmonary dysplasia. *Pediatrics*. 2018;141(5):e20173350.

71. Balinotti JE, Tiller CJ, Llapur CJ, et al. Growth of the lung parenchyma early in life. *Am J Respir Crit Care Med*. 2009;179:134-137.

72. Jarriel WS, Richardson P, Knapp RD, et al. A nonlinear regression analysis of nonlinear, passive-deflation flow-volume plots. *Pediatr Pulmonol*. 1993;15:175-182.

73. Gappa M, Pillow JJ, Allen J, et al. Lung function tests in neonates and infants with chronic lung disease: lung and chest-wall mechanics. *Pediatr Pulmonol*. 2006;41:291-317.

74. Tepper RS, Pagtakhan RD, Taussig LM. Noninvasive determination of total respiratory system compliance in infants by the weighted-spirometer method. *Am Rev Respir Dis*. 1984;130:461-466.

75. Greenough A, Pahuja A. Updates on functional characterization of bronchopulmonary dysplasia - the contribution of lung function testing. *Front Med (Lausanne)*. 2015;2:35.

76. Adams EW, Harrison MC, Counsell SJ, et al. Increased lung water and tissue damage in bronchopulmonary dysplasia. *J Pediatr*. 2004;145:503-507.

77. McEvoy CT, Schilling D, Go MD, et al. Pulmonary function in extremely low birth weight infants with bronchopulmonary dysplasia before hospital discharge. *J Perinatol*. 2021;41(1):77-83.

78. Moriette G, Gaudebout C, Clement A, et al. Pulmonary function at 1 year of age in survivors of neonatal respiratory distress: a multivariate analysis of factors associated with sequelae. *Pediatr Pulmonol*. 1987;3:242-250.

79. Farstad T, Brockmeier F, Bratlid D. Cardiopulmonary function in premature infants with bronchopulmonary dysplasia—a 2-year follow up. *Eur J Pediatr*. 1995;154:853-858.

80. Moschino L, Stocchero M, Filippone M, et al. Longitudinal assessment of lung function in survivors of bronchopulmonary dysplasia from birth to adulthood. The Padova BPD Study. *Am J Respir Crit Care Med*. 2018;198(1):134-137.

81. Miller AN, Kielt MJ, El-Ferzli GT, et al. Optimizing ventilator support in severe bronchopulmonary dysplasia in the absence of conclusive evidence. *Front Pediatr*. 2022;10:1022743.

82. Sindelar R, Shepherd EG, Ågren J, et al. Bronchopulmonary Dysplasia Collaborative. Established severe BPD: is there a way out? Change of ventilatory paradigms. *Pediatr Res*. 2021;90(6):1139-1146.

83. Mead J. Contribution of compliance of airways to frequency-dependent behavior of lungs. *J Appl Physiol*. 1969;26:670-673.

84. Hulskamp G, Pillow JJ, Dinger J, et al. Lung function tests in neonates and infants with chronic lung disease of infancy: functional residual capacity. *Pediatr Pulmonol*. 2006;41:1-22.

85. Stocks J, Godfrey S, Beardsmore C, et al. Plethysmographic measurements of lung volume and airway resistance. ERS/ATS Task Force on Standards for Infant Respiratory Function Testing. European Respiratory Society/ American Thoracic Society. *Eur Respir J*. 2001;17:302-312.

86. Morris MG, Gustafsson P, Tepper R, et al. The bias flow nitrogen washout technique for measuring the functional residual capacity in infants. ERS/ATS Task Force on Standards for Infant Respiratory Function Testing. *Eur Respir J*. 2001;17:529-536.

87. Hofhuis W, Huysman MW, van der Wiel EC, et al. Worsening of V'maxFRC in infants with chronic lung disease in the first year of life: a more favorable outcome after high-frequency oscillation ventilation. *Am J Respir Crit Care Med*. 2002;166:1539-1543.

88. Robin B, Kim YJ, Huth J, et al. Pulmonary function in bronchopulmonary dysplasia. *Pediatr Pulmonol*. 2004;37:236-242.

89. Filbrun AG, Popova AP, Linn MJ, et al. Longitudinal measures of lung function in infants with bronchopulmonary dysplasia. *Pediatr Pulmonol*. 2011;46:369-375.

90. Loi B, Vigo G, Baraldi E, et al. on behalf of the LUSTRE Study Group. Lung ultrasound to monitor extremely preterm infants and predict bronchopulmonary dysplasia. *Am J Respir Crit Care Med*. 2021;103:1398-1409.

91. Onland W, Hutten J, Miedema M, et al. Precision medicine in neonates: future perspectives for the lung. *Front Pediatr*. 2020;8:586061.

92. Lum S, Hulskamp G, Merkus P, et al. Lung function tests in neonates and infants with chronic lung disease: forced expiratory maneuvers. *Pediatr Pulmonol*. 2006;41:199-214.

93. Sly PD, Tepper R, Henschen M, et al. Tidal forced expirations. ERS/ATS Task Force on Standards for Infant Respiratory Function Testing. European Respiratory Society/American Thoracic Society. *Eur Respir J*. 2000;16:741-748.

94. Green M, Mead J, Turner JM. Variability of maximum expiratory flow-volume curves. *J Appl Physiol*. 1974;37:67-74.

95. Duke JW, Gladstone IM, Sheel AW, et al. Premature birth affects the degree of airway dysanapsis and mechanical ventilatory constraints. *Exp Physiol*. 2018;103:261-275.

96. Mead J. Dysanapsis in normal lungs assessed by the relationship between maximal flow, static recoil, and vital capacity. *Am Rev Respir Dis*. 1980;121:339-342.

97. Nelin LD, Kielt MJ, Jebbia M, et al. Bronchodilator responsiveness and dysanapsis in bronchopulmonary dysplasia. *ERJ Open Res*. 2022;8(3):00682-02021. doi:10.1183/23120541.00682-2021.

98. Talmaciu I, Ren CL, Kolb SM, et al. Pulmonary function in technology-dependent children 2 years and older with bronchopulmonary dysplasia. *Pediatr Pulmonol*. 2002;33:181-188.

99. Oppermann HC, Wille L, Bleyl U, et al. Bronchopulmonary dysplasia in premature infants. A radiological and pathological correlation. *Pediatr Radiol*. 1977;5:137-141.

100. Edwards DK, Colby TV, Northway Jr WH. Radiographic-pathologic correlation in bronchopulmonary dysplasia. *J Pediatr*. 1979;95:834-836.

101. Mahut B, De Blic J, Emond S, et al. Chest computed tomography findings in bronchopulmonary dysplasia and correlation with lung function. *Arch Dis Child Fetal Neonatal Ed*. 2007; 92:F459-F464.

102. Kubota J, Ohki Y, Inoue T, et al. Ultrafast CT scoring system for assessing bronchopulmonary dysplasia: reproducibility and clinical correlation. *Radiat Med*. 1998;16:167-174.

103. Raman P, Raman R, Newman B, et al. Development and validation of automated 2D-3D bronchial airway matching to track changes in regional bronchial morphology using serial low-dose chest CT scans in children with chronic lung disease. *J Digit Imaging*. 2010;23:744-754.

104. Vanhaverbeke K, Slaats M, Al-Nejar M, et al. Functional respiratory imaging provides novel insights into the long-term respiratory sequelae of bronchopulmonary dysplasia. *Eur Respir J*. 2021;57:2002110.

105. Hysinger EB, Higano NS, Critser PJ, et al. Imaging in neonatal respiratory disease. *Paediatr Respir Rev*. 2022;43:44-52.

106. Walkup LL, Higano NS, Woods JC. Structural and functional pulmonary magnetic resonance imaging in pediatrics-from the neonate to the young adult. *Acad Radiol*. 2019;26(3):424-430.

107. Dyke JP, Voskrebenzev A, Blatt LK, et al. Assessment of lung ventilation of premature infants with bronchopulmonary dysplasia at 1.5 Tesla using phase-resolved functional lung magnetic resonance imaging. *Pediatr Radiol*. 2023;53(6):1076-1084. doi:10.1007/s00247-023-05598-6.

108. Gouwens KR, Higano NS, Marks KT, et al. Magentic resonance imaging evaluation of regional lung vts in severe neonatal bronchopulmonary dysplasia. *Am J Respir Crit Care Med*. 2020; 202(7):1024-1031.

109. Kjellberg M, Sanchez-Crespo A, Jonsson B. First week of life respiratory management and pulmonary ventilation/perfusion matching in infants with bronchopulmonary dysplasia: a retrospective observational study. *J Perinatol*. 2023;43(3):317-323.

110. Kjellberg M, Björkman K, Rohdin M, et al. Bronchopulmonary dysplasia: clinical grading in relation to ventilation/perfusion mismatch measured by single photon emission computed tomography. *Pediatr Pulmonol*. 2013;48(12):1206-1213.

111. Abman SH. Pulmonary hypertension in chronic lung disease of infancy. Pathogenesis, pathophysiology, and treatment. In: Bland RD, Coalson JJ, eds. *Chronic Lung Disease of Infancy*. NY: Marcel Dekker; 2000:619-668.

112. Parker TA, Abman SH. The pulmonary circulation in bronchopulmonary dysplasia. *Semin Neonatol*. 2003;8:51-61.

113. Tomashefski Jr JF, Oppermann HC, Vawter GF, Reid LM. Bronchopulmonary dysplasia: a morphometric study with emphasis on the pulmonary vasculature. *Pediatr Pathol*. 1984;2:469-487.

114. Halliday HL, Dumpit FM, Brady JP. Effects of inspired oxygen on echocardiographic assessment of pulmonary vascular resistance and myocardial contractility in bronchopulmonary dysplasia. *Pediatrics*. 1980;65:536-540.

115. Gorenflo M, Vogel M, Obladen M. Pulmonary vascular changes in bronchopulmonary dysplasia: a clinicopathologic correlation in short- and long-term survivors. *Pediatr Pathol*. 1991;11: 851-866.

116. Khemani E, McElhinney DB, Rhein L, et al. Pulmonary artery hypertension in formerly premature infants with bronchopulmonary dysplasia: clinical features and outcomes in the surfactant era. *Pediatrics*. 2007;120:1260-1269.

117. Arjaans S, Haarman MG, Roofthooft MTR, et al. Fate of pulmonary hypertension associated with bronchopulmonary dysplasia beyond 36 weeks postmenstrual age. *Arch Dis Child Fetal Neonatal Ed*. 2021;106(1):45-50.

118. Bhatt AJ, Pryhuber GS, Huyck H, et al. Disrupted pulmonary vasculature and decreased vascular endothelial growth factor, Flt-1, and TIE-2 in human infants dying with bronchopulmonary dysplasia. *Am J Respir Crit Care Med*. 2001;164:1971-1980.

119. Abman SH. Bronchopulmonary dysplasia: "a vascular hypothesis". *Am J Respir Crit Care Med*. 2001;164:1755-1756.

120. De Paepe ME, Mao Q, Powell J, et al. Growth of pulmonary microvasculature in ventilated preterm infants. *Am J Respir Crit Care Med*. 2006;173:204-211.

121. Jakkula M, Le Cras TD, Gebb S, et al. Inhibition of angiogenesis decreases alveolarization in the developing rat lung. *Am J Physiol Lung Cell Mol Physiol*. 2000;279:L600-L607.

122. Menon RT, Shrestha AK, Shivanna B. Hyperoxia exposure disrupts adrenomedullin signaling in newborn mice: Implications for lung development in premature infants. *Biochem Biophys Res Commun*. 2017;487:666-671.

123. Perveen S, Patel H, Arif A, et al. Role of EC-SOD overexpression in preserving pulmonary angiogenesis inhibited by oxidative stress. *PloS One*. 2012;7:e51945.

124. Swier NL, Richards B, Cua CL, et al. Pulmonary vein stenosis in neonates with severe bronchopulmonary dysplasia. *Am J Perinatol*. 2016;33:671-677.

125. Mahgoub L, Kaddoura T, Kameny AR, et al. Pulmonary vein stenosis of ex-premature infants with pulmonary hypertension and bronchopulmonary dysplasia, epidemiology, and survival from a multicenter cohort. *Pediatr Pulmonol*. 2017;52:1063-1070.

126. Drossner DM, Kim DW, Maher KO, et al. Pulmonary vein stenosis: prematurity and associated conditions. *Pediatrics*. 2008; 122:e656-e661.

127. Abman SH, Warady BA, Lum GM, et al. Systemic hypertension in infants with bronchopulmonary dysplasia. *J Pediatr*. 1984; 104:928-931.

128. Anderson AH, Warady BA, Daily DK, et al. Systemic hypertension in infants with severe bronchopulmonary dysplasia: associated clinical factors. *Am J Perinatol*. 1993;10:190-193.

129. Mourani PM, Ivy DD, Rosenberg AA, et al. Left ventricular diastolic dysfunction in bronchopulmonary dysplasia. *J Pediatr*. 2008;152:291-293.

130. Guaman MC, Gien J, Baker CD, et al. Point prevalence, clinical characteristics, and treatment variation for infants with severe bronchopulmonary dysplasia. *Am J Perinatol*. 2015;32:960-967.

131. Murthy K, Porta NFM, Lagatta JM, et al. Inter-center variation in death or tracheostomy placement in infants with severe bronchopulmonary dysplasia. *J Perinatol*. 2017;37:723-727.

132. Davis S, Jones M, Kisling J, et al. Effect of continuous positive airway pressure on forced expiratory flows in infants with

tracheomalacia. *Am J Respir Crit Care Med*. 1998;158: 148-152.

133. Doull IJ, Mok Q, Tasker RC. Tracheobronchomalacia in preterm infants with chronic lung disease. *Arch Dis Child Fetal Neonatal Ed*. 1997;76:F203-F205.

134. McCoy KS, Bagwell CE, Wagner M, et al. Spirometric and endoscopic evaluation of airway collapse in infants with bronchopulmonary dysplasia. *Pediatr Pulmonol*. 1992;14:23-27.

135. Panitch HB, Allen JL, Alpert BE, et al. Effects of CPAP on lung mechanics in infants with acquired tracheobronchomalacia. *Am J Respir Crit Care Med*. 1994;150:1341-1346.

136. Andriolo BN, Andriolo RB, Saconato H, et al. Early versus late tracheostomy for critically ill patients. *Cochrane Database Syst Rev*. 2015;1:CD007271.

137. Holloway AJ, Spaeder MC, Basu S. Association of timing of tracheostomy on clinical outcomes in PICU patients. *Pediatr Crit Care Med*. 2015;16:e52-e58.

138. DeMauro SB, D'Agostino JA, Bann C, et al. Developmental outcomes of very preterm infants with tracheostomies. *J Pediatr*. 2014;164:1303-1310.e2.

139. Gien J, Kinsella J, Thrasher J, et al. Retrospective analysis of an interdisciplinary ventilator care program intervention on survival of infants with ventilator-dependent bronchopulmonary dysplasia. *Am J Perinatol*. 2017;34:155-163.

140. Baker CD, Martin S, Thrasher J, et al. A standardized discharge process decreases length of stay for ventilator-dependent children. *Pediatrics*. 2016;137:e20150637.

141. DeMauro SB, Wei JL, Lin RJ. Perspectives on neonatal and infant tracheostomy. *Semin Fetal Neonatal Med*. 2016;21:285-291.

142. Yallapragada S, Savani RC, Mūnoz-Blanco S, et al. Children's Hospital Neonatal Consortium severe bronchopulmonary dysplasia subgroup; Murthy K. Qualitative indications for tracheostomy and chronic mechanical ventilation in patients with severe bronchopulmonary dysplasia. *J Perinatol*. 2021;41(11): 2651-2657.

143. Smith MA, Steurer MA, Mahendra M, et al. Sociodemographic factors associated with tracheostomy and mortality in bronchopulmonary dysplasia. *Pediatr Pulmonol*. 2023;58(4):1237-1246.

144. Akangire G, Lachica C, Noel-MacDonnell J, et al. Outcomes of infants with severe bronchopulmonary dysplasia who received tracheostomy and home ventilation. *Pediatr Pulmonol*. 2023; 58(3):753-762.

145. Newton M, Johnson RF, Wynings E, et al. Pediatric tracheostomy-related complications: a cross-sectional analysis. *Otolaryngol Head Neck Surg*. 2022;167(2):359-365.

146. Sun L, Zhang H, Bao Y, et al. Long-term outcomes of bronchopulmonary dysplasia under two different diagnostic criteria: a retrospective cohort study at a Chinese Tertiary Center. *Front Pediatr*. 2021;9:648972.

147. Kugelman A, Reichman B, Chistyakov I, et al. Israel Neonatal Network. Post-discharge infant mortality among very low birth weight infants: a population-based study. *Pediatrics*. 2007; 120(4):e788-e794.

148. Geon JW, Oh M, Chang YS. Definitions of bronchopulmonary dysplasia and long-term outcomes of extremely preterm infants in Korean Neonatal Network. *Sci Rep*. 2021;11:24349.

149. House M, Nathan A, Bhuiyan MAN, et al. Morbidity and respiratory outcomes in infants requiring tracheostomy for severe bronchopulmonary dysplasia. *Pediatr Pulmonol*. 2021;56(8): 2589-2596.

150. Guirguis F, Chorney SR, Wang C, et al. Nationwide tracheostomy among neonatal admissions - a cross-sectional analysis. *Int J Pediatr Otorhinolaryngol*. 2022;152:110985.

151. Annesi CA, Levin JC, Litt JS, et al. Long-term respiratory and developmental outcomes in children with bronchopulmonary dysplasia and history of tracheostomy. *J Perinatol*. 2021; 41(11):2645-2650.

152. Jadcherla SR, Gupta A, Fernandez S, et al. Spatiotemporal characteristics of acid refluxate and relationship to symptoms in premature and term infants with chronic lung disease. *Am J Gastroenterol*. 2008;103:720-728.

153. Cotton R, Suarez S, Reese J. Unexpected extra-renal effects of loop diuretics in the preterm neonate. *Acta Paediatr*. 2012; 101:835-845.

154. Brion LP, Primhak RA, Ambrosio-Perez I. Diuretics acting on the distal renal tubule for preterm infants with (or developing) chronic lung disease. *Cochrane Database Syst Rev*. 2002: CD001817.

155. Rush MG, Engelhardt B, Parker RA, et al. Double-blind, placebo-controlled trial of alternate-day furosemide therapy in infants with chronic bronchopulmonary dysplasia. *J Pediatr*. 1990;117:112-118.

156. Stewart A, Brion LP. Intravenous or enteral loop diuretics for preterm infants with (or developing) chronic lung disease. *Cochrane Database Syst Rev*. 2011;2011:CD001453.

157. Stewart A, Brion LP, Ambrosio-Perez I. Diuretics acting on the distal renal tubule for preterm infants with (or developing) chronic lung disease. *Cochrane Database Syst Rev*. 2011; 2011:CD001817.

158. Bamat NA, Nelin TD, Eichenwald EC, et al. Loop diuretics in severe bronchopulmonary dysplasia: cumulative use and associations with mortality and age at discharge. *J Pediatr*. 2021; 231:43-49.e3.

159. Duijts L, van Meel ER, Moschino L, et al. European Respiratory Society guideline on long-term management of children with bronchopulmonary dysplasia. *Eur Respir J*. 2020;55:1900788.

160. Dawson SK, D'Andrea LA, Lagatta JM. Management of diuretics in infants with bronchopulmonary dysplasia discharged on home oxygen. *Pediatr Pulmonol*. 2023;58:522-529.

161. Clouse BJ, Jadcherla SR, Slaughter JL. Systematic review of inhaled bronchodilator and corticosteroid therapies in infants with bronchopulmonary dysplasia: implications and future directions. *PLoS One*. 2016;11:e0148188.

162. Sosulski R, Abbasi S, Bhutani VK, et al. Physiologic effects of terbutaline on pulmonary function of infants with bronchopulmonary dysplasia. *Pediatr Pulmonol*. 1986;2:269-273.

163. Wilkie RA, Bryan MH. Effect of bronchodilators on airway resistance in ventilator-dependent neonates with chronic lung disease. *J Pediatr*. 1987;111:278-282.

164. Koch A, Kreutzer KB, Poets C, et al. The impact of inhaled bronchodilators on bronchopulmonary dysplasia: a nonrandomized comparison from the NEuroSIS trial. *J Matern Fetal Neonatal Med*. 2020;33:4030-4032.

165. Euteneuer JC, Kerns E, Leiting C, et al. Inhaled bronchodilator exposure in the management of bronchopulmonary dysplasia in hospitalized infants. *J Perinatol*. 2021;41:53-61.

166. Henderson-Smart DJ, Davis PG. Prophylactic methylxanthines for endotracheal extubation in preterm infants. *Cochrane Database Syst Rev*. 2010:CD000139.

167. Doyle LW, Ehrenkranz RA, Halliday HL. Early (, 8 days) postnatal corticosteroids for preventing chronic lung disease in preterm infants. *Cochrane Database Syst Rev*. 2014:CD001146.

168. Doyle LW, Ehrenkranz RA, Halliday HL. Late (> 7 days) postnatal corticosteroids for chronic lung disease in preterm infants. *Cochrane Database Syst Rev*. 2014:CD001145.

169. Watterberg KL. Policy statement—postnatal corticosteroids to prevent or treat bronchopulmonary dysplasia. *Pediatrics*. 2010; 126:800-808.

170. Zhang ZQ, Zhong Y, Huang XM, et al. Airway administration of corticosteroids for prevention of bronchopulmonary dysplasia in premature infants: a meta-analysis with trial sequential analysis. *BMC Pulm Med*. 2017;17:207.

171. Shah SS, Ohlsson A, Halliday HL, et al. Inhaled versus systemic corticosteroids for the treatment of chronic lung disease in ventilated very low birth weight preterm infants. *Cochrane Database Syst Rev*. 2012:CD002057.

172. Cole CH, Colton T, Shah BL, et al. Early inhaled glucocorticoid therapy to prevent bronchopulmonary dysplasia. *N Engl J Med*. 1999;340:1005-1010.

173. Jonsson B, Eriksson M, Soder O, et al. Budesonide delivered by dosimetric jet nebulization to preterm very low birthweight infants at high risk for development of chronic lung disease. *Acta Paediatr*. 2000;89:1449-1455.

174. Kugelman A, Peniakov M, Zangen S, et al. Inhaled hydrofluoalkane-beclomethasone dipropionate in bronchopulmonary dysplasia. A double-blind, randomized, controlled pilot study. *J Perinatol*. 2017;37:197-202.

175. Beresford MW, Primhak R, Subhedar NV, et al. Randomised double blind placebo controlled trial of inhaled fluticasone propionate in infants with chronic lung disease. *Arch Dis Child Fetal Neonatal Ed*. 2002;87:F62-F63.

176. Halvorsen T, Skadberg BT, Eide GE, et al. Characteristics of asthma and airway hyper-responsiveness after premature birth. *Pediatr Allergy Immunol*. 2005;16:487-494.

177. Kim DK, Choi SH, Yu J, et al. Bronchial responsiveness to methacholine and adenosine 5'-monophosphate in preschool children with bronchopulmonary dysplasia. *Pediatr Pulmonol*. 2006;41:538-543.

178. Leiting C, Kerns E, Euteneuer JC, et al. Inhaled corticosteroid exposure in hospitalized infants with bronchopulmonary dysplasia. *Am J Perinatol*. 2022.

179. Abman SH, Hansmann G, Archer S, et al. American Heart Association and American Thoracic Society Joint Guidelines for Pediatric Pulmonary Hypertension. *Circulation*. 2015;132: 2037-2099.

180. Krishnan U, Feinstein JA, Adatia I, et al. Evaluation and management of pulmonary hypertension in children with bronchopulmonary dysplasia. *J Pediatr*. 2017;188:24-34.e1.

181. Johnson CE, Beekman RH, Kostyshak DA, et al. Pharmacokinetics and pharmacodynamics of nifedipine in children with bronchopulmonary dysplasia and pulmonary hypertension. *Pediatr Res*. 1991;29:500-503.

182. Mourani PM, Ivy DD, Gao D, et al. Pulmonary vascular effects of inhaled nitric oxide and oxygen tension in bronchopulmonary dysplasia. *Am J Respir Crit Care Med*. 2004;170:1006-1013.

183. Galie N, Ghofrani HA, Torbicki A, et al. Sildenafil citrate therapy for pulmonary arterial hypertension. *N Engl J Med*. 2005; 353:2148-2157.

184. Mourani PM, Sontag MK, Ivy DD, et al. Effects of long-term sildenafil treatment for pulmonary hypertension in infants with chronic lung disease. *J Pediatr*. 2009;154:379-384, 384. e1-e2.

185. Frank BS, Schafer M, Grenolds A, et al. Acute vasoreactivity testing during cardiac catheterization in Infants with BPD-associated pulmonary hypertension. *J Pediatr*. 2019;208:127-133.

186. Cristea AI, Carroll AE, Davis SD, et al. Outcomes of children with severe bronchopulmonary dysplasia who were ventilator dependent at home. *Pediatrics*. 2013;132:e727-e734.

187. Manimtim WM, Agarwal A, Alexiou S, et al. Respiratory outcomes for ventilator-dependent children with bronchopulmonary dysplasia. *Pediatrics*. 2023;151(5):e2022060651.

188. Vanhaverbeke K, Van Eyck A, Van Hoorenbeeck K, et al. Lung imaging in bronchopulmonary dysplasia: a systematic review. *Respir Med*. 2020;171:106101.

189. Aukland SM, Rosendahl K, Owens CM, et al. Neonatal bronchopulmonary dysplasia predicts abnormal pulmonary HRCT scans in long-term survivors of extreme preterm birth. *Thorax*. 2009;64:405-410.

190. Wong PM, Lees AN, Louw J, et al. Emphysema in young adult survivors of moderate-to-severe bronchopulmonary dysplasia. *Eur Respir J*. 2008;32:321-328.

191. Caskey S, Gough A, Rowan S, et al. Structural and functional lung impairment in adult survivors of bronchopulmonary dysplasia. *Ann Am Thorac Soc*. 2016;13:1262-1270.

192. Annesi CA, Levin JC, Litt JS, et al. Long-term respiratory and developmental outcomes in children with bronchopulmonary dysplasia and history of tracheostomy. *J Perinatol*. 2021; 41:2645-2650.

193. Cristea AI, Ackerman VL, Swigonski NL, et al. Physiologic findings in children previously ventilator dependent at home due to bronchopulmonary dysplasia. *Pediatr Pulmonol*. 2015;50:1113-1118.

194. Bonadies L, Papi A, Baraldi E. Is bronchopulmonary dysplasia in adult age a novel COPD endotype? *Eur Respir J*. 2022; 60(3):2200984.

195. Bardsen T, Roksund OD, Benestad MR, et al. Tracking of lung function from 10 to 35 years after being born extremely preterm or with extremely low birth weight. *Thorax*. 2022;77:790-798.

196. Bardsen T, Roksund OD, Eagan TM, et al. Impaired lung function in extremely preterm-born adults in their fourth decade of life. *Am J Respir Crit Care Med*. 2023.

197. Islam JY, Keller RL, Aschner JL, et al. Understanding the short- and long-term respiratory outcomes of prematurity and bronchopulmonary dysplasia. *Am J Respir Crit Care Med*. 2015; 192:134-156.

198. McGrath-Morrow SA, Collaco JM. Bronchopulmonary dysplasia: what are its links to COPD? *Ther Adv Respir Dis*. 2019; 13:1753466619892492.

Long-Term Pulmonary Outcome of Preterm Infants

Jeanie L.Y. Cheong and Lex W. Doyle

Chapter Outline

Controversies

What are the Long-Term Pulmonary Outcomes for Late Preterm Infants?

What are the Long-Term Pulmonary Outcomes for Very Preterm Infants, and What is the Effect of Having BPD on These Outcomes?

  Hospital Readmissions for Respiratory Illness

  Respiratory Health Problems

  Pulmonary Function in Childhood

  Pulmonary Function in Late Adolescence or Early Adulthood

Trends in Pulmonary Function With Increasing Age of Survivors

  Exercise Tolerance

Are We Improving Expiratory Airflow in Survivors Born Extremely Preterm Over Time in the Post-Surfactant Era?

What are the Effects of Cigarette Smoking?

Is There a Role for Caffeine in the Newborn Period?

What Further Research is Required?

Summary

Key Points

- Preterm infants are vulnerable to adverse long-term sequelae including pulmonary outcomes.
- Respiratory morbidities, including hospitalizations for respiratory infections, asthma, and wheezing illnesses, are higher in those born preterm compared with term. These risks decrease as the children get older.
- Expiratory flow is lower in children born preterm compared with controls and worse in children who had bronchopulmonary dysplasia compared with those who did not. These differences persist to adulthood.
- There is no convincing evidence that expiratory flow in preterm survivors is improving over time, despite advances in neonatal intensive care.
- More research is needed to determine the longer-term outcomes of preterm infants, especially into later adulthood, to determine the risk of early onset chronic obstructive airways disease.

Preterm birth continues to be a significant problem in the developed world. Preterm birth rates peaked at 13% in 2006 in the United States and have declined to approximately 10% currently.[1,2] "Late preterm" infants, with gestational ages from 34 to 36 completed weeks, form the majority—73% of preterm births in 2020.[2] Moreover, survival rates for preterm neonates, particularly those born very preterm (<32 completed weeks), have increased because of technologic and therapeutic advances, such as antenatal administration of corticosteroids and postnatal administration of exogenous surfactant, combined with a greater willingness to offer intensive care before and after birth. Unfortunately preterm infants are more susceptible to adverse sequelae than are term infants, and the lungs of preterm infants are particularly vulnerable to injury.[3] Despite advances in care, respiratory problems remain the major cause of mortality in extremely preterm (<28 completed weeks) infants in the surfactant era.[4] Of those who survive the neonatal period, some experience bronchopulmonary dysplasia (BPD), both "old"[5] and "new" forms,[3] with prolonged oxygen dependency, occasionally for years. Although most preterm survivors have no ongoing oxygen dependency or respiratory distress in early childhood, it is important to consider their pulmonary function, because they are more prone to respiratory ill health in late childhood and adulthood.

Controversies

Some of the controversies regarding pulmonary outcomes of preterm birth are as follows:
- What are the pulmonary outcomes for the late preterm infants, who make up the majority of preterm survivors?
- What are the pulmonary outcomes for the very preterm infants, including hospital readmissions, respiratory health problems, pulmonary function in childhood and later life, and exercise tolerance?
- What are the effects of having had BPD in the newborn period and of active cigarette smoking on outcomes in very preterm infants?
- Are we improving expiratory airflow in survivors born extremely preterm over time in the post-surfactant era?
- Is there a role for caffeine in the newborn period?
- What further research is required?

This chapter reviews long-term pulmonary outcomes for preterm infants. If data by gestational age are not available, data by birth weight are substituted, with the assumptions that birth weight <1500 g is approximately equivalent to gestational age <32 weeks, and birth weight <1000 g to gestational age <28 weeks.

What are the Long-Term Pulmonary Outcomes for Late Preterm Infants?

There are two published reviews of studies reporting long-term respiratory morbidity of late preterm infants.[6,7] Some studies have also included infants born "moderately preterm" (between 32 and 33 completed weeks of gestation). In total, there were 34 studies reporting respiratory outcomes of late preterm infants

between 2000 and 2014. Rates of readmission to hospital following first discharge home were higher in the late preterm group compared with term controls. Data from the UK Millenium cohort reported higher rates of hospital admissions for late preterm infants and children compared with controls born 39 to 41 weeks' gestation.[8] In the first 9 months after birth, the mean adjusted odds ratio (OR) for three or more hospital admissions for late preterm infants was 5.1 (95% confidence interval [CI] 3.0, 8.8) compared with controls. The hospital admission rates decreased with increasing age. However, late preterm children up to 5 years of age in that study were still at increased risk of hospital admissions compared with term-born children (adjusted OR 1.9 [1.3, 2.7]). The major reason for rehospitalization was for respiratory illnesses.[8] In a study enrolling infants born in Manitoba, Canada, during 1997 to 2001, preterm birth was a significant risk factor for readmission to hospital in the first 6 weeks after discharge: on the basis of birth weights, gestational ages for the majority of the infants in that study would have been 32 to 36 weeks.[9] The most common cause for readmission during the 6 weeks was respiratory illness (22%), which was more than twice as common as the next leading cause. Both reviews reported substantial respiratory morbidity caused by respiratory syncytial virus (RSV). One study reported that rates of hospital admission for RSV were 57 per 1000 in late preterm infants, which exceeded that of term controls (30 per 1000) but were close to that of very preterm infants (66–70 per 1000).[10] A similar trend was reported in a regional study of preterm children in the Netherlands, where the rates of hospitalizations in the first year due to RSV were 4% in those born between 32 and 36 weeks' gestation, compared with 3% in those born <32 weeks and 1% in the full term children.[11]

It has become clearer that respiratory morbidity for late preterm children persists beyond infancy. Many studies report increased prevalence of asthma, bronchiolitis, or wheezing illnesses in this group of children compared with term controls.[8,11-13] A large retrospective study of 7925 infants using electronic health data from 31 practices affiliated with an academic center in the United States reported associations between late preterm birth and persistent asthma to 18 months (adjusted OR 1.68, 95% CI 1.20, 2.29) and inhaled corticosteroid use (adjusted OR 1.66, 95% CI 1.01, 2.80). A large observational study between 1989 and 2008 in Finland also reported a similar increase in asthma risk with lower gestation at birth (adjusted OR 1.7, 95% CI 1.4, 2.0).[13] In the United Kingdom, the increased rates of asthma or wheezing illnesses persisted up to 5 years, with an adjusted OR of being prescribed any asthma-related medication of 2.2 (95% 1.6, 3.1).[8] However, data from the Third National Health and Nutrition Examination Survey (NHANES III, 1988–1994) did not show a significantly increased risk of asthma in late preterm infants.[14] Data were available from 6187 singletons of gestational ages 34 to 41 weeks who were between 2 and 83 months at the time of the survey; the 537 late preterm (34–36 weeks) children had a slightly higher rate of physician-diagnosed asthma than the 5650 children who were term, but the increase was not statistically significant (adjusted hazard ratio 1.3; 95% CI 0.8–2.0). In a systematic review and meta-analyses that included 52 studies,[15] there was a significant increase in hospital admissions for RSV or bronchiolitis in late preterm infants compared with term controls during infancy and early childhood (up to 6 years). Admissions for asthma were elevated until 6 years of age (hazard ratio [95% CI] of 1.22 [1.13, 1.32]) but not after that. Admissions for any respiratory problems fell with age, from a risk ratio (95% CI) of 2.25 (1.75, 2.89) within 28 days of hospital discharge to 1.24 (1.11, 1.40) from 12 to 18 years.

There are several registry studies from Scandinavia that report adult respiratory outcomes of infants born 32 to 36 weeks. There was heterogeneity of the gestational age range, and in the ascertainment of asthma in the different studies. Not all studies consistently reported an increased risk of asthma in adulthood. Damgaard et al.[16] reported outcomes of a national cohort in Denmark born between 1980 and 2009 in which those born at 32 to 36 weeks had an OR (95% CI) for purchase of asthma medication of 1.59 (1.43, 1.77) in infancy, 1.21 (1.12, 1.31) for 12 to 17 years, and persisting at 1.31 (1.25, 1.38) at 25 to 31 years. Crump et al.[17] reported outcomes of 25 to 35 years from the Swedish Medical Birth Register of births between 1973 and 1979. There were no associations between being born at 33 to 36 weeks and being prescribed asthma medications in adulthood.

There are now several reports of pulmonary function in late preterm children, all of which report more airway obstruction in late preterm infants compared with controls. One study from Brazil reported on 26 infants born with a mean gestational age of 32.7 weeks (range 30–34 weeks) who did not have substantial respiratory distress in the neonatal period. Pulmonary function tests performed at a mean age of 10 weeks and repeated at a mean of 64 weeks later showed more airway obstruction in these infants compared with 24 term controls, with no evidence of improvement between the two tests.[18] The investigators concluded that preterm birth per se resulted in abnormal lung development, but late preterm children clearly need to be reassessed later in childhood and into adulthood to determine whether early lung function abnormalities are permanent. A more recent study of 31 infants born at 33 to 36 weeks' gestation with no clinical respiratory disease and 31 race- and sex-matched term controls also reported abnormal pulmonary function at term-corrected age in the late preterm group compared with term controls.[19] The late preterm group had decreased respiratory compliance, decreased expiratory flow ratio, and increased respiratory resistance compared with term controls. A decrease in expiratory flow ratio in the newborn period is thought to be a reflection of expiratory airflow limitation and predicts subsequent wheezing. Kotecha et al. reported respiratory function at 8 to 9 years and 14 to 17 years from the Avon Longitudinal Study of Parents and Children.[20] Participants were divided into four gestational age groups, i.e., <32 weeks, 33 to 34 weeks, 35 to 36 weeks, and term. Of the 6705 children with lung function at 8 to 9 years, those born at 33 to 34 weeks had poorer spirometry measures (forced expiratory flow in 1 second [FEV_1], forced vital capacity [FVC], forced expiratory flow in the middle of the exhaled volume [FEF_{25-75}], and the ratio of FEV_1/FVC) than term children. There was attenuation of differences in FEV_1 and FVC between those born at 33 to 34 weeks and term controls by the time the children were reassessed at 14 to 17 years. Interestingly, the spirometry measures of the "late preterm group" (35–36 weeks' gestation) were similar to term controls at all time points. In a recent study from Sweden, lung function data of 149 children born at 32 to 36 weeks were compared with

2472 children born at term at 8 and 16 years of age. At 8 years of age, expiratory airflow (FEV_1) was lower only in preterm girls compared with girls born at term, but by 16 years of age, airflow was lower in both sexes compared with controls.[21] The 13- to 14-year follow-up of the LOLLIPOP study in the Netherlands reported only mild lung function abnormalities (lower peak expiratory flow, and maximum expiratory flow at 75% FVC) in the adolescents born at 32 to 36 weeks compared with controls.[22] However, the study was underpowered, with only a 47% follow-up (37 in the preterm group and 34 controls).

What Are the Long-Term Pulmonary Outcomes for Very Preterm Infants, and What Is the Effect of Having BPD on These Outcomes?

HOSPITAL READMISSIONS FOR RESPIRATORY ILLNESS

Rates of rehospitalization of very preterm infants are severalfold higher than in term controls, and rates of hospital readmission have risen as survival rates of more very preterm infants have increased over time.[23] For example, the UK Millenium cohort reported an adjusted OR of 13.7 (95% CI 6.5, 29.2) for three or more admissions to hospital for very preterm infants up to 9 months, which decreased with age (adjusted OR 6.0 [95% CI 3.2, 11.4] between 9 months and 5 years of age).[8] Respiratory illnesses are the most common cause of rehospitalization in these early years,[24-26] and they occur more frequently in preterm survivors who had BPD, especially those who were discharged home on oxygen.[24] However, as the rate of hospital readmission declines later in childhood, those who had BPD are no more likely to be readmitted to hospital for respiratory or other reasons by the time they reach mid adolescence.[27,28]

RESPIRATORY HEALTH PROBLEMS

Very preterm children have more ill health than term children over the first few years of life, particularly upper and lower respiratory illnesses.[23,29,30,31] Rates of morbidity are further increased in those who had BPD.[23,32-34] Asthma or recurrent wheezing is more prevalent later in life in those born very tiny or preterm than in those not born preterm or very tiny in some[35-37]

but not all studies.[27,38] Those who had BPD have even higher rates of asthma than those who did not.[39]

PULMONARY FUNCTION IN CHILDHOOD

In 2013, Kotecha et al.[40] published a systematic review of studies reporting on expiratory airflow, specifically the FEV_1, in preterm survivors, with or without term-born controls. The studies related to births from the 1960s through to births in the 1990s; most participants were born before surfactant was available. As such, they would have encompassed survivors who had the classical scarring and emphysematous BPD seen in the earliest survivors,[5] all the way through to the "new" BPD of the post-surfactant era,[3] characterized more by alveolar arrest.

In results from 22 studies (n = 2085 preterm; n = 3820 control), the FEV_1 was reduced by a mean of −8.7% of predicted for age, height, sex, and ethnicity in the preterm group compared with controls, with 95% CI −11.0%, −6.4%. Comparing the preterm group who had no BPD with term-born controls in 21 studies (n = 998 preterm, no BPD; n = 1347 control), the mean FEV_1 was reduced by −7.2% (95% CI −8.7%, −5.6%) of predicted.[40] Some studies defined BPD as oxygen dependency at 28 days after birth, and others defined it as oxygen dependency at or beyond 36 weeks' postmenstrual age. These definitions correspond with "any BPD" and "moderate-to-severe BPD," respectively, on the consensus definition of BPD established in 2001.[3] Comparing the preterm group with any BPD with term-born controls in 17 studies (n = 356 preterm, any BPD; n = 523 control), the mean FEV_1 was reduced by −16.2% (95% CI −19.9%, −12.4%) of predicted. Comparing the preterm group with moderate-to-severe BPD with term-born controls in 10 studies (n = 406 preterm, moderate-to-severe BPD; n = 1015 control), the mean FEV_1 was reduced by −18.9% (95% CI −21.1%, −16.7%) of predicted.[40]

Results from more recent studies that were not included in the systematic review are consistent with the results of Kotecha et al. Ronkainen et al.[41] reported the results of a systematic review of six studies; survivors born preterm had an increasing reduction in FEV_1, from −7.4% predicted for no BPD, to −10.5% predicted for any BPD, to −17.8% for moderate-to-severe BPD compared with term-born controls.

Simpson et al.[42] assessed a cohort of children at age 9 to 11 years born in the surfactant era. In addition to confirming airway obstruction, 92% of children born ≤32 weeks had structural abnormalities on CT scan, more pronounced in those with BPD. In a cohort of 35 survivors born extremely preterm (EP) in Norway in 1991 to 1992, Vollsæter et al.[43] found that expiratory airflow was worse in those who had moderate-to-severe BPD than in those who had mild BPD, who in turn were worse than those who had no BPD, at mean ages of 10.5 and 17.8 years. In a Swedish study of infants born <27 weeks' gestation between 2004 and 2007, Thunqvist et al.[44] reported that expiratory airflow at 6½ years was lower in 17 children who had severe BPD compared with 65 children who had moderate BPD; overall 90% of their cohort had either moderate or severe BPD.

PULMONARY FUNCTION IN LATE ADOLESCENCE OR EARLY ADULTHOOD

In an individual participant data meta-analysis of expiratory flow in late adolescence and early adulthood, individuals born very preterm (<32 weeks' gestation) or very low birth weight (<1500 g birth weight) were compared with term (37–42 weeks' gestation) or normal birth weight (>2499 g birth weight) controls; most individuals were born in the pre-surfactant era.[45] Eleven studies (n = 935 very preterm or very low birth weight, and 722 controls) were included, with a mean age of 21 years (range 16–33 years). The controls mostly had values for expiratory airflow in the expected range, with mean z-scores close to zero. Consistent with results in childhood, adults born preterm had substantial reductions in expiratory airflow as a group compared with controls; e.g., the mean difference for $zFEV_1$ was -0.78 (95% CI -0.96, -0.61) (Fig. 15.1). Similar trends were noted when considering clinically important reductions in airflow; e.g., the proportions with values for the FEV_1 <5th percentile were 24% in the preterm group and 7% in control group (OR 4.16, 95% CI 2.99, 5.78).

There have been three studies published since the individual participant data meta-analysis, two from cohorts born in the post-surfactant era, and one in the pre-surfactant era. Findings were similar to those of the individual participant data meta-analysis. Doyle et al.[46] measured expiratory airflows in 164 extremely preterm or extremely low-birth-weight participants

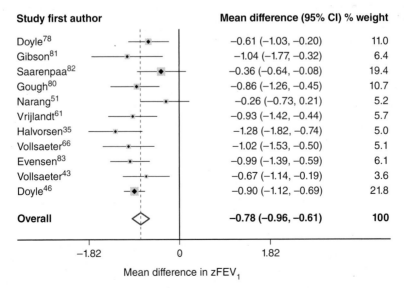

Study first author		Mean difference (95% CI)	% weight
Doyle[78]		−0.61 (−1.03, −0.20)	11.0
Gibson[81]		−1.04 (−1.77, −0.32)	6.4
Saarenpaa[82]		−0.36 (−0.64, −0.08)	19.4
Gough[80]		−0.86 (−1.26, −0.45)	10.7
Narang[51]		−0.26 (−0.73, 0.21)	5.2
Vrijlandt[61]		−0.93 (−1.42, −0.44)	5.7
Halvorsen[35]		−1.28 (−1.82, −0.74)	5.0
Vollsaeter[66]		−1.02 (−1.53, −0.50)	5.1
Evensen[83]		−0.99 (−1.39, −0.59)	6.1
Vollsaeter[43]		−0.67 (−1.14, −0.19)	3.6
Doyle[46]		−0.90 (−1.12, −0.69)	21.8
Overall		**−0.78 (−0.96, −0.61)**	**100**

−1.82   0   1.82

Mean difference in $zFEV_1$

Fig. 15.1 Forest plot of mean differences in z-scores for forced expired volume in 1 second *(zFEV₁)* between preterm groups and controls, for individual studies and overall. Superscript numbers indicate source of the data. *CI,* Confidence interval. (Reprinted with permission from Doyle et al Expiratory airflow in late adolescence and early adulthood in individuals born very preterm or with very low birthweight compared with controls born at term or with normal birthweight: a meta-analysis of individual participant data. *Lancet Respir Med.* 2019;7:677-686.)

born in 1991 to 1992 and 130 controls at age 25 years. As expected, the preterm group had clinically significant airflow limitation compared with the controls. The EPICURE study in the United Kingdom reported 19-year respiratory airflows for 129 extremely preterm (≤25 weeks' gestation) participants born in 1995 and 65 controls.[47] All spirometric measures were lower in the extremely preterm group, and reversibility with the bronchodilator was more common in the extremely preterm group than controls. Yang et al.[48] measured expiratory airflow of 224 survivors who were born <1500 g birth weight in New Zealand in 1986 at 26 to 30 years of age, and 100 controls who had not been admitted to an intensive care nursery in the newborn period. Those born very preterm (VP) had substantially reduced airflow compared with controls, as well as evidence of air trapping.

That BPD is associated with even lower values for expiratory airflow than not having BPD in preterm survivors compared with controls is clear in Table 15.1. Although most survivors with BPD have FEV_1 values within the normal range (means ≥80% predicted; z-score ≥−1.645), with the exceptions of the highly selected studies by Northway and colleagues[49] and the EPICure study[47] that recruited infants <26 weeks' gestation, they are worse than preterm controls without BPD and even worse relative to controls.

TRENDS IN PULMONARY FUNCTION WITH INCREASING AGE OF SURVIVORS

It is vital to have information about how lung function in preterm survivors may change as they grow up. In a regional Australian cohort of 297 extremely preterm or extremely low-birth-weight participants and

TABLE 15.1 FEV_1[a] for Studies With Respiratory Function Reported in Late Adolescence/Early Adulthood, Contrasting BPD With No BPD and Control Groups

Study (Year Published)	FEV₁ in Preterm Groups		FEV₁ in NBW Controls
	BPD	No BPD	
Northway et al.[49] (1990)	74.8 (14.5); n = 25[b]	96.6 (10.2); n = 26	100.4 (10.9); n = 53
Halvorsen et al.[35] (2004)	87.8 (13.8); n = 12[c]	97.7 (12.9); n =34	108.1 (13.8); n = 46
Doyle et al.[78] (2006)	81.6 (18.7); n = 33[b]	92.9 (12.8); n = 114	99.4 (9.5); n = 37
Vrijlandt et al.[61] (2006)	90.1 (19.8); n = 8[d]	99.2 (17.9); n = 12[d]	109.6 (13.4); n = 48
Wong et al.[79] (2008)	89.0 (22.6–121.9)[e]; n = 21		
Gough et al.[80] (2014)	81.9 (15.9); n = 72	97.0 (15.2); n = 57	101.2 (11.4); n = 78
Gibson et al.[81] (2015) (z-scores)	−1.37 (2.21); n = 24	−0.47 (1.30); n = 63	0.38 (0.79); n = 19
Vollsaeter et al.[66] (2015)	84.1 (75.8–92.3); n = 11	93.6 (85.0–102.3); n = 12	100.4 (95.5–105.3); n = 39
Caskey et al.[64] (2016)	88.2 (15.2); n = 25	102.0 (14.9); n = 24	109.4 (11.8); n = 25
Doyle et al.[50] (2017)	82.7 (13.7); n = 77	90.9 (11.4); n = 131	98.7 (10.7); n = 153
Saarenpaa et al.[82] (2015)	82.7 (14.4); n = 29	93.5 (14.3); n = 131	96.9 (12.8); n = 162
Vollsæter et al.[43] (2013)	n = 25	94.1 (85.8, 102.3); n = 58	99.9 (95.8, 104.0); n = 81
	Mild BPD: 88.3 (82.6, 93.9)		
	Moderate/severe BPD: 84.6 (76.9, 92.3)		
Doyle et al.[46] (2019)	83.6 (14.3); n = 65	91.6 (14.0); n = 99	100.3 (11.9); n = 130
Hurst et al.[47] (2020) (z-scores)	−1.83 (1.17); n = 87	−1.05 (0.99); n = 36	−0.29 (0.89); n = 64
Yang et al.[48] (2020) (z-scores)	−1.34 (1.41); n = 46	−0.50 (1.08); n = 178	−0.13 (1.17); n = 100

BPD, Bronchopulmonary dysplasia; *FEV1*, forced expiratory volume in 1 second; *NBW*, normal birth weight.
[a]Reported as percentage of predicted for age, height, and sex, with three exceptions.
[b]BPD determined by ventilator dependency, oxygen requirement >28 days, and chest radiograph findings consistent with Northway stage 3 or 4 changes.[5]
[c]BPD group had oxygen requirement at 36 weeks of gestation; the remainder of preterm subjects in this study are considered to have no BPD.
[d]Males only.
[e]Range: this study had no controls, either preterm or term.

260 term controls recruited in 1991 to 1992, Doyle et al. reported spirometry changes from age 8 to 18 years.[50] The preterm group had lower FEV_1 at both ages compared with controls (mean differences [95% CI] in z-score for FEV_1; 8 years −1.02 [−1.21, −0.82]; 18 years −0.92 [−1.14, −0.71]). The spirometry parameters declined with increasing age and were worse in those with BPD and in those who smoked. A follow-up study of the same cohort reported the trajectories from 18 to 25 years. Both extremely preterm or extremely low-birth-weight and control groups showed similar trajectories, unlike the earlier ages.[46] The EPICure study assessed participants at 11 and 19 years, and as per the Australian cohort, there was no evidence of "catch-up" growth with age.[47] Two other reports of survivors from the 1970s and 1980s did not find deterioration of lung function between mid-childhood and young adulthood.[51,52] This may reflect differences between pre- and post-surfactant cohorts and factors specific to the populations from different geographical regions.

EXERCISE TOLERANCE

Cardiopulmonary limitations may not be evident during standard respiratory function measurements conducted at rest, but may become apparent during an exercise test. In one study of 10-year-old children born in 1992 through 1994 weighing <1000 g and <32 weeks of gestation, the exercise capacity of the preterm group was approximately one-half that of term controls.[53] More recent studies have reported shorter walking distances using the 6-minute walk test in ex-preterm children with BPD compared with those without.[54-56] Some other studies,[57-60] but not all,[61-63] have also reported diminished peak oxygen consumption with exercise testing in preterm children. Not all of these studies were limited to very preterm subjects; one evaluated only infants <801 g birthweight,[59] another selected subjects <32 weeks' gestational age or <1500 g birthweight,[61] another included extremely preterm children born <28 weeks' gestation,[60] and the remainder studied only subjects with BPD and not complete cohorts of preterm children. Exercise limitation has also been reported in several studies in young adults where the preterm group had poorer exercise tolerance than term controls.[47,56,64]

Are We Improving Expiratory Airflow in Survivors Born Extremely Preterm Over Time in the Post-Surfactant Era?

The Victorian Infant Collaborative Study reported the changes in assisted ventilation and oxygen therapy in the neonatal nursery, and expiratory airflows at 7 to 8 years of age of three discrete cohorts of consecutive births <28 weeks' gestation in the post-surfactant era—1991 to 1992, 1997, and 2005.[65] They found that there was an increased consumption of all resources for assisted ventilation, especially nasal continuous positive airway pressure and oxygen, and in rates of BPD over time, particularly between the 1997 and 2005 cohorts. Moreover, these changes were accompanied by a substantial reduction in z-scores for FEV_1 at school age by approximately 0.75 SD between the 2005 and 1997 cohorts, suggesting that the increased use of resources for assisted ventilation that were thought to be less invasive in the newborn period was not associated with improved long-term lung function, but rather a deterioration, which is a disturbing trend.

There are limited data from other studies that contrast results over time within the surfactant era. Vollsæter et al.[66] from Norway reported expiratory flow data of 57 children aged 11 years born <28 weeks of gestation or with birth weight <1000 g in 1999 to 2000, and 35 children aged 10 years born <29 weeks of gestation or with birth weight <1001 g in 1991 to 1992, compared with controls born >37 weeks or >3000 g birth weight. The preterm groups had worse expiratory airflow than controls in both eras, but the gap was narrower in 1999 to 2000 (e.g., $zFEV_1$ mean difference −0.35, −0.70, 0.01) than in 1991 to 1992 (e.g., $zFEV_1$ mean difference −0.53, −1.07, 0.00), but there was little evidence for a statistically important difference between preterm groups and controls between the eras, due, in part, to the small sample sizes of the cohorts.

What Are the Effects of Cigarette Smoking?

Respiratory function in subjects of birth weight <1000 g who smoke in early adulthood has been reported to be worse than in those who do not smoke; Doyle and associates[67] reported the results of respiratory function at a mean age of 20.2 years in a cohort of

44 of 60 consecutive survivors born with <1000 g birth weight between 1977 and 1980 at the Royal Women's Hospital, Melbourne, Australia. Respiratory function had also been measured in 42 of the 44 subjects at 8 years. Respiratory function was compared in the 14 smokers and the 30 nonsmokers. Several respiratory function variables reflecting airflow were significantly diminished in smokers. The proportion with a clinically important reduction in airflow (FEV_1/FVC < 75%) was significantly higher in smokers (64%) than in nonsmokers (20%) ($\chi^2 = 8.3$; $P < 0.01$). There was a significantly larger decrease in the FEV_1/FVC ratio between ages 8 and 20 years in the smokers than in the nonsmokers (mean difference in rate of change: −8.2%; 95% CI −14.1% to −2.4%). Given that the rate of deterioration in respiratory function is more rapid in smokers <1000 g birth weight up to age 20 years and the fact that cigarette smoking is detrimental to respiratory function in all subjects in adulthood,[68,69] preterm-born adults who smoke should undergo respiratory function testing well into adulthood to establish whether chronic obstructive airway disease develops more rapidly and at earlier ages than in those who do not smoke. In a more contemporary cohort of extremely preterm or extremely low birth weight participants born in the state of Victoria in the post-surfactant era, those who smoked at 18 years of age had a decline in expiratory airflow between 8 and 18 years of age compared with nonsmokers.[50]

The individual participant data meta-analysis also identified perinatal and neonatal predictors of later airflow among those born preterm (Fig. 15.2). Notably, active smoking was not associated with changes in the FEV_1 (Fig. 15.2), but it was associated with higher scores in the FVC.[45] This finding was unexpected[45] and had been reported in another study[70] of almost 10,000 adolescents and young adults where smokers had higher FVC than nonsmokers, although gestational ages of the participants were not reported in that study. The reason for the elevated FVC level in smokers is unclear. In the individual participant data meta-analysis, there were negative associations between male sex and BPD with airflow variables; notably, the reduction for those who had BPD in the newborn period approached −1 SD for the FEV_1. However, antenatal corticosteroids were associated

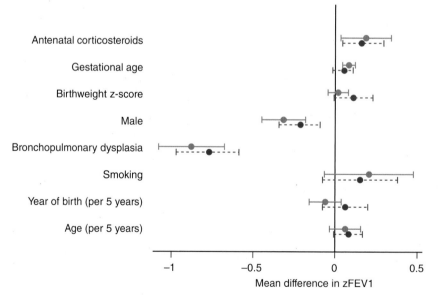

Fig. 15.2 Associations of z-scores for forced expired volume in 1 second *(zFEV₁)* with perinatal and demographic variables among participants born very preterm or with very low birth weight. Data are mean difference and 95% CI per change (indicated in brackets) in independent variable. *Solid lines* represent univariable analyses; *dashed lines* represent multivariable analyses. (Reprinted with permission from Doyle et al Expiratory airflow in late adolescence and early adulthood in individuals born very preterm or with very low birthweight compared with controls born at term or with normal birthweight: a meta-analysis of individual participant data. *Lancet Respir Med.* 2019;7:677-686.)

with better airflow. Gestational age, birth weight z-score, year of birth, and age at assessment were not independently associated with changes in the FEV_1 (Fig. 15.2). Since the peak of airway growth is achieved in the early 20s, this individual participant data meta-analysis highlights the concern that very preterm or very low birth weight individuals are not achieving their full airway growth potential and are destined for high rates of chronic obstructive pulmonary disease in later life.

Is There a Role for Caffeine in the Newborn Period?

Caffeine, a methylxanthine, is one of the most commonly prescribed medicines in the newborn nursery. Methylxanthines were first used in the 1970s to reduce apnea, but with little evidence about its long-term effects, either beneficial or harmful. The Caffeine for Apnea of Prematurity (CAP) study was designed to address the lack of long-term data, and its primary objective was to establish the long-term benefits and harms of neonatal caffeine therapy. In the CAP study, caffeine reduced ventilator and oxygen dependence, and BPD in the short term,[71] the combined rates of death or disability (cerebral palsy and cognitive delay) at 18 to 21 months of age,[72] and motor impairment at 5[73] and 11 years of age,[74] without any evidence of long-term neurological harm. In a subgroup studied at one of the CAP centers, caffeine in the newborn period improved $zFEV_1$ at 11 years by a mean of 0.56 SD (95% CI 0.15, 0.97), an effect that was related in part to its ability to prevent BPD in the newborn period.[75]

What Further Research Is Required?

Lower birth weight, and presumably increasing prematurity, is associated with worse respiratory health later in adulthood, including higher death rates from chronic obstructive airway disease and worse respiratory function, as reported in 1991 by Barker and coworkers[76] in a follow-up study of 5718 men born in Hertfordshire, England, from 1911 through 1930. The period of follow-up for very preterm survivors of modern perinatal/neonatal intensive care thus far has been only into the third decade and is clearly too short for accurate detection of chronic obstructive lung

disease, which typically occurs much later in life. Even less is known about the late preterm group. However, given the higher rates of respiratory ill health and clear reductions in airflow in preterm survivors in comparison with controls up to the third decade, follow-up until much later into adulthood is imperative. The other area of research that is vital is to repeat expiratory airflows in new cohorts of children born extremely preterm, to determine the long-term pulmonary impact of the increased use of less invasive methods for assisted ventilation, particularly nasal high-flow oxygen/air mixtures.[77]

Summary

- Late preterm (32–36 weeks of gestation) survivors, who greatly outnumber very preterm survivors, have more respiratory ill health in early childhood than term-born controls. However, the duration of follow-up has thus far been very short relative to total life expectancy.
- Very preterm (<32 weeks of gestation) survivors have more readmissions to hospital in early childhood, more upper and lower respiratory tract infections, and more asthma symptoms than term-born controls.
- Very preterm survivors have worse respiratory function than controls, particularly airway obstruction, both in childhood and in adolescence and early adulthood; they also have worse exercise tolerance than term-born controls.
- The detrimental effects of cigarette smoking on respiratory function are probably greater in preterm survivors, but more research is required.
- Having had BPD in the newborn period generally exacerbates all of these long-term respiratory problems.
- Respiratory function and respiratory health later in adult life for preterm infants must be determined, because they are more susceptible to earlier onset of chronic obstructive airway disease than controls.
- New cohorts of children born extremely preterm should have their lung function assessed at school age to ensure the long-term impact of the wide use of newer techniques of noninvasive assisted ventilation.

REFERENCES

1. Goldenberg RL, Culhane JF, Iams JD, Romero R. Epidemiology and causes of preterm birth. *Lancet*. 2008;371:75-84.
2. Osterman M, Hamilton B, Martin JA, Driscoll AK, Valenzuela CP. Births: final data for 2020. *Natl Vital Stat Rep*. 2021;70(17):1-50.
3. Jobe AH, Bancalari E. Bronchopulmonary dysplasia. *Am J Respir Crit Care Med*. 2001;163:1723-1729.
4. Doyle LW, Gultom E, Chuang SL, et al. Changing mortality and causes of death in infants 23-27 weeks' gestational age. *J Paediatr Child Health*. 1999;35:255-259.
5. Northway Jr WH, Rosan RC, Porter DY. Pulmonary disease following respirator therapy of hyaline-membrane disease. Bronchopulmonary dysplasia. *N Engl J Med*. 1967;276:357-368.
6. Colin AA, McEvoy C, Castile RG. Respiratory morbidity and lung function in preterm infants of 32 to 36 weeks' gestational age. *Pediatrics*. 2010;126:115-128.
7. Pike KC, Lucas JS. Respiratory consequences of late preterm birth. *Paediatr Respir Rev*. 2015;16:182-188.
8. Boyle EM, Poulsen G, Field DJ, et al. Effects of gestational age at birth on health outcomes at 3 and 5 years of age: population based cohort study. *BMJ*. 2012;344:e896.
9. Martens PJ, Derksen S, Gupta S. Predictors of hospital readmission of Manitoba newborns within six weeks postbirth discharge: a population-based study. *Pediatrics*. 2004;114:708-713.
10. Boyce TG, Mellen BG, Mitchel Jr EF, et al. Rates of hospitalization for respiratory syncytial virus infection among children in medicaid. *J Pediatr*. 2000;137:865-870.
11. Vrijlandt EJ, Kerstjens JM, Duiverman EJ, et al. Moderately preterm children have more respiratory problems during their first 5 years of life than children born full term. *Am J Respir Crit Care Med*. 2013;187:1234-1240.
12. Goyal NK, Fiks AG, Lorch SA. Association of late-preterm birth with asthma in young children: practice-based study. *Pediatrics*. 2011;128:e830-e838.
13. Harju M, Keski-Nisula L, Georgiadis L, et al. The burden of childhood asthma and late preterm and early term births. *J Pediatr*. 2014;164:295-299.e1.
14. Abe K, Shapiro-Mendoza CK, Hall LR, et al. Late preterm birth and risk of developing asthma. *J Pediatr*. 2010;157:74-78.
15. Isayama T, Lewis-Mikhael AM, O'Reilly D, et al. Health services use by late preterm and term infants from infancy to adulthood: a meta-analysis. *Pediatrics*. 2017;140:e20170266.
16. Damgaard AL, Hansen BM, Mathiasen R, et al. Prematurity and prescription asthma medication from childhood to young adulthood: a Danish national cohort study. *PLoS One*. 2015;10:e0117253.
17. Crump C, Winkleby MA, Sundquist J, et al. Risk of asthma in young adults who were born preterm: a Swedish national cohort study. *Pediatrics*. 2011;127:e913-e920.
18. Friedrich L, Pitrez PM, Stein RT, et al. Growth rate of lung function in healthy preterm infants. *Am J Respir Crit Care Med*. 2007;176:1269-1273.
19. McEvoy C, Venigalla S, Schilling D, et al. Respiratory function in healthy late preterm infants delivered at 33-36 weeks of gestation. *J Pediatr*. 2013;162:464-469.
20. Kotecha SJ, Watkins WJ, Paranjothy S, et al. Effect of late preterm birth on longitudinal lung spirometry in school age children and adolescents. *Thorax*. 2012;67:54-61.
21. Thunqvist P, Gustafsson PM, Schultz ES, et al. Lung function at 8 and 16 years after moderate-to-late preterm birth: a prospective cohort study. *Pediatrics*. 2016;137:e20152056.
22. Vrijlandt EJLE, Reijneveld SA, Aris-Meijer JL, et al. Respiratory health in adolescents born moderately-late preterm in a community-based cohort. *J Pediatr*. 2018;203:429-436.
23. Doyle LW, Ford G, Davis N. Health and hospitalisations after discharge in extremely low birth weight infants. *Semin Neonatol*. 2003;8:137-145.
24. Cunningham CK, McMillan JA, Gross SJ. Rehospitalization for respiratory illness in infants of less than 32 weeks' gestation. *Pediatrics*. 1991;88:527-532.
25. Hennessy EM, Bracewell MA, Wood N, et al. Respiratory health in pre-school and school age children following extremely preterm birth. *Arch Dis Child*. 2008;93:1037-1043.
26. Kitchen WH, Ford GW, Doyle LW, et al. Health and hospital readmissions of very-low-birth-weight and normal-birth-weight children. *Am J Dis Child*. 1990;144:213-218.
27. Doyle LW, Cheung MM, Ford GW, et al. Birth weight <1501 g and respiratory health at age 14. *Arch Dis Child*. 2001;84:40-44.
28. McCormick MC, Workman-Daniels K, Brooks-Gunn J, et al. Hospitalization of very low birth weight children at school age. *J Pediatr*. 1993;122:360-365.
29. O'Callaghan MJ, Burns Y, Gray P, et al. Extremely low birth weight and control infants at 2 years corrected age: a comparison of intellectual abilities, motor performance, growth and health. *Early Hum Dev*. 1995;40:115-128.
30. Chien YH, Tsao PN, Chou HC, et al. Rehospitalization of extremely-low-birth-weight infants in first 2 years of life. *Early Hum Dev*. 2002;66:33-40.
31. Skromme K, Leversen KT, Eide GE, et al. Respiratory illness contributed significantly to morbidity in children born extremely premature or with extremely low birthweights in 1999-2000. *Acta Paediatr*. 2015;104:1189-1198.
32. Yu VY, Orgill AA, Lim SB, et al. Bronchopulmonary dysplasia in very low birthweight infants. *Aust Paediatr J*. 1983;19:233-236.
33. Tammela OK. First-year infections after initial hospitalization in low birth weight infants with and without bronchopulmonary dysplasia. *Scand J Infect Dis*. 1992;24:515-524.
34. Korhonen P, Koivisto AM, Ikonen S, et al. Very low birthweight, bronchopulmonary dysplasia and health in early childhood. *Acta Paediatr*. 1999;88:1385-1391.
35. Halvorsen T, Skadberg BT, Eide GE, et al. Pulmonary outcome in adolescents of extreme preterm birth: a regional cohort study. *Acta Paediatr*. 2004;93:1294-1300.
36. Vrijlandt EJ, Boezen HM, Gerritsen J, et al. Respiratory health in prematurely born preschool children with and without bronchopulmonary dysplasia. *J Pediatr*. 2007;150:256-261.
37. Siltanen M, Savilahti E, Pohjavuori M, et al. Respiratory symptoms and lung function in relation to atopy in children born preterm. *Pediatr Pulmonol*. 2004;37:43-49.
38. Steffensen FH, Sorensen HT, Gillman MW, et al. Low birth weight and preterm delivery as risk factors for asthma and atopic dermatitis in young adult males. *Epidemiology*. 2000;11:185-188.
39. Ng DK, Lau WY, Lee SL. Pulmonary sequelae in long-term survivors of bronchopulmonary dysplasia. *Pediatr Int*. 2000;42:603-607.
40. Kotecha SJ, Edwards MO, Watkins WJ, et al. Effect of preterm birth on later FEV1: a systematic review and meta-analysis. *Thorax*. 2013;68:760-766.

41. Ronkainen E, Dunder T, Peltoniemi O, et al. New BPD predicts lung function at school age: Follow-up study and meta-analysis. *Pediatr Pulmonol*. 2015;50:1090-1098.

42. Simpson SJ, Logie KM, O'Dea CA, et al. Altered lung structure and function in mid-childhood survivors of very preterm birth. *Thorax*. 2017;72:702-711.

43. Vollsæter M, Røksund OD, Eide GE, et al. Lung function after preterm birth: development from mid-childhood to adulthood. *Thorax*. 2013;68:767-776.

44. Thunqvist P, Tufvesson E, Bjermer L, et al. Lung function after extremely preterm birth-A population-based cohort study (EX-PRESS). *Pediatr Pulmonol*. 2018;53:64-72.

45. Doyle LW, Andersson S, Bush A, et al. Expiratory airflow in late adolescence and early adulthood in individuals born very preterm or with very low birthweight compared with controls born at term or with normal birthweight: a meta-analysis of individual participant data. *Lancet Respir Med*. 2019;7: 677-686.

46. Doyle LW, Irving L, Haikerwal A, Lee K, Ranganathan S, Cheong J. Airway obstruction in young adults born extremely preterm or extremely low birth weight in the postsurfactant era. *Thorax*. 2019;74:1147-1153.

47. Hurst JR, Beckmann J, Ni Y, et al. Respiratory and cardiovascular outcomes in survivors of extremely preterm birth at 19 years. *Am J Respir Crit Care Med*. 2020;202:422-432.

48. Yang J, Kingsford RA, Horwood J, et al. Lung function of adults born at very low birth weight. *Pediatrics*. 2020;145:e20192359.

49. Northway Jr WH, Moss RB, Carlisle KB, et al. Late pulmonary sequelae of bronchopulmonary dysplasia. *N Engl J Med*. 1990;323:1793-1799.

50. Doyle LW, Adams AM, Robertson C, et al. Increasing airway obstruction from 8 to 18 years in extremely preterm/low-birthweight survivors born in the surfactant era. *Thorax*. 2017; 72:712-719.

51. Narang I, Rosenthal M, Cremonesini D, et al. Longitudinal evaluation of airway function 21 years after preterm birth. *Am J Respir Crit Care Med*. 2008;178:74-80.

52. Vollsaeter M, Clemm HH, Satrell E, et al. Adult respiratory outcomes of extreme preterm birth. A regional cohort study. *Ann Am Thorac Soc*. 2015;12:313-322.

53. Smith LJ, van Asperen PP, McKay KO, et al. Reduced exercise capacity in children born very preterm. *Pediatrics*. 2008;122: e287-e293.

54. Praprotnik M, Stucin Gantar I, Lucovnik M, et al. Respiratory morbidity, lung function and fitness assessment after bronchopulmonary dysplasia. *J Perinatol*. 2015;35:1037-1042.

55. Vardar-Yagli N, Inal-Ince D, Saglam M, et al. Pulmonary and extrapulmonary features in bronchopulmonary dysplasia: a comparison with healthy children. *J Phys Ther Sci*. 2015;27:1761-1765.

56. Cheong JLY, Haikerwal A, Wark JD, et al. Cardiovascular health profile at age 25 years in adults born extremely preterm or extremely low birthweight. *Hypertension*. 2020;76: 1838-1846.

57. Santuz P, Baraldi E, Zaramella P, et al. Factors limiting exercise performance in long-term survivors of bronchopulmonary dysplasia. *Am J Respir Crit Care Med*. 1995;152:1284-1289.

58. Pianosi PT, Fisk M. Cardiopulmonary exercise performance in prematurely born children. *Pediatr Res*. 2000;47:653-658.

59. Kilbride HW, Gelatt MC, Sabath RJ. Pulmonary function and exercise capacity for ELBW survivors in preadolescence: effect of neonatal chronic lung disease. *J Pediatr*. 2003;143:488-493.

60. MacLean JE, DeHaan K, Fuhr D, et al. Altered breathing mechanics and ventilatory response during exercise in children born extremely preterm. *Thorax*. 2016;71:1012-1019.

61. Vrijlandt EJ, Gerritsen J, Boezen HM, et al. Lung function and exercise capacity in young adults born prematurely. *Am J Respir Crit Care Med*. 2006;173:890-896.

62. Bader D, Ramos AD, Lew CD, et al. Childhood sequelae of infant lung disease: exercise and pulmonary function abnormalities after bronchopulmonary dysplasia. *J Pediatr*. 1987;110: 693-699.

63. Jacob SV, Lands LC, Coates AL, et al. Exercise ability in survivors of severe bronchopulmonary dysplasia. *Am J Respir Crit Care Med*. 1997;155:1925-1929.

64. Caskey S, Gough A, Rowan S, et al. Structural and functional lung impairment in adult survivors of bronchopulmonary dysplasia. *Ann Am Thorac Soc*. 2016;13:1262-1270.

65. Doyle LW, Carse E, Adams AM, et al. Victorian infant collaborative study group. ventilation in extremely preterm infants and respiratory function at 8 years. *N Engl J Med*. 2017;377: 329-337.

66. Vollsæter M, Skromme K, Satrell E, et al. Children born preterm at the turn of the millennium had better lung function than children born similarly preterm in the early 1990s. *PLoS One*. 2015;10:e0144243.

67. Doyle LW, Olinsky A, Faber B, Callanan C. Adverse effects of smoking on respiratory function in young adults born weighing less than 1000 grams. *Pediatrics*. 2003;112:565-569.

68. Higgins MW, Enright PL, Kronmal RA, et al. Smoking and lung function in elderly men and women. The Cardiovascular Health Study. *JAMA*. 1993;269:2741-2748.

69. Dockery DW, Speizer FE, Ferris BGJ, et al. Cumulative and reversible effects of lifetime smoking on simple tests of lung function in adults. *Am Rev Respir Dis*. 1988;137:286-292.

70. Gold DR, Wang X, Wypij D, et al. Effects of cigarette smoking on lung function in adolescent boys and girls. *N Engl J Med*. 1996;335:931-937.

71. Schmidt B, Roberts RS, Davis P, et al. Caffeine therapy for apnea of prematurity. *N Engl J Med*. 2006;354:2112-2121.

72. Schmidt B, Roberts RS, Davis P, et al. Long-term effects of caffeine therapy for apnea of prematurity. *N Engl J Med*. 2007;357:1893-1902.

73. Doyle LW, Schmidt B, Anderson PJ, et al. Reduction in developmental coordination disorder with neonatal caffeine therapy. *J Pediatr*. 2014;165:356-359.e2.

74. Schmidt B, Roberts RS, Anderson PJ, et al. Academic performance, motor function, and behavior 11 years after neonatal caffeine citrate therapy for apnea of prematurity: an 11-year follow-up of the CAP randomized clinical trial. *JAMA Pediatr*. 2017;171:564-572.

75. Doyle LW, Ranganathan S, Cheong JLY. Neonatal caffeine treatment and respiratory function at 11 years in children under 1,251 g at birth. *Am J Respir Crit Care Med*. 2017;196: 1318-1324.

76. Barker DJ, Godfrey KM, Fall C, et al. Relation of birth weight and childhood respiratory infection to adult lung function and death from chronic obstructive airways disease. *Brit Med J*. 1991;303:671-675.

77. Cheong JLY, Olsen JE, Huang L, et al. Changing consumption of resources for respiratory support and short-term outcomes in four consecutive geographical cohorts of infants born extremely preterm over 25 years since the early 1990s. *BMJ Open*. 2020;10:e037507.

78. Doyle LW, Faber B, Callanan C, et al. Bronchopulmonary dysplasia in very low birth weight subjects and lung function in late adolescence. *Pediatrics*. 2006;118:108-113.

79. Wong PM, Lees AN, Louw J, et al. Emphysema in young adult survivors of moderate-to-severe bronchopulmonary dysplasia. *Eur Respir J*. 2008;32:321-328.

80. Gough A, Linden M, Spence D, et al. Impaired lung function and health status in adult survivors of bronchopulmonary dysplasia. *Eur Respir J*. 2014;43:808-816.

81. Gibson AM, Reddington C, McBride L, et al. Lung function in adult survivors of very low birth weight, with and without bronchopulmonary dysplasia. *Pediatr Pulmonol*. 2015;50:987-994.

82. Saarenpää HK, Tikanmäki M, SipolaLeppänen M, et al. Lung function in very low birth weight adults. *Pediatrics*. 2015; 136:642-650.

83. Evensen KA, Steinshamn S, Tjønna AE, et al. Effects of preterm birth and fetal growth retardation on cardiovascular risk factors in young adulthood. *Early Hum Dev*. 2009;85:239-245.

Chapter 16

Perinatal Nutrition and the Lung

Cindy T. McEvoy and Cristina T. Navarrete

Chapter Outline

Introduction

Prenatal Nutrition and Lung Development

  Lung Development

Nutritional Interventions for Primary Prevention of Preterm Birth

Maternal Undernutrition

Maternal Over Nutrition

Maternal Intake of Micronutrients

  Vitamin C Supplementation to Pregnant Women Unable to Quit Smoking

  Vitamin D Supplementation

  Vitamin A Supplementation

  Vitamin E Supplementation

  Maternal Vitamin C and E Supplementation

Postnatal Nutrition and Respiratory Outcomes

Preterm Infant Nutrition

Undernutrition, Growth Failure & Pulmonary Consequences

Effect of Undernutrition on Lung Growth and Development

Effect of Undernutrition on Respiratory Muscle Function

Effect of Undernutrition on Lung Function

Effect of Undernutrition on the Antioxidant System

Effect of Undernutrition on Infection Susceptibility

Effect of Undernutrition on Alveolar Fluid Balance

Effect of Undernutrition on Control of Breathing

Effect of Undernutrition on Pulmonary Vascular Bed

Adequate Nutrition to Support Lung Growth and Function

  Macronutrients

  Micronutrients

  Trace Elements

  Other Nutrients

  Human Milk

Conclusion

Key Points

- Lung development is influenced by both prenatal and postnatal nutrient quality and quantity.
- The wide spectrum of maternal and preterm infant nutritional states has differing impacts on the trajectory of fetal-infant lung development.
- Specific nutrient supplements given during gestation or postnatally have been shown to affect pulmonary outcomes.

Introduction

The causes of altered fetal and neonatal lung development are numerous, but prematurity, which affects 10% to 12% of all infants born in the United States, is among the most important.[1] Since birth cohort studies have demonstrated that an individual (for the most part) follows a pulmonary function percentile established very early on in life,[2,3] optimizing maternal/perinatal nutrition and postnatal nutrition, especially to preterm infants, is critical to lifelong childhood respiratory health. As aptly stated by Dr. David Barker: "How do we build stronger people? By improving the nutrition of babies in the womb."[4] So simple but so profound with regard to the development of many organ systems, particularly the lung.

This chapter will present data from animal models and available clinical data of prenatal and early postnatal nutrition and potential interventions to optimize fetal and neonatal lung development, particularly in the context of preterm delivery. Optimal maternal nutrition is essential for adequate fetal nutrition to promote normal fetal lung development. This is comprised of maternal body mass index (BMI), weight gain during pregnancy, both macro- and micronutrient intakes, and adequate placental function to deliver the nutrients from the maternal circulation to the fetus. The interruption of gestation by preterm birth disrupts the maternal-fetal nutrient transfer and process of fuel store accumulation that prepares for birth and extrauterine life. The preterm infant will now depend on clinicians to provide the delicate balance of macro- and micronutrients needed for postnatal metabolic needs in addition to the demands of growth and development, while surmounting the metabolic limitations of immaturity.

Prenatal Nutrition and Lung Development

LUNG DEVELOPMENT

The development of human lung architecture starts in utero and continues through adolescence and early adulthood with the most substantial developments occurring during fetal life and the first year after birth. The airways form during early fetal life and are completed by 16 to 20 weeks of gestational age, while alveolar development begins around 20 weeks of gestational age and is largely completed by 3 years of age.[2] The outcome of altered lung development depends on the developmental stage when the insult occurs during fetal and early postnatal life, as well as its severity and duration.[2]

Nutritional Interventions for Primary Prevention of Preterm Birth

Since preterm birth is the most common cause of altered lung development,[1] preventing preterm birth (PTB) is a logical strategy to optimize lung development. A number of trials in unselected populations have evaluated diet, often in combination with increased physical activity. These studies have not consistently demonstrated a decrease in PTB.[5] A 2018 Cochrane review of randomized controlled trials (RCTs) of omega-3 long-chain polyunsaturated fatty acids (LCPUFAs), which are commonly found in fish, found an overall 11% reduction in preterm birth <37 weeks gestation and a 42% reduction in preterm birth <34 weeks. In low-risk pregnancies, it demonstrated a risk ratio of 0.31 (0.12, 0.79) in preterm births at <34 weeks.[6]

Maternal Undernutrition

Poor maternal nutrition/undernutrition/malnutrition is one of many potential causes of intrauterine growth restriction (IUGR) and/or small for gestational age (SGA), which is a common and important antecedent of altered fetal lung development.[2,7] IUGR is also a risk factor for reduced lung function and respiratory morbidity during infancy, childhood, and adulthood, and increases the odds of the development of bronchopulmonary dysplasia (BPD) in an infant delivered preterm.[8] Clinical trials to examine treatment versus nontreatment are obviously unethical, but the long-term effect of poor nutrition during pregnancy is demonstrated by the increased prevalence of chronic obstructive pulmonary disease (COPD) in those born to mothers exposed to the Dutch famine in 1944 to 1945 when caloric intake decreased to less than 800 kcal/day,[9] therefore supporting the concept that maternal nutrition should be optimized to ensure normal lung development.

In particular, IUGR in the first and second trimester has been associated with reduced vitamin E and abnormal lung function at 5 years of age and increased asthma risk.[10] Models of fetal growth restriction in animals, induced by calorie or protein restriction, have been associated with decreased lung weight and total DNA content, decreased maturation of type II cells and subsequent surfactant maturation, decreased alveoli numbers, and thickened airway walls.[11] Peroxisome proliferator-activated receptor gamma (PPARg) is a nuclear receptor transcription factor that is decreased in animal models of IUGR and is thought to contribute to lung development through its involvement in epithelial-mesenchymal interactions. Maternal supplementation with docosahexaenoic acid (DHA) in a rat model of IUGR increased PPARg levels and restored aberrant fetal lung development.[12] In a rat model of IUGR due to a low-calorie maternal diet, vitamin A supplementation reversed alveolar hypoplasia.[13] Maternal undernutrition is also often associated with other macro- and micronutrient deficits with potential ramifications as outlined in the following.

Maternal Over Nutrition

The worldwide incidence of obesity is projected to grow to 70% by 2025, so more women are entering pregnancy either overweight or obese, which exposes the fetus to an obesogenic intrauterine environment that impacts fetal lung development.[14] Overall, there is an increased risk of preterm delivery and adverse respiratory outcomes with obese pregnancies. There are many factors in the obese pregnancy that can affect fetal lung development.[14] Obese pregnancies lead to increased oxidative stress, which has implications for DNA, protein, and lipids in the maternal-placental-fetal unit.[15] Maternal obesity in pregnancy can change the maternal hypothalamic-pituitary-adrenal axis and lead to increased fetal cortisol exposure which may impair fetal lung growth.[16] Increased maternal cytokine production may also impact lung development.[17,18] The timing of weight gain during pregnancy may also be important for lung development outcomes. Several rat models of maternal high-fat diets have demonstrated increased airway hyperreactivity in the offspring[19] and human studies have associated pre-pregnancy maternal BMI with increased bronchodilator and steroid dispensing in early childhood, implying altered lung development.[20] The ideal time for intervention for maternal obesity is prior to pregnancy given concern for the growing fetus; however, intergenerational effects of fetal programing may still persist.

Maternal Intake of Micronutrients

Maternal micronutrients play a role in fetal lung development, protect against oxidant damage, are proangiogenic factors, and can modulate the inflammatory response that may impact lung development. Several micronutrients are outlined with regard to adverse in utero conditions in the following.

VITAMIN C SUPPLEMENTATION TO PREGNANT WOMEN UNABLE TO QUIT SMOKING

Fetal lung development is very sensitive to the effects of in utero smoke, and primarily to nicotine, the major toxin in cigarettes and electronic cigarettes. Smoking during pregnancy is the largest preventable cause of low birth weight, prematurity, and IUGR, all of which affect fetal lung development.[21,22] In addition, in a prospective study of preterm infants, smoking during pregnancy was shown to double the risk of developing BPD in preterm infants with a birth weight of 500 to 1250 g.[8] The incidence of smoking during pregnancy varies widely across the United States with at least 10% of pregnant women continuing to smoke,[23,24] and > 50% of smokers who become pregnant continue to smoke.[25,26] Smoking cessation during pregnancy remains the foremost goal, but a difficult intervention to improve fetal lung development.

Two separate randomized double-blind placebo-controlled trials (RCTs)[27-29] have shown that supplemental vitamin C (500 mg/day) to women unable to quit smoking during pregnancy significantly improves their offspring's pulmonary function tests (PFTs). In the first study, singleton pregnancies were randomized at <22 weeks of gestation. These offspring had significantly improved PFTs performed within 72 hours of birth with decreased airflow obstruction and increased passive respiratory compliance, and a 48% decrease in the incidence of wheeze through 12 months of age.[27] The second RCT demonstrated improved forced expiratory flows at 3 and 12 months of age in the offspring of pregnant smokers randomized to supplemental vitamin C (Fig. 16.1).[28,29] These results support the premise that in utero vitamin C supplementation to pregnant smokers improves fetal lung development and is associated with a persistent increase in pulmonary function early in life. These cohorts are in continued follow-up. Vitamin C may be an inexpensive and simple strategy in addition to smoking cessation efforts to decrease the effects of maternal smoking on infant lung function.

VITAMIN D SUPPLEMENTATION

The potential benefit of antenatal vitamin D supplementation on fetal lung growth and lung function has been demonstrated in animals and epidemiologic studies, but the long-term benefit from clinical trials is less clear. Lung maturation and airway smooth muscle differentiation have both been linked to paracrine effects of vitamin D and its metabolites, and vitamin D is known to play a role in alveolar growth in the embryo and fetus.[30] The functional and structural

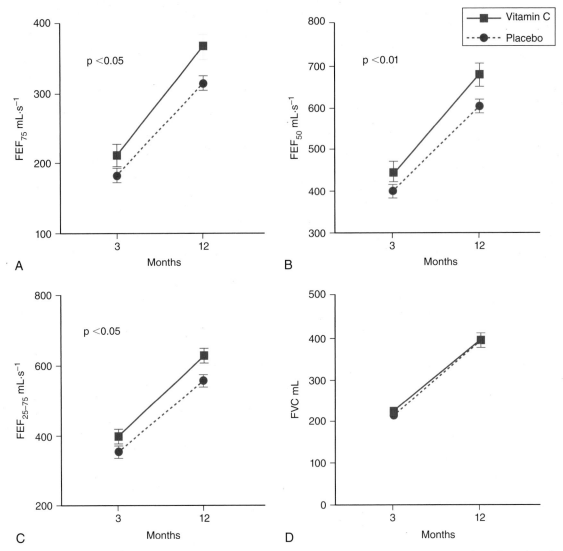

Fig. 16.1 Effect of vitamin C supplementation during pregnancy on infant airway function tests at 3 and 12 months of age. Plots of unadjusted means (expressed as mean ± SEM) for (A) forced expiratory flow at 75% of the expired volume (FEF75), (B) FEF at 50% of the expired volume (FEF50), (C) FEF at between 25% and 75% of the expired volume (FEF25–75), and (D) forced vital capacity *(FVC)*. FEF75, FEF50, and FEF25–75 were significantly improved in the vitamin C versus placebo group through 12 months of age by repeated measures analysis of covariance. There were no significant interactions for treatment group by study visit (3- and 12 months), suggesting effectively parallel differences between the treatment groups. (Reproduced with permission of the © ERS 2023. *Eur Respir J.* 2020;56(6):1902208. doi:10.1183/13993003.02208-2019.)

lung consequences of perinatal vitamin D deficiency have been effectively treated with vitamin D supplementation in animal models with improved alveolarization and decreased airway resistance.[31,32] Human epidemiological data have associated high dietary vitamin D intake during pregnancy with reduced risk of asthma/recurrent wheeze in the offspring, indicating a role of vitamin D during in utero lung and airway development.[33]

The Vitamin D Antenatal Asthma Reduction Trial (VDAART) randomized pregnant nonsmoking women with a history of asthma to daily 4000 IU vitamin D3 versus placebo. The women supplemented with vitamin D3 had significantly increased vitamin D levels and their offspring had a 6.1% lower incidence of asthma and recurrent wheeze at 3 years of age, but this was not statistically different between groups.[34] A combined analysis of VDAART with a second trial randomizing pregnant women to vitamin D3 versus placebo demonstrated a significant 26% reduced risk of asthma in the vitamin D versus control group: OR = 0.74 (95% CI 0.57–0.96), $P = 0.02$.[35] There was no effect of prenatal vitamin D on asthma at 6 years of age in the VDAART cohort, suggesting that postnatal vitamin D supplementation for continued improved respiratory outcomes may also be needed.[36]

VITAMIN A SUPPLEMENTATION

Vitamin A plays a key role in fetal lung development and is associated with hypoplastic lungs in a vitamin A–depleted rat model. In a double-blind RCT, maternal supplementation with vitamin A before, during, and after pregnancy in a malnourished population in Nepal was shown to significantly improve the spirometry measurements of the offspring at 9 to 13 years of age.[37]

VITAMIN E SUPPLEMENTATION

Vitamin E is thought to promote lung growth and airway modeling by increasing fetal antioxidant defenses. In a murine model of lung hypoplasia, vitamin E supplementation significantly increased lung weights, total DNA, and protein content.[38] A longitudinal cohort study demonstrated that maternal plasma alpha-tocopherol level during pregnancy was associated with improved fetal growth and with reduced reported respiratory symptoms at 5 years of age.[10]

MATERNAL VITAMIN C AND E SUPPLEMENTATION

Preeclampsia alters placental function and is associated with IUGR, preterm delivery, and is an independent factor for BPD aside from prematurity.[8] Altered placental function has been show to disrupt angiogenic signaling during early development with decreased proangiogenic factors, increased antiangiogenic factors, and decreased endothelial progenitor cells.[39] Therefore decreasing preeclampsia rate would improve fetal lung development on multiple levels. A multicenter RCT of vitamin C 1000 mg and vitamin E 400 IU/day versus placebo did not show a difference in preeclampsia, but a secondary analysis demonstrated vitamin C and E significantly decreased placental abruptions and decreased preterm births in pregnant smokers (RR 0.76; 95% CI 0.58, 0.99).[40]

Postnatal Nutrition and Respiratory Outcomes

The process of providing nutrients to maintain homeostasis in a premature infant, allowing similar in utero growth rates and body composition to continue, is complicated and not easily achieved in the clinical setting. Hurdles such as the lack of adequate and rapidly metabolizable energy stores, immaturity of the infant's metabolic capabilities, inability to immediately and fully utilize the gastrointestinal tract, lack of access to substantial amounts of mother's own milk (MOM), dependence on parenteral nutrition, and varying degrees of clinical illness make the provision of adequate nutrition challenging.[41]

Suboptimal nutrient delivery compromises the function of all organ systems and affects growth negatively. The respiratory system is no exception. Undernutrition has detrimental effects on lung growth and function, and its presence may be a further disadvantage to the already metabolically compromised premature infant. Preterm infant respiratory conditions, such as BPD, may be ameliorated by the provision of enough nutrients to support the process of ventilation, lung growth and repair, antioxidant defenses, and ability to ward off infections. The improved survival and extension of neonatal care to extremely low gestational age newborns, during the period when the most rapid phase of growth occurs, often creates a definition-challenged, common morbidity called extrauterine growth restriction (EUGR) or postnatal growth failure.[42,43] Progressively more preterm infants are being discharged from the neonatal intensive care unit with anthropometric measures that have crossed down growth chart percentiles or have low weight gain velocities,[42] and increasingly relationships between nutrition, early growth patterns, various morbidities, and longevity are being defined.

Pulmonary morbidity in the form of BPD is another major complication in the preterm infant population. While the epidemiology and degree of severity of this condition has changed over the years,[44] the incidence remains similar due to the increasing numbers of preterm births.[45] Among very low-birth-weight (VLBW, <1500 g) infants who are at greatest risk for this disease, the incidence of BPD ranges between 18% and 73% with a wide variability due to differing definitions of diagnostic criteria and diverse postnatal management styles.[46]

It is assumed that the growth and development of the respiratory system is largely programmed in utero and is interrupted by PTB. While there are multiple postnatal factors that influence lung growth and alveolar development,[47] some of these factors (e.g., adequate nutritional intake) are conveniently under the control of the medical professional. The following is a discussion of different nutritional approaches that may, in a positive or negative manner, influence respiratory outcomes.

Preterm Infant Nutrition

The target of human gestation is to produce a viable infant at birth. This objective is supported by the highly regulated active and facilitated transfer of nutrients from the mother through the placenta to the fetus for promotion of programmed growth and development. Because the rates of fetal nutrient transfer and consequent fetal growth for normal pregnancies are regarded as ideal, the current goal for optimal postnatal nutrition is the provision of nutrients to approximate the rate of growth and composition of weight gain for a normal fetus of the same postmenstrual age.[48] However, it is known that fetal nutrient transfer is not easily duplicated ex utero[49] and that metabolic demands are very different after birth. Thus, some experts believe that the standard of aiming for intrauterine growth rates may not be appropriate.[50] Fetal nutrient accretion is divided mostly between the energy costs of basal metabolism and growth of the fetus, but after birth, the infant has to allocate both exogenous nutrient supply and endogenous nutrient reserves for energy. Energy supplies in the newborn infant need to cover not just the higher basal metabolic needs but also the physical activity, thermogenesis, excretory losses, and, if present, the stress of illness (e.g., respiratory failure, sepsis). With the interruption of placental nutrient supply at birth, the premature infant is further disadvantaged by having limited endogenous energy reserves that are normally accumulated during the final trimester of gestation. From the seminal chemical analysis of fetuses by Widdowson, it is extrapolated that while a full-term infant has approximately 15% of the body weight represented by fat and about 2% as glycogen reserves, a 24-week preterm infant has only 1.7% fat by weight and an unmeasurable glycogen reserve.[51] Hence, this lack of energy reserve makes it vital to establish immediate postnatal nutritional intake or risk the onset of "metabolic" shock and recalcitrant nutrient deficits.[49] Hay and Thureen aptly declare that "the nutritional requirements of the preterm infant do not end with birth."[52] However, due to the perceived illness severity of these infants, nutritional needs are not always the highest priority of clinicians.[43,50]

Recommendations for preterm infant nutrition continue to evolve as perinatal care extends to lower gestational ages. In 1985, the American Academy of Pediatrics Committee on Nutrition produced recommendations for low birth weight (LBW, <2500 g) infant nutrition,[53] which was modified in 1999 by an NICHD workshop to extend the recommendations to the nutritional needs of the extremely low birth weight (ELBW, <1000 g) infant.[54] Because most of these recommendations are based on "healthy" preterm infants and designed to provide nutrients during the stable growing period, there is no clear recommendation on the nutritional support of the more immature, clinically unstable preterm infant. Until recently, these infants at birth were kept predominantly without enteral intake and started with an intravenous supply of plain dextrose in water or fluids containing very small amounts of dextrose, protein, and lipids that were gradually increased over the first week of life. The proportion of each macronutrient delivered is in contrast to normal fetal nutrient delivery (high glucose and lipid, and low amino acid).[52] Different investigators have suggested that the current nutritional recommendations and practices inevitably produce negative energy and protein balance and poor postnatal growth.[49,50] However, other researchers have reported that merely ensuring the adequate provision of early nutrition to VLBW infants would prevent early nutrient deficits and would consequently improve postnatal growth.[55] The mindful attention to early and "aggressive" (above current recommendations) nutritional strategies is increasingly becoming a top priority.[56]

Undernutrition, Growth Failure, and Pulmonary Consequences

EUGR has been widely defined as growth values less than or equal to the 10th percentile of intrauterine growth expectation based on estimated postmenstrual age in premature infants at the time of hospital discharge. Lately, this static definition has been challenged to focus more on the dynamic low growth trajectories or z-score deviations rather than an arbitrary time point that may place SGA or intrauterine growth–restricted infants at a disadvantage.[42] Despite semantic challenges, the incidence of postnatal growth failure in VLBW infants ranges between 43% and 97%,[42,45] with a wide variability due to the use of different reference growth charts and nonstandard nutritional strategies. Growth failure in VLBW infants results from the complex interaction of many factors, including morbidities affecting nutrient requirements, endocrine abnormalities, central nervous system damage, difficulties in suck and swallow coordination, and administration of drugs that affect nutrient metabolism.[57] However, inadequate nutrition (45%), especially during the first weeks of life, is largely responsible.[49] The consequences of EUGR are not fully known, in large part because it is difficult to separate the effects of the many other concurrent problems of prematurity (e.g., necrotizing enterocolitis, BPD, intraventricular hemorrhage [IVH]).

Malnutrition (or undernutrition), as defined by the World Health Organization, is the cellular imbalance between supply of nutrients and energy and the body's demand to ensure growth, maintenance, and specific functions. Malnutrition can be a consequence of inadequate or excessive nutrient quantity and/or quality. In the premature infant population, analysis of growth velocities during the initial NICU hospitalization of VLBW infants shows that after controlling for possible confounders (such as SGA, BPD, IVH, sepsis, and postnatal steroid exposure), poor rates of weight gain (presumably from suboptimal nutrition) exert a significant and independent effect on neurodevelopmental outcomes at 18 to 22 months corrected age.[50,58] The effects of malnutrition, however, are not limited to the brain. It can affect the entire body and its consequences on the respiratory system are substantial. In the developing VLBW infant, there are numerous potential pulmonary effects of undernutrition.

EFFECT OF UNDERNUTRITION ON LUNG GROWTH AND DEVELOPMENT

Growth, particularly weight gain, is traditionally the preferred means of assessing adequacy of nutritional support. To match intrauterine growth, a postnatal weight gain of 15 to 20 g/kg/day is conventionally accepted for the premature infant. The ultimate goal of adequate preterm infant weight gain is the body composition of a healthy term infant with proper distribution of lean body mass and fat mass. Growth of this metabolically active body mass (lean body mass component) needs an appropriate lung surface area to meet its needs for gas exchange. In humans, this is accomplished by increasing lung surface area, initially in terms of an increase in number of alveoli until early childhood[59] and later by an increase in alveolar size/dimension.

Different fetal and postnatal animal models of undernutrition consistently affect both somatic and lung growth.[60] Undernutrition in fetal sheep[61] and in mature and immature mice,[62,63] rats,[63] and rabbits[64] and starvation in adult humans[65] cause alveolar loss or enlargement, also called "nutritional" emphysema. This presentation of "nutritional" emphysema has similarities to the alveolar simplification seen in BPD. Slow postnatal growth rates in preterm sheep also result in reduced alveolar numbers and reduced surface area for gas exchange in relation to lung or body weight and this persists into maturity.[66] In preterm humans, the presence of IUGR independently increases the risk for BPD,[67] with VLBW infants growing at the lowest quartiles developing BPD and pulmonary hypertension (PH) more often than infants growing at the highest growth quartile.[58] Since EUGR may be analogous to intrauterine or fetal growth restriction, it is conceivable that EUGR per se may also increase the risk for BPD. Although the pathogenesis of BPD is multifactorial, it is plausible that inadequate energy secondary to undernutrition can limit the occurrence of biochemical and molecular events necessary for vital lung cell signaling, cell multiplication, differentiation and growth, and extracellular matrix structural protein deposition.

This may possibly explain the occurrence of BPD in some preterm infants who were minimally exposed to BPD-promoting factors like oxygen, mechanical ventilation, or infection/inflammation.[68]

As an alternative to the hypothesis that undernourishment leads to the development of an emphysema-like condition, the lung's response to caloric restriction could reflect an evolutionarily conserved adaptation to diminished oxygen consumption during food scarcity.[63,65] Whereas established BPD is frequently associated with poor somatic growth,[69] this poor growth may be merely a marker of disease severity, since infants that ultimately develop BPD are sicker and likely more undernourished.[50] Conversely, poor growth could be secondary to BPD per se, producing higher metabolic needs from increased work of breathing[70] and from episodes of hypoxemia that may be growth limiting.[71] If lung growth and surface area are limited, then the provision of adequate levels of oxygen systemically may be diminished, perpetuating the limitation of growth even further.

EFFECT OF UNDERNUTRITION ON RESPIRATORY MUSCLE FUNCTION

The energy source of muscle is either glycogen or fatty acids (FAs), from intrinsic stores or from circulating fuels like glucose and free FAs which are broken down to produce adenosine triphosphate (ATP). The diaphragm is the major muscle of respiration, utilizing 10% of basal metabolic rate in "healthy" preterm infants.[72] When energy supply is limited, muscle contractility may be compromised and lead to ineffective activity or, in the case of the diaphragm muscle, respiratory failure. In undernourished adult patients without lung disease, respiratory muscle strength, maximum voluntary ventilation, and vital capacity are reduced.[73] Undernutrition causes a decrease in diaphragm strength and endurance partially related to a loss of muscle mass.[73,74] In addition, two studies in rats found that undernutrition induces a significant decrease in mitochondrial oxygen consumption[75] and that a reduction in muscle insulin-like growth factor 1 (IGF-1) expression is associated with diaphragm muscle fiber atrophy.[76] Branched-chain amino acids (BCAAs) have been shown to improve diaphragm function in vitro, and when parenteral protein

solutions were enriched with BCAA, apnea events in preterm infants were decreased.[77]

Mechanical ventilation has been the basis of the respiratory care of the premature infant and prolonged dependence is associated with disuse atrophy of the diaphragm. In recent years, however, allowing infants to breathe spontaneously with minimal, noninvasive support in the form of continuous positive airway pressure (CPAP) has evolved as the preferred mode in select preterm infants (e.g., with good ventilatory drive).[44,45] CPAP alters the shape of the diaphragm and decreases its activity.[78] Hence, the provision of adequate energy substrate to sustain diaphragm and other respiratory muscle function may be more important than ever.

EFFECT OF UNDERNUTRITION ON LUNG FUNCTION

The extracellular matrix of the lung, composed mainly of collagen and elastin fibers, provides the template for normal parenchymal cell architecture on which efficient gas exchange depends. In addition, the organization and amount of this extracellular matrix influences the mechanical behavior of the lung parenchyma (tensile strength and lung elasticity) during the respiratory cycle. During lung growth, deposition of newly created connective tissue in this scaffold is essential. The preservation of this intricate connective tissue scaffold depends on the lung's capacity to prevent enzymatic disruption of the component matrix proteins. Specifically, the integrity of the normal connective tissue skeleton of the lung is determined by the maintenance of a balance between proteases (released by inflammatory cells) capable of cleaving these structural elements (e.g., matrix metalloproteinases) and specific protease inhibitors (e.g., tissue inhibitors of metalloproteinases).[79] The breakdown of connective tissue fibers leads to emphysema, and these same connective tissue fibers are affected by undernutrition. In a young rat starvation model, hydroxyproline (a collagen biomarker) and elastin levels in the lung are reduced with associated loss of tissue elastic forces, evident in pressure-volume curves.[74,80]

In addition to the connective tissue skeleton that contributes to lung function, surfactant is another very important contributor. Surfactant decreases surface tension at the air-liquid interface in the alveoli, provides lung stability (promotes expansion at inspiration and prevents collapse at expiration), and reduces the risk of infection. It contains about 80% phospholipids, 8% neutral lipids, and 12% protein.[81] The principal classes of phospholipids are saturated and unsaturated phosphatidylcholine compounds, phosphatidylglycerol, and phosphatidylinositol. FA moieties of the phospholipids may be derived from circulating long-chain free FAs or from de novo synthesis from glucose.[82] Different experimental animal models of undernutrition show reduced numbers of lamellar bodies, multilamellated structures, and lipid vacuoles in type II pneumocytes[74] and decreased dipalmitoylphosphatidylcholine content of lung lavage fluid[83] and lung phospholipid pool.[84] Despite the reduction in surfactant components, changes in lung mechanics were insignificant.

The rigid thoracic cage contains the lungs and together with the respiratory muscles generates the negative pressure and elastic recoil necessary for ventilation. Inadequate ossification of the bony skeleton, including the thoracic cage, is frequent after preterm birth. An easily distorted and compliant chest wall in combination with a poorly compliant lung parenchyma in association with significant lung disease sets the infant up for inefficient ventilation.[85] Normal bone calcium deposition and consequent improved rigidity is frequently impaired with the onset of metabolic bone disease (MBD) of prematurity. MBD is a frequent complication of preterm birth secondary to inadequate accretion and then inadequate provision of calcium and phosphorus in postnatal nutrition along with exposure to calcium-wasting medications like furosemide and glucocorticoids, which are commonly used in infants with BPD.[86,87] Complicating rib fractures in advanced disease makes breathing efforts even more inefficient,[88] increasing the risk for respiratory failure and prolonged ventilator dependence.

EFFECT OF UNDERNUTRITION ON THE ANTIOXIDANT SYSTEM

The balance between the production of reactive oxygen species (ROS) and the antioxidant defense system is important for homeostasis. Developmentally, the increase of various antioxidant enzymes and antioxidants (e.g., Cu-Zn-superoxide dismutase [SOD], Mn-SOD, and vitamins E and C) occurs late in gestation to prepare the infant for birth and exposure to the oxygen-rich environment ex utero.[89] The underdevelopment of both enzymatic and nonenzymatic (from interrupted maternal transfer) antioxidant defense systems in preterm infants tips the balance toward increased ROS-producing oxidant stress that is aggravated further by frequent exposure to ROS-generating conditions such as hyperoxia and inflammation.

The provision of supplemental oxygen continues to be an integral part of neonatal care although its use has become more judicious because of its association with oxygen toxicity and morbidities such as retinopathy of prematurity (ROP) and BPD.[44] BPD is considered among the oxygen radical diseases of the newborn. Lungs of infants with respiratory disorders have reduced staining for CuZnSOD.[89] High concentrations of oxygen induce lung inflammation, which may lead to chronic fibrotic and destructive changes, as the production of ROS and release of chemotactic factors lead to release of inflammatory mediators and proteolytic enzymes. In adult animal models of hyperoxia, fasting increased susceptibility to hyperoxic injury. Fasted mice had decreased lung concentrations of the tripeptide antioxidant glutathione,[90] of which cysteine, glutamate, and glycine are precursors. In newborn rat pups, the presence of undernutrition during hyperoxic exposure had an additive detrimental effect on somatic and lung growth and lethality (56% of the undernourished pups died in O_2 compared with 27% of the normally nourished pups).[60] Although elevations in antioxidant enzyme values were demonstrated in this study, it is speculated that protection from O_2-free radical toxicity is a complex phenomenon and that other vital factors (in addition to the endogenous antioxidant enzyme systems) are required to provide optimal protection against the detrimental effects of prolonged O_2 treatment.

EFFECT OF UNDERNUTRITION ON INFECTION SUSCEPTIBILITY

Undernutrition is known to alter pulmonary defense mechanisms, compromising epithelial cell integrity and clearance mechanisms, allowing easier access by pathogens, and jeopardizing cellular and humoral immune function. These changes lead to decreased ability of the host to eliminate pathogens and a predisposition to infections. Globally, undernourished children frequently succumb to repeated upper[91] and lower[92] respiratory tract infections. Animal models of malnutrition have also demonstrated decreased alveolar macrophage count,[93] phagocytosis, and microbial killing.[94] Newborn rats deprived of adequate protein antenatally were found to develop reduced alveolar macrophage function, which could be reversed by postnatal protein supplementation.[95]

Individual components of surfactant, specifically surfactant proteins A and D, have important roles in the innate immune response and in defense against microbes.[96] As already mentioned, undernutrition has an effect on surfactant, although whether it has any specific impact on surfactant proteins (or immunity) is unknown.

EFFECT OF UNDERNUTRITION ON ALVEOLAR FLUID BALANCE

Pulmonary edema is due to the movement of excess fluid into the interstitial space and alveoli as a result of the alteration in one or more of Starling's forces, either a change in hydrostatic or oncotic pressure gradients or in membrane permeability. In experimental animal models of hyperoxic or hypoxic exposure, anorexia, weight loss, and lung injury characterized by pulmonary edema and decreased lung water clearance developed.[97,98] The edema was partially or fully reversed by the provision of continuous enteral feeding,[97] refeeding, or treatment with the amino acid, glutamate.[99]

EFFECT OF UNDERNUTRITION ON CONTROL OF BREATHING

The incidence of sudden infant death syndrome is increased in individuals with evidence of IUGR[100]; however, there is little information on the postnatal effects of growth restriction or undernutrition on the control of breathing. In growth-restricted lambs, the ventilatory response to progressive hypoxia was related to birthweight, whereas the response to hypercapnia was not.[101] Respiratory center output was not modified by short-term intravenous supplementation of BCAAs.[102]

EFFECT OF UNDERNUTRITION ON PULMONARY VASCULAR BED

PH is a common comorbidity in infants with BPD and is associated with increased BPD severity.[103] Although difficult to associate with undernutrition clinically, rodent malnutrition models have shown that undernutrition causes different signs of PH such as right ventricular hypertrophy, decreased numbers of pulmonary arterioles, increased medial wall thickness of pulmonary arterioles, and increased ratio of pulmonary artery acceleration time to ejection time.[104] In addition, there is an emerging theory of a gut-lung axis, where malnutrition and its common association with intestinal dysbiosis or altered intestinal microbiota influence lung disease. When probiotics were administered to the same rodent malnutrition model earlier, PH was attenuated.[105]

Adequate Nutrition to Support Lung Growth and Function

The following paragraphs offer a brief description of the importance of each nutritional component on lung growth, pulmonary physiology, and pathophysiology (Table 16.1).

Energy: Energy is required for body function and growth and is obtained from food sources. In a preterm infant with negligible energy stores (as described earlier), energy is gained from nutritional intake, expended as needed, and then stored, if in excess. Energy expenditure is negatively related to gestational age and is positively related to energy intake, weight gain, and postnatal age.[106-108] Expert committees estimate that a daily energy intake of approximately 120 to 130 kcal/kg is sufficient to meet the metabolic demands of a healthy premature infant and to allow for growth rates comparable to intrauterine growth rates.[106] A review of nutritional intakes in a preterm infant cohort showed that for every 1-kcal/day increase in total energy intake, there was a 0.34-g/day increase in weight, a 0.003-cm/day increase in length, and a 0.002-cm/day increase in head circumference.[109]

It is unknown if these estimates of energy intake are also applicable to sick and unstable preterm infants. Whether energy expenditure changes during respiratory illness is unclear. Severity of illness was not found to correlate to energy expenditure in studies of some ventilated preterm infants,[107,108] but increased metabolic rates were observed in others.[110] No measures are available in nonventilator–dependent infants with respiratory distress, so the advantage of adjusting energy intake for increased respiratory distress is undefined. Because infants with established BPD have higher energy expenditure and poorer rates of weight gain,[69] energy intake targets are commonly raised. What is clear is that the process of respiration requires energy and deficient energy intakes impinge on respiration and may cause respiratory failure. Conversely, excessive intake may be counterproductive by increasing fat stores and energy expenditure for lipogenesis.

Water and fluid volume: Water is essential for life because it carries nutrients to cells, removes waste products, and makes up the physiochemical milieu that allows cellular work to occur.[111] Growth requires water intake into new tissues or cells. The ideal weight gain of 15 to 20 g/kg/day (new tissue generation) is comprised of 65% to 80% water mass (10–12 mL/kg/day).[111] Water is the major compound of enteral and parenteral nutrition. Daily recommended intakes vary according to gestational age, postnatal age, and fluid balance. Intakes are conventionally limited during the first few days of life when normal fluid shifts and weight loss occur. A large retrospective analysis showed that higher fluid intake and less weight loss during the first 10 days of life were associated with an increased risk of BPD.[112]

There is an association between the presence of a patent ductus arteriosus (PDA) and an increased risk for BPD. The acute pulmonary effects of a PDA include pulmonary edema (and occasionally hemorrhage), worsened lung mechanics, and deterioration in gas exchange with hypoxemia and hypercapnia.[113] Also, the greater pulmonary blood flow can trigger an inflammatory cascade that promotes BPD. One meta-analysis found that fluid restriction significantly reduced the risk of PDA and showed a trend towards reducing BPD risk.[114] Therefore, common clinical practice is to limit fluid intake when a PDA is suspected or when BPD is established. An unwanted consequence of limiting fluid intake is inadvertent delivery of insufficient calories because of inadequate caloric intake from unadjusted dilutions (continued provision of dilute or minimally concentrated fluids).

MACRONUTRIENTS

Macronutrients are the classes of chemical compounds that represent the largest quantities in the diet and which provide bulk energy. Carbohydrate and fat provide the energy needed to meet the demands of all organ systems, including the cardiorespiratory system.

When provided in adequate amounts, they spare proteins to support cell maturation, remodeling, growth, activity of enzymes, and transport proteins for all body organs.

Carbohydrates: Glucose, the primary circulating form of carbohydrate, is the major source of energy. It is the final pathway for the metabolism and oxidation of all carbohydrates and is an important carbon source for de novo synthesis of amino acids and FAs. The rates of endogenous hepatic glucose production are 8 to 9 mg/kg/min and 5 mg/kg/min in preterm and term infants, respectively.[115] These rates are considered to be sufficient to meet most of the energy requirements of the brain only. Consequently, those are the lower limit of glucose intakes that are aimed for initially. Levels required for energy needs plus growth may be as high as 12 to 13 mg/kg/min.

Oxidation of carbohydrates results in a higher rate of carbon dioxide production for the same amount of oxygen consumed (respiratory quotient [RQ] 1.0) when compared with fat (RQ 0.7) and protein (RQ 0.8).[116] Hence, administration of high-glucose loads should be made cautiously in conditions where there is difficulty in carbon dioxide elimination (e.g., respiratory failure, BPD). Also, high or excessive carbohydrate intake above the amount that can be oxidized for energy and stored as glycogen leads only to increased lipogenesis,[117] a process with inherent increased carbon dioxide production (RQ 5–8), altered fat deposition,[118] and obesity. Efforts should be made to maintain proper ratios of nonprotein energy to protein energy (20 to 40 nonprotein kcal for every gram of amino acid) to avoid weight gain secondary to fat mass rather than lean body mass and yet to avoid utilization of protein as an energy source and not for net protein growth, which can occur at low nonprotein caloric intakes (<60 kcal/kg/day).[119]

Fats: Lipids provide a concentrated form of energy and supply essential FAs, which are important for normal growth and development of the nervous system, retina, and immune system. Intravenous lipids commonly used in the clinical setting are composed of vegetable oil (single or a combination) and/or fish oil emulsified with egg phospholipids and glycerol. A 20% IV fat emulsion is typically started at 0.5 to 1 g fat/kg to as much as 2 g fat/kg on the first day of life, usually at the same time amino acids are started to prevent essential FA deficiency and provide a more generous source of calories. The lipid emulsion is advanced as tolerated in incremental rates of 0.5 to 1 g/kg/day to a typical maximum of 3 g/kg/day, infused over 24 hours. Excessive or rapid infusion of large doses of Intralipid has been correlated with an increase in alveolar-arteriolar diffusion gradient in adults but not in preterm infants when lipids are administered over 20 to 24 hours.[120]

LCPUFAs contained in lipid emulsions are readily incorporated in a dose-dependent manner into cell phospholipid membranes and other tissues, where they are involved in cell signaling, the production of eicosanoids involved in inflammation, blood vessel tone, platelet aggregation, and modulation of the immune system. The main LCPUFAs are the ω-6FAs (e.g., linoleic acid) and the ω-3FAs (linolenic). Mediators arising from ω-6FAs (thromboxane A2, leukotrienes B4, C4, D4, prostaglandins D2, E2, and F2, and prostacyclin I2) have a primarily proinflammatory effect, whereas those arising from ω-3FAs (thromboxane A3, leukotrienes B5, C5, D5, prostaglandinsD3, E3, and F3, and prostacyclin I3) are less potent and have reduced inflammatory activity.[121] ω-6FAs and ω-3FAs share metabolic pathways and thus interact with each other through a complex system involving substrate availability, competition for the same metabolic enzymes for synthesis, membrane incorporation, and powerful negative feedback of the end products.[122] Thus, DHA and eicosapentaenoic acid in the family of ω-3FAs interfere with arachidonic acid (ω-6FA) synthesis and downregulate associated inflammatory eicosanoids, making the ratio of ω-6FA to ω-3FA, the n6:n3 ratio, an important marker in the regulation of inflammatory mediators.[123]

Vegetable-derived oils (e.g., soybean oil in Intralipid and SMOFlipid) are rich in ω-6FA but not ω-3FA. Because of the antiinflammatory property of ω-3FAs, its potential role in different pathologies secondary to inflammation (including pulmonary disorders) is being defined.[124] In a hyperoxic lung injury model in neonatal rats, dams fed a diet rich in fat emulsion (Intralipid; high in ω-6FAs) produced newborn rats with high lung PUFA levels and marked protection against oxygen toxicity[125]; provision of fish oil (high in ω-3FAs) was shown to give the same protection.[126] Although not directly compared, the

clinicopathologic scores (combination of clinical status, histopathologic presence of lung edema, hemorrhage, and atelectasis) in the lungs were better in offspring of ω-3FA–fed mothers than in offspring of ω-6FA–fed mothers. In a different animal model, ω-3FAs resulted in decreased oxidative stress in the liver associated with lower activity of SOD and glutathione peroxidase.[127] Fish oil containing intravenous fat emulsions (e.g., Omegaven, SMOFlipid) and dietary preparations are now utilized to avoid the proinflammatory properties of ω-6FA–rich soy-based oils; however, their effect on inflammation-based neonatal pulmonary pathologies is still unknown, and the effect on prolongation of bleeding times may be a disadvantage.[128] In a retrospective cohort study, the increased use of ω-3FA–enriched fat emulsions (SMOFlipid) showed a trend of slightly higher rates of BPD, longer duration of invasive ventilation, and increased total days of pressure support and oxygen use.[129] Despite the advantage against hyperoxic damage, LCPUFAs are susceptible to lipid peroxidation and excessive intakes may reduce antioxidant capacity and enhance susceptibility to oxidative damage. Hence, newer approaches to lipid administration are leaning towards limiting lipid amounts to the minimum necessary to prevent essential FA deficiency and to provide just enough to meet caloric needs.

Proteins: Protein requirements for the neonate are inversely related to gestational age and size due to the more rapid growth rates and greater protein losses in the smaller, more premature infants.[130] The early provision of protein within the first minutes to hours after birth is critical to attainment of positive nitrogen balance and accretion, as premature babies lose ~1% of their protein stores daily.[131] Studies suggest that at least 1 g/kg/day of amino acids can decrease catabolism.[132] Current protein intake strategies include starting protein at rates appropriate for gestational age: 3.5 to 4 g/kg/day for infants <30 weeks' gestational age, 2.5 to 3.5 g/kg/day for infants 30 to 36 weeks' gestational age, and 2.5 g/kg/day for infants >36 weeks' gestational age.[130] Studies show that early and aggressive provision of protein and adequate nonprotein energy within the first few days of life is safe and effective at providing protein to meet accretion needs and facilitate intrauterine growth rates.[133] In addition, albumin synthesis is upregulated rapidly with amino acid administration immediately after birth.[134] Albumin is a key element in the regulation of plasma oncotic pressure and has antioxidant activity secondary to its ligand and free radical binding capacities.[135] Caution is necessary to avoid excessive protein intakes since this has been shown to induce metabolic stress from protein overload, impaired neurodevelopmental outcomes, and ironically growth failure.[136]

MICRONUTRIENTS

Micronutrients are substances that enable the body to produce enzymes, hormones, and other substances essential for proper metabolism of macronutrients. As tiny as the amounts are, however, the consequences of their absence are severe. Most of these micronutrients are transferred to the fetus late in gestation; thus, the preterm infant fails to receive them, and as a result, most preterm infants are born with micronutrient deficiencies. Although an adequate well-balanced nutritional intake is essential, specific manipulations of micronutrients that may be scarce in the preterm infant population may play a role in protecting them from developing BPD.

Vitamins

Vitamin A: Vitamin A is a fat-soluble micronutrient that is involved in the growth and differentiation of epithelial layers. It influences the orderly growth and differentiation of epithelial cells by regulating membrane structure and function. Retinol is the major circulating form and is among the substances transplacentally transferred late in gestation; hence preterm infants are born with low plasma retinol levels[137,138] and decreased stores in the liver and lungs.[139] In one study, infants who eventually progress to BPD were noted to have lower values of plasma retinol at birth and weeks later despite receiving the recommended intakes.[138] Initial clinical trials involving supplementation showed inconsistencies in pulmonary outcomes due to underdosage and loss by photodegradation and adherence to plastic tubing.[140] In a multicenter study reported by Tyson and colleagues,[141] retinol supplementation in ELBW ventilated infants, consisting of 5000 IU of vitamin A given intramuscularly three times per week for 4 weeks, resulted in a modest but significant decrease in oxygen requirement at 36 weeks postmenstrual age or death. For every 14 to 15 ELBW infants supplemented

in this study, 1 infant survived without chronic lung disease.[141] Current practice surveys reveal inconsistent application of vitamin A to clinical practice due to its perceived small benefit and the need for an intramuscular administration route.[142]

Vitamin D: Vitamin D is a fat-soluble vitamin with a primary function of maintaining serum calcium and phosphorus concentrations. Recent studies show it also has a role in lung maturation.[30] Furthermore, among the substances transferred late in gestation, it must be provided by dietary or parenteral supplementation because its production from sun exposure is not an option. Once enteral or parenteral supplemental vitamin D enters the circulation, it associates with vitamin D–binding protein. Depending on the preparation, hydroxylation has to occur first in the liver and then in the kidneys into the most active or hormonal form, 1,25(OH)2D. From 24 weeks of gestation, the infant is capable of enzymatic conversion to the active form of vitamin D.[30] The role of vitamin D in the multifactorial MBD of prematurity is still undefined. Animal and laboratory studies show substantial positive effects of vitamin D on the alveolar type II cell, fibroblast proliferation, surfactant synthesis, and alveolarization.[30] At birth, the newborn's serum 25(OH) D status is 50% to 70% of the maternal serum. Supplementation of the parent compound of vitamin D at 30 to 400 IU/kg/day results in substantial plasma 25(OH) D levels.[143] All infant formulas and human milk fortifiers in the United States are fortified with about 400 IU/L of vitamin D.

Vitamin E: Vitamin E (α- and γ-tocopherol) is a fat-soluble vitamin that has antioxidant properties that may reduce injury related to lipid peroxidation by scavenging free radicals. Vitamin E can be incorporated into cell membranes in proportion to the content of PUFAs, making cells more resistant to oxygen-induced injury.[144] Stored in the liver, adipose tissue, and skeletal muscles, vitamin E is integrated into lipid droplets and cell membranes at the cellular level. The limited proportion of adipose tissue in preterm infants limits total body vitamin E levels. The possibility that vitamin E may have a role in prevention of oxidation-related injury of pulmonary cell membranes has prompted clinical trials involving supplementation.[145,146] However, supplementation of vitamin E in preterm neonates does not prevent BPD.

Vitamin E plays a prominent role in respiratory and peripheral muscle function. Deficiency of vitamin E increases lipid peroxidation and glutathione oxidation in the rat diaphragm.[147] In addition, vitamin E deficiency is associated with impaired in vitro force generation of the diaphragm. Inspiratory resistive breathing (a technique for loading the respiratory muscles) induced impairment in in vitro force generation and increased oxidized glutathione levels in the diaphragm in vitamin E–deficient rats.[147] The provision of 2.8 to 3.5 IU/kg/day of vitamin E parenterally and 6 to 12 IU/kg/day enterally is recommended to maintain normal plasma levels and tissue stores.[148]

Vitamin C: Vitamin C (ascorbic acid) is a water-soluble vitamin with both antioxidant and prooxidant properties (when available in high amounts in the presence of free iron in vitro) and is essential in connective tissue formation. An RCT in VLBW infants receiving one of the three levels of ascorbic acid supplementation (low, low then high, or high) during the first 28 days of life showed no difference in pulmonary outcomes.[149] Although the difference was not statistically significant, the proportion of surviving infants with oxygen requirement at 36 weeks postmenstrual age in the high supplemented group (19%) was half that in the low supplementation group (41%).[149] Current recommended intake based on available parenteral multivitamin preparations is 32 mg/kg/day.

TRACE ELEMENTS

Important trace elements in human nutrition include zinc, copper, selenium, chromium, molybdenum, manganese, iodine, and iron. Although they quantitatively represent a small fraction of the total mineral content of the human body, they play a key role in several metabolic pathways. Preterm infants may have trace element deficiencies due to low stores at birth, even if clinical manifestations are absent, because major transfer of these substances occurs late in gestation. Very little is known about the metabolism of these trace elements in the nutrition of preterm infants and even less is known about their effect on the respiratory system.

Selenium functions partly as a component of proteins, including enzymes such as glutathione peroxidases, which play an important role in preventing free radical formation and oxygen toxicity. There are no data on fetal selenium accretion rates through direct chemical analysis of fetuses. Reduced selenium and glutathione peroxidase levels in VLBW infants were found to be associated with increased incidence of BPD.[150,151] Although a clinical trial of selenium supplementation (7 μg/kg/day parenterally or 5 μg/kg/day orally from week 1 to 36 weeks postmenstrual age or discharge home) did not improve outcomes, the investigators noted that lower maternal and neonatal prerandomization selenium levels were associated with increased respiratory morbidity.[152] Current recommendation is to provide 2 μg/kg/day. However, to maintain concentrations closer to umbilical cord blood levels, 3 μg/kg/day is suggested. To increase concentrations above umbilical cord blood levels and bring them closer to those of breastfed full-term infants, 5 to 7 μg/kg/day of selenium is recommended.[153] Manganese is a cofactor for the antioxidant enzyme mitochondrial SOD and is important in the activation of enzymes involved in synthesis of mucopolysaccharides necessary for growth and maintenance of connective tissue, cartilage, and bone.[154] Zinc is important for growth, cell differentiation, and the metabolism of proteins, carbohydrates, and lipids. It is also a cofactor, along with copper, in cytoplasmic SOD. Iron is important for brain development and erythropoiesis, although it is also a prooxidant. It has been shown that a greater cumulative dose of supplemental enteral iron exposure was associated with an increased risk of BPD (adjusted relative risk per 50-mg increase, 1.07; 95% CI, 1.02–1.11; $P = 0.002$).[155] Despite the demonstration of low levels of all trace elements, except for copper, in preterm infants receiving current suggested trace element doses in parenteral nutrition, there are no studies of the effect of giving higher doses to these preterm infants at risk for deficiencies.

OTHER NUTRIENTS

Calcium/phosphorus: Bone and rib cage formation requires protein and energy for collagen matrix synthesis, and an adequate intake of calcium and phosphorus is necessary for proper mineralization. Calcium is actively transported across the placenta to the fetus with a 1:4 maternal-to-fetal gradient so that calcium levels are higher in the fetus to meet the high demand of the developing skeleton. It has been estimated that fetal accretion in the last trimester is approximately 100 to 120 mg/kg/day for calcium and

50 to 65 mg/kg/day for phosphorus.[51,87] Interruption of placental supply of calcium at birth stimulates the release of parathyroid hormone (PTH) to maintain calcium homeostasis. PTH stimulates the reabsorption of calcium and excretion of phosphorus in the kidneys and bone reabsorption of calcium. Without any dietary intake, preterm infants are started on parenteral nutrition containing calcium in the form of inorganic salts and phosphorus as inorganic sodium or potassium phosphate. Owing to limits in solubility, the goal of parenteral calcium and phosphorus provision is to maintain normal serum levels and not to match in utero accretion rates. At best, about 60% of intrauterine mineralization is provided by 60 to 80 mg/kg/day of parenteral calcium and 58 to 60 mg/kg/day of parenteral phosphorus,[143] provided that amino acid intake is more than 2 to 2.25 g/kg/day and the volume of infusate is higher than 100 mL/kg/day. Rates closer to in utero accretion are attainable via assimilation from fortified human milk or preterm milk formula, explaining the urgency in the establishment of enteral nutrition. Current recommendations for the stable growing preterm are 100 to 160 mg/kg/day of calcium and 60 to 90 mg/kg/day of phosphorus[156] to account for the relative absorptive inefficiency of the developing gut. Preterm human milk contains 31 mg of calcium and 20 mg of phosphorus per 100 kcal; with 70% calcium and 80% phosphorus absorption, it provides about a third of in utero accretion rates.[157] Fortified preterm human milk provides 91 mg of calcium and 53 mg of phosphorus per 100 kcal, attaining about two-thirds of in utero accretion rates.

Surfactant precursors: Inositol is a six-carbon sugar present in several biologic compounds, such as in phosphatidylinositol found in surfactant and breast milk. Prior to the availability of exogenous surfactant, a trial of parenteral supplementation for preterm infants with respiratory distress showed that inositol supplementation (80 mg/kg/day of IV inositol for 5 days) was associated with longer survival and lower incidence of BPD.[158] A systematic review confirmed the same.[159] With the availability of exogenous surfactant replacement therapy, however, no subsequent randomized control trials have been conducted.

Individual amino acids: The supplementation of individual amino acids has not demonstrated positive results. Cysteine (glutathione precursor) supplementation in VLBW infants improved plasma levels but did not stimulate glutathione synthesis.[160] Supplementation using the cysteine-precursor, N-acetyl-L-cysteine, did not have any effect on the rates of death and BPD.[161,162] In fetal rat lung type II pneumocytes, glutamine is oxidized preferentially over glucose for energy metabolism.[163] Glutamine supplementation has been shown to reduce the risk of sepsis and mortality in critically ill adult surgical patients, although supplementation in VLBW infants had no effect.[164] It is unknown whether glutamine has any effect on pulmonary morbidity.

HUMAN MILK

The gold standard for complete infant nutrition provides a multitude of advantages. As far as its influence on preterm infant respiratory outcomes, a meta-analysis showed a reduction of BPD in exclusively MOM-fed infants (RR 0.74, 95% CI 0.57–0.96) but not in those who were supplemented.[165] Exclusive exposure to MOM is ideal; however, adequate maternal supply is a common limitation and the protein composition of preterm MOM declines over the first month of life. Adjustments using milk fortifiers show improvements in growth and a decrease of other preterm infant morbidities but no specific effect on pulmonary outcomes.

Human milk exposure influences the gut microbiome (premature infants are at increased risk for dysbiosis) and intestinal permeability (bacterial translocation may induce local and systemic inflammatory responses). There are increasing theories on how nutritional exposures qualitatively affect gut microbes and how this in turn influence systemic and, in particular, lung immune responses pointing to a gut-lung axis pathway origin of disease.

Conclusion

Nutrition is not only a basic need but also a therapeutic tool and a crucial aspect of prenatal and neonatal care. The lung is vulnerable to adverse exposures during fetal development. There are differing windows of susceptibility depending on the lung's developmental stage. Improved overall nutritional status of women, especially throughout gestation, is imperative to prime the development of fetuses. We are truly what we eat or in the case of the fetus, what the mother eats. Since preterm birth interrupts in utero lung development, as the lung continues to develop after birth, postnatal exposures, including nutrition, may significantly influence lung growth, especially since these exposures occur during the period of rapid alveolarization. Once the basic structure of the respiratory system has been realized during this critical phase, the development of lung function and anatomy follows a more or less fixed course and exhibits tracking well into adolescence and adulthood. As such, the lung function an individual is born with, or in the case of the preterm infant, the lung function developed through the NICU experience, will be a major determinant of lung function throughout life (Table 16.1).

TABLE 16.1	Selected Suggested Recommendations for Daily Nutrient Intakes for Preterm Infants					
	Current Recommendations[167]	Transitional Phase (2014 Recommendations)		Stable and Growing Phase (2014 Recommendations)		Comments
Source		Parenteral	Enteral	Parenteral	Enteral	
Energy (kcal/kg/d)	110–130	35–90	110–120	105–115	130–150	
Fluids (mL/kg/d)	135–200	80–140	80–140	120–150	150–200	
Carbohydrate: Glucose (mg/kg/min)		5–7 mg/kg/min initially, to progress to 10–11 mg/kg/min[52]		5–7 mg/kg/min initially, to progress to 10–11 mg/kg/min[52]		Plasma glucose target >60 and <120 mg/dL[52]
Carbohydrate (g/kg/d)	11–13	6–12	3.8–11.2	13–17	9–20	
Protein: Amino acids (g/kg/d)	3.5–4.5	3–4	3.6–3.8	3.5–4	3.8–4.4	
Fat: Lipids (g/kg/d)	4.55–8.1	0.5–1 up to 3[52]	1–3	3–4	6.2–8.4	Maintain serum triglyceride levels <150 to 250 mg/dL
Vitamin A (IU)	1332–3330	700–1500	700–1500	700–1500	700–1500	BPD prophylaxis 5000 IU IM 3×/week for 4 weeks for ventilated ELBW[141]
Vitamin D (IU)	400–1000	40–160	150–400	40–160	150–400	
Vitamin E (mg α-TE)	2.2–11	2.8–3.5	6–12	2.8–3.5	6–12[148]	
Vitamin C (mg/kg/d)	16.5–41	15–25	18–24	15–25	18–24	32[149]
Calcium (mg/kg/d)	120–220	60–90	120–230	60–80[166]	100–220	
Phosphorus (mg/kg/d)	70–120	47–70	60–140	45–60	60–140	
Zinc (mg/kg/d)	2–3	0.15	0.5–0.8	0.4	1–3	
Selenium (μg/kg/d)	7–10	0, 1.3	1.3	1.5–4.5	1.3–4.5	Up to 7 to approximate levels in breast-fed infants[153]
Copper (μg/kg/d)	120–230	0, 20	120	20	120–150	
Manganese (μg/kg/d)	1–15	0, 0.75	0.75	1	0.7–7.75	

BPD, Bronchopulmonary dysplasia; *ELBW*, extremely low birth weight.

Adapted from *American Academy of Pediatrics: Pediatric Nutrition Handbook*. 6th ed. 2009; Appendix in Tsang RC, Uauy R, Koletzko B, Zlotkin SH, eds. Nutrition of the Preterm Infant: Scientific Basis and Practical Guidelines. 2nd ed. Cincinnati, OH: Digital Education Publishing; 2005:417-418; and Koletzko, B., et al., Recommended Nutrient Intake Levels for Preterm Infants, in Nutritional Care of Preterm Infants: Scientific Basis and Practical Guidelines. 2021:191-197.

REFERENCES

1. Jordan BK, McEvoy CT. Trajectories of lung function in infants and children: setting a course for lifelong lung health. *Pediatrics*. 2020;146(4):e20200417.
2. Stocks J, Hislop A, Sonnappa S. Early lung development: lifelong effect on respiratory health and disease. *Lancet Respir Med*. 2013;1(9):728-742.
3. Agusti A, Faner R. Lung function trajectories in health and disease. *Lancet Respir Med*. 2019;7(4):358-364.
4. Barker DJP. Sir Richard Doll Lecture. Developmental origins of chronic disease. *Public Health*. 2012;126(3):185-189.
5. Matei A, Saccone G, Vogel JP, et al. Primary and secondary prevention of preterm birth: a review of systematic reviews and ongoing randomized controlled trials. *Eur J Obstet Gynecol Reprod Biol*. 2019;236:224-239.
6. Middleton P, Gomersall JC, Gould JF, et al. Omega-3 fatty acid addition during pregnancy. *Cochrane Database Syst Rev*. 2018; 11:CD003402.
7. Briana DD, Malamitsi-Puchner A. Small for gestational age birth weight: impact on lung structure and function. *Paediatr Respir Rev*. 2013;14(4):256-262.
8. Morrow LA, Wagner BD, Ingram DA, et al. Antenatal determinants of bronchopulmonary dysplasia and late respiratory disease in preterm infants. *Am J Respir Crit Care Med*. 2017;196(3):364-374.
9. Lopuhaa CE, Roseboom TJ, Osmond C, et al. Atopy, lung function, and obstructive airways disease after prenatal exposure to famine. *Thorax*. 2000;55(7):555-561.
10. Turner SW, Campbell D, Smith N, et al. Associations between fetal size, maternal {alpha}-tocopherol and childhood asthma. *Thorax*. 2010;65(5):391-397.
11. Kallapur SG, Ikegami M. Physiological consequences of intrauterine insults. *Paediatr Respir Rev*. 2006;7(2):110-116.
12. Joss-Moore LA, Wang Y, Baack ML, et al. IUGR decreases PPARgamma and SETD8 Expression in neonatal rat lung and these effects are ameliorated by maternal DHA supplementation. *Early Hum Dev*. 2010;86(12):785-791.
13. Londhe VA, Maisonet TM, Lopez B, Shin BC, Huynh J, Devaskar SU. Retinoic acid rescues alveolar hypoplasia in the calorie-restricted developing rat lung. *Am J Respir Cell Mol Biol*. 2013;48(2):179-187.
14. McGillick EV, Lock MC, Orgeig S, Morrison JL. Maternal obesity mediated predisposition to respiratory complications at birth and in later life: understanding the implications of the obesogenic intrauterine environment. *Paediatr Respir Rev*. 2017;21:11-18.
15. Malti N, Merzouk H, Merzouk SA, et al. Oxidative stress and maternal obesity: feto-placental unit interaction. *Placenta*. 2014;35(6):411-416.
16. Duthie L, Reynolds RM. Changes in the maternal hypothalamic-pituitary-adrenal axis in pregnancy and postpartum: influences on maternal and fetal outcomes. *Neuroendocrinology*. 2013;98(2):106-115.
17. Ramsay JE, Ferrell WR, Crawford L, Wallace AM, Greer IA, Sattar N. Maternal obesity is associated with dysregulation of metabolic, vascular, and inflammatory pathways. *J Clin Endocrinol Metab*. 2002;87(9):4231-4237.
18. Challier JC, Basu S, Bintein T, et al. Obesity in pregnancy stimulates macrophage accumulation and inflammation in the placenta. *Placenta*. 2008;29(3):274-281.
19. MacDonald KD, Moran AR, Scherman AJ, McEvoy CT, Platteau AS. Maternal high-fat diet in mice leads to innate airway hyperresponsiveness in the adult offspring. *Physiol Rep*. 2017;5(5):e13082.
20. MacDonald KD, Vesco KK, Funk KL, et al. Maternal body mass index before pregnancy is associated with increased bronchodilator dispensing in early childhood: a cross-sectional study. *Pediatr Pulmonol*. 2016;51(8):803-811.
21. Dietz PM, England LJ, Shapiro-Mendoza CK, Tong VT, Farr SL, Callaghan WM. Infant morbidity and mortality attributable to prenatal smoking in the U.S. *Am J Prev Med*. 2010;39(1):45-52.
22. Salihu HM, Aliyu MH, Pierre-Louis BJ, Alexander GR. Levels of excess infant deaths attributable to maternal smoking during pregnancy in the United States. *Matern Child Health J*. 2003; 7(4):219-227.
23. Tong VT, Dietz PM, Morrow B, et al. Trends in smoking before, during, and after pregnancy—Pregnancy Risk Assessment Monitoring System, United States, 40 sites, 2000-2010. *MMWR Surveill Summ*. 2013;62(6):1-19.
24. McEvoy CT, Spindel ER. Pulmonary effects of maternal smoking on the fetus and child: effects on lung development, respiratory morbidities, and life long lung health. *Paediatr Respir Rev*. 2017;21:27-33.
25. Filion KB, Abenhaim HA, Mottillo S, et al. The effect of smoking cessation counselling in pregnant women: a meta-analysis of randomised controlled trials. *BJOG*. 2011;118(12):1422-1428.
26. Schneider S, Huy C, Schütz J, Diehl K. Smoking cessation during pregnancy: a systematic literature review. *Drug Alcohol Rev*. 2010;29(1):81-90.
27. McEvoy CT, Schilling D, Clay N, et al. Vitamin C supplementation for pregnant smoking women and pulmonary function in their newborn infants: a randomized clinical trial. *JAMA*. 2014;311(20):2074-2082.
28. McEvoy CT, Shorey-Kendrick LE, Milner K, et al. Oral Vitamin C (500 mg/d) to Pregnant Smokers Improves Infant Airway Function at 3 Months (VCSIP). A Randomized Trial. *Am J Respir Crit Care Med*. 2019;199(9):1139-1147.
29. McEvoy CT, Shorey-Kendrick LE, Milner K, et al. Vitamin C to pregnant smokers persistently improves infant airway function to 12 months of age: a randomised trial. *Eur Respir J*. 2020: 1902208. doi:10.1183/13993003.02208-2019.
30. Lykkedegn S, Sorensen GL, Beck-Nielsen SS, Christesen HT. The impact of vitamin D on fetal and neonatal lung maturation: a systematic review. *Am J Physiol Lung Cell Mol Physiol*. 2015;308(7):L587-L602.
31. Yurt M, Liu J, Sakurai R, et al. Vitamin D supplementation blocks pulmonary structural and functional changes in a rat model of perinatal vitamin D deficiency. *Am J Physiol Lung Cell Mol Physiol*. 2014;307(11):L859-L867.
32. Sakurai R, Singh H, Wang Y, et al. Effect of perinatal vitamin D deficiency on lung mesenchymal stem cell differentiation and injury repair potential. *Am J Respir Cell Mol Biol*. 2021; 65(5):521-531.
33. Camargo Jr CA, Rifas-Shiman SL, Litonjua AA, et al. Maternal intake of vitamin D during pregnancy and risk of recurrent wheeze in children at 3 y of age. *Am J Clin Nutr*. 2007;85(3):788-795.
34. Litonjua AA, Carey VJ, Laranjo N, et al. Effect of prenatal supplementation with vitamin D on asthma or recurrent wheezing in offspring by age 3 years: the VDAART Randomized Clinical Trial. *JAMA*. 2016;315(4):362-370.
35. Wolsk HM, Chawes BL, Litonjua AA, et al. Prenatal vitamin D supplementation reduces risk of asthma/recurrent wheeze in early childhood: a combined analysis of two randomized controlled trials. *PLoS One*. 2017;12(10):e0186657.
36. Litonjua AA, Carey VJ, Laranjo N, et al. Six-year follow-up of a trial of antenatal vitamin D for asthma reduction. *N Engl J Med*. 2020;382(6):525-533.
37. Checkley W, West Jr KP, Wise RA, et al. Maternal vitamin A supplementation and lung function in offspring. *N Engl J Med*. 2010;362(19):1784-1794.

38. Cigdem MK, Kizil G, Onen A, Kizil M, Nergiz Y, Celik Y. Is there a role for antioxidants in prevention of pulmonary hypoplasia in nitrofen-induced rat model of congenital diaphragmatic hernia? *Pediatr Surg Int.* 2010;26(4):401-406.

39. Taglauer E, Abman SH, Keller RL. Recent advances in antenatal factors predisposing to bronchopulmonary dysplasia. *Semin Perinatol.* 2018;42(7):413-424.

40. Abramovici A, Gandley RE, Clifton RG, et al. Prenatal vitamin C and E supplementation in smokers is associated with reduced placental abruption and preterm birth: a secondary analysis. *BJOG.* 2015;122(13):1740-1747.

41. Ng DV, Brennan-Donnan J, Unger S, et al. How close are we to achieving energy and nutrient goals for very low birth weight infants in the first week? *JPEN J Parenter Enteral Nutr.* 2017;41(3):500-506.

42. Fenton TR, Cormack B, Goldberg D, et al. "Extrauterine growth restriction" and "postnatal growth failure" are misnomers for preterm infants. *J Perinatol.* 2020;40(5):704-714.

43. Hu F, Tang Q, Wang Y, et al. Analysis of nutrition support in very low-birth-weight infants with extrauterine growth restriction. *Nutr Clin Pract.* 2019;34(3):436-443.

44. Bancalari E, Jain D. Bronchopulmonary dysplasia: 50 years after the original description. *Neonatology.* 2019;115(4):384-391.

45. Stoll BJ, Hansen NI, Bell EF, et al. Neonatal outcomes of extremely preterm infants from the NICHD Neonatal Research Network. *Pediatrics.* 2010;126(3):443-456.

46. Lapcharoensap W, Gage SC, Kan P, et al. Hospital variation and risk factors for bronchopulmonary dysplasia in a population-based cohort. *JAMA Pediatr.* 2015;169(2):e143676.

47. Kotecha S. Lung growth: implications for the newborn infant. *Arch Dis Child Fetal Neonatal Ed.* 2000;82(1):F69-F74.

48. Kleinman RE ed. Pediatric Nutrition Handbook. 6th ed. Elk Grove Village, IL: American Academy of Pediatrics; 2009.

49. Embleton NE, Pang N, Cooke RJ. Postnatal malnutrition and growth retardation: an inevitable consequence of current recommendations in preterm infants? *Pediatrics.* 2001;107(2):270-273.

50. Ehrenkranz RA, Younes N, Lemons JA, et al. Longitudinal growth of hospitalized very low birth weight infants. *Pediatrics.* 1999;104(2 Pt 1):280-289.

51. Widdowson EM, McCance RA, Spray CM. The chemical composition of the human body. *Clin Sci.* 1951;10(1):113-125.

52. Thureen PJ, Hay WW. Nutritional requirements of the very low birth weight infant. In: Neu J, ed. *Gastroenterology and Nutrition: Neonatology Questions and Controversies.* Philadelphia, PA: Saunders Elsevier; 2008:208-222.

53. American Academy of Pediatrics Committee on Nutrition: Nutritional needs of low-birth-weight infants. *Pediatrics.* 1985;75(5):976-986.

54. Hay Jr WW, Lucas A, Heird WC, et al. Workshop summary: nutrition of the extremely low birth weight infant. *Pediatrics.* 1999;104(6):1360-1368.

55. Herrmann KR, Herrmann KR. Early parenteral nutrition and successful postnatal growth of premature infants. *Nutr Clin Pract.* 2010;25(1):69-75.

56. Graziano PD, Tauber KA, Cummings J, Graffunder E, Horgan MJ. Prevention of postnatal growth restriction by the implementation of an evidence-based premature infant feeding bundle. *J Perinatol.* 2015;35(8):642-649.

57. De Curtis M, Rigo J. Extrauterine growth restriction in very-low-birthweight infants. *Acta Paediatr.* 2004;93(12):1563-1568.

58. Ehrenkranz RA, Dusick AM, Vohr BR, Wright LL, Wrage LA, Poole WK. Growth in the neonatal intensive care unit influences neurodevelopmental and growth outcomes of extremely low birth weight infants. *Pediatrics.* 2006;117(4):1253-1261.

59. Balinotti JE, Tiller CJ, Llapur CJ, et al. Growth of the lung parenchyma early in life. *Am J Respir Crit Care Med.* 2009;179(2):134-137.

60. Frank L, Groseclose E. Oxygen toxicity in newborn rats: the adverse effects of undernutrition. *J Appl Physiol Respir Environ Exerc Physiol.* 1982;53(5):1248-1255.

61. Maritz GS, Cock ML, Louey S, Suzuki K, Harding R. Fetal growth restriction has long-term effects on postnatal lung structure in sheep. *Pediatr Res.* 2004;55(2):287-295.

62. Das RM. The effects of intermittent starvation on lung development in suckling rats. *Am J Pathol.* 1984;117(2):326-332.

63. Massaro D, Massaro GD. Hunger disease and pulmonary alveoli. *Am J Respir Crit Care Med.* 2004;170(7):723-724.

64. Mataloun MM, Rebello CM, Mascaretti RS, Dohlnikoff M, Leone CR. Pulmonary responses to nutritional restriction and hyperoxia in premature rabbits. *J Pediatr (Rio J).* 2006;82(3):179-185.

65. Coxson HO, Chan IH, Mayo JR, Hlynsky J, Nakano Y, Birmingham CL. Early emphysema in patients with anorexia nervosa. *Am J Respir Crit Care Med.* 2004;170(7):748-752.

66. Maritz G, Probyn M, De Matteo R, Snibson K, Harding R. Lung parenchyma at maturity is influenced by postnatal growth but not by moderate preterm birth in sheep. *Neonatology.* 2008;93(1):28-35.

67. Bose C, Van Marter LJ, Laughon M, et al. Fetal growth restriction and chronic lung disease among infants born before the 28th week of gestation. *Pediatrics.* 2009;124(3):e450-e458.

68. Laughon M, Bose C, Allred EN, et al. Antecedents of chronic lung disease following three patterns of early respiratory disease in preterm infants. *Arch Dis Child Fetal Neonatal Ed.* 2011;96(2):F114-F120.

69. Kurzner SI, Garg M, Bautista DB, et al. Growth failure in infants with bronchopulmonary dysplasia: nutrition and elevated resting metabolic expenditure. *Pediatrics.* 1988;81(3):379-384.

70. Kurzner SI, Garg M, Bautista DB, Sargent CW, Bowman CM, Keens TG. Growth failure in bronchopulmonary dysplasia: elevated metabolic rates and pulmonary mechanics. *J Pediatr.* 1988;112(1):73-80.

71. Groothuis JR, Rosenberg AA. Home oxygen promotes weight gain in infants with bronchopulmonary dysplasia. *Am J Dis Child.* 1987;141(9):992-995.

72. Guslits BG, Gaston SE, Bryan MH, England SJ, Bryan AC. Diaphragmatic work of breathing in premature human infants. *J Appl Physiol (1985).* 1987;62(4):1410-1415.

73. Arora NS, Rochester DF. Respiratory muscle strength and maximal voluntary ventilation in undernourished patients. *Am Rev Respir Dis.* 1982;126(1):5-8.

74. Dias CM, Pássaro CP, Antunes MA, et al. Effects of different nutritional support on lung mechanics and remodelling in undernourished rats. *Respir Physiol Neurobiol.* 2008;160(1):54-64.

75. Matecki S, Py G, Lambert K, et al. Effect of prolonged undernutrition on rat diaphragm mitochondrial respiration. *Am J Respir Cell Mol Biol.* 2002;26(2):239-245.

76. Lewis MI, Li H, Huang ZS, et al. Influence of varying degrees of malnutrition on IGF-I expression in the rat diaphragm. *J Appl Physiol (1985).* 2003;95(2):555-562.

77. Blazer S, Reinersman GT, Askanazi J, Furst P, Katz DP, Fleischman AR. Branched-chain amino acids and respiratory

pattern and function in the neonate. *J Perinatol.* 1994;14(4): 290-295.

78. Rehan VK, Laiprasert J, Nakashima JM, Wallach M, McCool FD. Effects of continuous positive airway pressure on diaphragm dimensions in preterm infants. *J Perinatol.* 2001;21(8):521-524.

79. Parks WC, Shapiro SD. Matrix metalloproteinases in lung biology. *Respir Res.* 2001;2(1):10-19.

80. Sahebjami H, MacGee J. Effects of starvation on lung mechanics and biochemistry in young and old rats. *J Appl Physiol (1985).* 1985;58(3):778-784.

81. Jobe AH. Pulmonary surfactant therapy. *N Engl J Med.* 1993; 328(12):861-868.

82. Batenburg JJ. Surfactant phospholipids: synthesis and storage. *Am J Physiol.* 1992;262(4 Pt 1):L367-L385.

83. Guarner V, Tordet C, Bourbon JR. Effects of maternal protein-calorie malnutrition on the phospholipid composition of surfactant isolated from fetal and neonatal rat lungs. Compensation by inositol and lipid supplementation. *Pediatr Res.* 1992;31(6):629-635.

84. Lechner AJ, Winston DC, Bauman JE. Lung mechanics, cellularity, and surfactant after prenatal starvation in guinea pigs. *J Appl Physiol (1985).* 1986;60(5):1610-1614.

85. Gerhardt T, Bancalari E. Chestwall compliance in full-term and premature infants. *Acta Paediatr Scand.* 1980;69(3):359-364.

86. Greenberg JM, Poindexter BB, Shaw PA, et al. Respiratory medication use in extremely premature (<29 weeks) infants during initial NICU hospitalization: Results from the prematurity and respiratory outcomes program. *Pediatr Pulmonol.* 2020;55(2):360-368.

87. Rigo J, De Curtis M, Pieltain C, Picaud JC, Salle BL, Senterre J. Bone mineral metabolism in the micropremie. *Clin Perinatol.* 2000;27(1):147-170.

88. Glasgow JF, Thomas PS. Rachitic respiratory distress in small preterm infants. *Arch Dis Child.* 1977;52(4):268-273.

89. Dobashi K, Asayama K, Hayashibe H, et al. Immunohistochemical study of copper-zinc and manganese superoxide dismutases in the lungs of human fetuses and newborn infants: developmental profile and alterations in hyaline membrane disease and bronchopulmonary dysplasia. *Virchows Arch A Pathol Anat Histopathol.* 1993;423(3):177-184.

90. Deneke SM, Lynch BA, Fanburg BL. Effects of low protein diets or feed restriction on rat lung glutathione and oxygen toxicity. *J Nutr.* 1985;115(6):726-732.

91. Zaman K, Baqui AH, Yunus M, Sack RB, Chowdhury HR, Black RE. Malnutrition, cell-mediated immune deficiency and acute upper respiratory infections in rural Bangladeshi children. *Acta Paediatr.* 1997;86(9):923-927.

92. Cunha AL. Relationship between acute respiratory infection and malnutrition in children under 5 years of age. *Acta Paediatr.* 2000;89(5):608-609.

93. Skerrett SJ, Henderson WR, Martin TR. Alveolar macrophage function in rats with severe protein calorie malnutrition. Arachidonic acid metabolism, cytokine release, and antimicrobial activity. *J Immunol.* 1990;144(3):1052-1061.

94. Martin TR, Altman LC, Alvares OF. The effects of severe protein-calorie malnutrition on antibacterial defense mechanisms in the rat lung. *Am Rev Respir Dis.* 1983;128(6):1013-1019.

95. Schuit KE, Krebs RE, Rohn D, Steele V. Effect of fetal protein malnutrition on the postnatal structure and function of alveolar macrophages. *J Infect Dis.* 1982;146(4):498-505.

96. Sano, H, Kuroki Y. The lung collectins, SP-A and SP-D, modulate pulmonary innate immunity. *Mol Immunol.* 2005;42(3):279-287.

97. Factor P, Ridge K, Alverdy J, Sznajder JI. Continuous enteral nutrition attenuates pulmonary edema in rats exposed to 100% oxygen. *J Appl Physiol (1985).* 2000;89(5):1759-1765.

98. Sakuma T, Hida M, Nambu Y, et al. Effects of hypoxia on alveolar fluid transport capacity in rat lungs. *J Appl Physiol (1985).* 2001;91(4):1766-1774.

99. Sakuma T, Zhao Y, Sugita M, et al. Malnutrition impairs alveolar fluid clearance in rat lungs. *Am J Physiol Lung Cell Mol Physiol.* 2004;286(6):L1268-L1274.

100. Oyen N, Skjaerven R, Little RE, Wilcox AJ. Fetal growth retardation in sudden infant death syndrome (SIDS) babies and their siblings. *Am J Epidemiol.* 1995;142(1):84-90.

101. Moss TJ, Davey MG, McCrabb GJ, Harding R. Development of ventilatory responsiveness to progressive hypoxia and hypercapnia in low-birth-weight lambs. *J Appl Physiol (1985).* 1996; 81(4):1555-1561.

102. Coloso VF, Gerhardt T, Suguihara C, et al. Branched-Chain Amino Acids (BCAA) and respiratory center function in the preterm neonate: a prospective, randomized, double-blind trial. *Pediatr Res.* 1997;41:249.

103. Al-Ghanem G, Shah P, Thomas S, et al. Bronchopulmonary dysplasia and pulmonary hypertension: a meta-analysis. *J Perinatol.* 2017;37(4):414-419.

104. Wedgwood S, Warford C, Agvateesiri SC, et al. Postnatal growth restriction augments oxygen-induced pulmonary hypertension in a neonatal rat model of bronchopulmonary dysplasia. *Pediatr Res.* 2016;80(6):894-902.

105. Wedgwood S, Warford C, Agvatisiri SR, et al. The developing gut-lung axis: postnatal growth restriction, intestinal dysbiosis, and pulmonary hypertension in a rodent model. *Pediatr Res.* 2020;87(3):472-479.

106. Hay Jr WW, Brown LD, Denne SC. Energy requirements, protein-energy metabolism and balance, and carbohydrates in preterm infants. *World Rev Nutr Diet.* 2014;110:64-81.

107. Bauer K, Laurenz M, Ketteler J, Versmold H. Longitudinal study of energy expenditure in preterm neonates ,30 weeks' gestation during the first three postnatal weeks. *J Pediatr.* 2003; 142(4):390-396.

108. DeMarie MP, Hoffenberg A, Biggerstaff SL, Jeffers BW, Hay Jr WW, Thureen PJ. Determinants of energy expenditure in ventilated preterm infants. *J Perinat Med.* 1999;27(6):465-472.

109. Collins CT, Gibson RA, Miller J, et al. Carbohydrate intake is the main determinant of growth in infants born <33 weeks' gestation when protein intake is adequate. *Nutrition.* 2008;24(5):451-457.

110. Wahlig TM, Gatto CW, Boros SJ, Mammel MC, Mills MM, Georgieff MK. Metabolic response of preterm infants to variable degrees of respiratory illness. *J Pediatr.* 1994;124(2):283-288.

111. Costarino AT, Baumgart S. Water as nutrition. In: Tsang RC, Lucas A, Uauy R, Zlotkin S, eds. *Nutritional Needs of the Preterm Infant.* Pawling, NY: Williams & Wilkins; 1993:1-14.

112. Oh W, Poindexter BB, Perritt R, et al. Association between fluid intake and weight loss during the first ten days of life and risk of bronchopulmonary dysplasia in extremely low birth weight infants. *J Pediatr.* 2005;147(6):786-790.

113. Bancalari E, Claure N, Gonzalez A. Patent ductus arteriosus and respiratory outcome in premature infants. *Biol Neonate.* 2005;88(3):192-201.

114. Bell EF, Acarregui MJ. Restricted versus liberal water intake for preventing morbidity and mortality in preterm infants. *Cochrane Database Syst Rev.* 2014;(12):CD000503.

115. Parimi P, Kalhan SC. Carbohydrates including oligosaccharides and inositol. In: Tsang RC, Uauy R, Koletzko B, Zlotkin S, eds.

Nutrition of the Preterm Infnat: Scientific Basis and Practical Guidelines. Cincinnati, OH: Digital Educational Publishing; 2005:81-95.

116. Sauer PJ, Van Aerde JE, Pencharz PB, Smith JM, Swyer PR. Glucose oxidation rates in newborn infants measured with indirect calorimetry and [U-13C]glucose. *Clin Sci (Lond).* 1986;70(6):587-593.

117. Van Aerde JE, Sauer PJ, Pencharz PB, Smith JM, Swyer PR. Effect of replacing glucose with lipid on the energy metabolism of newborn infants. *Clin Sci (Lond).* 1989;76(6):581-588.

118. Uthaya S, Thomas EL, Hamilton G, Doré CJ, Bell J, Modi N. Altered adiposity after extremely preterm birth. *Pediatr Res.* 2005;57(2):211-215.

119. Duffy B, Gunn T, Collinge J, Pencharz P. The effect of varying protein quality and energy intake on the nitrogen metabolism of parenterally fed very low birthweight (less than 1600 g) infants. *Pediatr Res.* 1981;15(7):1040-1044.

120. Brans YW, Dutton EB, Andrew DS, Menchaca EM, West DL. Fat emulsion tolerance in very low birth weight neonates: effect on diffusion of oxygen in the lungs and on blood pH. *Pediatrics.* 1986;78(1):79-84.

121. Waitzberg DL, Torrinhas RS. Fish oil lipid emulsions and immune response: what clinicians need to know. *Nutr Clin Pract.* 2009;24(4):487-499.

122. Arterburn LM, Hall EB, Oken H. Distribution, interconversion, and dose response of n-3 fatty acids in humans. *Am J Clin Nutr.* 2006;83(suppl 6):1467S-1476S.

123. Calder PC. n-3 polyunsaturated fatty acids, inflammation, and inflammatory diseases. *Am J Clin Nutr.* 2006;83(suppl 6): 1505S-1519S.

124. Schwartz J. Role of polyunsaturated fatty acids in lung disease. *Am J Clin Nutr.* 2000;71(suppl 1):393S-396S.

125. Sosenko IR, Innis SM, Frank L. Intralipid increases lung polyunsaturated fatty acids and protects newborn rats from oxygen toxicity. *Pediatr Res.* 1991;30(5):413-417.

126. Sosenko IR, Innis SM, Frank L. Menhaden fish oil, n-3 polyunsaturated fatty acids, and protection of newborn rats from oxygen toxicity. *Pediatr Res.* 1989;25(4):399-404.

127. Yeh SL, Chang KY, Huang PC, Chen WJ. Effects of n-3 and n-6 fatty acids on plasma eicosanoids and liver antioxidant enzymes in rats receiving total parenteral nutrition. *Nutrition.* 1997; 13(1):32-36.

128. Simopoulos AP. Summary of the NATO advanced research workshop on dietary omega 3 and omega 6 fatty acids: biological effects and nutritional essentiality. *J Nutr.* 1989;119(4): 521-528.

129. Choudhary N, Tan K, Malhotra A. Inpatient outcomes of preterm infants receiving omega-3 enriched lipid emulsion (SMOFlipid): an observational study. *Eur J Pediatr.* 2018;177(5): 723-731.

130. Hay WW, Thureen P. Protein for preterm infants: how much is needed? How much is enough? How much is too much? *Pediatr Neonatol.* 2010;51(4):198-207.

131. Denne SC, Poindexter BB. Evidence supporting early nutritional support with parenteral amino acid infusion. *Semin Perinatol.* 2007;31(2):56-60.

132. Thureen PJ, Hay Jr WW. Intravenous nutrition and postnatal growth of the micropremie. *Clin Perinatol.* 2000;27(1): 197-219.

133. Poindexter BB, Langer JC, Dusick AM, Ehrenkranz RA. Early provision of parenteral amino acids in extremely low birth weight infants: relation to growth and neurodevelopmental outcome. *J Pediatr.* 2006;148(3):300-305.

134. van den Akker CH, te Braake FW, Schierbeek H, et al. Albumin synthesis in premature neonates is stimulated by parenterally administered amino acids during the first days of life. *Am J Clin Nutr.* 2007;86(4):1003-1008.

135. Roche M, Rondeau P, Singh NR, Tarnus E, Bourdon E. The antioxidant properties of serum albumin. *FEBS Lett.* 2008; 582(13):1783-1787.

136. Kalhoff H, Manz F, Kiwull P, Kiwull-Schöne H. Food mineral composition and acid-base balance in preterm infants. *Eur J Nutr.* 2007;46(4):188-195.

137. Shenai JP, Chytil F, Jhaveri A, Stahlman MT. Plasma vitamin A and retinol-binding protein in premature and term neonates. *J Pediatr.* 1981;99(2):302-305.

138. Hustead VA, Gutcher GR, Anderson SA, Zachman RD. Relationship of vitamin A (retinol) status to lung disease in the preterm infant. *J Pediatr.* 1984;105(4):610-615.

139. Shenai JP, Chytil F. Vitamin A storage in lungs during perinatal development in the rat. *Biol Neonate.* 1990;57(2):126-132.

140. Silvers KM, Sluis KB, Darlow BA, McGill F, Stocker R, Winterbourn CC. Limiting light-induced lipid peroxidation and vitamin loss in infant parenteral nutrition by adding multivitamin preparations to Intralipid. *Acta Paediatr.* 2001;90(3):242-249.

141. Tyson JE, Wright LL, Oh W, et al. Vitamin A supplementation for extremely-low-birth-weight infants. National Institute of Child Health and Human Development Neonatal Research Network. *N Engl J Med.* 1999;340(25):1962-1968.

142. Ambalavanan N, Kennedy K, Tyson J, Carlo WA. Survey of vitamin A supplementation for extremely-low-birth-weight infants: is clinical practice consistent with the evidence? *J Pediatr.* 2004;145(3):304-307.

143. Atkinson SA, Tsang R. Calcium, magnesium, phosphorus and vitamin D. In: Tsang RC, Uauy R, Koletzko B, Zlotkin S, eds. *Nutrition of the Preterm Infant: Scientific Basis and Practical Guidelines.* Cincinnati, OH: Digital Educational Publishing; 2005: 245-275.

144. Burton GW, Traber MG. Vitamin E: antioxidant activity, biokinetics, and bioavailability. *Annu Rev Nutr.* 1990;10:357-382.

145. Watts JL, Milner R, Zipursky A, et al. Failure of supplementation with vitamin E to prevent bronchopulmonary dysplasia in infants less than 1,500 g birth weight. *Eur Respir J.* 1991;4(2):188-190.

146. Ehrenkranz RA, Ablow RC, Warshaw JB. Effect of vitamin E on the development of oxygen-induced lung injury in neonates. *Ann N Y Acad Sci.* 1982;393:452-466.

147. Anzueto A, Andrade FH, Maxwell LC, Levine SM, Lawrence RA, Jenkinson SG. Diaphragmatic function after resistive breathing in vitamin E-deficient rats. *J Appl Physiol (1985).* 1993; 74(1):267-271.

148. Greene HL, Hambidge KM, Schanler R, Tsang RC. Guidelines for the use of vitamins, trace elements, calcium, magnesium, and phosphorus in infants and children receiving total parenteral nutrition: report of the Subcommittee on Pediatric Parenteral Nutrient Requirements from the Committee on Clinical Practice Issues of the American Society for Clinical Nutrition. *Am J Clin Nutr.* 1988;48(5):1324-1342.

149. Darlow BA, Buss H, McGill F, Fletcher L, Graham P, Winterbourn CC. Vitamin C supplementation in very preterm infants: a randomised controlled trial. *Arch Dis Child Fetal Neonatal Ed.* 2005;90(2):F117-F122.

150. Sluis KB, Darlow BA, George PM, Mogridge N, Dolamore BA, Winterbourn CC. Selenium and glutathione peroxidase levels in premature infants in a low selenium community (Christchurch, New Zealand). *Pediatr Res.* 1992;32(2):189-194.

151. Darlow BA, Inder TE, Graham PJ, et al. The relationship of selenium status to respiratory outcome in the very low birth weight infant. *Pediatrics*. 1995;96(2 Pt 1):314-319.

152. Darlow BA, Winterbourn CC, Inder TE, et al. The effect of selenium supplementation on outcome in very low birth weight infants: a randomized controlled trial. The New Zealand Neonatal Study Group. *J Pediatr*. 2000;136(4):473-480.

153. Darlow BA, Austin NC. Selenium supplementation to prevent short-term morbidity in preterm neonates. *Cochrane Database Syst Rev*. 2003;(4):CD003312.

154. Zlotkin SH, Atkinson S, Lockitch G. Trace elements in nutrition for premature infants. *Clin Perinatol*. 1995;22(1):223-240.

155. Patel RM, Knezevic A, Yang J, et al. Enteral iron supplementation, red blood cell transfusion, and risk of bronchopulmonary dysplasia in very-low-birth-weight infants. *Transfusion*. 2019; 59(5):1675-1682.

156. Rigo J, Pieltain C, Salle B, Senterre J. Enteral calcium, phosphate and vitamin D requirements and bone mineralization in preterm infants. *Acta Paediatr*. 2007;96(7):969-974.

157. Abrams SA. In utero physiology: role in nutrient delivery and fetal development for calcium, phosphorus, and vitamin D. *Am J Clin Nutr*. 2007;85(2):604S-607S.

158. Hallman M, Bry K, Hoppu K, Lappi M, Pohjavuori M. Inositol supplementation in premature infants with respiratory distress syndrome. *N Engl J Med*. 1992;326(19):1233-1239.

159. Howlett A, Ohlsson A, Plakkal N. Inositol in preterm infants at risk for or having respiratory distress syndrome. *Cochrane Database Syst Rev*. 2019;7:CD000366.

160. te Braake FW, Schierbeek H, Vermes A, Huijmans JG, van Goudoever JB. High-dose cysteine administration does not increase synthesis of the antioxidant glutathione preterm infants. *Pediatrics*. 2009;124(5):e978-e984.

161. Sandberg K, Fellman V, Stigson L, Thiringer K, Hjalmarson O. N-acetylcysteine administration during the first week of life does not improve lung function in extremely low birth weight infants. *Biol Neonate*. 2004;86(4):275-279.

162. Ahola T, Lapatto R, Raivio KO, et al. N-acetylcysteine does not prevent bronchopulmonary dysplasia in immature infants: a randomized controlled trial. *J Pediatr*. 2003; 143(6):713-719.

163. Fox RE, Hopkins IB, Cabacungan ET, Tildon JT. The role of glutamine and other alternate substrates as energy sources in the fetal rat lung type II cell. *Pediatr Res*. 1996;40(1): 135-141.

164. Poindexter BB, Ehrenkranz RA, Stoll BJ, et al. Parenteral glutamine supplementation does not reduce the risk of mortality or late-onset sepsis in extremely low birth weight infants. *Pediatrics*. 2004;113(5):1209-1215.

165. Villamor-Martinez E, Pierro M, Cavallaro G, Mosca F, Villamor E. Mother's own milk and bronchopulmonary dysplasia: a systematic review and meta-analysis. *Front Pediatr*. 2019;7:224.

166. Atkinson SA, Tsang R. Calcium, Magnesium, Phosphorus and Vitamin D. In: Tsang RC, Uauy R, Koltzko B, Zlotkin S, eds. *Nutrition of the Preterm Infant: Scientific Basis and Practical Guidelines*. Cincinnati: Digital Educational Publishing, Inc; 2005: 245-275.

167. Koletzko B, Wieczorek S, Cheah FC, et al. Recommended nutrient intake levels for preterm infants. In: Koletzko B, ed, et al. *Nutritional Care of Preterm Infants: Scientific Basis and Practical Guidelines*. Basel, Switzerland: Karger; 2021:191-197.

Chapter 17

Caffeine—Respiratory Stimulant or Magic Bullet?

Barbara Schmidt

Chapter Outline

Introduction

Caffeine is the Respiratory Stimulant of Choice for Preterm Infants

Caffeine for Apnea of Prematurity (CAP) Trial
  Rationale for the CAP Trial
  Conduct of the CAP Trial
  Benefits of Caffeine in the CAP Trial
  What May Explain the Lasting Benefit of Caffeine on Motor Skills?
  Safety of Caffeine in the CAP Trial

Remaining Uncertainties About Neonatal Caffeine Therapy
  What is the optimal Caffeine Dosing Regimen?
  When to Start Caffeine
  When to Stop Caffeine

Is Caffeine a Magic Bullet?

Key Points

- Caffeine is the respiratory stimulant of choice to prevent or treat apnea of prematurity.
- The standard loading is 20 mg/kg of caffeine citrate, and the daily maintenance dose is 5 to 10 mg/kg.
- Beneficial effects of this caffeine regimen include reduced risks of motor impairment, bronchopulmonary dysplasia, and severe retinopathy of prematurity.
- Lasting harmful effects have not been detected with standard doses of caffeine up to 11 years after preterm birth.
- The safety of higher doses of caffeine remains uncertain.
- Initiation of caffeine therapy may be considered in all extremely preterm infants soon after birth unless they are fully ventilated and there are no immediate plans for a trial of extubation.
- Moderately and late preterm infants should not receive caffeine therapy unless they manifest apnea of prematurity.
- Termination of caffeine therapy should be individualized and guided by the infants' gestational age and their need for respiratory support.

Introduction

Apnea of prematurity is a common developmental disorder of respiratory control characterized by periodic breathing with pathological apnea. An apneic spell is defined as the cessation of respiratory air flow for at least 20 seconds, or any respiratory pause of shorter duration that is associated with cyanosis (desaturation), marked pallor, hypotonia, or bradycardia (<100 beats per minute).[1] Apnea can be central (no respiratory effort), obstructive (mostly due to upper airway obstruction), or mixed. Most apneic events are either mixed or obstructive.[1] The frequency, severity, and time to resolution of apnea are usually correlated inversely with gestational age at birth.[1,2] Apnea of prematurity resolves spontaneously by 44 weeks' postmenstrual age.[3] The two main treatment options are drug therapy with a respiratory stimulant, most commonly a methylxanthine, and the application of positive airway pressure.[1]

Caffeine is the Respiratory Stimulant of Choice for Preterm Infants

The methylxanthines theophylline, aminophylline, and caffeine appear to have similar beneficial effects on neonatal apnea.[4] Caffeine is the methylxanthine of choice because of its pharmacokinetic advantages over theophylline and aminophylline.[5] These advantages include the following:

- Longer plasma elimination half-life enabling once-per-day administration
- Wider therapeutic margin and lower risk of toxicity
- No need for routine therapeutic drug monitoring with standard doses
- Reliable enteral absorption that is unaffected by feedings

How big is the immediate caffeine treatment effect on apnea of prematurity? The largest and most recent placebo-controlled trial to address this question included 82 infants with gestational ages of 28 to 32 weeks who had experienced at least 6 apneas in a 24-hour period.[6] An intravenous loading dose of 20 mg/kg bodyweight caffeine citrate was followed by a daily maintenance dose of 5 mg/kg for a planned treatment period of 10 days. However, only 47% of infants in the caffeine group and 32% of infants in the placebo group completed 10 days of double-blind therapy. The remaining infants received open-label caffeine or were withdrawn from the study altogether.[6]

The US Food and Drug Administration (FDA) used these trial results in 1999 to approve caffeine for the treatment of apnea of prematurity. Table 17.1 summarizes the relevant endpoints in this study as tabulated in the FDA label.[7] At the doses used in this trial, caffeine reduced the frequency of apnea, but did not entirely eliminate apneic events in most patients.[7]

Caffeine for Apnea of Prematurity Trial

Over the past 15 years, caffeine has been transformed from a regularly used but insufficiently tested drug into one of the most evidence-based and commonly prescribed medications in neonatal medicine.[8] The Caffeine for Apnea of Prematurity (CAP) trial played a prominent role in this shift.[8,9]

RATIONALE FOR THE CAFFEINE FOR APNEA OF PREMATURITY TRIAL

By the late 1990s, more than a dozen randomized trials had been published in which a methylxanthine—caffeine, aminophylline, or theophylline—was tested against a comparator such as placebo or continuous positive airway pressure. Methylxanthines had been shown to reduce the frequency of apnea in preterm infants and their need for mechanical ventilation during the first 7 days of therapy.[10] In addition, methylxanthines were known to facilitate the removal of an endotracheal tube and to reduce the risk of postoperative apnea, bradycardia, and desaturation in infants born preterm.[10] However, beyond these short-term benefits, little was known about the clinical effects of methylxanthine therapy because of small sample sizes and a short median duration of follow-up of only 7 days. The effects of methylxanthines on clinically important outcomes such as mortality, common neonatal morbidities, growth, and child development remained unknown.[10]

TABLE 17.1 Effect of Caffeine on Apnea of Prematurity[7]			
Outcome	Caffeine N = 45	Placebo N = 37	P Value
Apnea rate on day 2 (mean per 24 h)	4.9	7.2	0.13
Patients with no apneas on day 2	27%	8%	0.03
Patients with 50% reduction of apneas from baseline on day 2	76%	57%	0.07

The lack of rigorous evaluation of neonatal caffeine therapy in randomized clinical trials (RCTs) was especially worrying because experimental evidence had accumulated suggesting that acute administration of methylxanthines may exacerbate hypoxemic and ischemic brain injury.[10,11] At standard treatment doses, caffeine and other methylxanthines are competitive inhibitors of A1 and A2$_A$ adenosine receptors.[5] By reducing the risk of energy failure and cell death, adenosine is neuroprotective during hypoxemia and ischemia in various animal models.[11] Extensive investigations of the adenosine receptor system and its inhibition in several species of laboratory animals had produced concerning but also conflicting results:

The physiological and pathophysiological roles of the adenosine receptor system in the immature brain are complex and, as yet, incompletely understood. Therefore, one cannot, at present, predict the in vivo effects of non-specific adenosine receptor blockade with methylxanthine therapy, either during times of oxygen sufficiency or during the brief hypoxic-ischaemic episodes that are so common in very preterm infants.[11]

This uncertainty about the safety of the routine use of methylxanthines in preterm infants became the rationale for the international CAP trial.[10]

CONDUCT OF THE CAFFEINE FOR APNEA OF PREMATURITY TRIAL

Concern about the safety of methylxanthine therapy at the time of the CAP trial design was reflected in the wording of the original study question:

Among infants with birth weights of 500 to 1250 g who are at risk of apnea of prematurity during the first 10 days of life, does the use of caffeine compared with placebo increase the risk of death or disability at a corrected age of 18 months?

Caffeine was chosen over aminophylline and theophylline because of its wider therapeutic margin.[5] The intravenous loading dose of 20 mg/kg of caffeine citrate was followed by a daily maintenance dose of 5 mg/kg. If apneas persisted, the daily maintenance dose could be increased to a maximum of 10 mg/kg of caffeine citrate. The maintenance doses were adjusted

weekly for changes in body weight and could be given orally once an infant tolerated full enteral feedings. Excerpts from the instructions in the CAP trial study aid are reproduced in Box 17.1.

Placebo was used to ensure masking of the assignment of the study drug. However, apneas that persisted despite optimal use of the study drug were treated if they required more than mild stimulation. Clinicians were instructed to control such apneas with all necessary nonpharmacologic therapies including various strategies of respiratory supports.[12] Apneas were not recorded in the CAP trial database because clinical records of apnea are known to be inaccurate.[1] For ethical reasons, the data center ensured that parent information and consent forms at all study sites included a statement that methylxanthines have been shown to reduce apnea and the need for assistance from a breathing machine.

The target sample size was enrolled between 1999 and 2004 in 9 high-income countries and 35 hospitals.

BOX 17.1 EXCERPTS FROM THE CAFFEINE FOR APNEA OF PREMATURITY (CAP) STUDY AID

HOW TO GIVE CAP STUDY DRUG?

- CAP Study Drug should be **used in lieu** of methylxanthines during the entire stay in the neonatal nursery.
- The **loading** dose of CAP Study Drug is 20 mg/kg caffeine citrate (equivalent to 10 mg/kg caffeine base) or normal saline placebo.
- The **maintenance** dose of CAP Study Drug is 5 mg/kg/day caffeine citrate (equivalent to 2.5 mg/kg/day caffeine base) or normal saline placebo. Doses should be **adjusted** once a week for changes in **body weight.**
- You can **increase** the **maintenance** dose to a maximum of 10 mg/kg/day caffeine citrate (equivalent to 5 mg/kg/day caffeine base) or normal saline placebo.
- You can give the Study Drug **orally** once the infant tolerates full enteral feeds.

WHEN TO STOP THE CAP STUDY DRUG?

- Remember to hold the Study Drug for any clinical symptoms and signs of **caffeine toxicity.**
- If you **temporarily** stop CAP Study Drug, for whatever reason, the need for partial or complete reloading doses is at your discretion.
- If you think your patient **no longer requires** methylxanthine therapy AND the infant has tolerated at least 5 consecutive days without positive airway pressure, you may permanently discontinue their CAP Study Drug.

Canadian study centers enrolled nearly half of the 2006 study participants. The second largest group of infants was recruited in Australia. Infants were randomly assigned to receive study drug until therapy for apnea of prematurity was no longer needed. The median postmenstrual age at the last dose in the caffeine group was 34.4 weeks (interquartile range 33.0–35.9 weeks).[12]

After ascertaining the primary outcome of death or disability at a corrected age of 18 months, the CAP trial investigators performed two additional comprehensive follow-up assessments, at 5 and 11 years, to detect lasting or previously unrecognized consequences of neonatal caffeine therapy.[13-15]

BENEFITS OF CAFFEINE IN THE CAFFEINE FOR APNEA OF PREMATURITY TRIAL

Earlier Weaning From Respiratory Supports

Caffeine facilitated weaning from respiratory supports. On average, endotracheal tubes, the use of any positive airway pressure, and the administration of supplemental oxygen were each discontinued approximately 1 week earlier for infants in the caffeine group than for infants in the placebo group (Fig. 17.1).[12]

Reduced Risk of Morbidities During Initial Hospital Stay

Caffeine reduced the risks of bronchopulmonary dysplasia (BPD), severe retinopathy of prematurity (ROP), and the use of surgical therapy to close a patent ductus arteriosus (Fig. 17.2).[12,13] In one large CAP trial center, the local risk reduction of BPD mostly explained why neonatal caffeine therapy improved the respiratory function of trial participants at age 11 years.[16] The caffeine treatment effect on the rate of BPD was greater in this local CAP trial subgroup than the average treatment effect in the study overall.[16] The rates of brain injury on cranial ultrasound and of necrotizing enterocolitis did not differ between the caffeine and placebo groups (Fig. 17.2).[12,13]

Reduced Risk of Motor Impairment Into Middle School Age

Caffeine improved the combined primary outcome of death or survival with neurodevelopmental disability at 18 months, corrected for prematurity. Most of this caffeine benefit could be attributed to a reduced risk of cerebral palsy.[13] In contrast, the rates of death were very similar in the caffeine and placebo groups, both at 18 months and 5 years (Fig. 17.3).[13,14] Beneficial caffeine effects on cognitive development were marginal at 18 months and no longer apparent at 5 years.[13,14]

Cerebral palsy is not the only adverse motor outcome after preterm birth. Many more former preterm children have developmental coordination disorder (DCD).[17,18] The motor skill difficulties associated with DCD interfere with activities of daily living and may adversely affect academic performance and behavior.[17,18] Caffeine reduced the risk of DCD (Fig. 17.3).[19] Although this

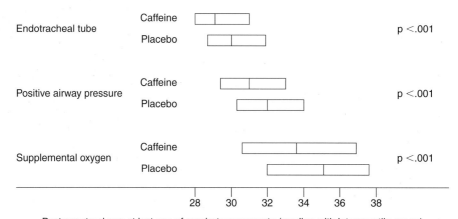

Postmenstrual age at last use of respiratory supports (median with interquartile range)

Fig. 17.1 Effect of caffeine on the postmenstrual age at last use of respiratory supports in the Caffeine for Apnea of Prematurity (CAP) trial.[12]

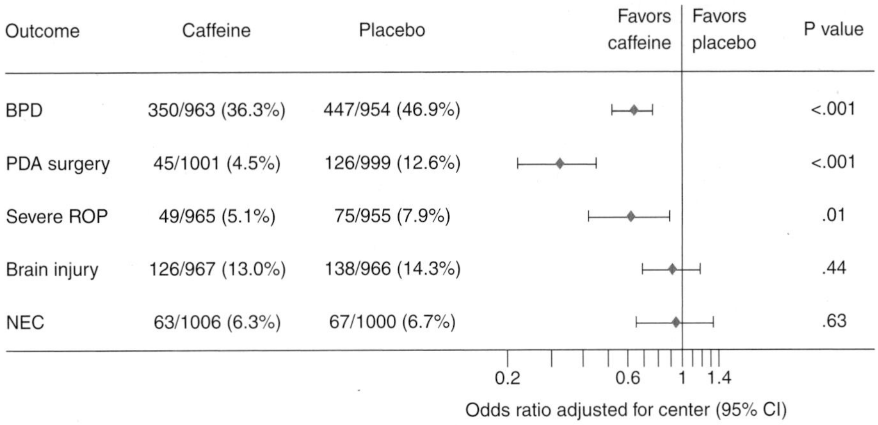

Outcome	Caffeine	Placebo	Favors caffeine	Favors placebo	P value
BPD	350/963 (36.3%)	447/954 (46.9%)			<.001
PDA surgery	45/1001 (4.5%)	126/999 (12.6%)			<.001
Severe ROP	49/965 (5.1%)	75/955 (7.9%)			.01
Brain injury	126/967 (13.0%)	138/966 (14.3%)			.44
NEC	63/1006 (6.3%)	67/1000 (6.7%)			.63

0.2   0.6   1 1.4
Odds ratio adjusted for center (95% CI)

Fig. 17.2 Effect of caffeine on selected morbidities in the Caffeine for Apnea of Prematurity (CAP) trial.[12,13] *BPD,* Bronchopulmonary dysplasia; *NEC,* necrotizing enterocolitis; *PDA,* patent ductus arteriosus; *ROP,* retinopathy of prematurity.

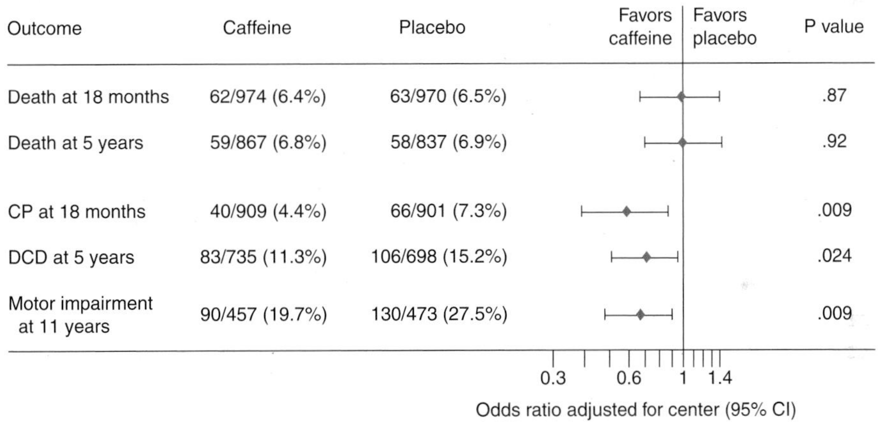

Outcome	Caffeine	Placebo	Favors caffeine	Favors placebo	P value
Death at 18 months	62/974 (6.4%)	63/970 (6.5%)			.87
Death at 5 years	59/867 (6.8%)	58/837 (6.9%)			.92
CP at 18 months	40/909 (4.4%)	66/901 (7.3%)			.009
DCD at 5 years	83/735 (11.3%)	106/698 (15.2%)			.024
Motor impairment at 11 years	90/457 (19.7%)	130/473 (27.5%)			.009

0.3   0.6   1 1.4
Odds ratio adjusted for center (95% CI)

Fig. 17.3 Effect of caffeine on death and motor impairment in survivors in the Caffeine for Apnea of Prematurity (CAP) trial.[13-16] *CP,* Cerebral palsy; *DCD,* Developmental Coordination Disorder.

CAP trial analysis was post hoc, the data necessary to assign the diagnosis of DCD had been collected prospectively during the 5-year follow-up visit.[14,19]

The risk of motor impairment remained lower in the caffeine than in the placebo group among selected CAP trial centers that participated in a final follow-up phase conducted when the children had reached the age of 11 years.[15] This benefit of caffeine on motor skills in middle school age was consistent with the earlier findings showing that caffeine reduced the risk of cerebral palsy at 18 months and DCD at 5 years.[13,14] Indeed, the relative treatment effects of caffeine (odds ratio adjusted for center with 95% confidence intervals) were remarkably similar at all three time points, despite substantial differences in the definitions of motor impairment and irrespective of the size of the follow-up cohorts (Fig. 17.3).

Caffeine also improved visuomotor, visuoperceptual, and visuospatial abilities at age 11 years.[20] There were no adverse effects on general intelligence, attention, and executive function.[20] Self-reported health-related quality of life was similar among the study participants who had been assigned to caffeine and placebo.[21]

WHAT MAY EXPLAIN THE LASTING BENEFIT OF CAFFEINE ON MOTOR SKILLS?

The [CAP] trial did not record the incidence of apnea in either arm of the study, but caffeine-treated infants received significantly less mechanical ventilation, oxygen therapy, and treatment with postnatal steroids, consistent with the decreased incidence of bronchopulmonary dysplasia. Apnea events are frequently associated with bradycardias and desaturations, which result in short-term interventions such as increased ventilatory support, increased oxygen exposure, increased stimulation, and interventions such as evaluation for infection. Thus, the benefits of caffeine result from prevention of interventions generally suspected of adverse long-term neurodevelopmental effects. Caffeine likely is not a direct brain or a lung drug but, rather, a drug that decreases adverse effects of interventions to treat apnea.[22]

Post hoc explanatory logistic regression analyses of the CAP trial data support this conclusion by Alan Jobe. During the initial hospitalization, study participants were weaned off all devices that deliver positive airway pressure (with or without an endotracheal tube) on average 1 week sooner in the caffeine group than in the placebo group.[12] This earlier discontinuation of any positive airway pressure alone explained 49% of the beneficial effect of caffeine on the combined outcome of death or disability at 18 months.[13] The postmenstrual age at last use of any positive airway pressure was by far the single most important of the following six potential explanatory variables that were examined:[13]

- postmenstrual age at last use of positive airway pressure through an endotracheal tube
- postmenstrual age at last use of any positive airway pressure
- postmenstrual age at last use of supplemental oxygen
- use of postnatal corticosteroids
- surgery to close a patent ductus arteriosus
- BPD, defined as receipt of supplemental oxygen at a postmenstrual age of 36 weeks.

When the children were 11 years old, a single post hoc logistic regression analysis was performed and showed that the postmenstrual age at the last use of any positive airway pressure explained 53% of the observed caffeine benefit on the outcome of motor impairment, with 95% confidence intervals of 22% to 100%.[15]

These explanatory analyses of possible mechanisms for the observed benefits at 18 months and 11 years are consistent with one another. They suggest that earlier discontinuation of all devices that deliver positive airway pressure—facilitated by neonatal caffeine therapy—may be responsible for much of the long-term treatment effect of caffeine in the CAP trial. The immediate respiratory stimulant action of caffeine in infants with apnea of prematurity thus appears to have clinical benefits that last into middle school age.

SAFETY OF CAFFEINE IN THE CAFFEINE FOR APNEA OF PREMATURITY TRIAL

Clinical Signs of Drug Toxicity

Clinical signs of caffeine toxicity were rare in CAP trial participants. Study drug doses were held or reduced for signs of suspected toxicity such as tachycardia, tachypnea, jitteriness, tremors, unexplained seizures, and vomiting in 2.3% of the infants in the caffeine group and 1.4% in the placebo group.[12] Plasma concentrations of caffeine were not measured because therapeutic drug monitoring is unnecessary at the caffeine doses used in the CAP trial.[5]

Growth

Although caffeine has been shown to increase oxygen consumption,[23] growth was not adversely affected in the CAP trial. Infants in the caffeine group gained less weight during the first 3 weeks after randomization than infants in the placebo group, but this difference disappeared during subsequent weeks.[12] Height, weight, and head circumference were similar in the caffeine and placebo groups at 18 months and 5 and 11 years.[13-15]

Behavior

Very preterm birth increases the risk of behavior problems later in childhood.[24] Concerns had been raised in the biomedical literature that methylxanthine therapy for apnea of prematurity may contribute to abnormal behaviors by altering the ontogeny of the adenosine receptor system in the developing brain.[11] However, the CAP trial findings did not suggest that exposure to caffeine increased behavior problems at early and middle school age.[14,15]

Sleep

Based on data in experimental animals, it had been hypothesized that exposure of the developing brain to caffeine may have persistent adverse effects on sleep.[25] Home sleep studies in 201 Canadian and Australian CAP trial participants at school age did not reveal any long-term detrimental effects of caffeine on sleep quality, quantity, or sleep disorders.[26] When compared with normative data obtained in children born at term, the prevalence of obstructive sleep apnea and periodic limb movements was increased in this CAP trial cohort of ex-preterm infants irrespective of their prior exposure to caffeine or placebo.[26]

Remaining Uncertainties About Neonatal Caffeine Therapy

WHAT IS THE OPTIMAL CAFFEINE DOSING REGIMEN?

Standard doses of caffeine citrate (20 mg/kg loading and 5–10 mg/kg/day maintenance) exert their pharmacodynamic action on respiratory control through interaction with adenosine receptors. Higher than standard doses will result in plasma concentrations at which the pharmacologic actions of caffeine become more complex and worrisome.[5]

Caffeine proved to be safe in the CAP trial. However, this conclusion should not be generalized to uses of caffeine that deviate substantially from the CAP trial protocol.

Sixty percent of the CAP trial participants had their daily maintenance dose of caffeine citrate increased above 5 mg/kg. The median drug dose throughout the treatment period in the caffeine group overall was 6.7 mg/kg per day (Unpublished data).

Some clinicians prescribe higher loading and maintenance doses than those tested in the CAP trial and recommended by the American Academy of Pediatrics.[1,12] According to a survey that was published in 2016, Australian neonatal consultants administer loading doses of caffeine citrate up to 80 mg/kg and daily maintenance doses up to 20 mg/kg.[27] Between 2010 and 2013, across 4 US neonatal intensive care units and 410 infants with gestational ages of 28 weeks or less, the median maximum daily maintenance dose of caffeine citrate was 16 mg/kg (interquartile range 10–20).[28]

There is insufficient evidence from RCTs comparing high with standard doses that this practice is effective and safe. The largest trial to date enrolled 287 infants less than 30 weeks' gestation at four Australian neonatal intensive care units between September 1996 and April 1999.[29] A total of 238 mechanically ventilated infants were randomly assigned to high or standard doses of caffeine within a "peri-extubation" stratum, and the remaining 49 infants were randomized within a "treatment of apnea" stratum.[29] Loading and maintenance doses of caffeine citrate were 80 mg/kg and 20 mg/kg per day in the high-dose group. Standard loading and maintenance doses of 20 mg/kg and 5 mg/kg per day were used in the comparison group.[29] This trial had a troubled publication history. Outcomes to hospital discharge and at 12 months were first reported in 2004, but only for the "peri-extubation" stratum.[30] Outcomes for the entire trial cohort between randomization and follow-up were reported 7 years later.[29] The time lag between the study reports and the duplicate publication of outcomes for infants in the larger peri-extubation stratum may have confounded some meta-analysts. Other limitations include 14% post-randomization exclusions and 13% attrition for the outcome of disability in survivors at one year.[29]

One other RCT reported outcomes beyond the initial hospital discharge, but the study was small and suffered from substantial loss to follow-up. Moreover, the contrast between the two dosing regimens was trivial, since only the loading dose but not the maintenance dose differed slightly between the comparison groups.[31]

Two teams of investigators reported outcomes to hospital discharge in the English language for RCTs in which doses of caffeine citrate were studied beyond those tested in the CAP trial.[32,33] After excluding the trial by McPherson et al., because it lacked a meaningful contrast between high and standard doses of caffeine, the pooled estimate of the three remaining trials shows that high-dose caffeine may reduce the risk of BPD at 36 weeks' postmenstrual age (Fig. 17.4).[29,32,33] The authors of recent systematic reviews reached the same conclusion, despite differing on the trials they included and the data they extracted from those trials for the outcome of BPD.[34-36] However, all review teams agreed that the evidence remains

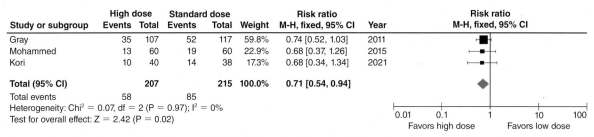

| Study or subgroup | High dose | | Standard dose | | Weight | Risk ratio | Year | Risk ratio |
	Events	Total	Events	Total		M-H, fixed, 95% CI		M-H, fixed, 95% CI
Gray	35	107	52	117	59.8%	0.74 [0.52, 1.03]	2011	
Mohammed	13	60	19	60	22.9%	0.68 [0.37, 1.26]	2015	
Kori	10	40	14	38	17.3%	0.68 [0.34, 1.34]	2021	
Total (95% CI)		**207**		**215**	**100.0%**	**0.71 [0.54, 0.94]**		
Total events	58		85					

Heterogeneity: Chi² = 0.07, df = 2 (P = 0.97); I² = 0%
Test for overall effect: Z = 2.42 (P = 0.02)

0.01   0.1   1   10   100
Favors high dose   Favors low dose

Fig. 17.4 Forest plot of randomized trials comparing high with standard doses of caffeine on bronchopulmonary dysplasia (BPD) at 36 weeks' postmenstrual age. Data were pooled using Review Manager (RevMan) 5.4.

weak for the clinical use of higher than standard doses, due to high risks of bias in the published trials, and imprecision of the observed treatment effects.[34-36]

Plasma elimination and clearance of caffeine are prolonged in the newborn but improve with increasing postnatal age and this may require dose adjustments over time.[5]

In the CAP trial, daily maintenance doses were adjusted weekly for changes in bodyweight.[12] Simulation studies have suggested that this adjustment for increasing weight may be insufficient to maintain stable drug levels throughout the first 8 weeks of life. It has been suggested further that dose adjustments by 1 mg/kg every 1 to 2 weeks may be required in response to the developmental changes in the pharmacokinetics of caffeine in preterm infants.[37] This hypothesis should be tested in a future RCT.

WHEN TO START CAFFEINE

In the CAP trial, infants could be enrolled up to 10 days after birth, but the median age at randomization was 3 days.[12] This means that the study drug was started soon after birth in half of the trial cohort, and that early starting of caffeine therapy in appropriately selected patients is an evidence-based practice. Furthermore, a post hoc subgroup analysis of the CAP trial raised the hypothesis that initiation of caffeine before 3 days may be associated with a greater reduction in time on respiratory support with or without an endotracheal tube.[38]

Who are appropriate candidates for neonatal caffeine therapy? In the CAP trial, 41% of all study participants were enrolled to treat documented apnea, 23% to prevent apnea and 36% to facilitate the removal of an endotracheal tube.[12] The incidence of apnea increases with decreasing gestational age and can be assumed to be universal in infants born before 29 weeks' gestation.[1] It is therefore reasonable to prescribe prophylactic caffeine for all extremely preterm infants soon after delivery unless they are fully ventilated and there are no immediate plans for a trial of extubation. Since problems with respiratory control are less pervasive in moderately and late preterm infants, caffeine therapy should only be prescribed for these more mature infants when apnea develops.[39]

It remains uncertain if fully ventilated extremely preterm infants would benefit from early initiation of caffeine therapy. Such infants cannot manifest overt apnea, and they were unlikely to be enrolled in the CAP trial soon after birth.[39] One recent single center RCT of earlier versus later caffeine in mechanically ventilated very preterm failed to show that early caffeine reduced the age at first successful extubation.[40] However, this trial should be considered inconclusive because of its small sample size and its early termination of recruitment.[40] Future trials in this small subgroup of very immature infants are needed.

WHEN TO STOP CAFFEINE

In the California Infant Functional Status Study of 865 infants with gestational ages between 24 and 32 weeks, the median postmenstrual age at the last recorded apnea was 35.6 (interquartile range 34.3–37.3) for infants born before 27 weeks and 33.3 (interquartile range 32.4–34.4) for infants born after 30 weeks.[41] BPD is associated with a delay in the maturation of respiratory control.[41,42] The most extremely premature infants may experience apnea beyond their term corrected age.[42] Therefore, the decision to stop caffeine should be individualized and the postmenstrual age at last use of caffeine should be expected to vary within and between neonatal intensive care units. A retrospective cohort study involving 304 US neonatal intensive care units during the years 2001 to 2016 did show that the timing of caffeine discontinuation varied from 32 to 37 weeks' postmenstrual age. However, this variability appeared to occur irrespective of the infants' gestational age, and the level of respiratory support at the time caffeine was stopped.[43]

No RCTs have compared different approaches to the termination of neonatal caffeine therapy. One ongoing trial explores whether prolonged administration of caffeine and continuation of therapy at home reduces the duration of hospitalization for moderately preterm infants.[44] A second trial is underway to examine the effect of prolonged caffeine therapy on the risk of intermittent hypoxemia.[45]

Is Caffeine a Magic Bullet?

Paul Ehrlich, a 1908 Nobel Prize winner for Physiology and Medicine and the "father" of chemotherapy, coined the term "Zauberkugel" (magic bullet) for a drug that eradicates microbes without damaging the host cells.[46] Since then, the term "magic bullet" has been used more generally in medicine to describe a perfect drug that has a desired main effect without harmful side effects.

Although caffeine is effective and safe when used as prescribed by the CAP trial protocol, it is not a magic bullet. Standard doses of caffeine reduce but do not eliminate the risks of apneas, BPD, severe ROP, and childhood motor impairment in very preterm infants. Referring to caffeine as a "magic bullet" is not only misleading but may also worsen the treatment creep that is evident in high-income countries and even encouraged by some national and regional guidelines.[47-49] At the same time, caffeine remains unavailable and unaffordable in many low- and middle-income countries including sub-Saharan Africa.[50-52]

REFERENCES

1. Eichenwald EC, Committee on Fetus and Newborn, American Academy of Pediatrics. Apnea of prematurity. *Pediatrics.* 2016;137(1). doi:10.1542/peds.2015-3757.
2. Erickson G, Dobson NR, Hunt CE. Immature control of breathing and apnea of prematurity: the known and unknown. *J Perinatol.* 2021;41(9):2111-2123.
3. Ramanathan R, Corwin MJ, Hunt CE, et al. Cardiorespiratory events recorded on home monitors: comparison of healthy infants with those at increased risk for SIDS. *JAMA.* 2001;285(17):2199-2207.
4. Henderson-Smart DJ, Steer PA. Caffeine versus theophylline for apnea in preterm infants. *Cochrane Database Syst Rev.* 2010;20(1):CD000273.
5. Aranda JV, Beharry KD. Pharmacokinetics, pharmacodynamics and metabolism of caffeine in newborns. *Semin Fetal Neonatal Med.* 2020;25(6):101183.
6. Erenberg A, Leff RD, Haack DG, et al. Caffeine citrate for the treatment of apnea of prematurity: a double-blind, placebo-controlled study. *Pharmacotherapy.* 2000;20(6):644-652.
7. Available at: https://www.accessdata.fda.gov/drugsatfda_docs/label/2020/020793s019lbl.pdf. Accessed December 15, 2021.
8. Dobson NR, Hunt CE. Caffeine: an evidence-based success story in VLBW pharmacotherapy. *Pediatr Res.* 2018;84(3):333-340.
9. Kreutzer K, Bassler D. Caffeine for apnea of prematurity: a neonatal success story. *Neonatology.* 2014;105(4):332-336.
10. Schmidt B. Methylxanthine therapy in premature infants: sound practice, disaster, or fruitless byway? *J Pediatr.* 1999;135(4):526-528.
11. Millar D, Schmidt B. Controversies surrounding xanthine therapy. *Semin Neonatol.* 2004;9(3):239-244.
12. Schmidt B, Roberts RS, Davis P, et al. Caffeine therapy for apnea of prematurity. *N Engl J Med.* 2006;354(20):2112-2121.
13. Schmidt B, Roberts RS, Davis P, et al. Long-term effects of caffeine therapy for apnea of prematurity. *N Engl J Med.* 2007;357(19):1893-1902.
14. Schmidt B, Anderson PJ, Doyle LW, et al. Survival without disability to age 5 years after neonatal caffeine therapy for apnea of prematurity. *JAMA.* 2012;307(3):275-282.
15. Schmidt B, Roberts RS, Anderson PJ, et al. Academic performance, motor function, and behavior 11 years after neonatal caffeine citrate therapy for apnea of prematurity: an 11-year follow-up of the CAP Randomized Clinical Trial. *JAMA Pediatr.* 2017;171(6):564-572.
16. Doyle LW, Ranganathan S, Cheong JLY. Neonatal caffeine treatment and respiratory function at 11 years in children under 1,251 g at birth. *Am J Respir Crit Care Med.* 2017;196(10):1318-1324.
17. Bolk J, Farooqi A, Hafström M, et al. Developmental coordination disorder and its association with developmental comorbidities at 6.5 years in apparently healthy children born extremely preterm. *JAMA Pediatr.* 2018;172(8):765-774.
18. Spittle AJ, Dewey D, Nguyen TN, et al. Rates of developmental coordination disorder in children born very preterm. *J Pediatr.* 2021;231:61-67.e2.
19. Doyle LW, Schmidt B, Anderson PJ, et al. Reduction in developmental coordination disorder with neonatal caffeine therapy. *J Pediatr.* 2014;165(2):356-359.
20. Mürner-Lavanchy IM, Doyle LW, Schmidt B, et al. Neurobehavioral outcomes 11 years after neonatal caffeine therapy for apnea of prematurity. *Pediatrics.* 2018;141(5):e20174047.

21. Schmidt B, Anderson PJ, Asztalos EV, et al. Self-reported quality of life at middle school age in survivors of very preterm birth: results from the caffeine for apnea of prematurity trial. *JAMA Pediatr.* 2019;173(5):487-489.

22. Jobe AH. Caffeine: a lung drug for all very low birth weight preterm infants? *Am J Respir Crit Care Med.* 2017;196(10):1241-1243.

23. Bauer J, Maier K, Linderkamp O, et al. Effect of caffeine on oxygen consumption and metabolic rate in very low birth weight infants with idiopathic apnea. *Pediatrics.* 2001;107(4):660-663.

24. Peralta-Carcelen M, Schwartz J, Carcelen AC. Behavioral and socioemotional development in preterm children. *Clin Perinatol.* 2018;45(3):529-546.

25. Montandon G, Horner RL, Kinkead R, et al. Caffeine in the neonatal period induces long-lasting changes in sleep and breathing in adult rats. *J Physiol.* 2009;587:5493-5507.

26. Marcus CL, Meltzer LJ, Roberts RS, et al. Long-term effects of caffeine therapy for apnea of prematurity on sleep at school age. *Am J Respir Crit Care Med.* 2014;190(7):791-799.

27. Gray PH, Chauhan M. Use of caffeine for preterm infants in Australia and New Zealand: a survey. *J Paediatr Child Health.* 2016;52(12):1121-1122.

28. Puia-Dumitrescu M, Smith PB, Zhao J, et al. Dosing and safety of off-label use of caffeine citrate in premature infants. *J Pediatr.* 2019;211:27-32.e1.

29. Gray PH, Flenady VJ, Charles BG, et al. Caffeine citrate for very preterm infants: effects on development, temperament and behaviour. *J Paediatr Child Health.* 2011;47(4):167-172.

30. Steer P, Flenady V, Shearman A, et al. High dose caffeine citrate for extubation of preterm infants: a randomised controlled trial. *Arch Dis Child Fetal Neonatal Ed.* 2004;89(6):F499-F503.

31. McPherson C, Neil JJ, Tjoeng TH, et al. A pilot randomized trial of high-dose caffeine therapy in preterm infants. *Pediatr Res.* 2015;78(2):198-204.

32. Mohammed S, Nour I, Shabaan AE, et al. High versus low-dose caffeine for apnea of prematurity: a randomized controlled trial. *Eur J Pediatr.* 2015;174(7):949-956.

33. Mohd Kori AM, Van Rostenberghe H, Ibrahim NR, et al. A randomized controlled trial comparing two doses of caffeine for apnoea in prematurity. *Int J Environ Res Public Health.* 2021;18(9):4509.

34. Vliegenthart R, Miedema M, Hutten GJ, et al. High versus standard dose caffeine for apnoea: a systematic review. *Arch Dis Child Fetal Neonatal Ed.* 2018;103(6):F523-F529.

35. Pakvasa MA, Saroha V, Patel RM. Optimizing caffeine use and risk of bronchopulmonary dysplasia in preterm infants: a systematic review, meta-analysis, and application of grading of recommendations assessment, development, and evaluation methodology. *Clin Perinatol.* 2018;45(2):273-291.

36. Brattström P, Russo C, Ley D, et al. High-versus low-dose caffeine in preterm infants: a systematic review and meta-analysis. *Acta Paediatr.* 2019;108(3):401-410.

37. Koch G, Datta AN, Jost K, et al. Caffeine citrate dosing adjustments to assure stable caffeine concentrations in preterm neonates. *J Pediatr.* 2017;191:50-56.e1.

38. Davis PG, Schmidt B, Roberts RS, et al. Caffeine for apnea of prematurity trial: benefits may vary in subgroups. *J Pediatr.* 2010;156(3):382-387.

39. Schmidt B, Davis PG, Roberts RS. Timing of caffeine therapy in very low birth weight infants. *J Pediatr.* 2014;164(5):957-958.

40. Amaro CM, Bello JA, Jain D, et al. Early caffeine and weaning from mechanical ventilation in preterm infants: a randomized, placebo-controlled trial. *J Pediatr.* 2018;196:52-57.

41. Bakewell-Sachs S, Medoff-Cooper B, Escobar GJ, et al. Infant functional status: the timing of physiologic maturation of premature infants. *Pediatrics.* 2009;123(5):e878-e886.

42. Eichenwald EC, Aina A, Stark AR. Apnea frequently persists beyond term gestation in infants delivered at 24 to 28 weeks. *Pediatrics.* 1997;100(3 Pt 1):354-359.

43. Ji D, Smith PB, Clark RH, et al. Wide variation in caffeine discontinuation timing in premature infants. *J Perinatol.* 2020;40(2):288-293.

44. Available at: https://clinicaltrials.gov/ct2/show/NCT03340727. Accessed January 13, 2022.

45. Available at: https://clinicaltrials.gov/ct2/show/NCT03321734. Accessed January 13, 2022.

46. Bosch F, Rosich L. The contributions of Paul Ehrlich to pharmacology: a tribute on the occasion of the centenary of his Nobel Prize. *Pharmacology.* 2008;82(3):171-179.

47. Bancalari E. Current management of apnea in premature infants: is caffeine the magic bullet? *Early Hum Dev.* 2014;90(suppl 2):S1-S2.

48. Available at: https://www.nice.org.uk/guidance/ng124/chapter/recommendations. Accessed January 16, 2022.

49. Available at: https://www.health.qld.gov.au/__data/assets/pdf_file/0033/846843/nmq-caffeine-citrate.pdf. Accessed January 16, 2022.

50. Schmidt B. Caffeine editorial. *Semin Fetal Neonatal Med.* 2020;25(6):101181.

51. Ekhaguere OA, Ayede AI, Ezeaka CV. Is caffeine available and affordable in low and middle-income countries? A survey in sub-Saharan Africa. *Semin Fetal Neonatal Med.* 2020;25(6):101182.

52. Nabwera HM, Ekhaguere OA, Kirpalani H, et al. Neonatal Nutrition Network (NeoNuNet). Caffeine for the care of preterm infants in sub-Saharan Africa: a missed opportunity? *BMJ Glob Health.* 2021;6(12):e007682.

Chapter 18

The Neonatal Lung: Lung Imaging Using Ultrasound and Electric Impedance Tomography

Arun Sett, David Gerald Tingay, and Daniele De Luca

Chapter Outline

Abbreviations

Introduction

Lung Ultrasound

  Background of Neonatal Lung Ultrasound

  Lung Ultrasound Technique

  Key Features of Neonatal Lung Ultrasound

  Scoring Systems

  The Learning Curve and Accuracy of Neonatal Lung
    Ultrasound

  Current Applications of Neonatal Lung Ultrasound

Electrical Impedance Tomography

  Principles of EIT

  EIT Image Acquisition and Reconstruction

  EIT Outcome Measures

  Current Neonatal Applications of Electrical
    Impedance Tomography

Conclusions And Future Directions

Key Points

- Lung ultrasound and electrical impedance tomography are point-of-care imaging modalities that provide continuous, radiation-free bedside lung imaging.
- Lung ultrasound relies on the interpretation of reproducible ultrasound artifact patterns that correspond to the degree of lung aeration. It has an established role in the diagnosis of numerous neonatal respiratory disorders.
- Electrical impedance tomography analyzes variations in electrical bioimpedance to provide detailed information on total and regional ventilation and aeration characteristics.
- Both tools have an established role in neonatal research and may improve the care of newborn infants by optimizing respiratory support.

Abbreviations

B-mode	Brightness mode
BPD	Bronchopulmonary dysplasia
CT	Computed tomography
CXR	Chest radiography
EEV	End-expiratory volume
EIT	Electrical impedance tomography
LU	Lung ultrasound
LUS	Lung ultrasound scoring system
M-mode	Motion mode
NICU	Neonatal intensive care unit
RDS	Respiratory distress syndrome
TTN	Transient tachypnea of the newborn

Introduction

Lung imaging is essential to guide neonatal respiratory support. Chest radiographs (CXRs) provide a static picture of the lung, expose infants to ionizing radiation, and correlate poorly with lung volume.[1] Lung ultrasound (LU) and electrical impedance tomography (EIT) are emerging point-of-care imaging modalities. Continuous, radiation-free images make these attractive tools to assess the newborn lung. This chapter will outline the principles, current research, and applications of both modalities.

Lung Ultrasound

HISTORY OF NEONATAL LUNG ULTRASOUND

The high acoustic impedance associated with the aerated lung initially relegated LU to a role as an adjunct to CXRs.[2] Despite early recognition that the presence of air and liquid influences ultrasound propagation, the diagnostic use of LU is a recent development.[3] Ultrasound interaction with the reflective pleura generates reproducible artifacts which vary proportionally with lung aeration. LU is easy to learn and concurs with CXR when distinguishing between the various causes of respiratory distress.[4] This has led to LU being adopted by adult, pediatric and most recently neonatal intensive care clinicians.

LUNG ULTRASOUND TECHNIQUE

High-frequency microlinear transducers are favored for LU due to their higher resolution and ability to scan the small newborn chest.[5] Detailed examination requires both longitudinal and transverse transducer orientation. Longitudinal orientation allows visualization across multiple intercostal spaces. In contrast, transverse orientation facilitates detailed assessment of pleural line integrity.

Homogeneous lung disorders including respiratory distress syndrome (RDS) secondary to primary surfactant deficiency and lung immaturity, where gravity-dependent aeration differences have not yet evolved, are accurately assessed by imaging only the anterior and lateral lung.[8] Posterior imaging improves the diagnostic accuracy for nonhomogeneous lung disorders such as bronchopulmonary dysplasia (BPD).[6-8]

KEY FEATURES OF NEONATAL LUNG ULTRASOUND

Lung Sliding

During real-time scanning, the pleural surface moves with respiration. This phenomenon known as "lung sliding" is an important indicator of pleural apposition and tidal ventilation.

M-Mode

B-mode (brightness mode) imaging is usually accompanied by M-mode (motion mode) confirmation of pleural sliding. The image acquired along a single line of sight is displayed over time, allowing for assessment of moving structures using a still image. Normal lung sliding produces the "seashore" sign (Fig. 18.1).[9]

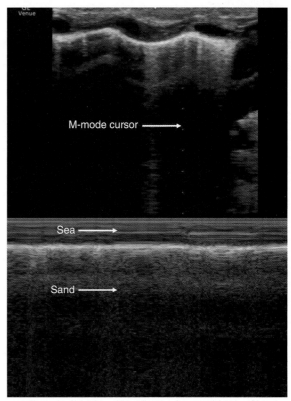

Fig. 18.1 The "seashore" sign. The M-mode cursor is positioned between the rib space and the corresponding M-mode trace is displayed below. The horizontal lines seen in the upper portion of the trace represent the static chest wall and are likened to waves in the sea. The grainy, sand-like appearance of the lower portion of the trace represents the lung ultrasound artifact moving within the M-mode plane.

This indicates apposition of the parietal and visceral pleura and when present, excludes pneumothorax.

A-Lines

A-lines result from a strong reverberation artifact between the pleura and ultrasound transducer. They are echogenic, horizontal lines which are equidistant from the pleura to the transducer (Fig. 18.2). A-lines occur in normal lung but are also dominant in pneumothorax.

B-Lines

B-lines are vertical, echogenic projections originating from the pleura (Fig. 18.3). B-lines move with respiration and originate from a tight reverberation artifact generated by increased lung water content or partial atelectasis.[10] B-lines commonly occur in healthy newborns[11] but the presence of three or more visualized per ultrasound field is considered pathological. With increasing disease severity, B-lines become more numerous and closely spaced. Eventually they become confluent, producing a "white lung" appearance known as the "interstitial-alveolar pattern."[12] B-lines assist evaluation of lung sliding and occur in transient tachypnea of the newborn (TTN), RDS, and other disorders characterized by nonspecific increases in

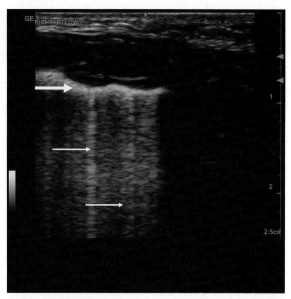

Fig. 18.3 B-lines *(small arrows)* are visualized as linear, vertical lines that originate from the pleural line *(large arrow)* and extend through the image.

lung water content secondary to inflammation or edema.[12-14]

SCORING SYSTEMS

Lung ultrasound scoring systems (LUS) have been developed whereby artifact patterns are categorized based on appearance. A simplified system (Fig. 18.4) using three distinct patterns accurately predicts ventilation requirements and the need for surfactant administration.[15-17] It is also used to monitor the initiation of breathing and transition after birth.[11,18]

Such scoring systems have the advantage of providing a rapid assessment of lung status. However, they do not provide assessments of all lung regions. In adults, detailed scoring systems interrogate multiple areas of the chest. These systems have been validated against computed tomography (CT), measures of lung mechanics, and gas washout techniques.[19] Similar comparisons are difficult in newborns, due to their smaller size and fragility.[5]

In order to overcome these problems, Brat et al. proposed a scoring system for use in newborns (Fig. 18.5).[20] Each lung is divided into three regions and a score of 0 to 3 (normal lung to extensive consolidation)

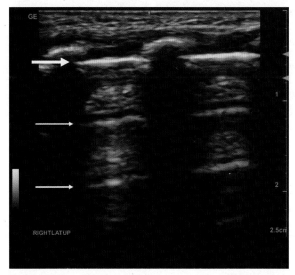

Fig. 18.2 A-lines. The pleural line is seen as a thin, bright, echogenic line *(large arrow)*. A-lines *(small arrows)* formed due to reverberation artifact are seen inferior to the pleural line.

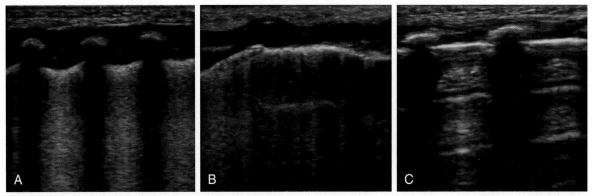

Fig. 18.4 Simplified scoring system proposed by Raimondi et al. (2012). **A,** Type 1 lung pattern, represented by coalescing B-lines forming a "white lung" image. **B,** Type 2 lung pattern represented by numerous B-lines which are not coalescing. **C,** Type 3 lung pattern, represented by predominantly A-lines. (Figure adapted from Raimondi F, Migliaro F, Sodano A, et al. Can neonatal lung ultrasound monitor fluid clearance and predict the need of respiratory support? *Crit Care.* 2012;16(6):R220.)

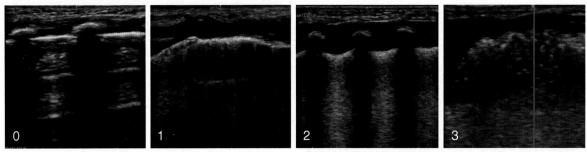

Fig. 18.5 The semi-quantitative scoring system proposed by Brat et al. For each examined area, a score of 0 to 3 is assigned. Scores correspond to four different patterns of lung aeration: 0, A-pattern (defined by A-lines only); 1, B-pattern (defined by ≥3 well-spaced B-lines); 2, severe B-pattern (defined by coalescing B-lines with or without consolidations limited to subpleural space); and 3, extensive consolidation. (Figure adapted from Brat R, Yousef N, Klifa R, et al. Lung ultrasonography score to evaluate oxygenation and surfactant need in neonates treated with continuous positive airway pressure. *JAMA Pediatr.* 2015;169(8):e151797.)

is assigned. This permits more detailed quantification of lung aeration, accounts for regional difference in LU findings, and correlates with oxygenation indices and endogenous surfactant function.[20-23] This scoring system is now widely used in newborn research to predict the need for respiratory support and surfactant administration and identify infants at risk of developing BPD.[7,21]

THE LEARNING CURVE AND ACCURACY OF NEONATAL LUNG ULTRASOUND

In comparison to other point-of-care ultrasound modalities such as echocardiography or cranial ultrasound, LU has a steep but short learning curve. In centers where LU is the preferred lung imaging modality, senior trainees were able to interpret LU to the same degree as experienced clinicians after 1 year of experience.[24] Numerous studies have detailed the accuracy for the LU diagnosis of common neonatal respiratory disorders, including RDS, pneumonia, and pneumothorax, which will be detailed in the remainder of this section.[16,17,20-22,25-27] Despite promising findings, the long-term impact of LU-guided therapies remains to be elucidated.

CURRENT APPLICATIONS OF NEONATAL LUNG ULTRASOUND

Lung Consolidation and Atelectasis

Progressive loss of aeration facilitates ultrasound propagation which reduces artifact formation and allows better imaging of lung tissue. Termed "hepatization,"

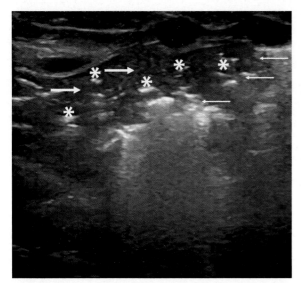

Fig. 18.6 Lung consolidation and atelectasis. The consolidated or atelectatic lung appears similar to liver tissue (hepatization; *large arrows*). Air bronchograms can be visualized *(asterisks)*. The pleural line is interrupted (shred sign; *small arrows*). Coalescing B-lines are seen below the consolidated lung.

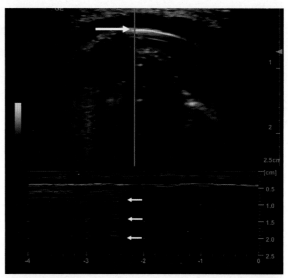

Fig. 18.7 Sonographic findings in pneumothorax. Transverse image of the lung demonstrating "lung point" *(large arrow)*. A sharp transition from a coalescing B-line pattern to a strong A-line profile is observed. Absent lung sliding *(barcode or stratosphere sign)* is demonstrated in the corresponding M-mode trace *(small arrows)*.

the unaerated lung has a similar ultrasound appearance to liver tissue (Fig. 18.6).[28] Interruption of the pleural line, coined the "shred sign" along with transmission of cardiac motion through consolidated lung, termed "lung pulse," aids diagnosis.[29,30] Further differentiation is possible by the visualization of air passing through the small airways (dynamic air bronchograms). However, this is difficult to observe in newborn infants. The reported sensitivity of LU diagnosis of pneumonia in the pediatric neonatal population ranges between 85% and 100%, although most studies were performed by highly experienced investigators.[31] For the diagnosis of atelectasis, LU may outperform CXR when compared to the gold standard of CT[32] and can discriminate gravity-dependent aeration loss.[6]

Pneumothorax

Pneumothorax occurs in up to 9.6% of extremely preterm infants.[33] Air between the parietal and visceral pleura produces an intense reverberation artifact forming a strong A-line profile. Lung sliding and B-lines disappear in the presence of pneumothorax (Fig. 18.7). The sharp transition from normal lung to pneumothorax is termed "lung point."[34] M-mode reveals absent lung sliding, termed the "barcode" or "stratosphere"

sign. The reported sensitivity for LU diagnosis of pneumothorax is 96% to 100% in symptomatic infants.[26,35-37] Rapid availability may expedite intervention in life-threatening situations.[26]

Pleural Effusion

LU is a well-established, accurate method of diagnosing pleural effusion.[38] Fluid attenuation of ultrasound beams leads to a hypoechoic appearance.[2] Fluid collection is gravity-dependent, corresponding to the lower lateral and posterior lung when supine. M-mode demonstrates the "sinusoid" sign; the lung is seen moving freely in extrapleural fluid (Fig. 18.8).[39]

Neonatal Respiratory Distress Syndrome and Surfactant Replacement Therapy

The sonographic appearance of RDS was first described over 20 years ago.[40] Numerous B-lines fuse to form a homogeneous "white lung" artifact with no areas of sparing (Fig. 18.9). This is often associated with subpleural consolidation.[10,41] Ultrasound findings worsen with the severity of RDS, and when used for monitoring disease progression, LU reduces the cumulative radiation exposure of serial chest x-rays.[22,42,43]

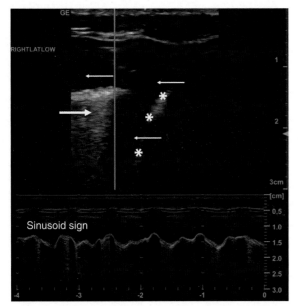

Fig. 18.8 Pleural effusion. Hypoechoic extrapleural fluid *(small arrows)* is seen between the lung *(large arrow)*, diaphragm *(asterisks)*, and chest wall. The corresponding M-mode trace demonstrates the "sinusoid sign."

The reported sensitivity of LU to predict surfactant therapy is 88% to 100%.[17,20,21,25,44] Delivery room LU performed between 5 and 10 minutes of age outperforms oxygen requirements in predicting surfactant need,[17] highlighting the potential of LU to improve the timeliness of surfactant administration.[41,45-47] Currently, studies addressing the long-term impact of LU-guided surfactant therapy are lacking.

Transient Tachypnea of the Newborn

Typical ultrasound findings of TTN include compact B-lines particularly in the hilar zones and relative sparing of nondependent regions, termed "double-lung point" (Fig. 18.10).[13] However, "double-lung point" is only present in approximately 50% of infants with TTN.[27] More importantly, when interpreted within the clinical context of the infant's presentation, LU can accurately distinguish TTN from RDS. Accurate diagnosis may allow clinicians to better allocate resources, initiate early respiratory support, and promptly transfer infants to tertiary centers for ongoing management.[27,48-50]

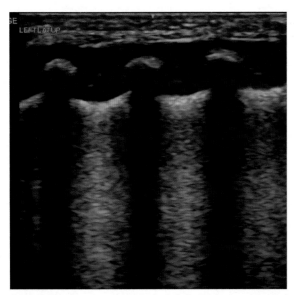

Fig. 18.9 Sonographic appearance of RDS. Numerous coalescing B-lines produce a "white lung" artifact pattern. *RDS,* Respiratory distress syndrome.

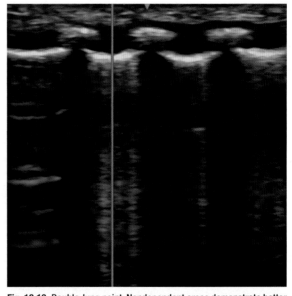

Fig. 18.10 Double-lung point: Nondependent areas demonstrate better aeration (left side, A-line predominant) compared to the more dependent lung (right side, numerous B-lines).

Bronchopulmonary Dysplasia

Despite advances in neonatal respiratory therapy, rates of BPD remain high.[51] The use of LU for early prediction of BPD is of interest as it allows for serial, noninvasive monitoring of lung aeration. Combined with early prediction of BPD, this may allow for more targeted, individualized interventions and monitoring of disease evolution.[52]

The non-homogeneous nature of BPD is captured using LU. Commonly, a heterogenous appearance comprising consolidation, coalescing B-lines, "white lung" artifact and normal lung is observed (Fig. 18.11). Recent studies have demonstrated promising accuracy for early diagnosis of BPD, with reported sensitivities between 70% and 93%.[7,53-55] The use of LU to allow targeted treatment of infants at risk of BPD requires further evaluation.

Electrical Impedance Tomography

EIT has been a lung imaging research tool for more than 30 years.[56] Interest in EIT has increased recently with the emergence of simple-to-use wearable electrode belts, accurate image reconstruction algorithms, and clinical devices for use in critical care, including infants.[57] These advances coincided with the first international consensus on the use of chest EIT, detailing the standards for execution of EIT imaging, analysis, and outcome measures.[56] This provided researchers and clinicians with a common framework to use EIT in the neonatal intensive care unit (NICU). Like LU, EIT is radiation-free, noninvasive and provides functional rather than static information about the lung. Compared to LU, EIT offers the ability to image the lungs in their entirety, calculate multiple measures

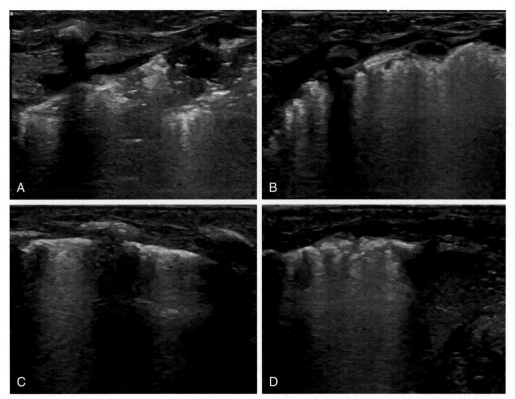

Fig. 18.11 Typical sonographic appearance of BPD. Images from the right anterior upper (A), left anterior upper (B), left lateral lower (C), and right lateral lower (D) regions are shown. A mixture of coalescing B-lines, pleural line abnormalities, and consolidation is observed. *BPD*, Bronchopulmonary dysplasia.

of aeration, ventilation, and mechanics, and can be applied over longer periods via wearable technology and bedside displays.[58]

PRINCIPLES OF ELECTRICAL IMPEDANCE TOMOGRAPHY

EIT is based on the principle that all tissues in the body alter electrical conductivity.[56] Within the chest, the high air content of lung tissue significantly "impedes" conductivity compared to other thoracic organs. EIT measures the changes in electrical conductivity in the lung during ventilation, allowing lung gas behavior within specific regions of the chest to be mapped.[56,59,60]

In infants, all devices use a small nonconstricting 16–32 electrode belt that measures the electrical voltages from repeated applications of very small alternating electrical currents through pairs of electrodes (Fig. 18.12). Belts minimize interoperator variability and improve accuracy of image reconstruction. Belts are usually placed at the nipple level. Current electrode belts are easy and quick to apply, with some incorporating electrode filaments woven into the primary material.[57] Most commercial infant belts can stay in place for at least 24 hours and can be used in most clinical situations.[58]

ELECTRICAL IMPEDANCE TOMOGRAPHY IMAGE ACQUISITION AND RECONSTRUCTION

Measures of electrical conductivity need to be contextualized to the pathophysiology being investigated.

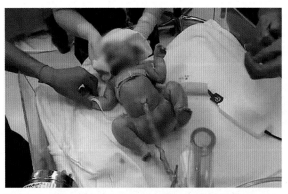

Fig. 18.12 An electrical impedance tomography (EIT) belt in situ on an infant during resuscitative management at birth. (Reproduced with permission from Tingay DG, Farrell O, Thomson J, et al. Imaging the respiratory transition at birth: unraveling the complexities of the first breaths of life. *Am J Respir Crit Care Med.* 2021;204(1):82-91.)

This is achieved by creating user-defined images, waves, or values of lung volumes and mechanics over time. The raw electrical activity is reconstructed into images of lung contents within a cross-sectional slice of the lungs (similar to CT) using age-specific mathematical models of the shape and contents of the chest.[56,59,61-63] EIT software allows clinicians to select different lung regions (such as a specific part of the right or left lung) and choose a suite of outcome measures to indicate lung function over single or multiple breaths.[56]

ELECTRICAL IMPEDANCE TOMOGRAPHY OUTCOME MEASURES

An advantage of EIT is the ability to generate many user-defined measures of lung function based on the clinical need. These include measures of tidal ventilation, aeration or end-expiratory volume (EEV), gas flow, and adverse events, such as atelectasis, overdistension, and air leak (Table 18.1).[56] Although electrical conductivity in the lung can be calibrated to absolute volumes, this is rarely undertaken in infants. EIT is generally used to describe relative changes in lung function. Lung function measures can be generated for the whole lung or individual regions that may be compared (measures of heterogeneity). Heterogeneity is particularly relevant in neonatal lung diseases. In many, the disease severity is defined by heterogeneity of lung volumes (such as RDS, pneumonia, and BPD).

CURRENT NEONATAL APPLICATIONS OF ELECTRICAL IMPEDANCE TOMOGRAPHY

Understanding Lung-Ventilator Interactions and Disease States

The attractiveness of EIT as a research tool is due to its ability to generate a diverse range of lung function measures simultaneously. This has allowed researchers to describe the lung's response to ventilatory changes at a level of resolution not currently available using other methods. EIT has been used to demonstrate how synchronization may improve lung function, describe response to surfactant, and lung ventilation-perfusion mismatching.[64-68] The ability to image different parts of the lung offers promise in complex neonatal lung diseases where evidence-based lung protective strategies are lacking, such as congenital diaphragmatic hernia.

TABLE 18.1 Commonly Used EI Measures and Terms

EIT Term	Abbreviation	Definition
Arbitrary units	A.U.	The measurement unit is commonly used in EIT to quantify the amplitude of impedance changes within EIT image pixels. As EIT data are rarely presented in units of volume, it is thus common to express the image units as "arbitrary." When A.U. data are presented, all differences are relative and an absolute change of 1 A.U. between two subjects should not be assumed to represent the same absolute volume change.
Functional EIT image	fEIT	An EIT image calculated from a time series of EIT images, designed to characterize a particular physiological feature. Each fEIT image pixel is calculated from that pixel's time series values. fEIT images can be based on the EIT data alone, such as tidal images, or based on EIT and additional monitoring data, such as images of regional opening pressures.
Global		A calculated EIT value or measure that represents the entire EIT cross-sectional area and thus the entire lung.
Pixel		The smallest element in a digital image and reflects the resolution of an EIT image. EIT images are reconstructed and displayed with an image size that depends on the algorithm and EIT system. The image size is based on the number of electrodes; 32 electrodes create 32×32 pixels along the horizontal rows and vertical columns.
Region of interest	ROI	An area within an EIT image on which further analysis is performed, such as part or whole of the right lung.

EIT Measure	Abbreviation	Definition
Ventilation Distribution		
Ventilation ratio	A/P or R/L ratio	The ratio of the sum of ventilation in one hemithorax to another, such as right and left, or gravity-dependent (anterior/posterior or ventral/dorsal). A value of 1.0 indicating equal ventilation. This ratio does not account for differing anatomical size of ROI. This can be accounted for if known (see relative distribution of aeration).
Center of ventilation	CoV	A fEIT measure used to quantify the distribution of ventilation in relation to the anteroposterior or right-to-left chest diameter and expressed as percentage. The geometric center of fEIT pixels is calculated and expressed as a fraction of the vertical (gravity-dependent) or horizontal (right-left) image size. In the former case, values lower than the ideal geometric center imply that ventilation is predominantly directed toward ventral (anterior) regions, and in the latter one towards the right lung. As the lungs are not equally sized in the chest, EIT systems usually provide information on the value that represents ideal CoV.
Global inhomogeneity index	GI	Difference between each pixel value and the median of all pixels. Similar to CoV provides a single numeric value to characterize the overall degree of spatial heterogeneity of ventilation, with a value of 1.0 representing uniform ventilation.[93]
Relative V_T in a ROI	%V_T or V_T (%)	The percentage of the entire V_T delivered to the lung during one or more inflations that is delivered to a user-selected ROI. If absolute V_T in mL is known, this value may be used for calibration.
Regional tidal variation	TV_{ROI}	The variation in tidal ventilation over time in a ROI.
Aeration Distribution		
Relative distribution of aeration		The ratio of the percentage of global EELV occurring within a specific ROI to the percentage of the lung within the cross-sectional slice included within the ROI anatomically. A value of 1.0 indicates homogenous aeration with the lung plane, for example, right and left lung. A value >1.0 suggests that aeration is relatively greater than the anatomical contribution of that ROI and may indicate overdistension and <1.0 atelectasis. This measure provides an indication of volume state of the lung.[89]

Continued on following page

TABLE 18.1	Commonly Used EI Measures and Terms (Continued)	
EIT Term	Abbreviation	Definition
Relative change in end-expiratory lung volume	$\Delta EELV_{ROI}$ or ΔEEV_{ROI}	The relative change in end-expiratory EIT signal between two points in time, expressed as a change in A.U., normalized to the distribution of all $\Delta EELV_{ROI}$ during the time series or calibrated to a known volume. The same measure can be used to calculate end inspiratory change (EILV or EIV).[82]
Others		
Time-difference EIT		The difference in the behavior of the time course signal in one ROI compared to another.
Percentage unventilated lung		The number of pixels within the global or ROI signal in which no tidal change in impedance is detected. This provides a measure of the amount of lung in which there was no apparent tidal ventilation (as a percentage of all pixels within the ROI). A pixel with no tidal impedance change may be due to atelectasis, overdistension, or sampling of non-lung tissue (especially common at the margins of image reconstruction models).
Relative measures of mechanics	C_{dynROI}	The change in lung impedance (A.U.) during an inflation or expiration relative to distending pressure (dynamic compliance; A.U./cm H_2O) or time (flow; A.U./s) or the time constant.
Relative Perfusion		Cyclical EIT data within the global signal or ROI related to raw EIT data filtered to the heart rate, and with exclusion of respiratory-related data. Provides an estimate of relative end-diastolic and end-systolic fluid status (e.g., blood) and thus perfusion.

EELV, End-expiratory lung volume; *EIT*, electrical impedance tomography.

More detailed information can be found in the online supplement of Frerichs I, Amato MB, van Kaam AH, et al. Chest electrical impedance tomography examination, data analysis, terminology, clinical use and recommendations: consensus statement of the TRanslational EIT developmeNt stuDy group. *Thorax*. 2017;72(1):83-93.

As EIT does not require constricting or complex measurement equipment, it is the only bedside method of measuring normal breathing patterns, body position, and lung function in neonates. EIT has repeatedly demonstrated that spontaneous breathing in both term and preterm infants preferentially ventilates the dependent lung.[65,69-73] This is contrary to the classic description of nondependent ventilation during acute RDS due to secondary lung injury.[64,74,75]

Electrical Impedance Tomography and Noninvasive Ventilation

A drawback of increased use of noninvasive ventilation is the loss of detailed respiratory function monitoring to guide care. EIT has been used to document the resultant EEV changes during and after extubation of preterm infants to noninvasive respiratory support,[71,74,76] consistently demonstrating a potential for greater heterogeneity of ventilation without oxygenation changes, even when EEV is maintained. This raises the potential for EIT to guide noninvasive ventilation settings. Changes in global and regional EEV have been identified when continuous positive airway pressure (CPAP) levels are altered. EIT may be used to describe the degree of lung hysteresis and identify the optimal pressure to apply.[76] EIT has also been used to describe the mechanistic impact of different modes of noninvasive support, including CPAP, nasal high-flow therapy, bilevel positive airway pressure, and nasal high-frequency ventilation.[69,77]

Electrical Impedance Tomography and Lung Recruitment

EIT was originally proposed as a method of guiding lung recruitment in the diseased lung. EIT-guided PEEP-based lung recruitment improved oxygenation in trials of adults with acute respiratory distress syndrome (ARDS) compared to standard approaches.[78,79] Promising benefits in clinical outcomes, including mortality, were reported; however, large clinical trials are still required. EIT can be used to map the volume response during open lung volume approaches during high-frequency oscillatory ventilation, including over-distension and derecruitment, as well as identify volume stability after a mean airway pressure change.[58,80-82]

Identifying Adverse Events

Respiratory adverse events such as air leak are unfortunately common in the NICU. EIT provides a simple visual display, ideal for rapidly evolving lung volume changes. Preclinical studies have shown that EIT can identify endotracheal tube placement in a main bronchus before clinical instability and without the need for chest radiography (Fig. 18.13).[83] Preclinical studies have also shown that EIT can identify and localize air leak before changes in oxygenation,[84-86] and more interestingly identify changes in the impacted lung region before the air leak occurred.[87] The CRADL project demonstrated that EIT can be used for continuous monitoring in the NICU.[58] This provides the potential to use EIT as continuous lung monitoring in high-risk infants, with LU to aid further diagnosis when needed.

Electrical Impedance Tomography in the Delivery Room

Cardiorespiratory monitoring is difficult in the delivery room and often limited to pulse oximetry and/or electrocardiograms. Detailed measures of lung function currently require the use of a facemask, the accuracy of which is often limited by mask leak or imposed stress on the neonate from application. EIT is ideal for assessing air-fluid interfaces and has been used to image the lung of healthy term infants at birth, providing the first detailed breath-by-breath images of concurrent aeration, ventilation, and gas flow within the lungs.[88] EIT was able to identify differences in the right, left, ventral, and dorsal lung during the respiratory transition. These unique breathing patterns may identify infants who require respiratory assistance and subsequently assess the effectiveness of resuscitative measures.

Electrical Impedance Tomography and Bronchopulmonary Dysplasia

Validated simple and reproducible measures of ventilation inhomogeneity, specifically center of ventilation (CoV) and global inhomogeneity (GI) index that are standard on current EIT systems, have been used to describe the multifactorial progressive processes that lead to and characterize BPD. In an observational study of 40 preterm infants, the magnitude of gravity-dependent ventilation inhomogeneity in the first month after birth was associated with a subsequent BPD diagnosis.[69] The same EIT measures have been shown to be closely correlated with molecular markers of acute injury in the lungs of preterm lambs—the first time any lung imaging tool has been related directly to lung injury at a molecular level.[89]

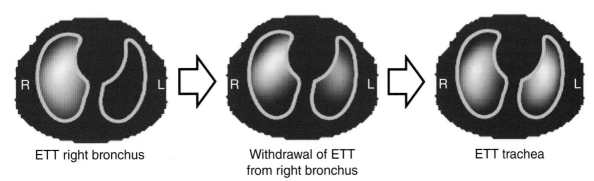

| ETT right bronchus | Withdrawal of ETT from right bronchus | ETT trachea |

Fig. 18.13 Functional electrical impedance tomography (fEIT) images of the distribution of tidal ventilation during three single inflations following intubation demonstrating the ease in which electrical impedance tomography (EIT) can identify inadvertent main bronchus intubation and correct location of an ETT. In these fEIT, the magnitude of tidal ventilation in each pixel of the lungs is given a sequentially uniform color scale from black (no ventilation) to lighter blues to white (highest ventilation). The first fEIT is an inflation immediately after intubation and shows all tidal ventilation in the right lung, indicating right main bronchus intubation. As the clinician withdraws the ETT during continuous EIT imaging increasing ventilation can be seen in the left lung (second fEIT), until the ETT is correctly placed in the trachea and even ventilation is demonstrated in both lungs.

Conclusions and Future Directions

Neonatal lung diseases, and the NICU setting, are ideally suited to bedside lung imaging. LU in neonatal intensive care has exponentially grown over the last decade.[90] Excellent interobserver agreement, comparatively easy learning, and ready availability have led to enthusiastic uptake by many international centers.[24,91,92] LU has demonstrated impressive diagnostic accuracy for a wide variety of neonatal respiratory conditions with potential to improve outcomes being demonstrated in early randomized controlled trials. EIT is an established research tool that has been fundamental to improving our understanding of neonatal lung diseases. The recent availability of clinical infant EIT systems provides an ideal synergy with LU, expanding the suite of respiratory measures available and offering continuous bedside monitoring. Future directions include more randomized controlled trials assessing the impact of both LU- and EIT-guided therapies on meaningful outcomes and standardized education programs to increase the use of these promising imaging modalities.

REFERENCES

1. Thome U, Töpfer A, Schaller P, et al. Comparison of lung volume measurements by antero-posterior chest X-ray and the SF6 washout technique in mechanically ventilated infants. *Pediatr Pulmonol.* 1998;26(4):265-272.
2. Wernecke K. Sonographic features of pleural disease. *AJR Am J Roentgenol.* 1997;168(4):1061-1066.
3. Sagar KB, Rhyne TL, Myers GS, et al. Characterization of normal and abnormal pulmonary surface by reflected ultrasound. *Chest.* 1978;74(1):29-33.
4. Corsini I, Parri N, Gozzini E, et al. Lung ultrasound for the differential diagnosis of respiratory distress in neonates. *Neonatology.* 2019;115(1):77-84.
5. Mongodi S, De Luca D, Colombo A, et al. Quantitative lung ultrasound: technical aspects and clinical applications. *Anesthesiology.* 2021;134(6):949-965.
6. Hoshino Y, Arai J, Hirono K, et al. Gravity-induced loss of aeration and atelectasis development in the preterm lung: a serial sonographic assessment. *J Perinatol.* 2022;42(2):231-236.
7. Loi B, Vigo G, Baraldi E, et al. Lung ultrasound to monitor extremely preterm infants and predict bronchopulmonary dysplasia: a multicenter longitudinal cohort study. *Am J Respir Crit Care Med.* 2021;203(11):1398-1409.
8. De Luca D, van Kaam AH, Tingay DG, et al. The Montreux definition of neonatal ARDS: biological and clinical background behind the description of a new entity. *Lancet Respir Med.* 2017;5(8):657-666.
9. Lichtenstein DA, Menu Y. A bedside ultrasound sign ruling out pneumothorax in the critically ill. Lung sliding. *Chest.* 1995;108(5):1345-1348.
10. Copetti R, Cattarossi L, Macagno F, et al. Lung ultrasound in respiratory distress syndrome: a useful tool for early diagnosis. *Neonatology.* 2008;94(1):52-59.
11. Blank DA, Kamlin COF, Rogerson SR, et al. Lung ultrasound immediately after birth to describe normal neonatal transition: an observational study. *Arch Dis Child Fetal Neonatal Ed.* 2018;103(2):F157-F162.
12. Lichtenstein D, Meziere G, Biderman P, et al. The comet-tail artifact. An ultrasound sign of alveolar-interstitial syndrome. *Am J Respir Crit Care Med.* 1997;156(5):1640-1646.
13. Copetti R, Cattarossi L. The 'double lung point': an ultrasound sign diagnostic of transient tachypnea of the newborn. *Neonatology.* 2007;91(3):203-209.
14. Yousef N, Vigo G, Shankar-Aguilera S, et al. Semiquantitative ultrasound assessment of lung aeration correlates with lung tissue inflammation. *Ultrasound Med Biol.* 2020;46(5):1258-1262.
15. Raimondi F, Migliaro F, Sodano A, et al. Can neonatal lung ultrasound monitor fluid clearance and predict the need of respiratory support? *Crit Care.* 2012;16(6):R220.
16. Raimondi F, Migliaro F, Sodano A, et al. Use of neonatal chest ultrasound to predict noninvasive ventilation failure. *Pediatrics.* 2014;134(4):e1089-e1094.
17. Badurdeen S, Kamlin COF, Rogerson SR, et al. Lung ultrasound during newborn resuscitation predicts the need for surfactant therapy in very- and extremely preterm infants. *Resuscitation.* 2021;162:227-235.
18. Blank DA, Rogerson SR, Kamlin COF, et al. Lung ultrasound during the initiation of breathing in healthy term and late preterm infants immediately after birth, a prospective, observational study. *Resuscitation.* 2017;114:59-65.
19. De Luca D. Semiquantititative lung ultrasound scores are accurate and useful in critical care, irrespective of patients' ages: the power of data over opinions. *J Ultrasound Med.* 2020;39(6):1235-1239.
20. Brat R, Yousef N, Klifa R, et al. Lung ultrasonography score to evaluate oxygenation and surfactant need in neonates treated with continuous positive airway pressure. *JAMA Pediatr.* 2015;169(8):e151797.
21. De Martino L, Yousef N, Ben-Ammar R, Raimondi F, Shankar-Aguilera S, De Luca D. Lung ultrasound score predicts surfactant need in extremely preterm neonates. *Paediatrics.* 2018;142(3):e20180463.
22. Raimondi F, Migliaro F, Corsini I, et al. Lung ultrasound score progress in neonatal respiratory distress syndrome. *Pediatrics.* 2021;147(4):e2020030528.
23. Autilio C, Echaide M, Benachi A, et al. A Noninvasive surfactant adsorption test predicting the need for surfactant therapy in preterm infants treated with continuous positive airway pressure. *J Pediatr.* 2017;182:66-73.e1.
24. Gomond-Le Goff C, Vivalda L, Foligno S, Loi B, Yousef N, De Luca D. Effect of different probes and expertise on the interpretation reliability of point-of-care lung ultrasound. *Chest.* 2020;157(4):924-931.
25. Raimondi F, Migliaro F, Corsini I, et al. Neonatal lung ultrasound and surfactant administration: a pragmatic, multicenter study. *Chest.* 2021;160(6):2178-2186.
26. Raimondi F, Rodriguez Fanjul J, Aversa S, et al. Lung ultrasound for diagnosing pneumothorax in the critically Ill neonate. *J Pediatr.* 2016;175:74-78.e1.
27. Raimondi F, Yousef N, Rodriguez Fanjul J, et al. A Multicenter lung ultrasound study on transient tachypnea of the neonate. *Neonatology.* 2019;115(3):263-268.

28. Weinberg B, Diakoumakis EE, Seife B, Zvi B. The air broncho-gram: sonographic demonstration. *AJR Am J Roentgenol.* 1986; 147(3):593-595.

29. Lichtenstein DA, Lascols N, Mezière G, Gepner A. Ultrasound diagnosis of alveolar consolidation in the critically ill. *Intensive Care Med.* 2004;30(2):276-281.

30. Lichtenstein DA, Mauriat P. Lung ultrasound in the critically Ill neonate. *Curr Pediatr Rev.* 2012;8(3):217-223.

31. Pereda MA, Chavez MA, Hooper-Miele CC, et al. Lung ultra-sound for the diagnosis of pneumonia in children: a meta-analysis. *Pediatrics.* 2015;135(4):714-722.

32. Liu J, Chen SW, Liu F, Li QP, Kong XY, Feng ZC. The diagnosis of neonatal pulmonary atelectasis using lung ultrasonography. *Chest.* 2015;147(4):1013-1019.

33. Bhatia R, Davis PG, Doyle LW, Wong C, Morley CJ. Identifica-tion of pneumothorax in very preterm infants. *J Pediatr.* 2011;159(1):115-120.e1.

34. Lichtenstein DA, Meziere G, Lascols N, et al. Ultrasound diag-nosis of occult pneumothorax. *Crit Care Med.* 2005;33(6): 1231-1238.

35. Cattarossi L, Copetti R, Brusa G, Pintaldi S. Lung ultrasound diagnostic accuracy in neonatal pneumothorax. *Can Respir J.* 2016;2016:6515069.

36. Liu J, Chi JH, Ren XL, et al. Lung ultrasonography to diagnose pneumothorax of the newborn. *Am J Emerg Med.* 2017;35(9): 1298-1302.

37. Dahmarde H, Parooie F, Salarzaei M. Accuracy of ultrasound in diagnosis of pneumothorax: a comparison between neonates and adults: a systematic review and meta-analysis. *Can Respir J.* 2019;2019:5271982.

38. Gryminski J, Krakówka P, Lypacewicz G. The diagnosis of pleu-ral effusion by ultrasonic and radiologic techniques. *Chest.* 1976;70(1):33-37.

39. Lichtenstein DA. Lung ultrasound in the critically ill. *Ann Inten-sive Care.* 2014;4(1):1.

40. Avni EF, Braude P, Pardou A, Matos C. Hyaline membrane dis-ease in the newborn: diagnosis by ultrasound. *Pediatr Radiol.* 1990;20(3):143-146.

41. Cattarossi L, Copetti R, Poskurica B, Miserocchi G. Surfactant administration for neonatal respiratory distress does not im-prove lung interstitial fluid clearance: echographic and experi-mental evidence. *J Perinat Med.* 2010;38(5):557-563.

42. Federici M, Federici PV, Feleppa F, et al. Pulmonary ultrasonog-raphy in the follow-up of respiratory distress syndrome on preterm newborns: reduction of X-ray exposure. *J Ultrasound.* 2011;14(2):78-83.

43. Escourrou G, De Luca D. Lung ultrasound decreased radiation exposure in preterm infants in a neonatal intensive care unit. *Acta Paediatr.* 2016;105(5):e237-e239.

44. Aldecoa-Bilbao V, Balcells-Esponera C, Herranz Barbero A, et al. Lung ultrasound for early surfactant treatment: development and validation of a predictive model. *Pediatr Pulmonol.* 2021; 56(2):433-441.

45. Raschetti R, Yousef N, Vigo G, et al. Echography-guided sur-factant therapy to improve timeliness of surfactant replace-ment: a quality improvement project. *J Pediatr.* 2019;212: 137-143.e1.

46. Rodriguez-Fanjul J, Jordan I, Balaguer M, Batista-Munoz A, Ra-mon M, Bobillo-Perez S. Early surfactant replacement guided by lung ultrasound in preterm newborns with RDS: the ULTRA-SURF randomised controlled trial. *Eur J Pediatr.* 2020;179(12): 1913-1920.

47. Perri A, Tana M, Riccardi R, et al. Neonatal lung ultrasonogra-phy score after surfactant in preterm infants: a prospective ob-servational study. *Pediatr Pulmonol.* 2020;55(1):116-121.

48. Liu J, Wang Y, Fu W, Yang CS, Huang JJ. Diagnosis of neonatal transient tachypnea and its differentiation from respiratory distress syndrome using lung ultrasound. *Medicine (Baltimore).* 2014;93(27):e197.

49. Liu J, Chen XX, Li XW, Chen SW, Wang Y, Fu W. Lung ultraso-nography to diagnose transient tachypnea of the newborn. *Chest.* 2016;149(5):1269-1275.

50. Ibrahim M, Omran A, AbdAllah NB, Ibrahim M, El-Sharkawy S. Lung ultrasound in early diagnosis of neonatal transient tachy-pnea and its differentiation from other causes of neonatal respi-ratory distress. *J Neonatal Perinatal Med.* 2018;11(3):281-287.

51. Doyle LW, Carse E, Adams AM, et al. Ventilation in extremely preterm infants and respiratory function at 8 years. *N Engl J Med.* 2017;377(4):329-337.

52. Steinhorn R, Davis JM, Gopel W, et al. Chronic pulmonary in-sufficiency of prematurity: developing optimal endpoints for drug development. *J Pediatr.* 2017;191:15-21.e1.

53. Alonso-Ojembarrena A, Serna-Guerediaga I, Aldecoa-Bilbao V, et al. The predictive value of lung ultrasound scores in develop-ing bronchopulmonary dysplasia: a prospective multicenter diagnostic accuracy study. *Chest.* 2021;160(3):1006-1016.

54. Oulego-Erroz I, Alonso-Quintela P, Terroba-Seara S, Jimenez-Gonzalez A, Rodriguez-Blanco S. Early assessment of lung aeration using an ultrasound score as a biomarker of develop-ing bronchopulmonary dysplasia: a prospective observational study. *J Perinatol.* 2021;41(1):62-68.

55. Mohamed A, Mohsen N, Diambomba Y, et al. Lung ultrasound for prediction of bronchopulmonary dysplasia in extreme pre-term neonates: a prospective diagnostic cohort study. *J Pediatr.* 2021;238:187-192.e2.

56. Frerichs I, Amato MB, van Kaam AH, et al. Chest electrical imped-ance tomography examination, data analysis, terminology, clinical use and recommendations: consensus statement of the TRansla-tional EIT developmeNt stuDy group. *Thorax.* 2017;72(1):83-93.

57. Sophocleous L, Frerichs I, Miedema M, et al. Clinical perfor-mance of a novel textile interface for neonatal chest electrical impedance tomography. *Physiol Meas.* 2018;39(4):044004.

58. Becher TH, Miedema M, Kallio M, et al. Prolonged continuous monitoring of regional lung function in infants with respiratory failure. *Ann Am Thorac Soc.* 2022;19(6):991-999.

59. Adler A, Arnold JH, Bayford R, et al. GREIT: a unified approach to 2D linear EIT reconstruction of lung images. *Physiol Meas.* 2009;30(6):S35-S55.

60. Adler A, Dai T, Lionheart WR. Temporal image reconstruction in electrical impedance tomography. *Physiol Meas.* 2007;28(7): S1-S11.

61. Tingay DG, Rajapaksa A, Zonneveld CE, et al. Spatiotemporal aeration and lung injury patterns are influenced by the first inflation strategy at birth. *Am J Respir Cell Mol Biol.* 2016; 54(2):263-272.

62. Grychtol B, Adler A. FEM electrode refinement for electrical impedance tomography. *Conf Proc IEEE Eng Med Biol Soc.* 2013;2013:6429-6432.

63. Ferrario D, Grychtol B, Adler A, Sola J, Bohm SH, Bodenstein M. Toward morphological thoracic EIT: major signal sources correspond to respective organ locations in CT. *IEEE Trans Biomed Eng.* 2012;59(11):3000-3008.

64. Miedema M, de Jongh FH, Frerichs I, van Veenendaal MB, van Kaam AH. Changes in lung volume and ventilation during

surfactant treatment in ventilated preterm infants. *Am J Respir Crit Care Med*. 2011;184(1):100-105.

65. Dowse G, Perkins E, Thomson J, Schinckel N, Pereira-Fantini P, Tingay D. Synchronized inflations generate greater gravity-dependent lung ventilation in neonates. *J Pediatr*. 2021;228: 24-30.e10.

66. Tingay DG, Waldmann AD, Frerichs I, Ranganathan S, Adler A. Electrical impedance tomography can identify ventilation and perfusion defects: a neonatal case. *Am J Respir Crit Care Med*. 2019;199(3):384-386.

67. Frerichs I, Dargaville PA, van Genderingen H, Morel DR, Rimensberger PC. Lung volume recruitment after surfactant administration modifies spatial distribution of ventilation. *Am J Respir Crit Care Med*. 2006;174(7):772-729.

68. Frerichs I, Hinz J, Herrmann P, et al. Regional lung perfusion as determined by electrical impedance tomography in comparison with electron beam CT imaging. *IEEE Trans Med Imaging*. 2002;21(6):646-652.

69. Thomson J, Ruegger CM, Perkins EJ, et al. Regional ventilation characteristics during non-invasive respiratory support in preterm infants. *Arch Dis Child Fetal Neonatal Ed*. 2021;106(4): 370-375.

70. Schinckel NF, Hickey L, Perkins EJ, et al. Skin-to-skin care alters regional ventilation in stable neonates. *Arch Dis Child Fetal Neonatal Ed*. 2021;106(1):76-80.

71. Bhatia R, Carlisle HR, Armstrong RK, Kamlin COF, Davis PG, Tingay DG. Extubation generates lung volume inhomogeneity in preterm infants. *Arch Dis Child Fetal Neonatal Ed*. 2022;107(1): 82-86.

72. Armstrong RK, Carlisle HR, Davis PG, Schibler A, Tingay DG. Distribution of tidal ventilation during volume-targeted ventilation is variable and influenced by age in the preterm lung. *Intensive Care Med*. 2011;37(5):839-846.

73. Hough J, Trojman A, Schibler A. Effect of time and body position on ventilation in premature infants. *Pediatr Res*. 2016;80(4): 499-504.

74. van der Burg PS, Miedema M, de Jongh FH, Frerichs I, van Kaam AH. Changes in lung volume and ventilation following transition from invasive to noninvasive respiratory support and prone positioning in preterm infants. *Pediatr Res*. 2015;77(3): 484-488.

75. Gattinoni L, D'Andrea L, Pelosi P, Vitale G, Pesenti A, Fumagalli R. Regional effects and mechanism of positive end-expiratory pressure in early adult respiratory distress syndrome. *JAMA*. 1993;269(16):2122-2127.

76. Bhatia R, Davis PG, Tingay DG. Regional volume characteristics of the preterm infant receiving first intention continuous positive airway pressure. *J Pediatr*. 2017;187:80-88.e2.

77. Gaertner VD, Waldmann AD, Davis PG, et al. Transmission of oscillatory volumes into the preterm lung during noninvasive high-frequency ventilation. *Am J Respir Crit Care Med*. 2021; 203(8):998-1005.

78. He H, Chi Y, Yang Y, et al. Early individualized positive end-expiratory pressure guided by electrical impedance tomography in acute respiratory distress syndrome: a randomized controlled clinical trial. *Crit Care*. 2021;25(1):230.

79. Heines SJH, Strauch U, van de Poll MCG, Roekaerts P, Bergmans D. Clinical implementation of electric impedance tomography in the treatment of ARDS: a single centre experience. *J Clin Monit Comput*. 2019;33(2):291-300.

80. Miedema M, de Jongh FH, Frerichs I, van Veenendaal MB, van Kaam AH. The effect of airway pressure and oscillation amplitude on ventilation in pre-term infants. *Eur Respir J*. 2012; 40(2):479-484.

81. Miedema M, de Jongh FH, Frerichs I, van Veenendaal MB, van Kaam AH. Regional respiratory time constants during lung recruitment in high-frequency oscillatory ventilated preterm infants. *Intensive Care Med*. 2012;38(2):294-299.

82. Miedema M, de Jongh FH, Frerichs I, van Veenendaal MB, van Kaam AH. Changes in lung volume and ventilation during lung recruitment in high-frequency ventilated preterm infants with respiratory distress syndrome. *J Pediatr*. 2011;159(2): 199-205.e2.

83. Schmolzer GM, Bhatia R, Davis PG, Tingay DG. A comparison of different bedside techniques to determine endotracheal tube position in a neonatal piglet model. *Pediatr Pulmonol*. 2013; 48(2):138-145.

84. Miedema M, McCall KE, Perkins EJ, et al. First real-time visualization of a spontaneous pneumothorax developing in a preterm lamb using electrical impedance tomography. *Am J Respir Crit Care Med*. 2016;194(1):116-118.

85. Miedema M, Frerichs I, de Jongh FH, van Veenendaal MB, van Kaam AH. Pneumothorax in a preterm infant monitored by electrical impedance tomography: a case report. *Neonatology*. 2011;99(1):10-13.

86. Bhatia R, Schmolzer GM, Davis PG, Tingay DG. Electrical impedance tomography can rapidly detect small pneumothoraces in surfactant-depleted piglets. *Intensive Care Med*. 2012;38(2): 308-315.

87. Miedema M, Adler A, McCall KE, Perkins EJ, van Kaam AH, Tingay DG. Electrical impedance tomography identifies a distinct change in regional phase angle delay pattern in ventilation filling immediately prior to a spontaneous pneumothorax. *J Appl Physiol*. 2019;127(3):707-712.

88. Tingay DG, Farrell O, Thomson J, et al. Imaging the respiratory transition at birth: unraveling the complexities of the first breaths of life. *Am J Respir Crit Care Med*. 2021;204(1):82-91.

89. Tingay DG, Pereira-Fantini PM, Oakley R, et al. Gradual aeration at birth is more lung protective than a sustained inflation in preterm lambs. *Am J Respir Crit Care Med*. 2019;200(5):608-616.

90. De Luca D, Autilio C, Pezza L, Shankar-Aguilera S, Tingay DG, Carnielli VP. Personalized medicine for the management of RDS in preterm neonates. *Neonatology*. 2021;118(2):127-138.

91. Brusa G, Savoia M, Vergine M, Bon A, Copetti R, Cattarossi L. Neonatal lung sonography: interobserver agreement between physician interpreters with varying levels of experience. *J Ultrasound Med*. 2015;34(9):1549-1554.

92. Singh Y, Tissot C, Fraga MV, et al. International evidence-based guidelines on Point of Care Ultrasound (POCUS) for critically ill neonates and children issued by the POCUS Working Group of the European Society of Paediatric and Neonatal Intensive Care (ESPNIC). *Crit Care*. 2020;24(1):65.

93. Zhao Z, Moller K, Steinmann D, Frerichs I, Guttmann J. Evaluation of an electrical impedance tomography-based Global Inhomogeneity Index for pulmonary ventilation distribution. *Intensive Care Med*. 2009;35(11):1900-1906.

Genetic Disorders of Alveolar Formation and Homeostasis

Daniel T. Swarr and Jeffrey A. Whitsett

Chapter Outline

Genetic Disorders of Lung Formation

Mutations in Genes in Pulmonary Mesenchyme

Mutations in Genes Expressed in the Embryonic Epithelium

Critical Role of Pulmonary Surfactant After Birth

Diffuse Pulmonary Disease Caused by Surfactant Dysfunction

Genetic Disorders of Surfactant Homeostasis

Inherited Disorders of Surfactant Homeostasis: SP-B, SP-C, and ABCA3

Surfactant Protein B (SP-B)

Surfactant Protein C (SP-C)

ABCA3: Disorder of Lipid Transport and Lamellar Body Formation

Clinical Perspectives

Key Points

- Lung morphogenesis begins with the formation of the tracheal and bronchial buds. Subsequent branching morphogenesis forms the respiratory tubules, the acini, and the alveolar regions of the lung required for gas exchange after birth.

- Lung morphogenesis is dependent upon precise paracrine signaling among pulmonary progenitor cells controlling gene transcription, which determines the precise numbers, positions, and functions of pulmonary cells.

- Interactions between the mesenchymal and endodermally derived pulmonary cells direct branching morphogenesis, sacculation, and alveolarization before birth.

- Mutations in genes expressed in pulmonary mesenchymal progenitors, including *FOXF1* and *TBX4*, disrupt lung morphogenesis and the formation and function of the pulmonary circulation.

- Mutations in genes expressed in endodermally derived cells, including *NKX2-1*, *ABCA3*, *SFTPB*, and *SFTPC*, cause respiratory failure after birth and childhood interstitial lung disorder in infancy.

- Lack of differentiation of the alveolar epithelium in preterm infants is associated with decreased production of surfactant lipids and proteins, resulting in respiratory distress after birth.

Genetic Disorders of Lung Formation

The human lung is comprised of more than 50 distinct cell types that differentiate from subsets of endodermal and mesodermally derived progenitors during embryogenesis.[2] Precisely orchestrated signaling pathways and transcriptional programs regulate cell proliferation, migration, and differentiation during morphogenesis of the lung. Epithelial cells from the foregut endoderm invade the splanchnic mesenchyme and are first distinguished from other foregut derivatives by the expression of NKX2-1 or thyroid transcription factor 1 (TTF-1), a nuclear transcription

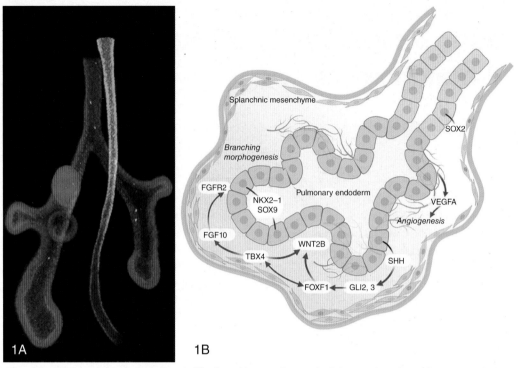

Fig. 19.1 The embryonic lung and gene network controlling branching morphogenesis. A, Lung and esophagus from embryonic day 11 mouse are stained with NKX2-1 (TTF-1) *(red)* and SOX2 *(blue)* showing early branching of the bronchial tubules and separation of the trachea. **B,** Gene network controlling embryonic mice lung formation. The peripheral lung buds grow into the splanchnic mesenchyme of the fetal lung. NKX2-1 is a transcription factor controlling formation of the respiratory epithelium from the embryonic foregut. Conducting (SOX2) versus acinar buds (SOX9) specify the airways from the peripheral regions. Epithelial cells secrete SHH, activating Gli2, 3, FOXF1, and TBX4 in the splanchnic mesenchyme together required for the production of FGF-10. FGF-10 activates FGFR2 in the epithelial cells to enhance the growth and migration of the lung tubules. VEGFA, produced by the epithelium, regulates the growth of the pulmonary capillaries. Gene mutations disrupting this epithelial-mesenchymal crosstalk cause pulmonary malformations and respiratory failure after birth.

factor expressed in the earliest lung progenitors (Fig. 19.1A). Epithelial cells lining conducting (airway) regions of the lung express SOX2, distinguishing them from the peripheral epithelial cells lining the acinar buds which express SOX9 and high levels of NKX2-1; the latter progenitors form the alveolar regions of the lung later in development. Paracrine signaling among epithelial cells lining the lung tubules and mesodermally derived cells of the splanchnic mesenchyme control the growth of differentiation of the embryonic lung during formation of the tracheal, bronchial, and pulmonary lung buds. The pulmonary vasculature and stromal cells including pericytes, fibroblasts, endothelial, mesothelial, and smooth muscle cells are derived from the splanchnic mesenchyme. Paracrine and juxtacrine interactions among the cells

direct branching morphogenesis, sacculation, and alveolarization required for the formation and function of the lung at birth. Identification of several genes critical for lung formation enables genetic diagnosis of respiratory disorders causing respiratory failure in newborn infants. Since lung organogenesis depends on precise cell–cell interactions, mutations in genes regulating critical processes in both epithelial and mesenchymal compartments of the lung cause severe lung dysfunction after birth.

Mutations in Genes in Pulmonary Mesenchyme

Epithelial cells of the lung tubules express and secrete sonic hedgehog (SHH), a signaling molecule which binds to smoothened (SMO) in subsets of pulmonary mesenchymal cells. This activates Gli2/3, which is required for the expression of TBX4 and FOXF-1, which in turn mediate the expression of FGF-10 and FGF-9. These FGFs activate their cognate receptor FGFR2 in epithelial cells in the acinar bud to control cell proliferation and migration during branching morphogenesis (Fig. 19.1B).[3-5] Expression of SOX2 in conducting airways and SOX9 in the peripheral acinar buds controls regiospecific proliferation and differentiation along the cephalocaudal axis of the lung. Mutations in the SHH, FOXF1, and TBX-FGF signaling networks cause acinar/alveolar hypoplasia resulting in a respiratory failure at birth (Fig. 19.2).[5] Loss of SHH signaling, either caused by defects in the cholesterol esterification of SHH (Smith-Lemli-Opitz syndrome) or mutations in Gli3 (Pallister Hall syndrome), causes pulmonary malformations in humans. Likewise, mutations disrupting normal FOXF-1 expression in the splanchnic mesenchyme cause alveolar capillary dysplasia with misalignment of pulmonary veins (ACDMPV). Newborn infants with ACDMVP develop respiratory failure and cyanosis after birth as a result of lung hypoplasia and severe defects in pulmonary vasculogenesis.[3] A majority of ACDMPV patients have point mutations or deletions (typically de novo) in the *FOXF-1* gene or in noncoding regions of the genome that impair expression of FOXF-1. The diagnosis of ACDMPV is made by gene sequencing or copy number analysis or by histopathological analysis of lung tissue. FOXF1

regulates TBX transcription factors expression in the splanchnic mesenchyme during lung formation. Mutations in the *TBX4* gene (MIM# 601719) cause acinar dysplasia/hypoplasia.[6] Less deleterious mutations in TBX4 cause the "small patellar syndrome" associated with pulmonary hypertension presenting in childhood.[7] Together TBX4 and FOXF1 regulate the expression of FGF-10 in lung mesenchyme, activating FGFR-2 in epithelial cells of the acinar buds required for branching of the lung tubules. Disruption of FGF-10 signaling caused by mutations in FGFR-2 is a rare cause of pulmonary hypoplasia and is associated with other organ malformations.[8,9]

Mutations in Genes Expressed in the Embryonic Epithelium (NKX2-1/TTF-1)

Mutations in genes critical for growth and differentiation of the embryonic respiratory epithelium cause respiratory disorders presenting in the newborn period.[10] NKX2-1 is a master transcription factor critical for growth and differentiation of the lung and is expressed in epithelial cells of the primordial lung buds as they invaginate into the splanchnic mesenchyme. Later in lung development, NKX2-1 controls lung maturation and surfactant protein and lipids synthesis. NKX2-1 is also expressed in the central nervous system and thyroid epithelium, thus mutations in the NKX2-1 may influence both CNS and thyroid function. While there is variability affecting each organ,

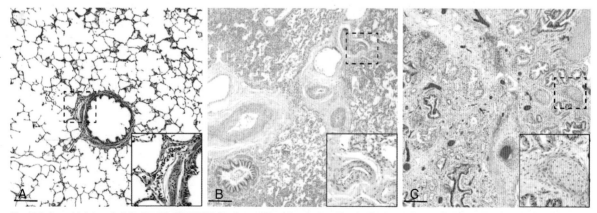

Fig. 19.2 Lung histology in infants with ACDMPV (alveolar capillary dysplasia with misalignment of the pulmonary veins) and acinar dysplasia. A, Hematoxylin-eosin staining of the normal lung from a 6-month-old infant. **B,** Lung tissue from a 9-month-old infant with ACDMPV caused by a mutation in *FOXF1*. *C,* Lung tissue from an infant with acinar dysplasia caused by a mutation in *TBX4.*

most patients with heterozygous mutations in NKX2-1 have clinical findings in the brain, thyroid, and lung. Diffuse lung disease, associated with primary hypothyroidism in newborn infants, supports the diagnosis of brain-thyroid-lung syndrome.[11] Approximately 60% of infants with TTF-1 mutations have alterations in lung function, often accompanied by altered expression of genes regulating surfactant homeostasis. Severely affected infants may present with respiratory failure caused by surfactant deficiency at birth. Hypothyroidism, ectopic or absent thyroid tissue, in concert with diffuse lung disease supports the diagnosis in newborn infants. The definitive diagnosis of brain-thyroid-lung syndrome is made by genetic analysis of the *NKX2-1* gene.[12-15]

Mutations in SOX2 and SOX9 Are Associated With Multiple Congenital Malformations

SOX2 is a transcription factor expressed in multiple tissues during embryogenesis and is more widely expressed than NKX2-1. Hemizygous mutations in SOX2 cause anophthalmia-microphthalmia associated with tracheal-esophageal, renal, and other malformations.[16] Lung abnormalities caused by disruption of SOX2 are consistent with the important role SOX2 plays during separation of the tracheal-esophageal tubes early in lung morphogenesis. SOX2 regulates differentiation of airway epithelial cells in conducting airways throughout lung development. Mutations in SOX9 have been associated with respiratory compromise caused by tracheobronchomalacia and campomelic dwarfism.[17]

Critical Role of Pulmonary Surfactant After Birth

Pulmonary surfactant is a complex mixture of lipids and associated proteins that are secreted by alveolar type 2 cells (AT2 cells) to prevent atelectasis during the respiratory cycle. Lack of pulmonary surfactant causes respiratory distress syndrome (RDS) in preterm infants and is required for adaptation of breathing after birth and throughout life. Surfactant-associated proteins and lipids are secreted by AT2 cells into the alveoli (Fig. 19.3). Surfactant lipids are produced by AT2 cells and are highly enriched in dipalmitoylphosphatidylcholine and phosphatidylglycerol. These lipids are packaged into

intracellular organelles termed lamellar bodies. Surfactant proteins B and C are small, hydrophobic proteins produced by proteolytic processing of proproteins encoded by the *SFTPB* and *SFTPC* genes. SP-B and SP-C are selectively expressed in AT2 cells, increasing prior to birth. Expression of surfactant proteins and lipids is regulated by a network of transcription factors within AT2 cells, including TTF-1, CEBPα, and SREBP. SP-B and SP-C are packaged with surfactant lipids and secreted into the alveoli in response to stretch, purinergic, and adrenergic signals. In the alveoli, lamellar bodies unwind and interact with SP-A and SP-D (encoded by *SFTPA* and *SFTPD* and secreted by AT2 cells) to form tubular myelin. Multilayered lipid films form from tubular myelin and spread over the alveolar surfaces reducing surface tension at the air-liquid interface. Lack of AT2 cell epithelial cell differentiation in preterm infants and the resultant paucity of surfactant lipids and proteins causes atelectasis and respiratory failure in preterm infants with RDS. Pulmonary maturation and accompanying pulmonary surfactant functions are enhanced by maternal antenatal glucocorticoid treatment, which is widely used to prevent RDS in preterm infants. Surfactant lipids and proteins are recycled after secretion by AT2 cells and are catabolized by alveolar macrophages. Secretion of surfactant is regulated by GPR-116, which is expressed on the surface of AT2 cells. GPR-116 inhibits surfactant secretion to maintain extracellular surfactant pool sizes.[18] Clearance and catabolism of surfactant by alveolar macrophages is dependent upon GM-CSF signaling. Lack of GM-CSF caused either by autoantibodies or mutations in the gene for GM-CSF receptor impairs surfactant clearance and causes pulmonary alveolar proteinosis (PAP).[19] Surfactant homeostasis is controlled by gene expression, protein processing, packaging, secretion, reuptake, and catabolism that work in concert to maintain alveolar surfactant concentrations throughout life (Fig. 19.3).

Diffuse Pulmonary Disease Caused by Surfactant Dysfunction

Mutations in genes affecting pulmonary surfactant function or production cause diffuse lung diseases in newborn infants (Table 19.1). Surfactant disorders usually present soon after birth and account for approximately 20% of diffuse interstitial lung disease in newborn infants. Surfactant proteins SP-B and SP-C

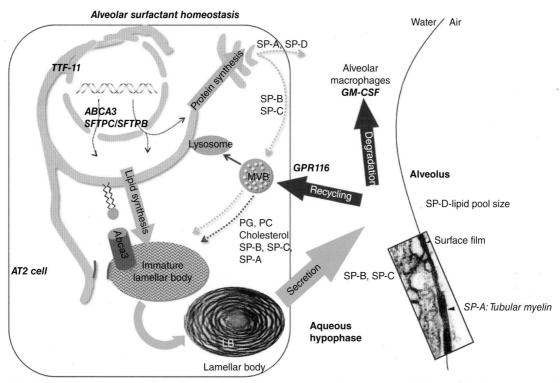

Fig. 19.3 Alveolar surfactant homeostasis. Surfactant lipids and proteins are produced by alveolar type 2 (AT2) cells. TTF-1, a master regulator of the respiratory epithelium, regulates lung morphogenesis in the embryonic lung and controls genes regulating surfactant lipid and protein synthesis, including *ABCA3*, *SFTPB*, and *SFTPC*, and other surfactant proteins (SP-A and SP-D). SP-B and SP-C are proteolytically processed and stored with surfactant lipids in lamellar bodies prior to secretion into the alveoli. SP-B and SP-C create multilayers that are required to reduce surface tension in the alveoli. SP-A and SP-D create tubular myelin and regulate surfactant lipid structures in the alveoli. GPR116 and SP-D regulate alveolar lipid pool sizes by modulating surfactant secretion and reuptake. GM-CSF regulates surfactant clearance by alveolar macrophages. Genetic disorders disrupting surfactant homeostasis cause respiratory distress in newborns and infants.

and the AT2 cell lipid transporter ABCA3 play important roles in surfactant metabolism and function, influencing lipid transport, packaging, formation of lamellar bodies, surfactant function, and its recycling. Surfactant proteins and ABCA3 are expressed at high levels in AT2 cells. Deleterious mutations in *SFTPB*

TABLE 19.1	Monogenic Diseases of Surfactant Homeostasis
ABCA3	Surfactant lipid transport in AT2 cells
SFTPB	Intracellular packaging and function of surfactant lipids
SFTPC	Misfolded protein, cell toxicity
SFTPA	Host defense, surfactant structure
NKX2-1	AT2 cell differentiation and function
CSFR1/2	Hereditary PAP

PAP, Pulmonary alveolar proteinosis.

and *ABCA3* genes usually cause respiratory failure soon after birth. Radiographic findings are consistent with surfactant deficiency, resulting in atelectasis, hypoxemia, and hypercapnia requiring assisted ventilation and oxygen that is generally refractory to intensive care treatment.[12]

Genetic Disorders of Surfactant Homeostasis

Four surfactant proteins, SP-A, SP-B, SP-C, and SP-D, are encoded by distinct genes: *SFTPA*, *SFTPB*, *SFTPC*, and *SFTPD*, and expression of each of the surfactant protein genes is controlled by TTF-1 in AT2 cells. Each surfactant protein plays distinct and important roles in alveolar homeostasis (Fig. 19.3). Surfactant proteins A and D (SP-A and SP-D) are structurally related members of the collectin family of host defense proteins that are highly expressed in the respiratory epithelium.[20,21] Two genes encoding SFTPA and one encoding SFTPD are located in close proximity on human chromosome 10. The pulmonary collectins share similar globular C-terminal lectin domains (termed CRDs or carbohydrate recognition domains) that bind to carbohydrate-rich surfaces on microbial pathogens. SP-A and SP-D share an NH_2 terminal domain consisting of an extended Gly-X-Y-Gly repeat motif that forms rigid, collagen-like trimeric structures that are cross-linked near the NH_2 terminus by sulfhydryl bonds. SP-A is synthesized by alveolar type II epithelial cells and nonciliated cells in conducting airways. SP-A is required for the formation of tubular myelin which is associated with phosphatidylcholine in pulmonary surfactant. SP-A–deficient mice lack tubular myelin but survive normally after birth, indicating that tubular myelin is not required for lung function. While surfactant function and metabolism are intact in SP-A–deficient mice, these animals are highly susceptible to infection and lung inflammation following intratracheal administration of various pulmonary pathogens and toxicants, including bacteria, fungus, endotoxin, and various respiratory viruses. SP-A is encoded by two genes in humans, both expressed in respiratory epithelial cells. Mutations in SFTPA have been associated with pulmonary fibrosis and adenocarcinoma in older individuals.[22]

SP-D is expressed in alveolar and airway epithelial cells and has also been detected in nonpulmonary tissues.[23,24] SP-D is weakly associated with surfactant lipids in the alveolus where it is enriched in small aggregate surfactant lipids. SP-D plays an important role in host defense, surfactant homeostasis, and in the regulation of lung inflammation. SP-D binds endotoxin, the surfaces of various fungi and bacteria, and viral pathogens, including RSV, influenza A, and coronavirus.[20,21] SP-D enhances the uptake and clearance of pulmonary pathogens by alveolar macrophages in the lung. Unlike SP-A, SP-D also plays a critical role in the regulation of surfactant lipid pool sizes and is required for the maintenance of normal, large, to small surfactant lipid aggregate forms and surfactant uptake by type II epithelial cells. Surfactant lipid ultrastructure is abnormal and lipid pool sizes are increased three- to fourfold in $Sftpd^{-/-}$ mice, demonstrating a critical role for SP-D in determining the structural forms of surfactant and its metabolism.[25]

Common genetic variations within the SFTPA and SFTPD genes have been associated with acute and chronic lung diseases.[26] However, these genetic associations are relatively weak, and the structural and functional basis for the susceptibility of individuals expressing certain SP-A and SP-D isoforms remains to be clarified. Human disease related to pathogenic variants in SFTPD has not been observed.

Inherited Disorders of Surfactant Homeostasis: SP-B, SP-C, and ABCA3

Hereditable disorders of surfactant homeostasis were initially recognized in term newborn infants with clinical features of RDS that did not respond to conventional therapies[27] and in infants with chronic lung diseases, generally termed *congenital alveolar proteinosis* (CAP) or *chronic pneumonitis of infancy* (CPI). In older individuals and children, these disorders have been associated with diffuse lung disease, often termed nonspecific interstitial pneumonitis (NSIP) or usual interstitial pneumonitis. Pathological findings in the lungs of infants are shown in Fig. 19.4. Mutations in SPTPB, SPTPC, and ABCA3 represent rare causes of the respiratory failure and chronic lung disease in infants but should be considered in full-term infants with acute RDS and chronic interstitial lung disease that fail to improve with conventional supportive therapies. A mutation in RAB5B, which regulates the intracellular transport of both pro–SP-B and pro–SP-C, was identified in a child with surfactant deficiency.[28]

Surfactant Protein B

Surfactant protein B (SP-B) is encoded by the *SFTPB* gene on the human chromosome 2. The active SP-B peptide is a 79 amino acid amphipathic peptide that is tightly associated with surfactant lipids (PC and PG) in lamellar bodies and pulmonary surfactant.[29] The active SP-B protein is selectively expressed in AT2 cells and is produced by proteolytic processing of a 381 amino acid precursor as it is transported through the cells to lamellar bodies. Nonciliated airway epithelial cells also express pro–SP-B but do not complete its processing. Expression of SP-B increases with advancing gestation in association with increasing surfactant

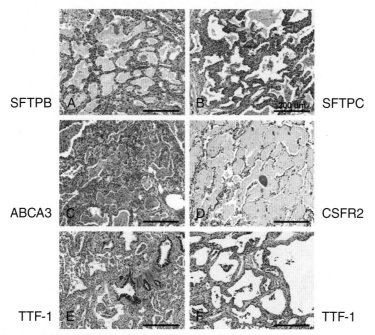

Fig. 19.4 Lung histopathology in an infant with genetic disorders of surfactant homeostasis. Lung biopsies were stained with hematoxylin-eosin and imaged by light microscopy to show histopathologic changes caused by genetic disorders of surfactant metabolism, including ABCA3, SFTPB, TTF-1 (NKX2-1), and hereditary pulmonary alveolar proteinosis (PAP), the latter caused by a mutation in the GM-CSF receptor. (Images courtesy of Susan E. Wert, Ph.D.)

lipids and other surfactant proteins (SP-A, SPD, and SP-C). Deletion of SP-B in mice (*Sftpb*[−/−] mice) and mutations in human *SFTPB* cause respiratory failure that presents at birth.[30,31] Studies in *Sftpb*[−/−] mice and in human infants demonstrated that SP-B is required for (1) surfactant activity, (2) formation of lamellar bodies and tubular myelin, (3) processing of pro–SP-C, and (4) the reuptake of surfactant proteins and lipids by type II cells.[32] Lack of SP-B (or pro–SP-B) profoundly disrupts intracellular and extracellular surfactant homeostasis. Since pro–SP-B and SP-B are required for the packaging of surfactant lipids in lamellar bodies and AT2 cell function, hereditary SP-B deficiency has not been successfully treated with surfactant replacement. Partial reduction of SP-B in mice and patients with ARDS, RDS, and BPD is associated with susceptibility to respiratory failure during lung injury and infection.[33-35]

Homozygous or compound heterozygous mutations in *SFTPB* have been associated with respiratory distress in term infants.[31,36] More than 50 distinct disease-causing mutations of *SFTPB* have been identified. A single mutation, 121 in 2 (c.397delCinsGAA), is seen in the majority of affected infants, which results in a truncated and unstable *SFTPB* mRNA. Infants generally present within hours after birth with respiratory distress, hypoxemia, and diffuse reticulogranular opacifications on chest radiography, similar to severe RDS. The active SP-B peptide is generally lacking in bronchoalveolar lavage (BAL) fluid from these infants. When *SFTPB* mutations result in the lack of synthesis of *SFTPB* RNA and pro–SP-B, immunohistochemical staining of lung tissue reveals the lack of pro–SP-B and SP-B staining. When SFTPB mutations are associated with the synthesis of a mutant pro–SP-B peptide, abnormal AT2 cell staining and aberrantly sized pro–SP-B peptides are detected by Western blot analysis or immunohistochemistry. At the ultrastructural level, lamellar bodies and tubular myelin are absent in lung tissues of patients with hereditary SP-B deficiency. Mutations in *SFTPB* affect mRNA and protein structure in multiple ways, including missense, stop codon, nonsense, deletion mutations, etc., that are identified by targeted gene sequencing.

Hereditary SP-B–associated disease is very rare, with an allele frequency of approximately 1/1000.[37] While heterozygous SP-B–deficient (Sftpb[+/−]) mice are susceptible to lung injury, clear clinical findings have not been associated with heterozygous carriers of *SFTPB* mutations. A definitive diagnosis of hereditary SP-B deficiency is made by the identification of mutations in the *SFTPB* gene. Respiratory failure associated with hereditary SP-B deficiency is refractory to conventional therapies, including surfactant replacement, mechanical ventilation, and ECMO. Several infants with SFTPB-related lung disease have survived the neonatal period.[38,39] Survival of infants with *SFTPB*-related disease has been extended by lung transplantation in a small number of infants.[40]

Surfactant Protein C

Surfactant protein C (SP-C) is a small hydrophobic peptide encoded by the *SFTPC* gene located on human chromosome 8. SP-C is produced from a precursor protein of 191 amino acids that is selectively expressed and processed by AT2 cells into a 33–35 amino acid, a peptide that is tightly associated with surfactant lipids in lamellar bodies and the alveolus.[29] SP-C is palmitoylated and is rich in hydrophobic amino acids to facilitate insertion into surfactant lipid membranes where it alters lipid packing. Like other surfactant proteins, SP-C is synthesized by the lung in increasing amounts with advancing gestation. Deletion of the *Sftpc* gene in mice perturbed surfactant function and caused severe chronic pulmonary inflammation and tissue remodeling in some strains of mice.[41] Consistent with these findings, mutations in *SFTPC* have been associated with acute respiratory failure in some newborn infants, but most patients present with lung disease later in childhood. SP-C–related lung diseases are usually recognized as diffuse interstitial lung disease in infants and children.[42] *SFTPC*-related lung disease is generally inherited as an autosomal dominant gene caused by the production of abnormal pro–SP-C peptides that cause AT2 cell toxicity. The abnormal processing of pro–SP-C is often mutation-specific, and the proteolytic products are mistrafficked and accumulate in AT2 cells. Lung disease is most commonly caused by mutations in the BRICHOS domain of the SP-C pro-protein. The p.I673Thr mutation in the BRICHOS domain accounts for the majority of disease alleles. Mutations in *SFTPC* are characterized by a high degree of variable expressivity, with the age of onset and disease severity varying greatly. This variability is likely influenced by both environmental and genetic modifiers. Lung histology is generally described as CPI or NSIP. Severe airspace loss and remodeling, mesenchymal thickening, fibrosis, epithelial cell hyperplasia, and accumulations of abnormal alveolar macrophages (often termed desquamating interstitial pneumonitis) are frequently reported in biopsies and pathological reports associated with this disorder. Both familial and de novo mutations in the *SFTPC* gene have been identified in approximately similar proportions. Partially or abnormally processed SP-C peptides accumulate within AT2 cells, causing cell stress that results in AT2 cell injury, inflammation, and tissue remodeling. Since subsets of AT2 cells serve as progenitor cells, the progressive loss of AT2 cells likely impairs alveolar repair. SP-C–related lung disease may be exacerbated by viral infections or other pulmonary stresses.

Mutations in *SFTPC* should be suspected in infants with or without a family history of neonatal or chronic lung disease who present with acute RDS or chronic lung disease in infancy that fails to resolve with standard therapies. Mutations in *SFTPC* are generally associated with the pathologic diagnosis of interstitial lung disease (Fig. 19.4). The active SP-C peptide is generally absent from BALF, and pro–SP-C (or abnormally sized pro–SP-C fragments) can be detected by immunohistochemistry or Western blot analysis of lung tissue. Mutations have been reported throughout the *SFTPC* gene, resulting in missense, nonsense, and stop mutations. Diagnosis of *SFTPC*-related lung disease should be considered in full-term infants with RDS or infants or children with chronic diffuse interstitial lung disease. A definitive diagnosis is made by the identification of *SFTPC* mutations by gene sequencing. Respiratory failure has been managed by lung transplantation in some infants. Although the precise incidence of this disorder is unknown at present, hereditary SP-C deficiency is a very rare cause of both acute and chronic lung disease in infants, children, and adults.

ABCA3: Disorder of Lipid Transport and Lamellar Body Formation

ABCA3 is a 1704 amino acid polypeptide that is a member of a family of transport proteins that share the Walker domains characteristic of other ABC transport proteins like the CFTR (cystic fibrosis transmembrane regulators). ABCA3 is present in limiting membranes of lamellar bodies in AT2 cells.[43] ABCA3 expression in AT2 cells increases in a manner similar to surfactant proteins and lipids throughout late gestation. ABCA3 is required for the formation of the lamellar bodies in AT2 cells and induces lamellar body-like organelles when transfected into cells in vitro. ABCA3 is encoded by the *ABCA3* gene located in human chromosome 16 and is expressed in other organs. Mutation in *ABCA3* and deletion of *Abca3* in mice cause respiratory failure at birth. ABCA3 plays a critical role in the ATP-dependent transport of phospholipids (hosphatidylcholine and phosphatidylglycerol) into the lamellar bodies. Its absence results in a lack of surfactant secretion and function, causing respiratory failure at birth. ABCA3-related lung disease was recognized in full-term infants with severe lung disease inherited as an autosomal recessive gene.[44] The carrier frequency for *ABCA3* mutations is estimated to be 1 in 33, predicting a disease frequency of 1 in 3500, although the number of infants diagnosed with this disease is much less.[45] Clinical findings of ABCA3 deficiency are similar to those of SP-B deficiency, causing diffuse alveolar disease, atelectasis, and respiratory failure in newborn infants. Light microscopy generally shows acute or chronic lung disease, "desquamating interstitial pneumonitis," and CAP, which is similar to that seen in *SFTPB*-related disease (Fig. 19.4). Ultrastructural abnormalities in AT2 cells are useful for the diagnosis of ABCA3-related disease. Lamellar bodies are absent, and small, abnormal vesicles with electron-dense inclusions are strongly suggestive of ABCA3 deficiency.[44] As seen in *SFTPB* mutations, tubular myelin is absent in the alveolar spaces in ABCA3 deficiency. A definitive diagnosis is made by identification of the mutations in the *ABCA3* gene. ABCA3 deficiency is inherited in an autosomal recessive fashion. Clinical findings are influenced by the nature of the mutation and resulting residual function of the protein. More than 400 distinct mutations have been associated with lung disease. Most infants with ABCA3-related disease present with severe respiratory failure refractory to clinical management. However, less severe mutations may present later in life as interstitial lung diseases with pathological diagnoses of NSIP. Heterozygous deleterious mutations in ABCA3 are associated with an increased risk of respiratory distress in preterm infants.[46] Mutations in ABCA3 are the most frequent cause of hereditary disorders of surfactant metabolism, accounting for 30% to 40% of cases.

Clinical Perspectives

Hereditary disorders disrupting lung morphogenesis or surfactant homeostasis should be suspected in full-term infants presenting with unexplained respiratory failure associated with clinical and radiographic findings typical of lung hypoplasia and diffuse lung disease consistent with surfactant dysfunction. Likewise, disorders of surfactant metabolism should be considered in infants with severe chronic lung disease, for example, CPI, nonspecific interstitial lung disease, or early-onset pulmonary fibrosis. A definitive genetic diagnosis of *FOXF1*, *TBX4*, *NKX2-1*, *ABCA3*, *SFTPC*, and *SFTPB* gene-related lung disease is useful for clinical decision-making and genetic counseling. Clinical care decisions can be guided by careful assessment of pulmonary function, lung imaging, and histopathology. Definitive diagnosis requires the identification of the mutations in the genes encoding the critical proteins. Definitive therapies have not been identified for any of the disorders presenting in the newborn period. Lung transplantation has helped the quality of life and extended survival in a number of infants with these severe lung diseases. In the United States, a number of laboratories have expertise in the diagnosis of monogenic diffuse lung disease, and opportunities to establish a genetic diagnosis have been greatly enhanced by the increasingly widespread use of high-throughput gene sequencing (whole exome or whole-genome sequencing) in critically ill neonates.[47] Considerable progress has been made in understanding the genetic basis of inherited disorders of surfactant metabolism and lung formation that cause severe lung disease in newborns, and our knowledge will likely continue to grow with the expanded use of WES/WGS in children with suspected inborn errors of lung morphogenesis and surfactant metabolism.

RECOMMENDED FOR REVIEW

Whitsett JA, Wert SE, Weaver TE. Diseases of pulmonary surfactant homeostasis. *Annu Rev Pathol*. 2015;10:371-93.

Griese M. Pulmonary surfactant in health and human lung diseases: state of the art. *Eur Respir J*. 1999;13(6):1455-1476.

Atochina-Vasserman EN, Beers MF, Gow AJ. Review: Chemical and structural modifications of pulmonary collectins and their functional consequences. *Innate Immun*. 2010;16(3):175-182.

Nogee LM, Ryan RM. Genetic testing for neonatal respiratory disease. *Children (Basel)*. 2021;8(3):216.

REFERENCES

1. Johansson HKL, Taxvig C, Olsen GPM, et al. Effects of the hedgehog signaling inhibitor itraconazole on developing rat ovaries. *Toxicol Sci*. 2021;182:60-69.
2. Sun X, Perl AK, Li R, et al. A census of the lung: CellCards from LungMAP. *Dev Cell*. 2022;57:112-145.e2.
3. Bishop NB, Stankiewicz P, Steinhorn RH. Alveolar capillary dysplasia. *Am J Respir Crit Care Med*. 2011;184:172-179.
4. Karolak JA, Gambin T, Szafranski P, et al. Potential interactions between the TBX4-FGF10 and SHH-FOXF1 signaling during human lung development revealed using ChIP-seq. *Respir Res*. 2021;22:26.
5. Vincent M, Karolak JA, Deutsch G, et al. Clinical, histopathological, and molecular diagnostics in lethal lung developmental disorders. *Am J Respir Crit Care Med*. 2019;200:1093-1101.
6. Suhrie K, Pajor NM, Ahlfeld SK, et al. Neonatal lung disease associated with TBX4 mutations. *J Pediatr*. 2019;206:286-292.e1.
7. Haarman MG, Kerstjens-Frederikse WS, Berger RMF. The ever-expanding phenotypical spectrum of human TBX4 mutations: from toe to lung. *Eur Respir J*. 2019;54:1901504.
8. Barnett CP, Nataren NJ, Klingler-Hoffmann M, et al. Ectrodactyly and lethal pulmonary acinar dysplasia associated with homozygous FGFR2 mutations identified by exome sequencing. *Hum Mutat*. 2016;37:955-963.
9. Prince LS. FGF10 and human lung disease across the life spectrum. *Front Genet*. 2018;9:517.
10. Nogee LM. Interstitial lung disease in newborns. *Semin Fetal Neonatal Med*. 2017;22:227-233.
11. Young LR, Deutsch GH, Bokulic RE, et al. A mutation in TTF1/NKX2.1 is associated with familial neuroendocrine cell hyperplasia of infancy. *Chest*. 2013;144:1199-1206.
12. Nogee LM. Genetic causes of surfactant protein abnormalities. *Curr Opin Pediatr*. 2019;31:330-339.
13. Nattes E, Lejeune S, Carsin A, et al. Heterogeneity of lung disease associated with NK2 homeobox 1 mutations. *Respir Med*. 2017;129:16-23.
14. Hamvas A, Deterding RR, Wert SE, et al. Heterogeneous pulmonary phenotypes associated with mutations in the thyroid transcription factor gene NKX2-1. *Chest*. 2013;144:794-804.
15. Galambos C, Levy H, Cannon CL, et al. Pulmonary pathology in thyroid transcription factor-1 deficiency syndrome. *Am J Respir Crit Care Med*. 2010;182:549-554.
16. Bakrania P, Robinson DO, Bunyan DJ, et al. SOX2 anophthalmia syndrome: 12 new cases demonstrating broader phenotype and high frequency of large gene deletions. *Br J Ophthalmol*. 2007;91:1471-1476.
17. Jo A, Denduluri S, Zhang B, et al. The versatile functions of Sox9 in development, stem cells, and human diseases. *Genes Dis*. 2014;1:149-161.
18. Bridges JP, Ludwig MG, Mueller M, et al. Orphan G protein-coupled receptor GPR116 regulates pulmonary surfactant pool size. *Am J Respir Cell Mol Biol*. 2013;49:348-357.
19. Trapnell BC, Nakata K, Bonella F, et al. Pulmonary alveolar proteinosis. *Nat Rev Dis Primers*. 2019;5:16.
20. McCormack FX, Whitsett JA. The pulmonary collectins, SP-A and SP-D, orchestrate innate immunity in the lung. *J Clin Invest*. 2002;109:707-712.
21. Wright JR. Immunoregulatory functions of surfactant proteins. *Nat Rev Immunol*. 2005;5:58-68.
22. Wang Y, Kuan PJ, Xing C, et al. Genetic defects in surfactant protein A2 are associated with pulmonary fibrosis and lung cancer. *Am J Hum Genet*. 2009;84:52-59.
23. Madsen J, Kliem A, Tornoe I, et al. Localization of lung surfactant protein D on mucosal surfaces in human tissues. *J Immunol*. 2000;164:5866-5870.
24. Stahlman MT, Gray ME, Hull WM, et al. Immunolocalization of surfactant protein-D (SP-D) in human fetal, newborn, and adult tissues. *J Histochem Cytochem*. 2002;50:651-660.
25. Korfhagen TR, Sheftelyevich V, Burhans MS, et al. Surfactant protein-D regulates surfactant phospholipid homeostasis in vivo. *J Biol Chem*. 1998;273:28438-28443.
26. Haataja R, Hallman M. Surfactant proteins as genetic determinants of multifactorial pulmonary diseases. *Ann Med*. 2002;34:324-333.
27. Nogee LM. Alterations in SP-B and SP-C expression in neonatal lung disease. *Annu Rev Physiol*. 2004;66:601-623.
28. Huang H, Pan J, Spielberg DR, et al. A dominant negative variant of RAB5B disrupts maturation of surfactant protein B and surfactant protein C. *Proc Natl Acad Sci U S A*. 2022;119:e2105228119.
29. Weaver TE, Conkright JJ. Function of surfactant proteins B and C. *Annu Rev Physiol*. 2001;63:555-578.
30. Clark JC, Wert SE, Bachurski CJ, et al. Targeted disruption of the surfactant protein B gene disrupts surfactant homeostasis, causing respiratory failure in newborn mice. *Proc Natl Acad Sci U S A*. 1995;92:7794-7798.
31. Nogee LM, Garnier G, Dietz HC, et al. A mutation in the surfactant protein B gene responsible for fatal neonatal respiratory disease in multiple kindreds. *J Clin Invest*. 1994;93:1860-1863.
32. Whitsett JA, Weaver TE. Hydrophobic surfactant proteins in lung function and disease. *N Engl J Med*. 2002;347:2141-2148.
33. Melton KR, Nesslein LL, Ikegami M, et al. SP-B deficiency causes respiratory failure in adult mice. *Am J Physiol Lung Cell Mol Physiol*. 2003;285:L543-L549.
34. Ballard PL, Nogee LM, Beers MF, et al. Partial deficiency of surfactant protein B in an infant with chronic lung disease. *Pediatrics*. 1995;96:1046-1052.
35. Gregory TJ, Longmore WJ, Moxley MA, et al. Surfactant chemical composition and biophysical activity in acute respiratory distress syndrome. *J Clin Invest*. 1991;88:1976-1981.
36. Nogee LM, Wert SE, Proffit SA, et al. Allelic heterogeneity in hereditary surfactant protein B (SP-B) deficiency. *Am J Respir Crit Care Med*. 2000;161:973-981.
37. Cole FS, Hamvas A, Rubinstein P, et al. Population-based estimates of surfactant protein B deficiency. *Pediatrics*. 2000;105:538-541.
38. Dunbar AE III, Wert SE, Ikegami M, et al. Prolonged survival in hereditary surfactant protein B (SP-B) deficiency associated with a novel splicing mutation. *Pediatr Res*. 2000;48:275-282.
39. Lopez-Andreu JA, Hidalgo-Santos AD, Fuentes-Castello MA, et al. Delayed presentation and prolonged survival of a child with surfactant protein B deficiency. *J Pediatr*. 2017;190:268-270.e1.

40. Hamvas A, Nogee LM, Mallory Jr GB, et al. Lung transplantation for treatment of infants with surfactant protein B deficiency. *J Pediatr*. 1997;130:231-239.
41. Glasser SW, Detmer EA, Ikegami M, et al. Pneumonitis and emphysema in sp-C gene targeted mice. *J Biol Chem*. 2003;278: 14291-14298.
42. Nogee LM, Dunbar AE III, Wert SE, et al. A mutation in the surfactant protein C gene associated with familial interstitial lung disease. *N Engl J Med*. 2001;344:573-579.
43. Mulugeta S, Gray JM, Notarfrancesco KL, et al. Identification of LBM180, a lamellar body limiting membrane protein of alveolar type II cells, as the ABC transporter protein ABCA3. *J Biol Chem*. 2002;277:22147-22155.
44. Shulenin S, Nogee LM, Annilo T, et al. ABCA3 gene mutations in newborns with fatal surfactant deficiency. *N Engl J Med*. 2004;350:1296-1303.
45. Wambach JA, Casey AM, Fishman MP, et al. Genotype-phenotype correlations for infants and children with ABCA3 deficiency. *Am J Respir Crit Care Med*. 2014;189:1538-1543.
46. Wambach JA, Wegner DJ, Depass K, et al. Single ABCA3 mutations increase risk for neonatal respiratory distress syndrome. *Pediatrics*. 2012;130:e1575-e1582.
47. Nogee LM, Ryan RM. Genetic testing for neonatal respiratory disease. *Children (Basel)*. 2021;8:216.

Chapter 20

Fetal Intervention in Congenital Malformations of the Respiratory System

Rodrigo Ruano and Oluwateniayo O. Okpaise

Chapter Outline

Introduction
Congenital Diaphragmatic Hernia
    Embryology and Etiology
    Prenatal Diagnosis
    Prenatal Fetal Therapy

Congenital Lung Masses Or Congenital Pulmonary Malformations
    Types of Congenital Pulmonary Malformations
    Fetal Therapy for the Congenital Pulmonary Malformations
Conclusions

Key Points

- Congenital malformations of the respiratory system consist of a wide range of fetal anomalies that can affect the developing of the fetal lungs.
- Most congenital malformations of the respiratory system can be diagnosed prenatally by identifying hyperechoic lung masses on ultrasonography.
- Once the prenatal diagnosis of congenital malformations of the respiratory system is made, it is crucial to have these patients referred to a specialized center with multidisciplinary teams.
- The main congenital malformations of the respiratory system are congenital diaphragmatic hernia (CDH), congenital bronchial atresia (BA), congenital pulmonary airway malformation (CPAM), bronchopulmonary sequestrations (BPS), and congenital high airway obstruction syndrome (CHAOS).
- Congenital malformations of the respiratory system in the fetus can be associated with different severity of pulmonary hypoplasia and pulmonary arterial hypertension.
- Fetal interventions are specifically performed for each disease following precise indications.

- The main objectives of the fetal interventions for congenital malformations of the respiratory system are to prevent severe pulmonary hypoplasia and severe pulmonary arterial hypertension.
- Fetal endoscopic tracheal occlusion (FETO) is a fetal intervention for severe CDH performed between 22 and 30 weeks' gestation with the objective of promoting fetal lung growth.
- Ultrasound-guided laser ablation seems to be the best option to treat BPSs complicated with hydrops.
- Ultrasound-guided ablation can also be used for congenital microcystic adenomatoid malformation.
- Fetal tracheostomy during EXIT is the treatment of choice for CHAOS.

The authors confirm that there is no conflict of interest.

Introduction

Congenital malformations of the respiratory system encompass a wide range of fetal defects that can affect the developing fetal lung vasculature, airways, and parenchyma.[1] These abnormalities account for approximately

5% to 18% of fetal abnormalities and thus are considered rare.[2] Although infrequent, congenital pulmonary malformations (CPMs) can be detected in the prenatal period or remain asymptomatic and be diagnosed coincidentally later on in childhood.[3] The possible complications associated with pulmonary malformations can lead to long-term secondary complications after birth or demise in the neonatal period due to severe respiratory failure. As the likelihood of death is high in some of these conditions, in utero surgical interventions are increasingly being used to improve outcomes.

The present chapter reviews the main etiologies, clinical presentations, diagnosis, and prognosis of conditions that impair normal fetal pulmonary development, as well as highlight various fetal therapeutic procedures used to correct them.

Congenital Diaphragmatic Hernia

Congenital diaphragmatic hernia (CDH) results from an embryological closure defect resulting in diaphragmatic discontinuity.[4] The loss of diaphragmatic continuity allows for the protrusion of the abdominal contents in the thoracic cavity, which limits the development of the fetal lungs.[5] As it is associated with abnormal lung development, including airways, vascular, and alveolar structures, pulmonary hypoplasia can be significant and can lead to severe respiratory failure and death after birth.[6] Due to the abnormal branching architecture and decreased surfactant production, CDH is associated with high mortality rates and lifelong morbidity.[4,7]

EMBRYOLOGY AND ETIOLOGY

In the normal embryological process, the diaphragm is derived from various contributors, including the septum transversum, body wall, dorsal mesentery, and pleuroperitoneal folds, which are meant to fuse.[4] CDH can develop as early as 8 weeks of gestation when one or more of these structures fail to fuse; 90% of CDH presentations are posterolateral, known as Bochdalek hernias, while the anterolateral Morgagni hernias make up the remainder.[8,9]

The development of CDHs is thought to be influenced by both genetic and environmental factors.[10] Genetic aspects of disease development are highly varied and include aneuploidies, cytogenic abnormalities,

and single-gene mutations; common aneuploidies associated with CDH are trisomy 18, 13, and 21.[10] In rare cases, CDH can have inheritance patterns such as X-linked recessive or dominant traits.[9] These can run in families and present with herniation of both sides of the thoracic cavity; a subtype known as *familial diaphragmatic agenesis* is inherited in an autosomal recessive manner and has a poorer prognosis than typical posterolateral herniations.[9] While a majority of the cases of CDH are isolated, approximately 40% are syndromic in their origin (WAGR [Wilms tumor, aniridia, genitourinary anomalies, and intellectual disability], Denys-Drash, and Wolf-Hirschhorn syndromes).[7,11] Environmental causative factors are associated with maternal exposure to substances like tobacco and alcohol, advanced maternal age, a history of diabetes, and high maternal BMI.[12]

CDH can be isolated or associated with other anomalies, which can increase mortality and morbidity of the infant.[13] Cardiac anomalies are the most commonly associated with CDHs, with a prevalence of 30% in live births; these heart defects can have a vast spectrum of presentation, with more severe defects having a higher rate of mortality.[13] The development of pulmonary hypertension in the postnatal period is another complication associated with diaphragmatic herniation. CDH causes aberrant airway branching and impaired alveolarization, disrupting the pulmonary vascularization, leading to high pulmonary vascular resistance that persists after delivery.[9]

The bulk of fetuses with congenital diaphragmatic herniations present with the defect on the left side of the thorax, whereas right-sided defects account for approximately 15% of the cases; bilateral presentations account for less than 1%.[14] Right-sided CDH presentations can be associated with hepatopulmonary fusion, in which an unidentifiable plane of separation is seen between the lung and herniated liver.[15] This rare malformation allows the merging of fetal lung and liver, leading to indistinguishable histopathological findings; hepatopulmonary fusion can also provoke pulmonary bronchial and vascular pathologies as well.[15]

PRENATAL DIAGNOSIS

The diagnosis of CDH is typically made prenatally, as the displacement of abdominal organs into the thoracic cavity can be seen on multiple imaging modalities, including routine ultrasound investigations, typically around a gestational age of 24 weeks.[5,11]

Although ultrasound is the most common mode of diagnosis, three-dimensional (3D) imaging, fetal MRI, and echocardiography can aid in determining not only the severity but prognosis as well.[5] Ruano et al.[16] showed that 3D sonography and MRI measurements could accurately determine fetal lung volumes and thus can be used to diagnose pulmonary hypoplasia in fetuses with CDH. While the direct measurement of the lung volume is a sound way of predicting neonatal outcomes, Metkus et al.[17] were the first to demonstrate that lung-to-head ratio (LHR) could be used to accurately determine the size of the lung contralateral to the side of the hernial defect.[18]

PRENATAL FETAL THERAPY

Fetal endoscopic tracheal occlusion (FETO) is a minimally invasive procedure (no need for a hysterotomy to perform the procedure) that is now one of the surgical options for CDH.[19] It involves the percutaneous placement of instruments under sonographic guidance and fetoscopic placement of a tracheal balloon to improve fetal lung development. Several studies, including a recent randomized controlled trial, have shown that tracheal occlusion reduces perinatal morbidity and mortality rates and decreases the need for ECMO.[20-26] FETO can promote lung regrowth and pulmonary vascular development in the fetus and may decrease the severity of pulmonary arterial hypertension.[21,22]

FETO is typically used in fetuses with severe herniation without other major congenital malformations.[20] Before FETO, fetal congenital diaphragmatic herniations were treated via Fetendo tracheal clipping, but this was associated with damage to the fetal vocal cords and trachea; thus, FETO is now the preferred approach.[23]

The gestational timeframe for FETO intervention is typically between 22 and 30 weeks of gestation.[23] In this procedure, a trocar is inserted through the maternal abdominal wall and into the amniotic cavity under ultrasonic guidance. Following this, a fetoscope is inserted into the fetus' mouth to reach the trachea and advanced until the carina is seen. At that point, the tracheal balloon is deployed.[23] Preferably, the balloon should remain in the trachea until at least the 34th week of gestation when the plug is removed. Until that time,

frequent monitoring is needed to ensure deflation or other complications do not occur.[24] The procedure typically lasts an average of 15 minutes and is performed using local maternal anesthesia and fetal intramuscular anesthesia to minimize the risk of complications during the procedure.[21]

The time frame for balloon removal depends on a myriad of factors, including the surgeon's level of expertise, stability of mother and fetus, and balloon accessibility. However, it is usually removed at 34 weeks' gestation when a maximal fetal lung response is seen.[24-26] Multiple methods can be used for the removal, such as fetoscopic retrieval, percutaneous puncture, and removal via the ex utero intrapartum treatment (EXIT procedure). Following removal, the pregnancy can be managed expectantly; however, if removal is not possible during pregnancy, immediate removal after delivery must occur.[24] In a trial performed by Ruano et al.,[27] the EXIT procedure was used to remove tracheal balloons in all subjects involved. Once this removal occurred, the umbilical cord was cut, and delivery occurred.[27] Ruano et al.[28-31] also demonstrated that the maximal fetal pulmonary response is achieved at approximately 34 weeks of gestation. Removing the fetal tracheal balloon at this time frame may allow for a more effective transition of type I alveolar cells to type II cells.[32]

FETO is not without complications, the most prevalent being preterm delivery and premature rupture of the membranes (PROM).[33] These complications are related to the size of the fetoscope used during the procedure, with larger fetoscopes associated with more side effects.[22] Furthermore, the duration of the procedure also increases the risk of premature rupture of membranes, so fetal surgeons should strive to perform FETO in the shortest time possible.[22] While intraamniotic hemorrhage due to trocar insertion is possible, its incidence decreases with surgical expertise.[22]

Attempts to close the CDH in utero via open fetal thoracotomy and maternal hysterotomy have failed so far. Open fetal repair of the diaphragmatic hernia in utero has a higher risk for maternal morbidity and premature delivery and showed no overall improvement in fetal survival.[21,32] Furthermore, open repair is not possible in fetuses that present with liver herniation as attempts at reduction can damage the umbilical vein.[32]

Future applications of FETO to reduce the prevalence of possible complications include integrating smart balloon technology.[21] This was first described by Sananes et al.[34] who developed the "Smart-TO" composed of latex and a magnetic valve. The application of a magnetic field can open the valve and deflate the balloon, reducing the need for the traditional methods of removing the balloon.[34]

Congenital Lung Masses or Congenital Pulmonary Malformations

CPMs are a group of relatively uncommon disorders that can result in abnormal fetal lung development and respiratory failure in the postnatal period.[35] These rare conditions can affect a wide range of pulmonary structures, allowing for a spectrum of pathological and clinical presentations.[1]

Various etiological factors may explain the development of CPMs, but the four main theories at present are defective foregut budding and differentiation, genetic causes, vascular abnormalities, and airway obstruction.[3] Most CPMs are identified prenatally during routine ultrasound checkups, particularly in the second trimester.[36] Mediastinal shift and evidence of thoracic compression detected on sonographic examination is associated with a poorer prognosis; fetuses with these features are at higher risk for needing postnatal surgical correction.[36]

TYPES OF CONGENITAL PULMONARY MALFORMATIONS

Congenital Pulmonary Airway Malformation

Congenital pulmonary airway malformations (CPAMs), previously known as congenital cystic adenomatoid malformations (CCAMs), are a group of diverse conditions that cause the formation of cystic and noncystic pulmonary lesions in early fetal development.[37] This condition affects the lower respiratory tract, and the cystic appearance is thought to be secondary to the abnormal airway branching during organogenesis.[38] CPAM accounts for over 90% of fetal cystic lung lesions and is typically diagnosed around the 18th to 20th gestational week.[38]

Triggering factors of CPAMs are controversial, but a proposed hypothesis is an imbalance between cell proliferation and apoptosis during organogenesis.[39] A study by Hsu et al.[39] showed that CPAM is genetically heterogeneous and requires more than 1 gene mutation for the disease to manifest.

Based on their appearance, CPAM was historically classified into three groups based on their histopathological presentation by Stocker et al.[40]

- Type 1 is characterized by cysts larger than 2 cm, covered by bronchial epithelium overlying fibromuscular stroma.
- Type 2 has smaller cysts, less than 2 cm, covered by bronchiolar epithelium, which is associated with airway obstruction.
- Type 3 does not appear as a cystic lesion but has a macroscopically solid appearance.[41]

Types 0 and 4 have been added to this classification with an overall improvement.[38] Type 0 is characterized by acinar dysplasia in the trachea and bronchi, while type 4 describes predominantly large air-filled cysts in the distal acini.[3]

CPAM can also present with abnormal connections to the airway and pulmonary vasculature[37] and studies with ultrasound, magnetic resonance imaging, and even computerized tomography may be needed.[37]

Bronchial Atresia

Bronchial atresia is an unusual congenital malformation that results in the dysplastic formation of the fetal bronchi in the main, lobar, or segmental bronchi.[42] These malformations will result in either the hyperinflation and hyperplasia of the lung parenchyma or normal formation, depending on the anatomical level of the obstruction. Eventually, there will be an accumulation of mucus behind the obstruction.[3,42] The exact cause is unknown, but proposed hypotheses include intrauterine ischemia and secondary atresia due to obstructions like herniations or mucosal hypertrophy.[43] Prenatal imaging will show fluid-filled lung distal to the atretic lesion; MRI and CT imaging can demonstrate the complex lung mass.[37]

Segmental Bronchial Atresia

Segmental bronchial atresia is the most common presentation and occurs when the segmental bronchi are affected.[44] It has been suggested that segmental bronchial atresia can be associated with other pulmonary malformations, including CPAM and BPS.[45]

Mainstem Bronchial Atresia

Mainstem bronchial atresia (MBA) is a rare congenital abnormality incompatible with postnatal life, as it involves the entire lung parenchyma distal to the atresia.[46,47] As it is a lethal condition, prompt differential diagnosis from other pathological states is important. MBA seems to have a predilection for developing in the right bronchus with presentations of hyperplasia, mediastinal shift, fetal hydrops, and even death.[45] Survival rate in fetuses with MBA is very low.[45,46]

Bronchopulmonary Sequestration

BPS is a rare congenital disorder in which unaerated tissue is located outside the tracheobronchial tree but receives blood supply directly from the systemic circulation; these masses may be intralobular or extralobular in their origin.[48,49] BPS is thought to be due to accessory lung buds forming below the normal lung bud of the primitive foregut. This accessory mass will continually move caudally as the esophagus elongates, allowing it to derive blood supply from systemic vessels during migration.[50]

Intralobular lesions are located within the visceral pleura of the functioning lung, while the extralobular lesions have a separate visceral pleura altogether.[51] Intralobular sequestrations are more common than their extralobular counterparts, making up more than 70% of the presenting cases, and most are found in the lower lobes.[52] The relation of these masses to the normal lung parenchyma also determines their venous drainage, with intralobular masses draining directly into the pulmonary veins and extralobular draining to the systemic venous circulation.[51] Their size can vary from unremarkable to large enough to cause complications in utero, including mediastinal shifts, cardiac dysfunction, hydrops fetalis, and fetal demise.[49] It is also possible for BPS to have an abnormal connection to the gastrointestinal tract, particularly the esophagus. Extralobular sequestrations are associated with other congenital anomalies like CDHs.[51,52]

Prenatal diagnosis of BPS is based on the presence of hyperechogenic lung masses seen by a standard two-dimensional ultrasound investigation.[48] Aberrant blood supply to the mass can also be detected using color Doppler sonography, but this is not a very sensitive mode of investigation.[48] Compared to ultrasonography, fetal MRI can better distinguish the accessory lobe from normal fetal lung tissue.[53]

Congenital High Airway Obstruction Syndrome

Congenital high airway obstruction syndrome, also known as CHAOS, is a unique fetal condition in which an intrinsic upper airway obstruction develops.[54] This blockage can be partial or complete, and result from a variety of causes including laryngeal cysts, tracheal atresia/stenosis, laryngeal stenosis, and laryngeal atresia that is the most frequent cause.[55,56]

Blockades in the upper airway will cause distal accumulation and entrapment of pulmonary fluid, which cause secondary pulmonary hyperplasia and flattening of the diaphragm.[57] The enlarged fetal lungs can then compress adjacent organs, like the heart and vena cava, ultimately leading to heart failure in utero.[58] Associated findings with this fetal heart failure include placentomegaly, ascites, and fetal hydrops, which can all lead to fetal demise.[58]

While the etiology of CHAOS is unknown and its occurrence is sporadic, there have been associations with certain genetic syndromes and chromosomal abnormalities.[59] The most common genetic syndrome associated with CHAOS is Fraser syndrome, an autosomal recessive disorder characterized by laryngeal atresia, renal agenesis, polydactyly, and microphthalmia.[59] The chromosomal anomalies cri-du-chat and DiGeorge syndrome, which are due to deletions in chromosomes 5p and 22q11.2 respectfully, can also present with CHAOS.[60]

Most cases of CHAOS are diagnosable in utero, which is essential as stillbirth and death in the postnatal period are likely complications of this condition.[61] Typical findings on prenatal sonographic examination include large lungs, displaced heart, flattened diaphragm, and increased amounts of amniotic fluid.[61] While ultrasonography is the initial diagnostic method for CHAOS, MRI can offer additional information, which is essential for surgical planning and correction.[61] Unfortunately, while these modalities can confirm the prenatal diagnosis of CHAOS, they can be limited in determining the severity and complexity of the obstruction.[54]

FETAL THERAPY FOR THE CONGENITAL PULMONARY MALFORMATIONS

The main indication for in utero fetal therapy for CPMs is the presence of fetal hydrops and/or fetal cardiac dysfunction.[62] There are different modalities of fetal therapy, including (1) open fetal tumor resection,

(2) ultrasound-guided laser vascular ablation of the feeding tumor vessels, and (3) interstitial radiofrequency ablation of the fetal lung mass.[63] We will discuss next the specific therapeutic modality for each disease.

Fetal Therapy for Congenital Pulmonary Airway Malformation and Segmental Bronchial Atresia

While CPAM can be treated in the postnatal period, there are various methods of managing CPAM in the prenatal period to improve the outcome of the fetus and prevent secondary complications. Fetal hydrops and/or fetal cardiac dysfunction[64] occurs in less than 5% of cases but is associated with extremely high perinatal mortality (>90%). The first step is always to administer maternal corticosteroids, 12 mg given intramuscularly.[65] If this therapy is not successful in reversing the fetal hydrops in 48 to 72 hours, the next step is to offer fetal surgery, including open fetal surgery or minimally invasive procedures.[38] The first reported case of open surgical resection was described by Harrison et al.[66] Since this report, different intervention methods have been implemented to correct CPAMs surgically, including the use of EXIT. EXIT is a procedure used to secure the fetal airway while the fetus remains attached to the uteroplacental circulation.[67] The EXIT procedure can be done in the case of large CPAMs with secondary consequences such as pulmonary hypoplasia, mediastinal shift, and fetal hydrops.[38,68]

Minimally invasive procedures are preferred over open surgical procedures as they allow for fewer side effects for the mother and fetus. Ruano et al.[69] described the treatment of CCAM by using a process known as interstitial laser ablation. This is performed under ultrasound guidance and uses laser wire to coagulate the lesion using heat, leading to eventual cell death.[69,70] Sclerotherapy has also shown success in treating microcystic CPAMs complicated by fetal hydrops; however, complications like the intravascular dissemination of the sclerotherapeutic agent and fetal death are possible.[70]

Fetal Therapy for Mainstem Bronchial Atresia

Bronchial atresia can cause many secondary complications that can lead to fetal demise, including pulmonary hyperplasia, mediastinal shift, and fetal hydrops.[71] While fetal surgery is potentially lifesaving, it is not always indicated, as both the risks and benefits of the procedure should be considered. Smaller peripherally located atresias typically do not need intervention, while centrally located ones frequently need some sort of resection.[71,72] Fetuses selected for this procedure should have a normal karyotype and no associated severe anatomical abnormalities.[72] After an incision is made in the wall of the uterus, the fetal arm is exposed, and a thoracotomy is performed to remove the obliterated bronchial segment and the accompanying mucocele.[42] Once the obstructing mass is removed, the resolution of fetal hydrops and mediastinal shift will occur, and growth of the contralateral lung will be possible.[46]

Martinez et al.[47] first described fetoscopic surgery as an alternative to open resection for treating bronchial atresia. In this procedure, an endoscope is placed into the fetal mouth and down the trachea to view the stenotic region; a laser guidewire is used to perforate the mucocele and allow for drainage.[73]

Bronchopulmonary Sequestration

Ultrasound-guided ablation of the abnormal feeding vessels that develop in association with BPS decreases the chances of perinatal death.[49,74] A case report by Ruano et al.[74] described the laser ablation of pulmonary sequestration in a woman at 29 gestational weeks complicated by fetal hydrops. This procedure was done under maternal and fetal anesthesia using a 20-gauge needle and 600 μm laser fiber to disrupt the abnormal connection between this pulmonary mass and the fetal aorta.[74] Once the blood supply was cut off, the pulmonary mass decreased, allowing for an increase in fetal lung volumes and a complete resolution of the hydrops.

As BPS can be associated with other fetal congenital malformations, minimally invasive intervention, like laser ablation, may not be enough to ensure complete correction; in cases such as this, open surgery may be the better option. The resection of BPS also depends on their location; extralobular sequestrations are excised using sequestrectomies as they have their own pleural lining, while lobectomies are used to remove intralobular sequestrations due to their more complex vasculature and loss of defined intersegmental planes.[35,49]

Congenital High Airway Obstruction Syndrome

Although rare, CHAOS was once thought to be a certain fatal condition; however, due to surgical advancements, fetal demise is no longer inevitable.

The EXIT procedure has been used before delivery to allow an airway to be established while the fetus remains attached to the placental circulation.[75] Peiro et al.[76] and Ruano et al.[54] have suggested using fetoscopic laser ablation to treat congenital high airway obstruction as an alternative to EXIT procedures.[76] While fetal complications may improve following laser ablation of the obstructed fetal airway, additional procedures may be needed.[76,77]

Conclusions

Congenital malformations of the respiratory system represent a group of heterogeneous abnormalities that can present with overlapping findings on imaging. Although the prenatal diagnosis of some conditions that fall into the spectrum of CPMs can be difficult, the use of ultrasound and magnetic resonance imaging can identify specific distinguishing factors to aid sonographers and surgeons in their diagnosis. Once a diagnosis and disease severity have been determined, surgeons can then establish which mode of surgical intervention would be most appropriate. The main indication for in utero fetal therapy is the presence of fetal hydrops and/or fetal cardiac dysfunction. There are different modalities of fetal interventions with specific approaches determined by the type of congenital malformations of the respiratory system. These procedures should only be performed in a highly specialized tertiary fetal therapy center with an experienced multidisciplinary team.

REFERENCES

1. Nadeem M, Elnazir B, Greally P. Congenital pulmonary malformation in children. *Scientifica (Cairo)*. 2012;2012:209896.
2. Annunziata F, Bush A, Borgia F, et al. Congenital lung malformations: unresolved issues and unanswered questions. *Front Pediatr.* 2019;7:239.
3. Lee EY, Dorkin H, Vargas SO. Congenital pulmonary malformations in pediatric patients: review and update on etiology, classification, and imaging findings. *Radiol Clin North Am.* 2011;49(5):921-948.
4. Kosiński P, Wielgoś M. Congenital diaphragmatic hernia: pathogenesis, prenatal diagnosis and management: literature review. *Ginekol Pol.* 2017;88(1):24-30.
5. Chandrasekharan PK, Rawat M, Madappa R, et al. Congenital diaphragmatic hernia: a review. *Matern Health Neonatol Perinatol.* 2017;3(1):6.
6. Ruano R, Martinovic J, Aubry MC, et al. Predicting pulmonary hypoplasia using the sonographic fetal lung volume to body weight ratio: how precise and accurate is it. *Ultrasound Obstet Gynecol.* 2006;28(7):958-962.
7. Wynn J, Yu L, Chung WK. Genetic causes of congenital diaphragmatic hernia. *Semin Fetal Neonatal Med.* 2014;19(6):324-330.
8. Juretschke LJ. Congenital diaphragmatic hernia: update and review. *J Obstet Gynecol Neonatal Nurs.* 2001;30(3):259-268.
9. Baerg J, Thirumoorthi A, Hazboun R. Congenital diaphragmatic hernia. In: Derbel F, ed. *Hernia.* 2017. Available at: https://www.intechopen.com/chapters/56039. doi:10.5772/intechopen.69362.
10. Kardon G, Ackerman KG, McCulley DJ, et al. Congenital diaphragmatic hernias: from genes to mechanisms to therapies. *Dis Model Mech.* 2017;10(8):955-970.
11. Tovar JA. Congenital diaphragmatic hernia. *Orphanet J Rare Dis.* 2012;7(1):1.
12. Mesas Burgos C, Ehrén H, Conner P, et al. Maternal risk factors and perinatal characteristics in congenital diaphragmatic hernia: a nationwide population-based study. *Fetal Diagn Ther.* 2019;46(6):385-391.
13. Ruano R, Javadian P, Kailin JA, et al. Congenital heart anomaly in newborns with congenital diaphragmatic hernia: a single-center experience. *Ultrasound Obstet Gynecol.* 2014;45(6):683-688.
14. DeKoninck P, Gomez O, Sandaite I, et al. Right-sided congenital diaphragmatic hernia in a decade of fetal surgery. *BJOG.* 2015;122(7):940-946.
15. Saleem A, Alnaqi AAA, Taqi EA. Right-sided congenital diaphragmatic hernia associated with hepatopulmonary fusion and congenital pulmonary malformation. *J Pediatr Surg Case Rep.* 2021;72:101958.
16. Ruano R, Aubry MC, Dumez Y, et al. Predicting neonatal deaths and pulmonary hypoplasia in isolated congenital diaphragmatic hernia using the sonographic fetal lung volume-body weight ratio. *AJR Am J Roentgenol.* 2008;190(5):1216-1219.
17. Metkus AP, Filly RA, Stringer MD, et al. Sonographic predictors of survival in fetal diaphragmatic hernia. *J Pediatr Surg.* 1996;31(1):148-151; discussion 151-152.
18. Cordier AG, Russo FM, Deprest J, et al. Prenatal diagnosis, imaging, and prognosis in Congenital Diaphragmatic Hernia. *Semin Perinatol.* 2020;44(1):51163.
19. Braga AFA, da Silva Braga FS, Nascimento SP, et al. Oclusão traqueal por fetoscopia em hérnia diafragmática congênita grave: estudo retrospectivo [Fetoscopic tracheal occlusion for severe congenital diaphragmatic hernia: retrospective study]. *Rev Bras Anestesiol.* 2017;67(4):331-336.
20. Belfort MA, Olutoye OO, Cass DL, et al. Feasibility and outcomes of fetoscopic tracheal occlusion for severe left diaphragmatic hernia. *Obstet Gynecol.* 2017;129(1):20-29.
21. Ruano R, Vega B. Fetal surgery: how recent technological advancements are extending its applications. *Expert Rev Med Devices.* 2019;16(8):643-645.
22. Ruano R, Ali RA, Patel P, et al. Fetal endoscopic tracheal occlusion for congenital diaphragmatic hernia: indications, outcomes, and future directions. *Obstet Gynecol Surv.* 2014;69(3):147-158.
23. Helal AA. Principles of fetal surgery. In: *Pediatric Surgery, Flowcharts and Clinical Algorithms.* ntechOpen. https://www.intechopen.com/books/8463; 2019.
24. Perrone EE, Deprest JA. Fetal endoscopic tracheal occlusion for congenital diaphragmatic hernia: a narrative review of the history, current practice, and future directions. *Transl Pediatr.* 2021;10(5):1448-1460.
25. Deprest JA, Nicolaides KH, Benachi A, et al. Randomized trial of fetal surgery for severe left diaphragmatic hernia. *N Engl J Med.* 2021;385(2):107-118.

26. Deprest JA, Benachi A, Gratacos E, et al. Randomized trial of fetal surgery for moderate left diaphragmatic hernia. *N Engl J Med.* 2021;385(2):119-129.

27. Ruano R, Yoshisaki CT, da Silva MM, et al. A randomized controlled trial of fetal endoscopic tracheal occlusion versus postnatal management of severe isolated congenital diaphragmatic hernia. *Ultrasound Obstet Gynecol.* 2012;39(1):20-27.

28. Ruano R, da Silva MM, Campos JA, et al. Fetal pulmonary response after fetoscopic tracheal occlusion for severe isolated congenital diaphragmatic hernia. *Obstet Gynecol.* 2012;119(1): 93-101.

29. Ruano R, Peiro JL, da Silva MM, et al. Early fetoscopic tracheal occlusion for extremely severe pulmonary hypoplasia in isolated congenital diaphragmatic hernia: preliminary results. *Ultrasound Obstet Gynecol.* 2013;42(1):70-76.

30. Ruano R, Klinkner DB, Balakrishnan K, et al. Fetoscopic therapy for severe pulmonary hypoplasia in congenital diaphragmatic hernia: a first in prenatal regenerative medicine at mayo clinic. *Mayo Clin Proc.* 2018;93(6):693-700.

31. Trad ATA, Czeresnia R, Ibirogba E, et al. Sonographic pulmonary response after tracheal occlusion in fetuses with severe isolated congenital diaphragmatic hernia. *J Clin Ultrasound.* 2022;50(2):185-190.

32. Deprest J, Gratacós E, Nicolaides KH. Fetoscopic tracheal occlusion (FETO) for severe congenital diaphragmatic hernia: evolution of a technique and preliminary results. *Ultrasound Obstet Gynecol.* 2004;24:121-126.

33. Araujo Júnior E, Tonni G, Martins WP, et al. Procedure-related complications and survival following Fetoscopic Endotracheal Occlusion (FETO) for severe congenital diaphragmatic hernia: systematic review and meta-analysis in the FETO era. *Eur J Pediatr Surg.* 2016;27(04):297-305.

34. Sananès N, Regnard P, Mottet N, et al. Evaluation of a new balloon for fetal endoscopic tracheal occlusion in the nonhuman primate model. *Prenat Diagn.* 2019;39(5):403-408. Available at: https://doi.org/10.1002/pd.5445.

35. Shanmugam G, MacArthur K, Pollock JC. Congenital lung malformations: antenatal and postnatal evaluation and management. *Eur J Cardiothorac Surg.* 2005;27(1):45-52.

36. Ruchonnet-Metrailler I, Leroy-Terquem E, Stirnemann J, et al. Neonatal outcomes of prenatally diagnosed congenital pulmonary malformations. *Pediatrics.* 2014;133(5):e1285-e1291.

37. Biyyam DR, Chapman T, Ferguson MR, et al. Congenital lung abnormalities: embryologic features, prenatal diagnosis, and postnatal radiologic-pathologic correlation. *RadioGraphics.* 2010;30(6):1721-1738.

38. David M, Lamas-Pinheiro R, Henriques-Coelho T. Prenatal and postnatal management of congenital pulmonary airway malformation. *Neonatology.* 2016;110:101-115.

39. Hsu JS, Zhang R, Yeung F, et al. Cancer gene mutations in congenital pulmonary airway malformation patients. *ERJ Open Res.* 2019;5(1):00196-2018.

40. Stocker JT, Madewell JE, Drake RM. Congenital cystic adenomatoid malformation of the lung. Classification and morphologic spectrum. *Hum Pathol.* 1977;8(2):155-171.

41. Popper H, Murer B. Congenital Pulmonary Airway Malformation (CPAM) Types 1–4. In: *Pulmonary Pathology Essentials of Diagnostic Pathology.* Springer, Cham; 2020. https://doi.org/10.1007/978-3-030-22664-0_21

42. Keswani SG, Crombleholme TM, Pawel BR, et al. Prenatal diagnosis and management of mainstem bronchial atresia. *Fetal Diagn Ther.* 2005;20(1):74-78.

43. Wang Y, Dai W, Sun Ye, et al. Congenital bronchial atresia: diagnosis and treatment. *Int J Med Sci.* 2012;9(3):207-212.

44. Hartman T. Bronchial atresia. In: Hartman T, ed. *Pearls and Pitfalls in Thoracic Imaging: Variants and Other Difficult Diagnoses.* Cambridge University Press; 2011. doi:10.1017/CBO9780511977701.

45. Abitayeh G, Ruano R, Martinovic J, et al. Prenatal diagnosis of main stem bronchial atresia using 3-dimensional ultrasonographic technologies. *J Ultrasound Med.* 2010;29(4):633-638.

46. Zamora IJ, Sheikh F, Olutoye OO, et al. Mainstem bronchial atresia: a lethal anomaly amenable to fetal surgical treatment. *J Pediatr Surg.* 2014;49(5):706-711.

47. Martínez JM, Prat J, Gómez O, et al. Decompression through tracheobronchial endoscopy of bronchial atresia presenting as massive pulmonary tumor: a new indication for fetoscopic surgery. *Fetal Diagn Ther.* 2013;33(1):69-74.

48. Ruano R, Benachi A, Aubry MC, et al. Prenatal diagnosis of pulmonary sequestration using three-dimensional power Doppler ultrasound. *Ultrasound Obstet Gynecol.* 2005;25(2):128-133. Available at: https://doi.org/10.1002/uog.1797.

49. Ruano R, Ibirogba ER, Wyatt MA, et al. Sequential minimally invasive fetal interventions for two life-threatening conditions: a novel approach. *Fetal Diagn Ther.* 2021;48(1):70-77.

50. Chakraborty RK, Modi P, Sharma S. *Pulmonary Sequestration.* Treasure Island, FL: StatPearls Publishing; 2022.

51. Newman B. Congenital bronchopulmonary foregut malformations: concepts and controversies. *Pediatr Radiol.* 2006;36(8):773-791.

52. Abbey P, Narula MK, Anand R. Congenital malformations and developmental anomalies of the lung. *Curr Radiol Rep.* 2014;2(11):71.

53. Li Z, Lv YD, Fang R, et al. Usefulness of prenatal magnetic resonance imaging in differential diagnosis of fetal congenital cystic adenomatoid malformation and bronchopulmonary sequestration. *World J Clin Cases.* 2021;9(4):822-829.

54. Ruano R, Cass DL, Rieger M, et al. Fetal laryngoscopy to evaluate vocal folds in a fetus with congenital high airway obstruction syndrome (CHAOS). *Ultrasound Obstet Gynecol.* 2014;43(1):102-103. Available at: https://doi.org/10.1002/uog.13191.

55. Werner H, Lopes J, Ribeiro G, et al. Congenital High Airway Obstruction Syndrome (CHAOS): virtual navigation in the fetal airways after intrauterine endoscopic treatment. *J Obstet Gynaecol Can.* 2021;43(7):879-883.

56. Wang Y, Zhao L, Li X. Congenital high airway obstruction with tracheoesophageal fistula: a case report. *Medicine (Baltimore).* 2018;97(51):e13709.

57. Sharma R, Dey AK, Alam S, Mittal K, Thakkar H. A series of congenital high airway obstruction syndrome: classic imaging findings. *J Clin Diagn Res.* 2016;10(3):TD07-TD09.

58. Lim FY, Crombleholme TM, Hedrick HL, et al. Congenital high airway obstruction syndrome: natural history and management. *J Pediatr Surg.* 2003;38(6):940-945.

59. D'Eufemia MD, Cianci S, Di Meglio F, et al. Congenital high airway obstruction syndrome (CHAOS): discussing the role and limits of prenatal diagnosis starting from a single-center case series. *J Prenat Med.* 2016;10(1-2):4-7.

60. Mudaliyar US, Sreedhar S. Chaos syndrome. *BJR Case Rep.* 2017;3(3):20160046.

61. Artunc Ulkumen B, Pala HG, Nese N, Tarhan S, Baytur Y. Prenatal diagnosis of congenital high airway obstruction syndrome: report of two cases and brief review of the literature. *Case Rep Obstet Gynecol.* 2013;2013:728974.

62. Crombleholme TM, Coleman B, Hedrick HL, et al. Cystic adenomatoid malformation volume ratio predicts outcome in

prenatally diagnosed cystic adenomatoid malformation of the lung. *J Pediatr Surg.* 2002;37(3):331-338.

63. Klinkner DB, Atwell T, Teles Abrao Trad A, et al. Innovative fetal therapy for a giant congenital pulmonary airway malformation with hydrops. *Fetal Diagn Ther.* 2022;49(5-6):250-255. doi:10.1159/000521690.

64. Cass DL, Olutoye OO, Ayres NA, et al. Defining hydrops and indications for open fetal surgery for fetuses with lung masses and vascular tumors. *J Pediatr Surg.* 2012;47(1):40-45.

65. Curran PF, Jelin EB, Rand L, et al. Prenatal steroids for microcystic congenital cystic adenomatoid malformations. *J Pediatr Surg.* 2010;45(1):145-150.

66. Harrison MR, Adzick NS, Jennings RW, et al. Antenatal intervention for congenital cystic adenomatoid malformation. *Lancet.* 1990;336(8721):965-967.

67. Dighe MK, Peterson SE, Dubinsky TJ, et al. EXIT Procedure: technique and indications with prenatal imaging parameters for assessment of airway patency. *RadioGraphics.* 2011;31(2):511-526.

68. Steiner H, Boemers T, Forstner R, et al. Ex-Utero Intrapartum Treatment (EXIT) in a giant case of Congenital Cystic Adenomatoid Malformation (CCAM) of the lung. *Ultraschall Med.* 2007;28(6):626-628.

69. Ruano R, da Silva MM, Salustiano EM, et al. Percutaneous laser ablation under ultrasound guidance for fetal hyperechogenic microcystic lung lesions with hydrops: a single center cohort and a literature review. *Prenat Diagn.* 2012;32(12):1127-1132.

70. Abbasi N, Morency A-M, Langer JC, et al. Fetal sclerotherapy for hydropic congenital cystic adenomatoid malformations of the lung refractory to steroids: a case report and review of the literature. *Fetal Diagn Ther.* 2020;47:24-33.

71. Peranteau WH, Moldenhauer JS, Khalek N, et al. Open fetal surgery for central bronchial atresia. *Fetal Diagn Ther.* 2014;35(2):141-147.

72. Adzick NS, Harrison MR, Crombleholme TM, et al. Fetal lung lesions: management and outcome. *Am J Obstet Gynecol.* 1998;179(4):884-889.

73. Cruz-Martinez R, Méndez A, Perez-Garcilita O, et al. Fetal bronchoscopy as a useful procedure in a case with prenatal diagnosis of congenital microcystic adenomatoid malformation. *Fetal Diagn Ther.* 2015;37(1):75-80.

74. Ruano R, de APEJ, Marques da Silva M, et al. Percutaneous intrauterine laser ablation of the abnormal vessel in pulmonary sequestration with hydrops at 29 weeks' gestation. *J Ultrasound Med.* 2007;26(9):1235-1241.

75. Kanamori Y, Takezoe T, Tahara K, et al. Congenital high airway obstruction syndrome (CHAOS) combined with esophageal atresia, tracheoesophageal fistula and duodenal atresia. *J Pediatr Surg Case Rep.* 2017;26:22-25.

76. Peiro JL, Nolan HR, Alhajjat A, et al. A technical look at fetoscopic laser ablation for fetal laryngeal surgical recanalization in congenital high airway obstruction syndrome. *J Laparoendosc Adv Surg Tech A.* 2020;30(6):695-700.

77. Martinez JM, Castañón M, Gómez O, et al. Evaluation of fetal vocal cords to select candidates for successful fetoscopic treatment of congenital high airway obstruction syndrome: preliminary case series. *Fetal Diagn Ther.* 2013;34(2):77-84.

INDEX

Note: Page numbers followed by "f" refer to figures; page numbers followed by "t" refer to tables; page numbers followed by "b" refer to boxes.

A

ABCA3. *see* Adenosine triphosphate-binding cassette transporter 3
Acidosis, effect of, 173–174
Acinetobacter spp., ventilator-assisted pneumonia and, 96b
Acute pulmonary hypertension, in preterm infants, 63–64
Adenosine receptor system, 315, 318
Adenosine triphosphate-binding cassette transporter 3
  disorder of lipid transport and lamellar body formation, 343f, 345
  roles in surfactant metabolism and function, 340–341
Adolescence, pulmonary function in, 283–284, 283f, 284t
Adulthood, early, pulmonary function in, 283–284, 283f, 284t
Adult stem cells, 222–223
AEC1. *see* Alveolar type 1 epithelial cells
AEC2. *see* Alveolar type 2 epithelial cells
Aerosolization, 135–136, 135t
Aerosolized steroids
  postnatal, 215
  prenatal, 215
Airway
  devices, 39–40
  laryngeal mask, 38–40
    delivery of surfactant by, 136–137
Airway microbial community turnover, 79
  in sequentially sampled tracheal aspirates, 79
Airway microbiome of newborn lung, 75–87
Alcohol abuse, maternal, lung development and, 23
Alveolar capillary dysplasia (ACD), 56, 63
Alveolar capillary dysplasia with misalignment of pulmonary veins (ACDMPV), 338–339, 339f
Alveolar fluid balance, undernutrition effect on, 300
Alveolar macrophage, 16–17, 17f
Alveolar stem cells, in cell-based therapy, 223
Alveolar type 1 epithelial cells (AEC1), 223
Alveolar type 2 epithelial cells (AEC2), 223
Alveolar ventilation, oxygen delivery to tissues, 182, 182f
Androgen and estrogen biosynthesis, 80
Angiogenesis, in severe bronchopulmonary dysplasia, 259–260

Antenatal corticosteroids, 206–212
  in current population, 208–209
  historical overview of, 206
  mechanism of action, on fetal lungs, 207–208, 208f
  nonrandomized controlled trial for, 209–210, 209f, 210f
  pharmacokinetics of, 206–207, 207f
  randomized controlled trials for, 208–209, 209t
Antenatal ductal closure, vascular development, 61
Antenatal infection models, 84
Antenatal inflammation/infection, 4–21
  fetal exposure to, 7–9, 7f, 8t, 10f
    early gestational responses, 13–14
    experimental results, 9–12, 11f, 12f
    immune response and modulation, 16–18, 17f
  overview, 4–5
Antenatal steroids
  after 34 weeks' gestational period, 211
  drug and dose choices for, 211–212
  before elective cesarean section, 211
  long-term outcomes after, 212
  in low-resource environments, 212
  repeated, 210–211
Antibiotics, for ventilator-associated pneumonia, 98–101
Antimicrobials, for ventilator-associated pneumonia, 102
Antioxidant defense system, undernutrition effect on, 299
Apnea
  neonates, clinical challenges in, 153–154
Apnea of prematurity, 37, 108, 313–314
  caffeine for, 314–319
    benefits of, 316–317
    conduct of, 315–316
    excerpts from, 315, 315b
    rationale for, 314–315
    study drug, 315, 315b
    treatment effect of, 314, 314t
  characteristics, 313–314
  treatment effect on, 314, 314t
Arabella NCPAP Infant Flow System, 111
Arachidonic acid-prostacyclin pathway, 58
Arterial oxygenation, BPD and, 246
  targets, impact of, 241–243
Asphyxia, 178
  defined, 40
  hypotension in, 42

Asphyxia-induced hypotension, 45
Assist control (A/C) ventilation, 193–194
Assisted ventilation modes, choice of, 194–195
Asthma, 76
  after preterm birth, 280–281
Atelectasis, BPD and, 236
Atelectrauma, 190
Atrial septal defects, in severe bronchopulmonary dysplasia, 260–261
Avoid Mechanical Ventilation trial, 138

B

Bacterial clearance, 85
Bacterial lipopolysaccharide (LPS) exposure, 80
Bacterial overgrowth, ventilator-assisted pneumonia and, 103
Bacteroidetes, 76
Bags for positive-pressure ventilation, 37–38
Barker, Dr. David, 291
Barotrauma, 190
BASCs. *see* Bronchoalveolar stem cells
Betamethasone, 206
  lung maturation and, 19–21, 20f
Betamethasone acetate, 206
Betamethasone phosphate, 206, 211–212
Betamethasone phosphate plus betamethasone acetate, 211–212
Biotrauma, 190
Birth, cardiorespiratory interactions at, 166–169, 167t
Birth weight, ventilator-associated pneumonia, 95, 97–98
Biventricular systolic and diastolic dysfunction, 178–179
Blood transfusions, neonatal respiratory control, 160
Body mass index (BMI), 291–292
Bone marrow (BM)-derived mesenchymal stem cells, for bronchopulmonary dysplasia, 224–225
Bone morphogenic protein receptor type 2 (BMPR2), 60
BPD. *see* Bronchopulmonary dysplasia
BPS. *see* Bronchopulmonary sequestration
Bradycardia
  neonatal respiratory control, 155–157
  tracheal catheterization, surfactant administration, 144
Bradycardia model, 45

Brain injury, during early transition and potential clinical implication, 181
Branched-chain amino acids (BCAAs), 298
Breast milk, ventilator-associated pneumonia and, 102
Bronchial atresia (BA)
　dysplastic formation of fetal bronchi, 352
　mainstem, 353
　　fetal therapy for, 354
　prenatal imaging, 352
　segmental, 352
　　fetal therapy for, 354
Bronchoalveolar lavage (BAL) of single lung segment, 76
Bronchoalveolar stem cells (BASCs), 223
Bronchopulmonary dysplasia (BPD), 18–19, 55–56, 189–190
　antenatal corticosteroids and, 19–21, 19t
　caffeine reduced risk of, 316, 317f, 319–320, 320f
　cell-based therapy for, 224–230
　　barriers and opportunities for implementation, 227–230
　　evidence from clinical trial, 226–227
　　evidence from preclinical studies, 224–225, 225f
　　mechanisms of repair, 225–226
　　optimal cells for, 227–228
　chorioamnionitis and, 19–21, 19t
　clinical and research implications, 235–247
　clinical presentation of, 236–237
　definition of, 235–236
　　National Institutes of Health Workshop, 239t
　diagnosis of, 237–238
　　impact of timing on, 243–244
　　2019 NICHD Neonatal Research Network, 239–240, 240t
　electrical impedance tomography for, 333
　future research, 246–247
　incidence of, 295–296
　long-term outcomes in, 282–285
　lung ultrasound for, 329, 329f
　new, 282
　outcomes of, 244
　pathogenesis of, 18
　populations at risk for, 244–245
　postdelivery corticosteroid treatments for, 205–206
　in preterm infants, 292, 293, 295–298, 300, 301
　prognosis for long-term impairment, 245–246
　pulmonary morbidity, 295–296
　severe
　　cardiovascular system in, 259–261
　　chest radiograph showing, 251f
　　definitions and scope of, 250–253
　　evaluation and treatment of, 261–271, 261t
　　forced flows in, 258

Bronchopulmonary dysplasia (Continued)
　incidence of, 253
　long-term outcomes of, 271–272
　lung imaging in, 258–259, 259f
　lung mechanics in, 256–257
　lung volumes in, 257–258
　pathogenesis of, 253–255
　pathophysiology of, 255–261
　physiology-based approach, 249–272
　respiratory function in, 255–256
　ventilator-dependent, 251f
　ventilator strategies in, 261t
　severity graded diagnostic criteria, 238–240
　　to changing respiratory support practices, 239, 240t
　　cumulative oxygen supplementation, combined with oxygen requirement, at 36 weeks postmenstrual age, 238–239, 239t
　　mode of respiratory support only, 239–240, 240t, 241f, 242f
　　supplemental oxygen criteria for, 238
　Ureaplasma species, 83–85
Bronchopulmonary dysplasia–associated pulmonary hypertension, 64
Bronchopulmonary sequestration (BPS)
　associated with fetal congenital malformations, 354
　extralobular lesions, 353
　imaging studies, 353
　intralobular lesions, 353
　location, 353
　prenatal diagnosis of, 353
Bubble CPAP, 111
Budesonide, 215

C

Caffeine
　advantages, 314
　CAP trial, 314–319
　citrate, 314, 315, 315b, 319
　as magic bullet, 321
　methylxanthine, 314
　respiratory stimulant for preterm infants, 314
　role in newborn period, 287
　standard doses of, 319–320, 320f
　treatment effect on apnea of prematurity, 314, 314t
Caffeine for apnea of prematurity (CAP) trial, 287, 314–319
　benefits of, 316–317
　　on motor skills, 318
　　reduced risk of morbidities during initial hospital stay, 316, 317f
　　reduced risk of motor impairment into, 316–317, 317f
　　weaning from respiratory supports, 316, 316f
　conduct of, 315–316
　effect of, 314, 314t

Caffeine for apnea of prematurity (CAP) trial (Continued)
　excerpts from, 315, 315b
　rationale for, 314–315
　safety of caffeine in, 318–319
　　adverse effects on sleep, 319
　　clinical signs of drug toxicity, 318
　　growth, 318
　　increased behavior problems, 318
　　study drug, 315, 315b
Caffeine therapy, neonatal respiratory control, 157–158, 158t
Calcium, 304–305
Capnography, during cardiac compressions, 43
Carbohydrates, 301
Carbon dioxide (CO_2), during early transition and potential clinical implication, 181
Cardiac catheterization, for pulmonary hypertension, in bronchopulmonary dysplasia, 269t
Cardiac development and function, abnormalities of, 63
Cardiac output, impact of lung disease and ventilator support on components of, 167t
Cardiorespiratory interactions, at birth, 166–169, 167t
Cardiorespiratory system, 166
Cardiovascular interaction, physiology of, 169–171
　afterload, 170t, 171
　contractility, 170t, 171
　preload, 170–171, 170f, 170t
Cardiovascular system
　effect, on respiratory system, 174–180
　in severe bronchopulmonary dysplasia, 259–261
Catheterization, tracheal, surfactant administration via, 137–140, 137t
　bradycardia in, 144
　catheter positioning methods, 146–147
　clinical trials of, 137t, 138–140, 141f
　　Avoid Mechanical Ventilation Trial in, 138
　　NINSAPP Trial in, 138–139
　　OPTIMIST-A trial, 139
　　summation of, 139–140
　　Take Care Study, 137t
　depth of catheter insertion for, 138
　effectiveness of, 140, 142f
　future research directions for, 146–147
　hypoxia in, 144
　infant selection, 144–146
　　exclusion criteria, 145–146, 145t
　　gestation range, 144
　　inclusion criteria, 144–145, 145t
　laboratory studies of, 140–143
　longer-term outcomes, 146
　observational and cohort studies of, 138
　optimal premedication, different gestation ranges, 146

Catheterization, tracheal, surfactant administration via (Continued)
premedication for, 143–144
avoidance of bradycardia, 143–144
minimization of discomfort, 143
respiratory effort maintenance, 143–144
procedural complications of, 144
recommendations for, 144–146
repeated, 144
scientific and practical considerations for, 140–144
spontaneous breathing, 146
surfactant reflux in, 144
videolaryngoscopy, role of, 147
Catheter positioning methods
tracheal catheterization, surfactant administration, 146–147
CDH. see Congenital diaphragmatic hernia (CDH)
Celestone, 206, 211–212
Cell-based therapy, for neonatal lung disease, 221–230
alveolar stem cells in, 223
for bronchopulmonary dysplasia, 224–230
barriers and opportunities for implementation, 227–230
evidence from clinical trial, 226–227
evidence from preclinical studies, 224–225, 225f
mechanisms of repair, 225–226
optimal cells for, 227–228
endogenous lung stem cells in, 223–224
lung endothelial progenitors in, 224
lung mesenchymal stem cells in, 224
stem cells in, 221–223, 222f
Central chemosensitivity, 152–153
Central respiratory control, 152
Cerebral blood flow, during early transition and potential clinical implication, 181
cGMP-specific phosphodiesterase (PDE5), 57
CHAOS. see Congenital high airway obstruction syndrome (CHAOS)
Chest compressions, 41–43
blood pressure during, 42
capnography during, 43
compression-to-ventilation ratio in, 42
compression-ventilation coordination in, 42–43
ETCO$_2$ capnography during, 43
heart rate response, 43
initiation, 41
technique of, 41
two-finger technique, 42
two-thumb compression technique, 42, 42f
ventilation, Coordination of, 42–43
Chest radiograph, of severe bronchopulmonary dysplasia (BPD), 251, 251f, 258–259
Chest radiographs (CXRs), 323–324, 333
Chorioamnion, 5–6, 12–13

Chorioamnionitis
antenatal corticosteroids and, 19–21, 19t, 20f
bronchopulmonary dysplasia and, 18–19
clinical, 5–6, 10f
diagnosis of, 5–7, 6f
experimental chronic, 14–16, 16f
funisitis and, 5
histologic, 5, 6f
in preterm infants, 18
severe bronchopulmonary dysplasia (BPD) and, 253–254
Chromosome 21, 60
Chronic obstructive pulmonary disease (COPD), 76, 292
Chronic pneumonitis of infancy (CPI), 342
Cigarette smoking. see Smoking
Citrobacter spp., ventilator-assisted pneumonia and, 96b
Clinical chorioamnionitis, 5–6, 10f
Cold stress in nonasphyxiated newborns, 35
Collateral vessels, severe bronchopulmonary dysplasia and, 260–261
Color, in initial assessment, 34
Congenital alveolar proteinosis (CAP), 342
Congenital cystic adenomatoid malformations (CCAMs), 352
Congenital diaphragmatic hernia (CDH), 62–63, 178–179
associated with abnormal lung development, 350
causes of, 350
development of, 350
diagnosis of, 350–351
embryology and etiology, 350
fetal endoscopic tracheal occlusion, 351–352
mortality rates, 350
Congenital heart disease, 179
Congenital high airway obstruction syndrome (CHAOS), 353
diagnosis, 353
etiology of, 353
EXIT procedure, 355
fetal heart failure, 353
fetal therapy, 354–355
Fraser syndrome, 353
intrinsic upper airway obstruction development, 353
prenatal diagnosis of, 353
secondary pulmonary hyperplasia, 353
sonographic examination, 353
in utero, 353
Congenital malformations of respiratory system
congenital diaphragmatic hernia, 350–352. see also Congenital diaphragmatic hernia (CDH)
congenital pulmonary malformations, 349–350, 352–355
in abnormal fetal lung development, 352
bronchial atresia, 352–353

Congenital malformations of respiratory system (Continued)
bronchopulmonary sequestration, 353
CHAOS, 353. see also Congenital high airway obstruction syndrome (CHAOS)
congenital pulmonary airway malformations, 352
etiological factors, 352
fetal therapy for, 353–355
Congenital pulmonary airway malformation (CPAM), 352
with abnormal connections to airway and pulmonary vasculature, 352
classification, 352
fetal cystic lung lesions, 352
fetal therapy for, 354
imaging studies, 352
triggering factors, 352
Congenital pulmonary malformations (CPMs), 349–350
in abnormal fetal lung development, 352
etiological factors, 352
fetal therapy for, 353–355
bronchopulmonary sequestration, 354
CHAOS, 354–355
mainstem bronchial atresia, 354
modalities of, 353–354
segmental bronchial atresia, 354
types, 352–353
bronchial atresia, 352–353
bronchopulmonary sequestration, 353
congenital high airway obstruction syndrome, 353
congenital pulmonary airway malformations, 352
Constrictors, 57
Continuous distending pressure, for respiratory distress syndrome, 111–112
Continuous oxygen, BPD and, 238
Continuous positive airway pressure (CPAP), 134, 191–193, 298
bubble, 111
effects of, 172–173
nasal high flow vs., 123, 124f, 125f
nasal interfaces, 109–110, 110f
in resuscitation, 37
role of, in preterm infants, 108–109
settings, 118
for surfactant, 113–114
with early intubation, 113
era, 112
INSURE technique and, 113
with nasal, 113
weaning, 115–116
Coronary perfusion pressure, in resuscitation, 43–44
Corrected age, BPD and, 243
Corticosteroids
antenatal, 1–2, 8t, 19–21, 19t, 20f, 206–212
chorioamnionitis and, 19–21, 19t, 20f

Corticosteroids (*Continued*)
  in current population, 208–209
  historical overview of, 206
  mechanism of action, on fetal lungs,
    207–208, 208f
  non-randomized controlled trial for,
    209–210, 209f, 210f
  pharmacokinetics of, 206–207, 207f
  randomized controlled trials
    for, 208–209, 209t
  for severe bronchopulmonary dysplasia,
    268, 269
CPAM. *see* Congenital pulmonary airway
    malformation (CPAM)
CPAP. *see* Continuous positive airway
    pressure
CPMs. *see* Congenital pulmonary
    malformations (CPMs)
Culture-independent molecular
    methods, 76
Cumulative oxygen supplementation,
    combined with oxygen requirement,
    at 36 weeks postmenstrual age,
    238–239, 239t
"CURPAP" trial, 113
Cysteine (glutathione precursor)
    supplementation, 305

D
DART study. *see* Dexamethasone:
    A Randomized Trial (DART) study
Delivery room
  respiratory and cardiovascular support
    in, 29–46
  stabilization, 191–192
Developmental coordination disorder
    (DCD), 316–317, 317f
Developmental deficiencies in innate
    immunity
  dysregulated inflammation, 85–86
  Ureaplasma species, 85–86
Dexamethasone: A Randomized Trial
    (DART) study, 214
Dexamethasone phosphate
  antenatal, 206, 211–212
  postnatal, 214
Diaphragmatic hernia, congenital,
    178–179
Distal airway stem cells, 223
Diuretics, for severe bronchopulmonary
    dysplasia, 267–268
Docosahexaenoic acid (DHA), 292–293
Dopamine, 67–68
Dose, for mesenchymal stem cell
    transplantation, 230
Double-lung point, 328, 328f
Down syndrome (trisomy 21), 60
Doxapram, 160
Drying and stimulation, in resuscitation, 34
Ductal closure
  antenatal, vascular development, 61
Ductal-dependent cyanotic heart disease, 179

Dysplasia
  bronchopulmonary, 189–190
    antenatal corticosteroids and, 19–21, 19t
    cell-based therapy for, 224–230
    chorioamnionitis and, 19–21, 19t
    clinical and research implications,
      235–247
    clinical presentation of, 236–237
    definition of, 235–236, 239t
    diagnosis of, 237–238
    future research, 246–247
    incidence of, 295–296
    long-term outcomes in, 282–285
    new, 282
    outcomes of, 244
    pathogenesis of, 18
    populations at risk for, 244–245
    postdelivery corticosteroid treatments
      for, 205–206
    in preterm infants, 292, 293,
      295–298, 300, 301
    prognosis for long-term impairment,
      245–246
    pulmonary morbidity, 295–296
    severe. *see* Severe bronchopulmonary
      dysplasia
    severity graded diagnostic criteria,
      238–240
    supplemental oxygen criteria for, 238
    time point to diagnosis of, 243–244

E
ECFCs. *see* Endothelial colony-forming cells
Echocardiography, for pulmonary
    hypertension, in bronchopulmonary
    dysplasia, 269t
Electrical impedance tomography (EIT),
    329–333
  advantage of, 330
  and bronchopulmonary dysplasia, 333
  CRADL project, 333
  in delivery room, 333
  electrode belt in situ on infant, 330, 330f
  functional, 333, 333f
  image acquisition and reconstruction, 330
  and lung recruitment, 332–333
  vs. lung ultrasound, 329–330
  lung-ventilator interactions and disease
    states, 330–332
  neonatal applications of, 330–333
  and noninvasive ventilation, 332
  outcome measures, 330, 331–332t
  principles of, 330
  respiratory adverse events, 333, 333f
  uses of, 329–330
Embryonic stem cells, 222
EME Infant Flow Nasal CPAP device, 111
Endogenous lung stem cells, in cell-based
    therapy, 223–224
Endogenous serotonin (5-HT) production, 57
Endothelial colony forming cells (ECFCs),
    224, 228

Endothelial progenitor cells (EPCs), 56, 224
  in cell-based therapy, 224
Endotoxin, intraamniotic
  betamethasone and, 19–21, 20f
  lung maturation and, 14, 15f, 16f
Endotracheal intubation. *see also*
    Mechanical ventilation
  after failed nasal CPAP, 115
  noninvasive respiratory support *vs.*, 109
  routine, *vs.* nasal CPAP, 112
  for surfactant administration, nasal CPAP
    vs., 114
Endotracheal tube (ETT), 45, 45t, 189–190
  surfactant administration without,
    135–137, 135t
  ventilator-assisted pneumonia and, 94
End-tidal CO_2 ($ETCO_2$), during cardiac
    compressions, 43
Energy, 300–301
Enterobacter spp., ventilator-assisted
    pneumonia and, 96, 96b
EPCs. *see* Endothelial progenitor cells
Epinephrine, in resuscitation, 44, 45
Erythromycin therapy, 86
Escherichia coli, ventilator-assisted
    pneumonia and, 96b
ETT. *see* Endotracheal tube
Excitatory neurotransmitters and
    neuromodulators, 152
Exercise tolerance, pulmonary function
    and, 285
Experimental pneumonia models, 84
Extrauterine growth restriction
    (EUGR), 295
  consequences of, 297
  definition, 297
Extremely low-birth-weight (ELBW),
    296–297
  infants, 76–79
Ex-utero intrapartum treatment (EXIT
    procedure), 351

F
Face mask, 39–40
Familial diaphragmatic agenesis, 350
Fats, 301–302
Fetal alcohol syndrome, lung development
    and, 23
Fetal endoscopic tracheal occlusion
    (FETO), 351–352
  for CDH, 351
  complications, 351
  EXIT procedure, 351
  in fetuses with severe herniation, 351
  future applications of, 352
  gestational timeframe for, 351
  lung regrowth and pulmonary vascular
    development, 351
  timeframe for balloon removal, 351
Fetal growth restriction, 21, 22–23
Fetal inflammatory response syndrome,
    chorioamnionitis and, 9t

Fetal lung development
  maternal over nutrition, 293
  maternal undernutrition, 292–293
  micronutrients, 293–295
    preeclampsia alters placental function, 295
    vitamin A supplementation, 295
    vitamin C supplementation to pregnant women unable to quit smoking, 293, 294f
    vitamin D supplementation, 293–295
    vitamin E supplementation, 295
  prenatal nutrition and, 292
  undernutrition effect on, 297–298
FETO. *see* Fetal endoscopic tracheal occlusion (FETO)
Fetoscopic surgery, for bronchial atresia, 354
Fisher & Paykel system, 122, 122f
Flow-inflating bags, for positive-pressure ventilation, 37–38
Fluorescent in situ hybridization (FISH) on alveolar epithelia, 79
Fluoxetine, 61
Fluticasone propionate, for severe bronchopulmonary dysplasia, 269
Forced flows, in severe bronchopulmonary dysplasia, 258
FOXF-1 gene, 63, 338–339, 345
Funisitis, 5
Furosemide, for severe bronchopulmonary dysplasia, 267–268

G
GABA. *see* Gamma-aminobutyric acid
Gammaaminobutyric acid (GABA), 152
Gastric bacteria, ventilator-assisted pneumonia and, 96–97
gCap cells, 224
Gene mutations
  in embryonic epithelium (NKX2-1/TTF-1), 339–340
  in pulmonary mesenchyme, 338–339, 338f, 339f
  pulmonary surfactant, 340–341
  in SOX2 and SOX9, 340
Genetic disorders
  of lung formation, 337–338, 338f
  mutations in
    ABCA3, 345
    genes expressed in the embryonic epithelium (NKX2-1/TTF-1), 339–340
    genes in pulmonary mesenchyme, 338–339, 339f
    SFTPB, 343–344
    SFTPC, 344
    SOX2 and SOX9, associated with multiple congenital malformations, 340
  of surfactant homeostasis, 341–342, 341f
    ABCA3, 343f, 345
    lung histopathology in infant, 342, 343f

Genetic disorders (*Continued*)
    SP-A, 341–342
    SP-B, 342–344
    SP-C, 343f, 344
    SP-D, 341–342
Global inhomogeneity (GI) index, 333
Glutamine supplementation, 305
Glutathione sulfonamide (GSA), ventilatorassisted pneumonia and, 104
Glycine, 152
Group B *Streptococcus,* ventilator-assisted pneumonia and, 96b
GSA. *see* Glutathione sulfonamide

H
Hand hygiene, ventilator-associated pneumonia and, 102, 103, 104b
Heart disease, congenital, 179
Heart rate
  in initial assessment, 43
  in positive-pressure ventilation, 37
Hematopoietic stem cells, 221
HFNC. *see* High-flow nasal cannula
HFNV. *see* High-frequency nasal ventilation
HFOV. *see* High-frequency oscillatory ventilation
HFV. *see* High-frequency ventilation
High-flow nasal cannula (HFNC), for severe bronchopulmonary dysplasia, 250–251, 261–262
High-frequency jet ventilation (HFJV), in severe bronchopulmonary dysplasia (BPD), 254
High-frequency nasal ventilation (HFNV), noninvasive
  clinical studies, 119
  gas exchange during, 118
  mechanisms of action, 118–119
  observational and crossover studies, 119
  randomized controlled trials, 119, 120t
  settings during, 119–121
High-frequency oscillatory ventilation (HFOV), in severe bronchopulmonary dysplasia (BPD), 254
High-frequency ventilation (HFV), 197–199
High-resolution computed tomography (HRCT), for severe bronchopulmonary dysplasia (BPD), 258–259, 259f
Histologic chorioamnionitis, 5, 6f
Homogeneous lung disorders, 324
HRCT. *see* High-resolution computed tomography
Human Microbiome Project, 76
Human milk, 305
Hydrocortisone, 215
  infusions, 215
Hypercapnia, permissive, effect of, 173–174
Hyperoxia, severe bronchopulmonary dysplasia (BPD) and, 253–254
Hyperoxygenation, maternal with face mask oxygen, 52

Hypertension, pulmonary, 175–176, 175f
  echocardiography for, in severe bronchopulmonary dysplasia, 269t
  in severe bronchopulmonary dysplasia, 259–260
  treatment of, 269–270, 269t
Hyperthermia, 35
Hypotension, management of, 45
Hypothermia, prevention of, 35
Hypovolemia, in resuscitation, 45
Hypoxemia, neonatal respiratory control, 155–157
Hypoxemic respiratory failure, 61–62
Hypoxia inducible factors (HIFs), 53–55

I
ILCOR neonatal life support task force, 35–37
Immature innate immunity, ventilator-assisted pneumonia and, 96
Immune response and modulation, from fetal exposures to inflammation, 16–18, 17f
Induced pluripotent stem cells (iPSCs), 222, 228
Infant Flow Driver, 111
Infants
  BPD and, 236–237
  electrode belt in situ on, 330, 330f
  selection of, for surfactant delivery via tracheal catheterization, 144–146, 145t
Infant selection
  tracheal catheterization, surfactant administration, 144–146
    exclusion criteria, 145–146, 145t
    gestation range, 144
    inclusion criteria, 144–145, 145t
Infection-related preterm birth, 79
Infection, severe bronchopulmonary dysplasia (BPD) and, 253–254
Inflammation, severe bronchopulmonary dysplasia (BPD) and, 253–254
Inhaled nitric oxide (iNO)
  pulmonary hypertension, 65–67, 66f
  therapy, 52
Inhibitory neurotransmitters and neuromodulators, 152
In-line suctioning devices, ventilator-associated pneumonia and, 101–102
Innate immune tolerance, 18
Innate immunity
  developmental deficiencies in, *Ureaplasma* species, 85–86
  ventilator-assisted pneumonia and, 96
Inositol, 305
INSURE technique, 134
Interdisciplinary care, in severe bronchopulmonary dysplasia, 270–271
Intermittent hypoxia, 156–157
International Liaison Committee on Resuscitation (ILCOR) guidelines, 191–192

Intrauterine growth restriction (IUGR), 292
  bronchopulmonary dysplasia and, 21–23, 22f
  severe bronchopulmonary dysplasia (BPD) and, 253–254
Intrauterine infection, *Ureaplasma* species, 80–85
Intrauterine inflammation, *Ureaplasma* species, 81–82
Intraventricular hemorrhage (IVH), chorioamnionitis and, 19, 19t

K

Kangaroo care, neonatal respiratory control, 159
Kinesthetic stimulation using oscillating mattresses, 160
Klebsiella spp., ventilator-assisted pneumonia and, 96, 96b

L

Laryngeal mask airway, 39–40, 40f
  delivery of surfactant by, 136–137
Left ventricular (LV)
  afterload, effects of intrathoracic pressure on, 169f
  hypertrophy, in severe bronchopulmonary dysplasia, 260–261
Liggins and Howie trial, 206, 212
Linezolid, for ventilator-associated pneumonia, 99–100
Lipid mediators, 57
Lipopolysaccharide (LPS) exposure, 80
Long-chain polyunsaturated fatty acids (LCPUFAs), 292, 302
Long-term pulmonary outcomes, 279–287
  caffeine role in, 287
  controversies in, 280
  for late preterm infants, 280–282
  pulmonary function in
    in adolescence or early adulthood, 283–284, 283f, 284t
    in childhood, 282–283
    with increasing age of survivors, 284–285
  research requirements for, 287
  for very preterm infants, 282–285
    cigarette smoking and, 285–287, 286f
    exercise tolerance, 285
    expiratory airflow in survivors born extremely preterm over time in post-surfactant era, 285
    rehospitalization rates, 282
Low birth weight (LBW), 296–297
Low-resource environments, antenatal steroids in, 212
Lung compression, 62–63
Lung development, 1–24
  adverse events, 2–3, 3f
  alveolar, 52, 53f
  canalicular, 52, 53f
  embryonic, 52, 53f

Lung development (*Continued*)
  fetal. *see* Fetal lung development
  Foxf1, 56
  inflammatory responses, 12–13, 13t
  lung maturation and, 3–4
  overview, 1–2, 2f
  perinatal and, 1–2
  pseudoglandular, 52, 53f
  saccular, 52, 53f
  stages, 52, 53f
  transcription factors, 56
Lung disease
  environmental factors and, 23
  impact of, 167t
Lung formation, genetic disorders of, 337–338, 338f
Lung growth and function, nutritional support to, 300–305
  calcium/phosphorus, 304–305
  energy, 300–301
  human milk, 305
  individual amino acids, 305
  macronutrients, 301–303
    carbohydrates, 301
    fats, 301–302
    LCPUFAs, 302
    proteins, 302–303
    vegetable-derived oils, 302
  micronutrients, 303–304
    vitamin A, 303
    vitamin C, 304
    vitamin D, 303
    vitamin E, 303, 304
  surfactant precursors, 305
  trace elements, 304
  water and fluid volume, 301
Lung imaging
  electrical impedance tomography, 329–333. *see also* Electrical impedance tomography (EIT)
  ultrasound. *see* Lung ultrasound (LU)
Lung injury, 3, 4, 8
  fetal exposure to inflammation, 9–10
  severe bronchopulmonary dysplasia (BPD) and, 253–254
  ventilation strategies for, 189–200
Lung maturation, 3–4
  environmental factors and, 23
  inflammation-mediated, 14, 15f
Lung microbiota, 79, 80
Lungs
  function, BPD and, 245–246
  function measures, 330
  histology in infants
    with ACDMPV, 339f
    genetic disorders of surfactant homeostasis, 343f
  imaging, in severe bronchopulmonary dysplasia, 258–259, 259f
  mechanics, in severe bronchopulmonary dysplasia, 256–257
  volume in severe bronchopulmonary dysplasia, 257–258

Lung sliding, 324
Lung-to-head ratio (LHR), 351
Lung transplantation, 345
Lung ultrasound (LU)
  A-lines, 325, 325f
  B-lines, 325, 325f
  vs. EIT, 329–330
  future directions, 334
  history of, 324
  learning curve and accuracy of, 326
  lung sliding, 324
  M-mode cursor, 324–325, 324f
  neonatal applications of, 326–329
    for bronchopulmonary dysplasia, 329, 329f
    lung consolidation and atelectasis, 326–327, 327f
    pleural effusion, 327, 328f
    pneumothorax, 327, 327f
    respiratory distress syndrome, 327–328, 328f
    surfactant replacement therapy, 328
    transient tachypnea of newborn, 328, 328f
  in neonatal intensive care, 334
  scoring systems, 325–326, 326f
  technique, 324

M

Macronutrients, 301–303
Magnetic resonance imaging (MRI), 355
  for BPS, 353
  for bronchial atresia, 352
  for CHAOS, 353
  for congenital diaphragmatic hernia, 351
  for CPAM, 352
Mainstem bronchial atresia, 353
  fetal therapy for, 354
Malnutrition/undernutrition
  consequences of, 297
  definition, 297
  effect on
    alveolar fluid balance, 300
    antioxidant system, 299
    control of breathing, 300
    infection susceptibility, 299–300
    lung function, 298–299
    lung growth and development, 297–298
    pulmonary vascular bed, 300
    respiratory muscle function, 298
  maternal, 292–293
Manganese, 304
MAP. *see* Mean airway pressure
Masks, face, 39–40
Maternal exposures, vascular development, 61
Maternal smoking, severe bronchopulmonary dysplasia (BPD) and, 253–254
Maternal vascular underperfusion, pulmonary development, 60–61
Mean airway pressure (MAP), effects of, 172–173

Mechanical ventilation (MV), 168–169, 171–172
  adverse effects of, 108–109
  bronchopulmonary dysplasia (BPD) due to, 254
  duration of, pneumonia and, 93
  evidence-based approach to, 199–200
  historical perspective on, 109
  hypoxemia in. *see also* Hypoxemia
  noninvasive respiratory support and, 192–193
  respiratory care of premature infant, 298
  for severe bronchopulmonary dysplasia and, 262–267, 262t, 263f, 264f, 265f, 266f
  strategies, 193
  synchronized, 193
  ventilator-associated lung injury and, 190
Mechanosensory stimulation, neonatal respiratory control, 160
Meconium aspiration syndrome (MAS), 35–37
Meconium in utero, 178
Meconium-stained amniotic fluid (MSAF), 35–37
Mesenchymal stem cell (MSC)
  in cell-based therapy, 224
  transplantation
    dose, 230
    in hyperoxia-induced alveolar simplification, 225f
    for preterm infants, 226–229
    route, 229–230
    timing of administration of, 229
Metabolic bone disease (MBD), 299
Methicillin-resistant *S. aureus* (MRSA), as cause of ventilator-associated pneumonia, 99–100
Methylxanthine therapy, 287, 313–314, 318
Microbial diversity, 75
Micronutrients, 303–304
  fetal lung development, 293–295
    preeclampsia alters placental function, 295
    vitamin A supplementation, 295
    vitamin C supplementation to pregnant women unable to quit smoking, 293, 294f
    vitamin D supplementation, 293–295
    vitamin E supplementation, 295
Microvascular pulmonary endothelial cells, 56
Minimally invasive surfactant therapy, 113–114, 113f
Mother's own milk (MOM), 295
MRSA. *see* Methicillin-resistant *S. aureus*
Multipotent stem cells, 221, 222f
Mutations
  ABCA3, 345
  in genes expressed in the embryonic epithelium (NKX2-1/TTF-1), 339–340
  in genes in pulmonary mesenchyme, 338–339, 339f

Mutations *(Continued)*
  in *SFTPB,* 343–344
  in *SFTPC,* 344
  in SOX2 and SOX9, associated with multiple congenital malformations, 340
Mycoplasma species, chorioamnionitis and, 5–6

N
Nasal cannulas, for nasal CPAP, 111
Nasal continuous positive airway pressure (NCPAP). *see also* Noninvasive ventilation
  BPD and, 239
  complications of, 115
  devices for, 110–111
  failure of, 115
  for postextubation support, 114–115
    with nasal IPPV, 114–115
  pressure in, 111
  prophylactic surfactant and, 112
  for respiratory distress syndrome, 111–112
    brief, early intubation for surfactant *vs.,* 113
    continuous distending pressure and, 111–112
    surfactant administration and, 113–114
    in surfactant era, 112
  routine intubation *vs.,* 112
  for severe bronchopulmonary dysplasia, 254–255, 261–262
  trauma from, 115
  weaning from, 115–116
Nasal high flow (nHF), for preterm infants, 121–126, 122f
  as an alternative treatment, 125–126
  CPAP *vs.,* 123, 124f, 125f
  evidence from randomized trial for, 122–123
    delivery room, stabilization in, 122–123
    for extubation failure prevention, 123
    as primary respiratory support, 123
  function of, 122
  mechanisms, 122
  NIPPV *vs.,* 123
  potential concerns with use of, 124–125
  safety of, 123–124
Nasal high-frequency oscillatory ventilation (HVOF), 192–193
Nasal intermittent positive-pressure ventilation (NIPPV), 116–118, 192–193. *see also* Noninvasive ventilation
  in apnea of prematurity, 118
  mechanisms of, 116
  with nasal CPAP, 114–115
  nasal high flow *vs.,* 123, 124f, 125f
  postextubation mode, 117–118
  for primary respiratory support, 117
  in respiratory distress syndrome, 116–118
  synchronized *versus* unsynchronized, 116–117

National Institute of Child Health and Human Development (NICHD)
  Neonatal Research Network, 236–237, 239–240
National Institutes of Health (NIH), defined severe bronchopulmonary dysplasia (BPD), 250–253
NAVA. *see* Neurally adjusted ventilatory assist
NCPAP. *see* Nasal continuous positive airway pressure
Neonatal apnea, clinical challenges in, 153–154
Neonatal caffeine therapy, 315, 319–321
  appropriate candidates for, 320
  dosage, 319–320, 320f
  long-term benefits and harms of, 287
  in randomized clinical trials, 315
  starting of, 320
  when to stop, 320–321
Neonatal intensive care units (NICUs), nasal CPAP, 111
Neonatal lung disease, cell-based therapy for, 221–230
  alveolar stem cells in, 223
  for bronchopulmonary dysplasia, 224–230
    barriers and opportunities for implementation, 227–230
    evidence from clinical trial, 226–227
    evidence from preclinical studies, 224–225, 225f
    mechanisms of repair, 225–226
    optimal cells for, 227–228
  endogenous lung stem cells in, 223–224
  lung endothelial progenitors in, 224
  lung mesenchymal stem cells in, 224
  stem cells in, 221–223, 222f
Neonatal lung injury, 75–87
  Ureaplasma species, 83, 83b
Neonatal lung ultrasound. *see* Lung ultrasound (LU)
Neonatal respiratory control
  biological challenges in characterizing, 151–152
  inflammatory mechanisms, 153
  intermittent hypoxemia and bradycardia, association between, 155–157
  mechanistic insights into morbidity, 157
  pharmacological and nonpharmacological therapies, 157
  prone positioning, 159
  routine home monitoring, 160
Neonatal Resuscitation Program (NRP), 191–192
Neonatal sepsis, 179–180
Neurally adjusted ventilatory assist (NAVA), 198–199
Newborn life, transition to, 29–32, 30f, 31f, 32f
Newborn lung microbiome, 76–80, 77f, 78f
Newborn mortality, chorioamnionitis and, 19t

NIPPV. *see* Nasal intermittent positive-pressure
NIV. *see* Noninvasive ventilation
NKX2-1, 337–340
NOMID. *see* Neonatal-onset multisystem inflammatory diseases
Nonintubated Surfactant Application (NINSAPP) trial, for tracheal catheterization, 138–139
Noninvasive high-frequency ventilation (NIHFV)
  clinical studies, 119
  mechanisms of action, 118–119
  observational and crossover studies, 119
  randomized controlled trials, 119, 120t
  settings during, 119–121
Noninvasive respiratory support, 192–193
  neonatal respiratory control, 158–159
  of preterm infants, 107–126
    for apnea of prematurity, 108
    brief history of, 109
    future directions in, 126
    intubation *vs.*, 108–109
    for respiratory failure, 108–109
Noninvasive respiratory support, EIT and, preterm infants to
Noninvasive ventilation (NIV)
  of preterm infants
    nasal CPAP in. *see* Nasal continuous positive airway pressure (NCPAP)
    nasal IPPV in. *see* Nasal intermittent positive-pressure ventilation (NIPPV)
Nonspecific interstitial pneumonitis (NSIP), 342
NRP. *see* Neonatal Resuscitation Program
Nutrition, 291–306
  interventions for primary prevention of preterm birth, 292
  and lung development, prenatal, 292
  maternal micronutrients, 293–295
    preeclampsia alters placental function, 295
    vitamin A supplementation, 295
    vitamin C supplementation to pregnant women unable to quit smoking, 293, 294f
    vitamin D supplementation, 293–295
    vitamin E supplementation, 295
  maternal over, 293
  maternal undernutrition, 292–293
  postnatal nutrition and respiratory outcomes, 295–296
  preterm infant, 296–297
  support lung growth and function, 300–305
    energy, 300–301
    human milk, 305
    macronutrients, 301–303
    micronutrients, 303–304
    other nutrients, 304–305
    trace elements, 304
    water and fluid volume, 301
Nutritional emphysema, 297–298

O
Obesity
  adverse respiratory outcomes during pregnancy, 293
  incidence of, 293
Olfactory sensitivity, neonatal respiratory control, 159
Open lung strategy, importance of, 196–197
Optimal cells, for bronchopulmonary dysplasia, 227–228
OPTIMIST-A trial, 139
Oral secretions, removal of, ventilator-assisted pneumonia and, 103
Oxidative stress, severe bronchopulmonary dysplasia (BPD) and, 253–254
Oxygen
  administration, neonatal respiratory control, 159
  delivery device, impact of, 243
  delivery to tissues, alveolar ventilation and oxygenation, 182, 182f
  instability in premature infants, 151–160
  supplemental, for severe bronchopulmonary dysplasia, 261–262
  at 36 weeks postmenstrual corrected age, 238
Oxygenation
  instability, mechanisms, 154–155, 155f
  oxygen delivery to tissues, 182, 182f
  pulse oximetry in, 34
Oxygen hood, nasal CPAP for postextubation support *vs.*, 114–115
Oxygen saturation (SpO$_2$), in oxygen therapy, 34, 36f
Oxygen toxicity, 40–41

P
Pallister Hall syndrome, 338–339
Patent ductus arteriosus (PDA), 61, 166–167, 176–178, 316, 317f
  acute pulmonary effects of, 301
Patient positioning, ventilator-assisted pneumonia and, 96
PAV. *see* Proportional assist ventilation
PBF. *see* Pulmonary blood flow
PDA. *see* Patent ductus arteriosus
PEEP. *see* Positive end-expiratory pressure
Perinatal asphyxia, 62
Peripheral chemosensitivity, 152–153
Periventricular/intraventricular hemorrhage (P/ IVH), 181
Permissive hypercapnia, 182
  effect of, 173–174
  mild, mechanical ventilation and, 199–200
Peroxisome proliferator-activated receptor gamma (PPARg), 292–293
Persistent pulmonary hypertension of the newborn (PPHN), 57, 61–62, 167, 167t
Pharyngeal instillation, 135t, 136

Phosphorus, 304–305
P/IVH. *see* Periventricular/intraventricular hemorrhage
Placental insufficiency
  vascular development, 60–61
Pleural effusion, lung ultrasound for, 327, 328f
Pluripotent stem cells, 221, 222f
PMA. *see* Postmenstrual age
Pneumonia, ventilator-associated, 93–104
  birth weight and, 95, 97–98
  definition of, 94, 95b
  epidemiology of, 95–96
  future research directions for, 104
  outcomes in, 103–104
  pathogenesis of, 96–98, 96b, 97f, 98f
  prevention of, 101–103, 104b
  risk factors for, 95–98
  treatment of, 98–101, 100b
  ventilation duration and, 99–101
Pneumothorax
  lung ultrasound for, 327, 327f
  from nasal CPAP, 123–124
Point-of-care ultrasound, 326
Polymicrobial disease, 79
Positive end-expiratory pressure (PEEP), 30, 30f, 31f, 191–192
  effects of, 172–173
Positive pressure respiratory support, BPD and, 238–239, 243
Post-ligation cardiac syndrome, 177
Postmenstrual age (PMA), severe bronchopulmonary dysplasia (BPD) in, 250–251
Postnatal growth failure, 295
Postnatal pulmonary vascular development, 57–58
Postnatal steroids, 212–216
  alternatives to early systemic, 215–216
  for bronchopulmonary dysplasia, 213–214
  drug, dose, route, and duration of therapy with, 214
  future directions, 216
  historical review, 212–213, 213f
  meta-analyses of early and late treatments of, 214
  pulmonary outcomes of, 205–216
  use of, 216
Postnatal vascular disease, 60–61
Post-surfactant era, 285
PPHN. *see* Persistent pulmonary hypertension
Pre-Bötzinger complex, 152
Preeclampsia, severe bronchopulmonary dysplasia (BPD) and, 253–254
Pregnancy
  maternal obesity in, 293
  poor nutrition during, 292–293
  vitamin C supplementation effect during, 293, 294f
Premature infants
  BPD and, 245, 246

Premature infants (*Continued*)
respiratory control and oxygen instability in, 151–160
Prematurity, ventilator-associated pneumonia, 95
Premedications, tracheal catheterization, 143–144
avoidance of bradycardia, 143–144
minimization of discomfort, 143
respiratory effort maintenance, 143–144
Prenatal fetal therapy, 351–352
Prenatal steroids
early use of, 215, 216t
future directions, 216
pulmonary outcomes of, 205–216
Pressure-support ventilation (PSV), 194
Preterm birth (PTB), 292
Ureaplasma species, 81–82
Preterm infants
birth rates, 279–280
chorioamnionitis in, 18
long-term pulmonary outcomes, 279–287
caffeine role in, 287
controversies in, 280
for late preterm infants, 280–282
research requirements for, 287
for very preterm infants, 282–285
mortality in, 279–280
nutrition, 296–297. *see also* Nutrition
daily nutrient intakes for, 305–306, 306t
rate of fetal nutrient transfer, 296
recommendations for, 296–297
pulmonary function in, long-term pulmonary outcomes
in adolescence or early adulthood, 283–284, 283f, 284t
in childhood, 282–283
with increasing age of survivors, 284–285
for very preterm infants, long-term pulmonary outcomes
cigarette smoking and, 285–287, 286f
exercise tolerance, 285
expiratory airflow in survivors born extremely preterm over time in post-surfactant era, 285
rehospitalization rates, 282
Preterm premature rupture of membranes (pPROM), 81
Prolyl hydroxylase (PHD2), 64
Proportional assist ventilation, 197–198
Prostacyclin (PGI2), 57
Proteins, 302–303
Proteobacteria, 76
Proteus spp., ventilator-assisted pneumonia and, 96b
Pseudomonas aeruginosa, ventilator-assisted pneumonia and, 96, 96b
PSV. *see* Pressure-support ventilation
Pulmonary artery, 52, 56, 57
changes in, 52–53, 54f
hypertension, 351

Pulmonary artery (*Continued*)
pressure in severe bronchopulmonary dysplasia, 259–260
Pulmonary blood flow (PBF), 29
Pulmonary-cardiovascular interaction, 165–182
after transition and potential clinical implications, 181–182
cardiorespiratory interactions at birth, 166–169, 167t
cardiovascular system on respiratory system, effect of, 174–180
congenital heart disease and, 179
physiology of, 169–171
afterload, 170t, 171
contractility, 170t, 171
preload, 170–171, 170f, 170t
respiratory system on cardiovascular system, effect of, 171–174
during transition and potential clinical implications, 180–181
Pulmonary circulation
development of, 52
endothelium-derived vasodilator, 52–53, 54f
physiology of, 52–53
pulmonary arterial and venous resistance, 52–53, 54f
Pulmonary edema, 300
Pulmonary endothelial cells, 57
Pulmonary endothelial NO production, 57–58
Pulmonary function, in very preterm infants
in adolescence or early adulthood, 283–284, 283f, 284t
in childhood, 282–283
with increasing age of survivors, 284–285
Pulmonary function tests (PFTs), 293
Pulmonary hypertension, 51–69, 175–176, 175f
acute, in preterm infants, 63–64
adjunctive and alternative therapies, 67
blood pressure management, 67–68
bronchopulmonary dysplasia–associated, 64
cAMP-specific phosphodiesterases, 67
cGMP-specific phosphodiesterase (PDE5), 67
echocardiography for, in severe bronchopulmonary dysplasia, 269t
endothelin blockade, 67
inhaled nitric oxide, 65–67, 66f
oxygen targets, 65
PGI2-cAMP pathway, 67
plasma ET-1 levels, 67
pulmonary vasoconstriction, 67–68
right ventricular dysfunction, 67–68
in severe bronchopulmonary dysplasia, 259–260
treatment of, 269–270, 269t
treatment, 65–69
weaning protocol, 66f, 67

Pulmonary hypertension (PH), 52, 297–298, 300
Pulmonary hypoplasia, 178, 350, 351, 354
Pulmonary outcomes, long-term, of preterm infants, 279–287
caffeine role in, 287
controversies in, 280
for late preterm infants, 280–282
pulmonary function in
in adolescence or early adulthood, 283–284, 283f, 284t
in childhood, 282–283
with increasing age of survivors, 284–285
research requirements for, 287
for very preterm infants, 282–285
cigarette smoking and, 285–287, 286f
exercise tolerance, 285
expiratory airflow in survivors born extremely preterm over time in post-surfactant era, 285
rehospitalization rates, 282
Pulmonary surfactant
gene mutations in, 340–341
role after birth, 340
Pulmonary vascular development
adventitia, 58, 59f
angiogenic factor dysregulation, 60
antenatal ductal closure, 61
cord blood angiogenic factors, 60–61
endothelin, 59–60
extrauterine environment, 58–59
genetic factors, 60
histological features, 58
hypoxic conditions, in utero, 53–55, 55f
maternal exposures, 61
maternal vascular underperfusion, 60–61
mediators, 53–57
placental insufficiency, 60–61
signaling abnormalities, 59
Pulmonary vascular disease, 178
Pulmonary vasculature, development of, 52
Pulmonary vasodilation, 57
Pulmonary vasodilator therapy in neonates, 65–66
Pulmonary vasoreactivity, in severe bronchopulmonary dysplasia, 259–260
Pulmonary veins, 52–53
Pulmonary vein stenosis (PVS), 64–65, 65f
severe bronchopulmonary dysplasia and, 260
Pulmonary venous return, 166–167, 169, 170
Pulse oximetry, 41
in resuscitation, 34
Pulse pressure variation, 169

R
Radiant warmers, 34, 35
Raised volume rapid thoracic compression (RVRTC) method, in severe bronchopulmonary dysplasia, 257

Randomized clinical trials (RCTs)
  doses of caffeine citrate, 319–320
  neonatal caffeine therapy, 315
Randomized controlled trials (RCTs)
  of LCPUFAs, 292
  vitamin C supplementation to pregnant
    woment unable to quit smoking,
    293, 294f
Rapid thoracic compression (RTC), in severe
    bronchopulmonary dysplasia, 258
RDS. see Respiratory distress syndrome
Reactive oxygen species (ROS), 299
Resident microvascular EPCs, 56–57
Respiratory assessment
  initial, 35–37
  in positive-pressure ventilation, 37
Respiratory control, in premature infants,
    151–160
Respiratory distress syndrome (RDS),
    108, 134
  chorioamnionitis and, 9t
  lung maturation, 1–2
  lung ultrasound for, 327–328, 328f
  nasal IPPV for, 116–118
  nasal NCPAP for, 111–112. see also Nasal
    continuous positive airway pressure
    (NCPAP)
    brief, early intubation for surfactant
      vs., 113
    continuous distending pressure and,
      111–112
    surfactant administration and, 113–114
    in surfactant era, 112
    treatment of, surfactant in, 112
Respiratory function, severe
    bronchopulmonary dysplasia and,
    255–256
Respiratory health problems, after preterm
    birth, 282
Respiratory interaction, physiology
    of, 169–171
  afterload, 170t, 171
  contractility, 170t, 171
  preload, 170–171, 170f, 170t
Respiratory morbidities associated with
    preterm birth, 156
Respiratory muscle function,
    undernutrition effect on, 298
Respiratory support, continuous distending
    pressure in, 111–112
Respiratory syncytial virus infection, after
    late preterm birth, 280
Respiratory system
  congenital malformations of
    congenital diaphragmatic hernia,
      350–352. see also Congenital
      diaphragmatic hernia (CDH)
    congenital pulmonary malformations.
      see Congenital pulmonary
      malformations (CPMs)
Respiratory system, effect, on
    cardiovascular system, 171–174

Resuscitation
  algorithm, 35, 36f
  anticipating need for, 32–34
  chest compressions in, 41–43
  coronary perfusion pressure in, 43–44
  CPAP in, 37
  discontinuing efforts, 45–46
  epinephrine in, 44, 45
  initial assessment in, 34–35
  intubation in, 40
  medications for, 43–45, 45t
  positive-pressure ventilation in, 37–41
    assessment, 39
    inflation pressure in, 37–38
    inflation rate, 37–38
  risk factors, 33t
  steps in, 35–37, 36f
    airway, 34–35
    dried and stimulated, 34
    maintain normal temperature, 33–34
    tactile stimulation, 37
    warming, 35
  volume infusion in, 45
Retinopathy of prematurity (ROP), 299
  caffeine reduced risk of, 316, 317f
Rhesus macaque model, 82
ROCK pathway, 61
ROP. see Retinopathy of prematurity

S
sBPD. see Severe bronchopulmonary
    dysplasia
Sclerotherapy, for CPAMs, 354
Scoring systems, lung ultrasound,
    325–326, 326f
"Seashore" sign, 324–325, 324f
Segmental bronchial atresia, 352
  fetal therapy for, 354
Selenium, 304
Self-inflating bags, for positive-pressure
    ventilation, 37–38
Semi-quantitative scoring system, 326f
Sepsis, 179–180
  fluid management, 180
Severe bronchopulmonary dysplasia (sBPD)
  cardiovascular system in, 259–261
  chest radiograph showing, 251f
  definitions and scope of, 250–253
  evaluation and treatment of,
    261–271, 261t
    drug therapies in, 267–269
    interdisciplinary care in, 270–271
    mechanical ventilation in, 262–267,
      262t, 263f, 264f, 265f, 266f
    pulmonary hypertension in, 269–270,
      269t
  forced flows in, 258
  incidence of, 253
  long-term outcomes of, 271–272
  lung imaging in, 258–259, 259f
  lung mechanics in, 256–257
  lung volumes in, 257–258

Severe bronchopulmonary
    dysplasia (Continued)
  pathogenesis of, 253–255
  pathophysiology of, 255–261
  physiology-based approach, 249–272
  respiratory function in, 255–256
  ventilator-dependent, 251f
  ventilator strategies in, 261t
Sildenafil, 69
Sildenafil, for pulmonary hypertension, in
    bronchopulmonary dysplasia, 269t
Sildenafil TheRapy In Dismal prognosis
    Early-onset intrauterine growth
    Restriction (STRIDER) consortium, 69
SIMV. see Synchronized intermittent
    mandatory ventilation
Single-cell RNA-seq study in fetal rhesus
    macaques, 10–11
"Sinusoid" sign, 327, 328f
Sleep, caffeine effects on, 319
Sleep disordered breathing (SDB), 155–156
Small for gestational age,
    bronchopulmonary dysplasia
    and, 21–23, 22f
Smith-Lemli-Opitz syndrome, 338–339
Smoking
  maternal, lung maturation and, 23
  pulmonary function and, 285–287, 286f
Spironolactone, for severe
    bronchopulmonary dysplasia, 267–268
SpO₂. see Oxygen saturation
Spontaneous breathing
  in surfactant distribution, 146
  tracheal catheterization, surfactant
    administration, 146
Staphylococcus aureus, ventilator-assisted
    pneumonia and, 96, 96b
Staphylococcus epidermidis, 104
Stem cells
  adult, 222–223
  in cell-based therapy, 221–223, 222f
  division, 222–223, 222f
  embryonic, 222
  multipotent, 221
  potency, 221, 222f
Stenotrophomonas maltophilia, ventilator-
    assisted pneumonia and, 96b
Steroids
  antenatal
    after 34 weeks' gestational period, 211
    drug and dose choices for, 211–212
    before elective cesarean section, 211
    long-term outcomes after, 212
    in low-resource environments, 212
    repeated, 210–211
  postnatal, 212–216
    alternatives to early systemic, 215–216
    for bronchopulmonary dysplasia,
      213–214
    drug, dose, route, and duration of
      therapy with, 214
    historical review, 212–213, 213f

Steroids (*Continued*)
  meta-analyses of early and late
      treatments of, 214
  use of, 216
  prenatal, early use of, 215, 216t
  for severe bronchopulmonary dysplasia,
      267, 269
Stimulation, in resuscitation, 37
Suctioning
  in meconium staining, 35–37
  routine, 34–35
Sudden infant death syndrome, 300
Supplemental oxygen
  BPD and
    at day 28, 238
    diagnosis based on, 238
    indications for, 238
SUPPORT. *see* Surfactant, Positive Pressure,
    and Oxygenation Randomized Trial
Surfactant, 113–114, 180–181, 298–299
  administration of
    invasive or minimally invasive,
        113–114, 113f
  antenatal corticosteroids and, 3–4
  CPAP in, 113–114
    with early intubation, 113
    era, 112
    INSURE technique and, 113
    with nasal, 113
  individual components of, 300
  precursors, 305
Surfactant delivery, newer strategies for,
    133–147
  aerosolization, 135–136, 135t
  to infants treated by CPAP, 134
  by laryngeal mask airway, 136–137
  pharyngeal instillation, 135t, 136
  techniques for, without endotracheal
      tube, 135–137, 135t
  via brief tracheal catheterization,
      137–140, 137t
    avoidance of bradycardia in, 143–144
    bradycardia in, 144
    clinical trials of, 137t, 138–140, 141f
    depth of catheter insertion for, 138
    effectiveness of, 140, 142f
    future research directions for, 146–147
    hypoxia in, 144
    laboratory studies of, 140–143
    observational and cohort studies
        of, 138
    premedication for, 143–144
    procedural complications of, 144
    recommendations for, 144–146
    repeated, 144
    scientific and practical considerations
        for, 140–144
    surfactant reflux in, 144
  via thin catheter, 137, 145t
Surfactant homeostasis
  alveolar, 341f
  clinical perspectives, 345

Surfactant homeostasis (*Continued*)
  genetic disorders of, 341–342, 341f
    lung histopathology in infant, 342, 343f
    SP-A, 341–342
    SP-D, 341–342
  hereditable disorders of, 342
    ABCA3, 345
    SP-B, 342–344
    SP-C, 344
  monogenic diseases of, 340–341, 341t
Surfactant, Positive Pressure, and
    Oxygenation Randomized Trial
    (SUPPORT), 112
  in severe bronchopulmonary dysplasia
      (BPD), 254–255
Surfactant protein A (SP-A), 85
Surfactant protein B (SP-B), 342–344
Surfactant protein C (SP-C), 344
Surfactant reflux
  tracheal catheterization, surfactant
      administration, 144
Sustained lung inflation, effect of, 173
Synchronized intermittent mandatory
    ventilation (SIMV), 193
Synchronized ventilation, modes of, 193
  assist control, 193–194
  assisted ventilation modes, 194–195
  high-frequency ventilation, 197–199
  open lung strategy, 196–197
  pressure-support ventilation, 194
  synchronized intermittent mandatory
      ventilation, 193
  volume-targeted ventilation, 195–196,
      196t
Systemic hypertension, in severe
    bronchopulmonary dysplasia, 260–261
Systemic-to-pulmonary collateral vessels, in
    severe bronchopulmonary dysplasia,
    260–261

T

T-box transcription factor 4 gene (*TBX4*),
    60, 338–339, 345
Thiazides, for severe bronchopulmonary
    dysplasia, 267–268
Tidal volume (V_T)
  effect of, 173
  severe bronchopulmonary dysplasia
      (BPD) and, 254
TLRs. *see* Toll-like receptors
Toll-like receptors (TLRs), 85–86
  endotoxins and, 12–13
Totipotent stem cells, 221, 222f
Trace elements, 304
Tracheal aspirates, ventilator-assisted
    pneumonia and, 94, 96
Tracheal catheterization, surfactant
    administration via, 137–140, 137t
  bradycardia in, 144
  catheter positioning methods, 146–147
  clinical trials of, 137t, 138–140, 141f
    Avoid Mechanical Ventilation Trial in, 138

Tracheal catheterization, surfactant
    administration via (*Continued*)
    NINSAPP Trial in, 138–139
    OPTIMIST-A trial, 139
    summation of, 139–140
    Take Care Study, 137t
  depth of catheter insertion for, 138
  effectiveness of, 140, 142f
  future research directions for, 146–147
  hypoxia in, 144
  infant selection, 144–146
    exclusion criteria, 145–146, 145t
    gestation range, 144
    inclusion criteria, 144–145, 145t
  laboratory studies of, 140–143
  longer-term outcomes, 146
  observational and cohort studies of, 138
  optimal premedication for babies at
      different gestation ranges, 146
  premedication for, 143–144
    avoidance of bradycardia, 143–144
    minimization of discomfort, 143
    respiratory effort maintenance, 143–144
  procedural complications of, 144
  recommendations for, 144–146
  repeated, 144
  scientific and practical considerations for,
      140–144
  spontaneous breathing, 146
  surfactant reflux in, 144
  videolaryngoscopy, role of, 147
Tracheobronchomalacia, in severe
    bronchopulmonary dysplasia, 255–256
Transient tachypnea of newborn (TTN),
    lung ultrasound for, 328, 328f
Transitional circulation, 57–58
Tricuspid regurgitation (TR), for estimating
    pressure gradient, 181–182
Two-finger technique, 42
Two-thumb compression technique, 42, 42f

U

Ultrasound
  for congenital diaphragmatic hernia, 351
  for CPMs, 352
Ultrasound-guided ablation for BPSs, 354
Umbilical cord blood (UCB)–derived
    mesenchymal stem cells, for
    bronchopulmonary dysplasia, 224–227
Umbilical cord clamping in newborn
    transition, 166–167
Umbilical cord (UC)-derived mesenchymal
    stem cells, for bronchopulmonary
    dysplasia, 227, 228
Umbilical cord milking, 168
Undernutrition
  consequences of, 297
  definition, 297
  effect on
    alveolar fluid balance, 300
    antioxidant system, 299
    control of breathing, 300

Undernutrition (*Continued*)
infection susceptibility, 299–300
lung function, 298–299
lung growth and development, 297–298
pulmonary vascular bed, 300
respiratory muscle function, 298
maternal, 292–293
Ureaplasma parvum, 76, 80–81, 84–85
Ureaplasma species
in bronchopulmonary dysplasia, 83–85
chorioamnionitis and, 5–6
on cytokine release, 85
developmental deficiencies in innate
immunity, 85–86
eradication, 86–87
experimental models, 82
intraamniotic, lung maturation
and, 13, 13t
intrauterine infection, 84–85
in intrauterine infection, 80–85
in intrauterine inflammation, 81–82
microbial isolate in upper genital tract, 82
in neonatal lung injury, 83, 83b
in preterm birth, 81–82
species- or serovar-specific virulence
factors, 80–81
U. parvum, 76, 80–81, 84–85
U. urealyticum, 76, 80–81, 85
ventilator-assisted pneumonia and, 97–98
very low birth weight, 81
in vitro studies, 82
in vitro susceptibility of, 86
Ureaplasma urealyticum, 76, 80–81, 85

V

VALI. *see* Ventilator-associated lung injury
Vancomycin, for ventilator-associated
pneumonia, 99–100, 100b
Vapotherm Precision Flow, 122
Variable-flow nasal CPAP device, 111
Vascular development. *see also* Lung
development; Pulmonary vascular
development
Vascular endothelial growth factor (VEGF),
55–56

Vascular endothelial growth factor receptor
2 (VEGFR2), 224
Vascular remodeling in neonatal pulmonary
hypertension, 58, 59f
Vascular underperfusion, maternal
pulmonary development, 60–61
Vegetable-derived oils, 302
VEGF. *see* Vascular endothelial growth
factor
VEGF-induced lung angiogenesis, 56
VEGFR2. *see* Vascular endothelial growth
factor receptor 2
Venous return, cardiorespiratory
interactions and, 166–167
Ventilation, synchronized, modes of, 193
assist control, 193–194
assisted ventilation modes, 194–195
high-frequency ventilation, 197–199
open lung strategy, 196–197
pressure-support ventilation, 194
synchronized intermittent mandatory
ventilation, 193
volume-targeted ventilation, 195–196, 196t
Ventilator-associated lung injury (VALI), 190
delivery room stabilization for, 191–192
mechanism of injury in, 190, 191f
reduction, 190–191
Ventilator-associated pneumonia, 93–104
birth weight and, 95, 97–98
definition of, 94, 95b
epidemiology of, 95–96
future research directions for, 104
outcomes in, 103–104
pathogenesis of, 96–98, 96b, 97f, 98f
prevention of, 101–103, 104b
risk factors for, 95–98
treatment of, 98–101, 100b
ventilation duration and, 99–101
Ventilator-induced lung injury, severe
bronchopulmonary dysplasia (BPD)
and, 253–254
Ventilator strategies, 182
Vermont Oxford Network trial, 112

Very low birth weight (VLBW), 295–296
Very low-birth-weight (VLBW)
infants, antenatal steroids in, 209
Victorian Infant Collaborative Study, 285
Videolaryngoscopy
tracheal catheterization, surfactant
administration, 147
Vitamin A, in fetal lung development,
295, 303
Vitamin C (ascorbic acid)
in fetal lung development, 304
to pregnant women unable to quit
smoking, 293, 294f
Vitamin D Antenatal Asthma Reduction
Trial (VDAART), 294–295
Vitamin D, in fetal lung development,
293–295, 303
Vitamin E (α- and γ-tocopherol), in fetal
lung development, 295, 303, 304
Vitamins, 303–304
Volume guarantee (VG) ventilation, 195–196
Volume infusion, in resuscitation, 45
Volume-targeted ventilation (VTV), 195–196,
196t
Volutrauma, 190
severe bronchopulmonary dysplasia
(BPD) and, 254
VTV. *see* Volume-targeted ventilation

W

Water and fluid volume, 301
Weaning, from nasal CPAP, 115–116
Weight, birth, ventilator-associated
pneumonia, 95, 97–98
White lung artifact pattern, 327, 328f, 329
Wilms tumor, aniridia, genitourinary
anomalies, and intellectual disability
(WAGR), 350

Z

Zauberkugel (magic bullet), 321
Zinc, 304